GROWTH FACTORS AND THE OVARY

SERONO SYMPOSIA, USA

A Continuation Order Plan is available for this series. A continuation order will bring delivery of each new volume immediately upon publication. Volumes are billed only upon actual shipment. For further information please contact the publisher.

GROWTH FACTORS AND THE OVARY

Edited by
Anne N. Hirshfield
University of Maryland
Baltimore, Maryland

PLENUM PRESS • NEW YORK AND LONDON

Library of Congress Cataloging in Publication Data

Ovarian Workshop on Paracrine Communication in the Ovary, Ontogenesis and Growth Factors (1988: Tacoma, Wash.)
  Growth factors and the ovary / edited by Anne N. Hirshfield.
     p.   cm.
  ''Proceedings of the Seventh Ovarian Workshop on Paracrine Communication in the Ovary, Ontogenesis and Growth Factors, sponsored by Serono Symposia, USA, held July 30–August 1, 1988, in Tacoma, Washington''—T.p. verso.
  Includes bibliographies and indexes.
  ISBN-13: 978-1-4684-5690-5   e-ISBN-13: 978-1-4684-5688-2
  DOI: 10.1007/978-1-4684-5688-2

  1. Ovaries—Physiology—Congresses. 2. Ovaries—Growth—Congresses. 3. Growth factors—Physiological effect—Congresses. I. Hirshfield, Anne Newman. II. Serono Symposia, USA. III. Title.
  [DNLM: 1. Growth Substances—physiology—congresses. 2. Ovary—physiology—congresses. WP 540 0945g]
  QP261.0853 1988
  599'.0166—dc20
  DNLM/DLC   89-15976
  for Library of Congress   CIP

The views expressed in this volume are the responsibility of the named authors. Great care has been taken to maintain the accuracy of the information contained in the volume. However, neither Plenum Press, Serono Symposia, USA, nor the editors can be held responsible for errors or any consequences arising from the use of information contained herein.

Some of the names of products referred to in this book may be registered trademarks or proprietary names, although specific references to this fact may not be made; however, the use of a name without designations is not to be construed as a representation by the publisher or editors that it is in the public domain. In addition, the mention of specific companies or of their products or proprietary names does not imply any endorsement or recommendation on the part of the publisher or editors.

Proceedings of the Seventh Ovarian Workshop on Paracrine Communication in the Ovary, Ontogenesis and Growth Factors, sponsored by Serono Symposia, USA, held July 30–August 1, 1988, in Tacoma, Washington

Ovarian Workshop

Board of Directors

Preface

The First Ovarian Workshop was held in June 1976; its goal was to achieve a collective understanding of current thought on ovarian follicular development and function, and to generate clear definitions of the most important areas to be explored in the future. The Ovarian Workshops quickly became a major biennial event for the community of reproductive biologists and their students studying ovarian function. As a young graduate student, I gave my first scientific presentation at the First Ovarian Workshop and I have attended all but one of the subsequent meetings. The Workshops provided a unique forum for the sharing of ideas with colleagues studying closely related problems. I was therefore especially pleased to have been asked to organize the Seventh Ovarian Workshop and to be given an opportunity to help perpetuate these important meetings.

The Seventh Ovarian Workshop was held on the campus of the University of Puget Sound in Tacoma, Washington on July 31 and August 1, 1988. Serono Symposia USA generously financed and coordinated the meeting. I would like to express my particular thanks to Dr. L. Lisa Kern and Dr. James Posillico for their invaluable help prior to, during, and after the meeting.

I would also like to thank Mary Benson and her staff at the University of Puget Sound who made us feel at home in every way. The Board of Directors of the Seventh Ovarian Workshop consisted of Eli Adashi, Joanne Fortune, Geula Gibori, Aaron Hsueh, William LeMaire, Gordon Niswender, and Harold Papkoff. Their valuable advice is gratefully acknowledged. James Hammond, David Schomberg, and Waldemar Schmidt not only contributed outstanding talks and served as chairmen of the sessions, but they also played central roles in planning the scientific program. Thanks also go to all the invited speakers, poster presenters, and discussion participants who provided the substance of this workshop and the enthusiasm that made it such a memorable event.

Anne N. Hirshfield

Contents

I. Ontogeny of the Ovary

II. Keynote Speakers

III. Growth Factors and the Ovary

IV. Poster Presentation Manuscripts

I. Ontogeny of the Ovary

Mesenchymal-Epithelial Interactions in the Growth and Development of the Urogenital Tract

G. R. Cunha

Department of Anatomy, University of California
San Francisco, CA 94143

Introduction

Mesenchymal-epithelial interactions are known to be of prime importance during development. In many developing organs, mesenchyme influences epithelial growth, induces specific patterns of ductal branching morphogenesis, specifies epithelial morphology and spatial organization, and elicits specific patterns of epithelial cytodifferentiation and functional activity (1-5). In the genital tract, mesenchymal-epithelial interactions are also known to regulate the expression of specific hormone receptors (6-7). Although it has been formerly thought that hormonal effects on epithelial cells are elicited directly by intra-epithelial receptors, investigation of androgenic and estrogenic responses in male and female genital tracts, respectively, suggests that a spectrum of hormonal effects elicited by sex steroids in epithelial cells are elicited via indirect processes regulated by mesenchyme. While all organogenetic processes are initiated prenatally, organs of the reproductive system are rudimentary at birth, and most of the developmental processes as well as the onset of functional activity occur over extended periods postnatally. In laboratory rodents, organogenesis of the reproductive tract takes place in the period from the latter third of gestation to about 2 months postpartum, during which time new tissue architecture forms. It is likely that postnatal morphogenesis proceeds by the same fundamental developmental mechanisms that are operative during earlier prenatal periods. However, the question arises as to the exact role of mesenchymal-epithelial interactions in adulthood after morphological and functional maturity is attained.

For all adult reproductive organs, epithelial morphology and functional activity must be sustained as epithelial cells continually senesce, die, and are replaced. As epithelial cells turn over, cellular proliferation must be regulated to maintain normal morphology and function. Morphogenetic events in adult reproductive organs closely resemble the primary developmental events that occur in the perinatal period. This is particularly true of seasonal breeders in which morphogenetic processes occur cyclically in both sexes, but also applies to females during estrous and menstrual cycles, pregnancy, and lactation. During all types of reproductive cycles, parenchymal and stromal components of organs may be degraded and later regenerated from rudimentary precursors. Periods of morphogenesis and growth are usually followed by expression of functional activity. In this review, we will explore the role of mesenchymal-epithelial interactions during fetal and postnatal periods, including adulthood. For the purposes of this review, the term stroma will be used to indicate loose fibrous connective tissue of the adult which contains fibroblasts and smooth muscle cells as the predominant cell types. Mesenchyme is defined as undifferentiated embryonic connective tissue and is the precursor of stroma.

Mesenchymal-Epithelial Interactions in Prostatic Development

Mesenchyme of the developing male genital tract elicits the formation of a variety of epithelial morphologies: simple tubular organs, e.g., ductus deferens (8); branched ductal architecture, e.g., prostate (9-11); or elaborately folded and branched mucosa, e.g., seminal vesicle (12). Experimental separation and recombination of epithelium and mesenchyme from the same organ (homotypic tissue recombinants) has established that in the absence of mesenchyme the epithelium fails to undergo organogenesis or differentiation, thus indicating that mesenchyme is required for epithelial morphogenesis (9,11,13). In heterotypic tissue recombinants, in which mesenchyme and epithelium are derived from different organ rudiments, mesenchyme may induce and specify new patterns of epithelial morphology and cytodifferentiation. Analysis of prostatic induction in tissue recombinants composed of urogenital sinus mesenchyme (UGM) recombined with embryonic or adult urinary bladder epithelium (BLE) reveals the profound effect that mesenchyme can have on epithelium (10,11,14). In UGM + BLE tissue recombinants, the mesenchyme evokes the development of solid prostatic epithelial ducts that exhibit a high rate of cellular proliferation (15). These elongating solid ducts subsequently branch, canalize, and the epithelial cells undergo secretory cytodifferentiation (1,10,11,13-15). The secretory phenotype induced in the epithelium of the adult urinary bladder is unmistakably prostatic by several criteria, including the expression of prostate-specific antigens, prostatic secretory proteins, androgen receptors, and the expression of androgen dependency for DNA synthesis (1,7). Thus, urogenital sinus mesenchyme plays a seminal role in many aspects of prostatic epithelial morphogenesis, growth and cytodifferentiation.

Recently, tissue recombination techniques have also been used to investigate androgen-dependent morphogenesis of the seminal vesicles. This system has demonstrated conclusively that normal functional differentiation accompanies morphogenesis. In mature males, the seminal vesicle epithelium produces large amounts of androgen-dependent, tissue-specific proteins (16-18). These proteins may be detected using polyclonal antibody probes utilizing a variety of immunological approaches (17,19). Species-specific immunologic probes have allowed us to distinguish the seminal vesicle secretory proteins of rats and mice in adult seminal vesicle tissue and in homotypic seminal vesicle tissue recombinants (17). Thus, when neonatal (0-1 day) seminal vesicle mesenchyme (SVM) and epithelium (SVE) were separated, recombined, and grown for 3-5 weeks as subcapsular renal grafts in adult male hosts, the recombinants exhibited normal seminal vesicle morphology and produced proteins antigenically similar to those of normal seminal vesicle (12). Denaturing polyacrylamide gel electrophoresis (SDS-PAGE) and immunoblotting of the secretion derived from these homotypic tissue recombinants demonstrated that the full complement of proteins characteristic of seminal vesicle were expressed in SVM+SVE tissue recombinants. Furthermore, when rat and mouse tissues were recombined, i.e., rat SVM + mouse SVE or mouse SVM + rat SVE, the secreted proteins were characteristic of the species from which the epithelium was derived, thus ruling out any contamination of the mesenchyme with its epithelium as the source of the secreted proteins.

Normal functional differentiation was also observed in instructive inductions. For instance, the upper portion of the fetal wolffian duct, which normally forms the epididymis when combined with SVM, was induced to differentiate into seminal vesicle tissue. As with the homotypic seminal vesicle recombinants, use of the antibodies to seminal vesicle secretory proteins demonstrated that the mesenchyme-induced change in epithelial histodifferentiation was accompanied by a parallel change in functional differentiation. The SVM + upper WDE tissue recombinants produced the full complement of seminal vesicle secretory proteins characteristic of the species from which the wolffian duct epithelium had been derived (12). In addition, other antibody probes were used to show that secretory glycoproteins normally produced by mature epididymis (20,21) were absent, indicating that these tissue recombinants did not represent a hybrid between seminal vesicle and epididymis.

Role of Mesenchyme as a Mediator of Androgenic Effects upon Epithelium

For years it has been tacitly assumed that effects of testosterone or its metabolites on target epithelial cells result from binding of the hormone to androgen receptors within the responding cells themselves. This idea is derived from the following observations: (a) androgen receptors are detectable in extracts of whole prostate as well as in prostatic epithelial and stromal cells (22-29); and, (b) androgens evoke growth of the prostate and specifically stimulate prostatic epithelial proliferation (30-34). Thus, androgenic stimulation of prostatic epithelial DNA synthesis has been thought to result from the receptor-mediated action of androgens within prostatic epithelial cells themselves. It must be recognized that this simple correlation between androgen-induced epithelial proliferation and epithelial androgen receptors does not, by any means, establish a causal relationship. An alternate mechanism by which androgens might induce epithelial proliferation in target organs has been posed in which androgens act upon mesenchymal or stromal cells which elaborate regulatory substances influencing epithelial proliferation (35-37). This model has evolved in part from experiments with the androgen-insensitive Tfm (testicular feminization) mouse. The insensitivity to androgens of Tfm mice (or humans) is based upon abnormal androgen receptors which may be undetectable, present in reduced levels, or may be thermally unstable (38-42). Despite the insensitivity of Tfm tissues to androgens, Tfm epithelial cells from either the urinary bladder or urogenital sinus can be induced to form prostatic ducts when recombined with urogenital sinus mesenchyme (UGM) derived from androgen-receptor-positive wild-type fetuses, provided androgens are present (11,13-15,43-45). Conversely, when Tfm mesenchyme is utilized, prostatic tissue never develops regardless of the genotype of the epithelium. These observations demonstrate that the mesenchyme is the actual target and mediator of androgenic effects upon the epithelium, a concept proposed earlier from comparable studies on androgen-induced regression of the embryonic mouse mammary anlagen (46,47). During prostatic development in tissue recombinants composed of wild-type UGM + Tfm bladder epithelial cells (UGM + Tfm BLE), ductal morphogenesis, epithelial growth, and secretory cytodifferentiation take place and are comparable to that observed in tissue recombinants prepared solely with wild-type tissues. All of these events are induced by androgens, but are expressed in androgen-insensitive Tfm epithelium lacking androgen receptors (15,45). This suggests that androgenic effects upon the epithelium are mediated by the mesenchyme, an interpretation supported by the presence of nuclear 3H-DHT binding sites in mesenchymal cells of fetal androgen target organs (26,48,49).

While the concept of mesenchymal mediation of androgenic effects is derived from investigation of developing organs, it also appears to be applicable to the mature prostate. However, since the adult prostate has androgen receptors in both epithelial and stromal cells (23-29), proliferation of prostatic epithelial cells could be elicited by direct androgenic action. Nonetheless, evidence reveals that the presence of intra-epithelial androgen receptors is neither necessary nor sufficient for regulation of prostatic growth by androgens. This conclusion is based on three lines of evidence. First, incorporation of 3H-thymidine into DNA in tissue recombinants composed of UGM + Tfm BLE is induced by androgens administered to the hosts. The kinetics of this effect are similar to that reported for wild-type prostate (13,45). Second, when tissue recombinants composed of wild-type UGM plus a single adult wild-type prostatic duct (UGM + PR) are grown for 1 month in an intact male host, prostatic ductal mass expands several hundredfold. By contrast, if a wild-type prostatic duct is grown under similar conditions but in association with Tfm UGM (Tfm UGM + PR), the duct is maintained but does not grow (50). Third, proliferation of primary cultures of normal prostatic epithelium (free of stroma) occurs at similar rates in the presence or absence of androgens (51,52). This has lead McKeehan (52) to suggest that testosterone is not a direct mitogen for prostatic epithelium.

More recently, these findings have been refined and extended through autoradiographic analysis utilizing 3H-thymidine labelling index in prostatic epithelial cells of UGM + Tfm BLE tissue recombinants. Prostatic epithelial proliferation (labelling index) is androgen dependent and similar in mature prostatic ducts in both UGM + wild-type BLE and UGM + Tfm BLE recombinants (45). Since Tfm epithelial cells of UGM + Tfm BLE recombinants are devoid of androgen receptors (15,45), prostatic epithelial proliferation cannot be attributed to mechanisms involving intra-epithelial androgen receptors. Instead, these data suggest an indirect mechanism involving trophic factors or regulators produced by androgen-receptor-positive stromal cells.

Role of Stroma in Morphogenesis and Growth of Estrogen-Target Epithelia

While many lines of evidence support an indirect, stroma-mediated mechanism of androgen action, for estrogen target epithelia a comparable approach has not been possible due to the lack of an estrogen insensitive mutant. Nonetheless, several parallel observations suggest that mesenchyme plays an important role in the biology of estrogen target epithelia. As in males, development of the epithelial parenchyma of female estrogen target organs is induced and specified by the mesenchyme (53,54). For example, vaginal stroma (VS) induces neonatal uterine epithelium (UtE) to undergo vaginal differentiation, while uterine stroma (UtS) induces neonatal vaginal epithelium (VE) to undergo uterine differentiation (53-55). Grafts that express vaginal differentiation (VS + UtE) make proteins that, when analyzed by two-dimensional SDS-PAGE, give a protein map that is very similar to that produced by the vagina. Likewise, UtS + VE recombinants (which express uterine differentiation) synthesize a uterine profile of proteins (56). Moreover, the induced vaginal epithelium of VS + UtE recombinants when grown in intact cycling female hosts produces alternating layers of cornified and mucified cells through the estrous cycle in concert with the host's vaginal epithelium (53,55,56). This cyclic change in epithelial phenotype is one of the unique functional characteristics of vaginal epithelium (55). Thus, in developing estrogen-target organs, the mesenchyme induces specific patterns of epithelial morphogenesis, cytodifferentiation, and functional activity.

Although estrogens are not required for development of the female genital tract, the fetal and neonatal female genital tracts of many species are responsive to exogenous estrogens, and a vast array of teratogenic effects and many epithelial abnormalities are elicited by estrogenic compounds in the developing female genital tract of humans as well as laboratory animals. In addition, exogenous estrogens have been shown to elicit significant increases in uterine and vaginal epithelial proliferation in neonatal mice (57-60), vaginal epithelial cornification (61-63), and uterine epithelial hypertrophy (64). These effects have been elicited by diethylstilbestrol, estradiol, and triphenylethylene compounds such as tamoxifen, nafoxidine, and clomiphene citrate as well as the phytoestrogen, coumestrol (61,63-68). Thus, the estrogenic sensitivity of epithelial cells of the developing female genital tract is well documented. These estrogenic effects upon uterine and vaginal epithelium of neonatal mice appear to be mediated via the mesenchymal cells because during the early neonatal period in mice, estrogen receptors are undetectable in the uterine epithelium but are present in the uterine mesenchyme (60,69,70). As an aside, it should be noted that the timing of expression of estrogen receptors in neonatal mouse uterine epithelium appears about 2 to 3 days earlier in outbred CD-1 mice than in inbred strains (60,71). Nonetheless, even though the uterine epithelium of 4-day-old Balb/c mice is devoid of estrogen receptors, these cells respond to exogenous estrogen in vivo by increasing the rate of proliferation. The lag between estrogen administration and increased DNA synthesis is similar to that of ovariectomized adult mice (72). In addition, neonatal uterine epithelial cells at the peak of estrogen-induced proliferation also lack estrogen receptors (60). These results suggest that in the neonatal mouse estrogen-induced proliferation of uterine epithelium is mediated by estrogen-receptor-positive mesenchymal cells. Since the time course of estrogen response is equivalent to that of the adult, it is possible that the proliferative response of adult uterine epithelium is also mediated by a similar indirect mechanism even though adult uterine epithelium has estrogen receptors.

Numerous reports of cultures of normal vaginal and uterine epithelial cells are consistent with such a stroma-mediated process because it has not been possible to show direct mitogenic effects of estrogens on primary epithelial cultures in vitro (73-80), although some neoplastic epithelial cells are mitogenically responsive to estrogen in culture (81-83). The single report by Ishiwata et al. (76), in which estradiol stimulated the proliferation of normal endometrial epithelial cells in culture, suffers from the lack of any demonstration of steroid specificity and the requirement of nearly micromolar concentrations of estradiol for effectiveness. Thus, epithelial cells, normally responsive to estrogens in vivo, usually do not respond mitogenically to estrogens in vitro. However, there are a few reports demonstrating that estrogen stimulates DNA synthesis and cellular proliferation when the epithelia are grown as mixed stromal and epithelial cell cultures or as tissue explants in organ culture.

These sporadic and seldom repeated reports suggest that an estrogenic effect (proliferation) is more likely to occur if the stroma is present in the culture system.

Several hypotheses have been proposed to explain the inability of estradiol to stimulate normal epithelial cell proliferation in vitro. Culture conditions may selectively encourage the proliferation of estrogen-independent cells, or the epithelium may become altered in culture so that it no longer requires estradiol for growth. Alternatively, estrogens and other sex steroids may elicit epithelial growth by acting indirectly via stroma-derived growth regulators not present in pure epithelial cultures. To examine some of these possibilities, we have investigated the ability of cultured vaginal and uterine epithelium to reexpress normal morphology and hormone responsiveness when recombined with homologous stroma. In this regard, uterine and vaginal epithelia from ovariectomized 40-day-old mice were grown under serum-free conditions in collagen gels for 1 to 2 weeks (80). Total DNA content of the vaginal and uterine epithelial cultures increased fourfold and four- to eightfold, respectively, in the absence of estradiol. Moreover, proliferation of these epithelia was not stimulated by estradiol or diethylstilbestrol in vitro (79,80,84). The vaginal epithelium in serum-free culture did not keratinize or mucify normally. Nonetheless, these epithelial cells did possess functional estrogen receptors insofar as exposure of these epithelia to estradiol in vitro reduced cytosolic estrogen receptor content, increased nuclear estrogen receptor levels, and increased cytosolic progesterone receptor levels (84). Therefore, the lack of a proliferative response to estradiol in vitro was not due to an inactive estrogen receptor system (84).

In an attempt to restore differentiation and growth responses absent in vitro, cultured vaginal epithelium was recombined with fresh vaginal stroma and the resultant tissue recombinants grown under the renal capsule of intact female hosts for 4 weeks (85). Under these conditions the cultured vaginal epithelium reexpressed its normal histotypic features, including the characteristic change from keratinization to mucification during the estrous cycle. The epithelium in recombinants composed of uterine stroma and cultured uterine epithelium was also histologically normal (85). In these tissue recombinants, estrogen-dependent proliferation of both uterine and vaginal epithelium was also restored. While these observations do not prove that estrogens evoke their effects upon target epithelial cells via stromal mediators, it is evident that loss of differentiated features in uterine and vaginal epithelia in vitro and loss of growth responsiveness to estrogens in vitro can be recovered following reassociation with homologous stroma and transplantation of the tissues in vivo. These observations underscore the importance of stroma since direct grafting of cultured uterine and vaginal epithelia in vivo is incompatible with continued epithelial survival (85).

Conclusion

In summary, in both the male and female genital tracts mesenchymal or stromal cells appear to play central roles in regulating a variety of androgenic and estrogenic effects upon epithelium. Clearly, mesenchymal cells induce and specify patterns of epithelial morphology and cytodifferentiation as well as function. Mitogenic effects of androgens and estrogens appear to also have strict stromal requirements. Studies utilizing serum-free in vitro approaches are now underway in several laboratories to define the mechanism of these interactions between epithelium and mesenchyme.

Acknowledgments

The authors would like to thank Ron Feavyear for typing the manuscript. This study was supported in part by the following grants: March of Dimes No. 1-837; NIH grants AM 32157; HD 17491; CA 05388; HD 21919.

References

1. Cunha GR, Fujii H, Neubauer BL, Shannon JM, Sawyer LM, Reese BA. Epithelial-mesenchymal interactions in prostatic development. I. Morphological observations of prostatic induction by urogenital sinus mesenchyme in epithelium of the adult rodent urinary bladder. J Cell Biol 1983; 96:1662-70.
2. Sengel P. Morphogenesis of skin. New York: Cambridge University Press, 1976.
3. Ekblom P. Basement membrane proteins and growth factors in kidney differentiation. In: Trelstad RL, ed. The role of extracellular matrix in development. New York: AR Liss, 1984:173-206.
4. Haffen K, Kedinger M, Simon-Assman P. Mesenchyme-dependent differentiation of epithelial progenitor cells in the gut. J Pediatr Gastroenterol Nutr 1987; 6:14-23.
5. Bernfield MR, Banerjee SD, Koda JE, Rapraeger AC. Remodeling of the basement membrane as a mechanism of morphogenetic tissue interaction. In: Trelstad RL, ed. The role of extracellular matrix in development. New York: AR Liss, 1984:545-96.
6. Cunha GR, Reese BA, Sekkingstad M. Induction of nuclear androgen-binding sites in epithelium of the embryonic urinary bladder by mesenchyme of the urogenital sinus of embryonic mice. Endocrinology 1980; 107:1767-70.
7. Neubauer BL, Chung LWK, McCormick K, Taguchi O, Thompson TC, Cunha GR. Epithelial-mesenchymal interactions in prostatic development. II. Biochemical observations of prostatic induction by urogenital sinus mesenchyme in epithelium of the adult rodent urinary bladder. J Cell Biol 1983; 96:1671-6.
8. Cunha GR. Alterations in the developmental properties of stroma during the development of the urogenital ridge into ductus deferens and uterus in embryonic and neonatal mice. J Exp Zool 1976; 197:375-88.
9. Cunha GR. Epithelio-mesenchymal interactions in primordial gland structures which become responsive to androgenic stimulation. Anat Rec 1972; 172:179-96.
10. Cunha GR, Chung LWK, Shannon JM, Taguchi O, Fujii H. Hormone-induced morphogenesis and growth: role of mesenchymal-epithelial interactions. Recent Prog Horm Res 1983; 39:559-98.
11. Cunha GR, Lung B. The possible influences of temporal factors in androgenic responsiveness of urogenital tissue recombinants from wild-type and androgen-insensitive (Tfm) mice. J Exp Zool 1978; 205:343-2.
12. Cunha GR, Higgins SJ, Young PF. Seminal vesicle mesenchyme induces heterotypic Wolffian duct derived epithelium to express seminal vesicle differentiation and to secrete seminal vesicle secretory proteins. Endocrinology 1988; 122:189.
13. Cunha GR, Chung LWK. Stromal-epithelial interactions: induction of prostatic phenotype in urothelium of testicular feminized (Tfm/Y) mice. J Steroid Biochem 1981; 14:1317-21.
14. Cunha GR, Donjacour AA, Cooke PS, et al. The endocrinology and developmental biology of the prostate. Endocr Rev 1987; 8:338-62.

15. Shannon JM, Cunha GR. Characterization of androgen binding and deoxyribonucleic acid synthesis in prostate-like structures induced in testicular feminized (Tfm/Y) mice. Biol Reprod 1984; 31:175-83.
16. Fawell SE, MacDonald CJ, Higgins SJ. Comparison of seminal vesicle secretory proteins of rodents using antibody and nucleotide probes. Mol Cell Endocrinol 1987; 50:107-14.
17. Fawell SE, Higgins SJ. Tissue distribution, developmental profile and hormonal regulation of androgen responsive secretory proteins of rat seminal vesicles studied by immunocytochemistry. Mol Cell Endocrinol 1986; 48:39-49.
18. Higgins SJ, Burchell JM, Mainwaring WI. Androgen dependent synthesis of basic secretory proteins by the rat seminal vesicle. Biochem J 1976; 158:271-82.
19. Fawell SE, Pappin DJ, Higgins SJ. Androgen regulated protein of rat seminal vesicle secretion constitute a structurally related family present in the copulatory plug. Mol Cell Endocrinol 1986; 45:205-13.
20. Brooks DE, Higgins SJ. Characterization and androgen dependence of proteins associated with luminal fluid and spermatozoa in the rat epididymis. J Reprod Fertil 1980; 59:363-75.
21. Brooks DE, Tiver K. Localization of epididymal secretory proteins on rat spermatozoa. J Reprod Fertil 1983; 69:651-7.
22. Fang S, Anderson KM, Liao S. Receptor proteins for androgens. On the role of specific proteins in the retention of 17B-hydroxy-5a-androstan-3-one by the rat ventral prostate in vivo and in vitro. J Biol Chem 1969; 244:6584-95.
23. Jung-Testas I, Groyer M-T, Bruner-Lorand J, Hechter O, Baulieu E-E, Robel P. Androgen and estrogen receptors in rat ventral prostate epithelium and stroma. Endocrinology 1981; 109:1287-9.
24. Krieg M, Schlenker A, Voigt K-D. Inhibition of androgen metabolism in stroma and epithelium of the human benign prostatic hyperplasia by progesterone, estrone, and estradiol. Prostate 1985; 6:233-40.
25. Lahtonen R, Bolton NJ, Konturri M, Vihko R. Nuclear androgen receptors in the epithelium and stroma of human benign prostatic hypertrophic glands. Prostate 1983; 4:129-39.
26. Shannon JM, Cunha GR. Autoradiographic localization of androgen binding in the developing mouse prostate. Prostate 1983; 4:367-73.
27. Sirett DAN, Cowan SK, Janeczko AE, Grant JK, Glen ES. Prostatic tissue distribution of 17B-hydroxy-5a-androstan-3-one and of androgen receptors in benign hyperplasia. J Steroid Biochem 1979; 13:723-8.
28. Stumpf WE, Sar M. Autoradiographic localization of estrogen, androgen, progestin, and glucocorticosteroid in "target tissues" and "non-target tissues." In: Pasqualini JR, ed. Receptors and mechanism of action of steroid hormones. New York: Marcel Dekker, Inc., 1976:41-84.
29. Tilley WD, Horsfall DJ, McGee MA, Henderson DW, Marshall VR. Distribution of oestrogen and androgen receptors between the stroma and epithelium of the guinea pig prostate. J Steroid Biochem 1985; 22:713-9.
30. Bruchovsky N, Lesser B, van Doorn EV, Craven S. Hormonal effects on cell proliferation in rat prostate. Vitam Horm 1975; 33:61-102.
31. Coffey DS. The effects of androgens on DNA and RNA synthesis in sex accessory tissue. In: Brandes D, ed. Male accessory sex organs, structure and function. New York: Academic Press, 1974:303-28.

32. Evans GS, Chandler JA. Cell proliferation studies in rat prostate I. The proliferative role of basal and secretory epithelial cells during normal growth. Prostate 1987; 10:163-78.

33. Tuohimaa P, Niemi M. Cell renewal and mitogenic activity of testosterone in male sex accessory glands. In: Brandes D, ed. Male accessory sex organs, structure and function. New York: Academic Press, 1974:329-43.

34. Tuohimaa P. Control of cell proliferation in male accessory sex glands. In: Spring-Mills E, Hafez ESE, eds. Male accessory sex glands. New York: Elsevier/North Holland, 1980:131-53.

35. Cunha GR. Epithelial-stromal interactions in development of the urogenital tract. Int Rev Cytol 1976; 47:137-94.

36. Cunha GR, Shannon JM, Taguchi O, Fujii H, Chung LWK. Mesenchymal-epithelial interactions in hormone-induced development. J Animal Science 1982; 55(suppl):14-31.

37. Cunha GR, Chung LWK, Shannon JM, Reese BA. Stromal-epithelial interactions in sex differentiation. Biol Reprod 1980; 22:19-42.

38. Attardi B, Ohno S. Cytosol androgen receptor from kidney of normal and testicular feminized (Tfm) mice. Cell 1974; 2:205-12.

39. Bardin CW, Bullock LP, Sherins RJ, Mowszowicz I, Blackburn WR. Androgen metabolism and mechanism of action in male pseudohermaphroditism: a study of testicular feminization. Recent Prog Horm Res 1973; 29:65-109.

40. Ohno S. Major sex determining genes. New York: Springer-Verlag, 1979.

41. Wilson JD, Griffin JE, George FW, Leshin M. Recent studies on the endocrine control of male phenotypic development. In: Serio M, Zanisi M, Motta M, Martini L, eds. Sexual differentiation: basic and clinical aspects. New York: Raven Press, 1984:223-32.

42. Wilson JD, Griffin JE, Leshin M, George FW. Role of gonadal hormones in development of the sexual phenotypes. Hum Genet 1981; 58:78-84.

43. Cunha GR, Donjacour AA, Sugimura Y. Stromal-epithelial interactions and heterogeneity of proliferative activity within the prostate. Biochem Cell Biol 1986; 64:608-14.

44. Lasnitzki I, Mizuno T. Prostatic induction and interaction of epithelium and mesenchyme from normal wild-type and androgen-insensitive mice with testicular feminization. J Endocrinol 1980; 85:423-8.

45. Sugimura Y, Cunha GR, Bigsby RM. Androgenic induction of deoxyribonucleic acid synthesis in prostate-like glands induced in the urothelium of testicular feminized (Tfm/y) mice. Prostate 1986; 9:217-25.

46. Drews U, Drews U. Regression of mouse mammary gland anlagen in recombinants of Tfm and wild-type tissues: testosterone acts via the mesenchyme. Cell 1977; 10:401-4.

47. Kratochwil K, Schwartz P. Tissue interaction in androgen response of the embryonic mammary rudiment of mouse: identification of target tissue of testosterone. Proc Natl Acad Sci USA 1976; 73:4041-4.

48. Takeda H, Mizuno T, Lasnitzki I. Autoradiographic studies of androgen-binding sites in the rat urogenital sinus and postnatal prostate. J Endocrinol 1985; 104:87-92.

49. Wasner G, Hennermann I, Kratochwil K. Ontogeny of mesenchymal androgen receptors in the embryonic mouse mammary gland. Endocrinology 1983; 113:1771-80.

50. Norman JT, Cunha GR, Sugimura Y. The induction of new ductal growth in adult prostatic epithelium in response to an embryonic prostatic inductor. Prostate 1986; 8:209-20.

51. Peehl DM, Stamey TA. Serum-free growth of adult human prostatic epithelial cells. In Vitro Cell Dev Biol 1986; 22:82-90.
52. McKeehan WL, Adams PS, Rosser MP. Direct mitogenic effects of insulin, epidermal growth factor, glucocorticoid, cholera toxin, unknown pituitary factors and possibly prolactin, but not androgen, on normal rat prostate epithelial cells in serum-free, primary cell culture. Cancer Res 1984; 44:1998-2010.
53. Cunha GR. Stromal induction and specification of morphogenesis and cytodifferentiation of the epithelia of the Mullerian ducts and urogenital sinus during development of the uterus and vagina in mice. J Exp Zool 1976; 196:361-70.
54. Cunha GR, Fujii H. Stromal-parenchymal interactions in normal and abnormal development of the genital tract. In: Herbst A, Bern HA, eds. Developmental effects of diethylstilbestrol (DES) in pregnancy. New York: Thieme-Stratton, Inc., 1981:179-93.
55. Cooke PS, Fujii DK, Cunha GR. Vaginal and uterine stroma maintain their inductive properties following primary culture. In Vitro Cell Dev Biol 1987; 23:159-66.
56. Cunha GR, Shannon JM, Taguchi O, Fujii H, Meloy BA. Epithelial-mesenchymal interactions in hormone-induced development. In: Sawyer RH, Fallon JF, eds. Epithelial-mesenchymal interactions in development. New York: Praeger Scientific Press, 1983:51-74.
57. Forsberg J-G. An estradiol mitotic rate inhibiting effect in the Mullerian epithelium in neonatal mice. J Exp Zool 1970; 175:369-74.
58. Kimura T, Kawashima S, Nishizuka Y. Effects of prenatal treatment with estrogen on mitotic activity of vaginal anlage cells in mice. Endocrinol Jpn 1980; 27:739-45.
59. Eide A. The effect of oestradiol on DNA synthesis in the neonatal mouse uterus and cervix. Cell Tissue Res 1975; 156:551-5.
60. Bigsby RM, Cunha GR. Estrogen stimulation of DNA synthesis in epithelium lacking estrogen receptors. Endocrinology 1986; 119:390-6.
61. Takasugi N. Cytological basis for permanent vaginal changes in mice treated neonatally with steroid hormones. Int Rev Cytol 1976; 44:193-224.
62. Cunha GR, Lee AK, Lung B. Electron microscopic observations of vaginal development in untreated and neonatally estrogenized Balb/c Crgl mice. Am J Anat 1978; 152:343-82.
63. Burroughs CD, Bern HA, Stoksdtad ELR. Prolonged vaginal cornification and other changes in mice treated neonatally with coumestrol, a plant estrogen. J Toxicol Environ Health 1985; 15:51-61.
64. Mc Cormack S, Clark JH. Clomid administration to pregnant rats causes abnormalities of the reproductive tract in offspring and mothers. Science 1979; 204:629-31.
65. Forsberg J-G, Kalland T. Neonatal estrogen treatment and epithelial abnormalities in the cervicovaginal epithelium of adult mice. Cancer Res 1981; 41:721-34.
66. McLachlan JA, Newbold RR, Bullock BC. Long term effects on the female mouse genital tract associated with prenatal exposure to diethylstilbestrol. Cancer Res 1980; 40:3988-99.
67. Taguchi O, Nishizuka Y. Reproductive tract abnormalities in female mice treated neonatally with tamoxifen. Am J Obstet Gynecol 1985; 151:675-8.
68. Burroughs CD, Williams BA, Mills KT, Bern HA. Genital tract abnormalities in female C57BL/Crgl mice exposed neonatally to phytoestrogens (cuomestrol and zearalenone). Cancer Res 1986; 27:220.
69. Cunha GR, Shannon JM, Vanderslice KD, Sekkingstad M, Robboy SJ. Autoradiographic analysis of nuclear estrogen binding sites during postnatal development of the genital tract of female mice. J Steroid Biochem 1982; 17:281-6.

70. Stumpf WE, Narbaitz R, Sar M. Estrogen receptors in the fetal mouse. J Steroid Biochem 1980; 12:55-64.
71. Korach KS, Horigome T, Tomooka Y, Yamashita S, Newbold RR, McLachlan JA. Inmmnodetection of estrogen receptor in epithelial and stromal tissues of neonatal mouse uterus. Proc Natl Acad Sci USA 1988; 85:3334-7.
72. Martin L, Finn CA, Trinder G. Hypertrophy and hyperplasia in the mouse uterus after oestrogen treatment: an autoradiographic study. J Endocrinol 1973; 56:133-44.
73. Flaxman BA, Chopra DP, Newman D. Growth of mouse vaginal epithelial cells in vitro. In Vitro 1973; 9:194-201.
74. Shannon JM, Cunha GR. Characterization of androgen binding and deoxyribonucleic acid synthesis in prostate-like structures induced in testicular feminized (Tfm/Y) mice. Biol Reprod 1984; 31:175-83.
75. Kirk D, King RJB, Heyes J, Peachey L, Hirsch PJ, Taylor WT. Normal human endometrium in cell culture. In Vitro 1978; 14:651-62.
76. Ishiwata I, Okumura H, Nozawa S, Kurihara S, Yamada KI. Effects of estradiol-17B on growth and differentiation of benign and malignant human uterine cervical squamous cells in vitro. Acta Cytol 1978; 22:555-61.
77. Casimiri V, Rath NC, Parvez H, Psychoyos A. Effect of sex steroids on rat endometrial epithelium and stroma cultured separately. J Steroid Biochem 1980; 12:293-8.
78. Lippman ME, Huff KK, Jakesz R, et al. Estrogens regulate production of specific growth factors in hormone-dependent human breast cancer. Ann NY Acad Sci 1986; 464:11-6.
79. Tomooka Y, DiAugustine RP, McLachlan JA. Proliferation of mouse uterine epithelial cells in vitro. Endocrinology 1986; 118:1011-8.
80. Iguchi T, Uchima FDA, Ostrander PL, Hamamoto ST, Bern HA. Proliferation of normal mouse uterine luminal epithelial cells in serum-free collagen gel culture. Proc Japan Acad 1985; 61:292-5.
81. Lippman ME, Huff KK, Jakesz R, et al. Estrogens regulate production of specific growth factors in hormone-dependent human breast cancer. Ann NY Acad Sci 1986; 464:11-6.
82. Soto AM, Sonnenschein D. Mechanism of estrogen action on cellular proliferation: evidence for indirect and negative control on cloned breast tumor cells. Biochem Biophys Res Commun 1984; 122:1097-103.
83. Holinka CF, Hata H, Kuramoto H, Gurpide E. Responses to estradiol in a human endometrial adenocarcinoma cell line (Ishikawa). J Steroid Biochem 1986; 24:85-9.
84. Uchima FDA, Edery M, Iguchi T, Bern HA. Estrogen induces progesterone receptor but not proliferation of mouse vaginal epithelium in vitro. Cancer Res 1984; 25:206.
85. Cooke PS, Uchima FA, Fujii DK, Bern HA, Cunha GR. Restoration of normal morphology and estrogen responsiveness in cultured vagina and uterine epithelia transplanted with stroma. Proc Natl Acad Sci USA 1986; 83:2109-13.

2

Overview of Embryological and Fetal Development of the Ovary and Testis

Luciano Zamboni

Department of Pathology, Harbor-UCLA Medical Center
Torrance, California 90509

The events that take place in the urogenital region during mammalian embryonal and fetal life represent ideal subjects of study for those interested in cellular differentiation and organogenesis. Within a short period of time, from a few hours in species with short gestational periods to no more than several days in those with longer ones, the urogenital region witnesses the arrival of the primordial germ cells (PGCs), their colonization of the genital folds, and the concomitant "activation" of the cells preexisting in the area, major phenomena that culminate in the development of a sexually indifferent gonad. The subsequent differentiation of the latter into a testis or an ovary is accompanied by the maturation of the PGCs into germinal elements with distinct sexually dimorphic characteristics, the development of a complex system of blood vessels and nerves, the differentiation of interstitial elements with important endocrine functions, the sexually dimorphic involution/transformation of the mesonephros, and the organization of the metanephros as the definitive excretory organ.

Of these phenomena, the migration of the PGCs to, and their colonization of, the genital ridges, the origin of the somatic cells which at first contribute to the formation of the blastema of the sexually indifferent gonad together with the germinal cells and later differentiate into the definitive testicular and ovarian sustentacular elements, and the sexually dimorphic patterns of male and female germinal cell differentiation with emphasis on the time of initiation of meiosis are those that have been most intensively studied. While many of the issues related to the evolution of these phenomena and their regulatory mechanisms have been clarified, others remain unsettled and require further study.

In all mammals, onset of gonadal development is heralded by the arrival of the PGCs to the gonadal folds following a migratory journey that initiates in the yolk sac and takes the germ cells through the primitive intestine and its mesentery. In mammals, PGC migration is exclusively extravascular, sporadic reports to the contrary (1, for example) being based on the erroneous interpretation, mostly due to similarities in size and overall appearance, of circulating megakaryocytes as primordial germinal cells. It has been firmly established that the PGCs cover the distance separating the yolk sac from the gonadal folds primarily by ameboidism (2,3; see 4 for a review), a functional characteristic that they retain also in vitro (5); additionally, recent studies have emphasized the role of fibronectin (6) and laminin (De Felici; personal communication) as important coadjuvants of germ cell movements. The factor(s) that may be responsible for the targeted directionality of PGC migration are still unidentified (for a review, see 4). Chemotaxis has been postulated most frequently; however, this hypothesis makes it difficult to explain why significant numbers of germ cells fail to attain the gonadal folds and instead seed ectopic sites (*vide infra*). Throughout the migratory phase, the PGCs are constantly associated with somatic cells (3), the author being unaware of any instance in which migrating germ cells were not seen in contact with the latter. The type of somatic cells involved in this associative relationship obviously varies depending upon the sites; the degree of germinal-somatic cell association also varies from very close, as in the primitive gut where the PGCs are completely surrounded by the intestinal epithelial cells to focal and ephemeral, as in the mesentery where contact between the two involves only narrow areas of the cellular surfaces and, due to their ameboidal movements, the PGCs rapidly switch from one somatic cell to another (3). The association with the somatic cells appears to be essential not only for successful completion of PGC migration, but also for the viability of the germ cells and their ability to divide; in fact, the rapid loss of viability that they display in culture where they fail to survive longer than a few hours, and the cessation of mitotic activity (De Felici, personal communication), may well be related to their being separated from the somatic cells.

The morphology and the functional attitudes of the PGCs change drastically following their arrival in the gonadal folds. The cells lose their ameboidal features (3,7) and assume regular spheroidal outlines. In the cytoplasm, one of the most evident changes is the disappearance of the lipid and glycogen reserves that were so prominent throughout migration when they represented major sources of the energy required for ameboidal activity. Due to these changes and the acquisition of features usually associated with increasing degrees of differentiation such as a reduced number of free ribosomes, more mature type mitochondria, prominent Golgi complexes, etc., the germinal cells are now identified as gonocytes all displaying identical morphologic characteristics, irrespective of their genetic sex. Another distinctive feature of the germinal cells in the gonadal folds is the tendency to aggregate to one another forming clusters of variable number of elements. Contributing significantly to this phenomenon is the cessation of movements; the germinal cells continue to divide, but being stationary, their progeny accumulates locally. The patterns by which the germinal cells associate with the somatic cells in the gonadal folds also are markedly different from those characteristic of the migratory period. Due to the absence of movements, the association is no longer saltatory, as it was, for example, during their ascent through the mesentery (3), but permanent and stable; due to the high cellularity of the area (*vide infra*), they are now completely surrounded by the somatic cells rather than only focally as during migration.

In all species, the arrival of the PGCs to the gonadal folds coincides with "activation" of the somatic cells indigenous to the area; this activation is expressed prevalently by intense cell proliferation and by profound tissue organizational changes. The contemporaneity of the two phenomena, PGC arrival in the genital ridges and somatic cell "activation," strongly suggests that the former is responsible for the induction of the latter, evidence notwithstanding that proliferation of the somatic cells of the genital region can occur also in the absence of germinal cells such as in embryos from mothers treated with 1.4 butanediol dimetosul-phonate, a drug that selectively destroys the primordial germ cells (8).

While the concomitant occurrence of germ cell arrival in the gonadal folds and the proliferation and reorganization of the indigenous somatic cells is a consistent feature of all animals so far studied, profound differences exist among species with regard to the type and origin of the somatic cells that undergo "activation" as a result of, or simultaneously with, colonization of the gonadal area by the PGCs. This is an important point because, in subsequent stages of gonadal development, these cells at first will represent the somatic components of the gonadal cords, and then will differentiate into the definitive sustentacular elements of the mature gonad, i.e., the Sertoli cells of the testis and the granulosa cells of the ovary. The importance of this aspect of gonadal development is best demonstrated by the attention paid to it by past and present investigators and the controversies that it has generated. The most frequently postulated origins (reviewed in 9) are: *mesothelial*, i.e., the precursors of the gonadal sustentacular cells would differentiate from the coelomic mesothelium lining the surface of the genital ridges; *mesenchymal*, i.e., they would derive from the cells of the genital ridge stroma; and *mixed*, i.e., they would be an admixture of mesothelial- and mesenchymal-derived elements. A fourth hypothesis, i.e., that they would be of mesonephric origin, was advanced by a few classic investigators but, until recently, it was paid only sporadic and marginal attention. This controversial topic was restudied in recent years in a few laboratories, including our own, utilizing refined methods of mor-phologic analysis such as high resolution light microscopy and electron microscopy. These studies have considerably improved our understanding of this aspect of gonadal develop-ment; they also have explained, at least in part, the reasons for the different opinions expressed on this point in the past by demonstrating that the origin of the somatic cells that, together with the germinal cells, contribute to the assembly of the developing gonad differs among species. In rodents, animals with rudimentary, nonfunctional mesonephroi (10), they are of mesonephric origin and derive from the epithelial cells of the tubules situated dorsal to the genital ridge (11). In ruminants, the somatic elements of the gonads are also mesonephric in origin but they differentiate from the cellular elements of the glomerulus of the "giant nephron," (12,13) a singular structure which is a peculiarity of the mesonephroi of these animals. In primates, instead, the somatic cells of the gonad are of mesothelial origin (9) and do derive from the coelomic mesothelial cells lining the surface of the genital folds as originally reported by several classic investigators; in primates, thus, the mesonephros shares in the organization of the gonads only with regard to the assembly of the gonadal rete and, in the male, of the more distal segments of the testicular excretory system (*vide infra*), whereas in rodents and ruminants, it participates in the organization of both the gonad and its excretory pathways. In a recent article (9), we explained these differences on the basis of the differences that exist among species concerning not only degrees of organization and functionality of their mesonephroi, but also the relationship between the time when the PGCs arrive in the gonadal folds and stages of mesonephric development or involution. In animals where the mesonephros is rudimentary and nonfunctional such as rodents, or is already undergoing physiologic regression at the time the PGCs arrive in the genital ridges as in ruminants, its role in the assembly of the gonad is pivotal, whereas in animals such as primates in which it performs important excretory functions and is still developing at the time "activation" of the somatic cells of the genital ridge is to occur, nonmesonephric elements are the source of the somatic cell population of the gonad.

In spite of these major differences, the "activation" of the somatic cells, their organizational changes, and the relationship that they establish with the germinal cells are identical in all species. The first expression of their activated state is an intense and sustained proliferation associated with an invasive process, whereby the multiplying cells escape from their original territorial boundaries, breaking through basal laminae, and invade the genital ridge area. In ruminants, they break through the Bowman's capsule of the giant glomerulus and its basement membrane (12,13); in rodents, they traverse the basement membrane delimiting the ventral extremities of the mesonephric tubules (11), and in primates, separating the coelomic mesothelium from the underlying stroma (9). As a result of these proliferative and invasive processes, the originally sparsely cellular gonadal folds become crowded by increasing numbers of somatic cells which rapidly outnumber the germinal cells continuing for a while to arrive in the area. The much enlarged genital ridge eventually becomes completely "filled" by a compact cell mass consisting of somatic cells and, to a much lesser degree, germinal cells. This mixed cell mass, referred to as the "blastema," typifies the organization of the sexually indifferent gonad of all mammals; ventrally, it blends with the coelomic surface of the organ and dorsally, it continues with the mesonephric elements, be they the remnants of involuting glomeruli and/or tubules, or the Bowman's capsules of fully functional glomeruli. At this stage, the sexually indifferent gonad lacks evident stromal, vascular, and nervous elements.

In all mammals so far studied, the sexual differentiation of the male gonad precedes that of the female, the interval varying from a few hours to a few days depending upon species; throughout this time the female gonad is identifiable as such solely because it retains the organizational characteristics typical of the sexually indifferent period. Ovarian development is a gradual process which is heralded by the appearance of stromal elements and blood capillaries at the dorsal margin of the gonad. Rapidly, these become organized into septa of stromal and vascular tissue that deepen into the blastema along a dorso-ventral direction cleaving it into a complex, ramified system of interconnected ovigerous cords. As they become gradually incorporated within the progressively elongating tips of the ovigerous cords, the gonocytes begin to undergo a sequence of differentiative steps, a process referred to as oogenesis and resulting in their rather rapid evolution into oocytes. In all mammals, except prosimians, these changes reach completion prior to the end of fetal life or, in a few species such as lagomorphs, at the latest within the first few days of neonatal life, at which time the oogenetic process is over and the ovary contains oocytes exclusively. In the prosimians, instead, oogenesis is not synchronized and thus not restricted to the fetal period; it continues instead throughout most of the animal's life, i.e., through puberty and adulthood until the end of the reproductive period (14,15). For the objectives of this review, however, the unique oogenesis of these animals will be ignored and only the conventional process typical of all other mammals will be considered.

In the first phase of the oogenetic process, the oocytes enter a period of intense mitotic activity assuming at the same time features of oogonia (16,17). The most evident of these features is the presence of intercellular bridges linking the oogonia to one another and resulting in the formation of syncytia-like oogonial clusters. These bridges are the structural expression of the incomplete mitoses that are typical of this phase of the differentiation of the female germinal cell, whereby karyokinesis is not followed by cytokinesis. Very likely, due to the presence of these bridges through which there is continuous flow of organelles and information from one cell to another, the maturation of the germinal cells within individual clusters proceeds in a synchronized fashion, at least for a while (17,18); the germinal cells undergo subsequent mitoses together and, together, they enter meiotic prophase at the end of the oogonial period of differentiation. In most mammals, prosimians again being the exception, the first meiotic (maturational) division of the female germinal cells does not reach completion in a continuous manner, but becomes interrupted at the diplotene stage of prophase; the oocytes remain in this suspended state of meiotic animation (arrest) until meiosis is resumed shortly before either ovulation or atresia. Obviously, the duration of meiotic arrest differs among species depending upon the length of the interval separating birth from onset of reproductive life (from a few weeks in rodents to more than a decade in humans), as well as among individual oocytes depending as to when their follicles begin to mature or undergo atretic involution (in the woman, for example, the resumption of meiosis in the last oocyte to be ovulated occurs approximately 40 years after that of the first).

Fetal ovarian germinal cell differentiation adheres to timetables that are typical of the species. In rodents, the oogonial phase of differentiation lasts only 24 or, at the most, 36 h occurring on or about the 15th-16th of the 20-21 day long intrauterine development, all oocytes entering meiotic prophase and then becoming meiotically arrested between day 17 and 18; in the human, in contraposition, a few weeks separate the time when the first and the last oocytes enter meiosis and then become arrested. Thus, even though restricted to a short period of fetal development and occurring synchronously in the syncytially linked germinal cells, oogonial and oocytic phases of differentiation do not involve simultaneously all the germinal cells of a given ovary, their occurrence being a function of the time when the gonocytes become incorporated within the developing cords. Together with the directionality of ovigerous cord development, this accounts for the fact that, during the period between the appearance of the first stromal septa at the dorsal margin of the gonad and birth, the ovary typically exhibits evident organizational and germinal cell differentiational gradients. At any given time during this period, the innermost segments of the ovigerous cords are always more organized and more developmentally advanced, and contain germinal cells more differentiated, than the outermost ones; for example, they may contain meiotic oocytes or oocytes already arrested in meiotic prophase while the outermost segments still display mitotic oogonia. However, at the end of fetal life or, at the latest, after the first few days of neonatal life, all ovarian germinal cells have differentiated into oocytes arrested in the diplotene stage of meiotic prophase. Meiotic arrest is accompanied by morphologic changes, whereby the oocytes assume characteristics that they will retain for most of their intrafollicular life until resumption of meiosis. The intercellular bridges disappear and the oocytes regain independence from one another. They increase considerably in size, becoming 6 or 7 times larger than the premeiotic cells. Their nuclei are large and regular in outline and contain one or two prominent nucleoli and chromatin with typical (dyctiate) aggregational patterns. Their cytoplasms are expanded and characterized by prominent and elaborate Golgi complexes in juxtanuclear position (the Balbiani or vitelline body of classic investigators), sparse and short ergastoplasmic reticulum cisternae, and scattered mitochondria. Due to the volumetric increase of the oocytes, the segment of the cord where each is contained becomes expanded with consequent flattening of the originally cuboidal or columnar somatic cells; consequently, these dilated segments of the cords assume follicle-like features, i.e., a spheroidal outline with a single layer of attenuated somatic (pregranulosa) cells resting on a basal lamina and radially arranged around the centrally located oocyte. These dilated, follicle-like segments are positioned along the extension of the original ovigerous cords like the beads of a rosary, the intervening segments, those not containing oocytes, being narrow and cylindrical. Having developed within the context of a cord system, at this stage all follicles are connected to one another, a phenomenon that was first reported by us (19). They remain in this condition for variable periods of time; in the mouse, for example, they become individualized only at the end of the third week of life when, as a result of the encroachment of the mature interstitium, the interfollicular segments of the cords become progressively thinner and eventually disappear (19).

It is evident from the above that, albeit far from being fully mature, at the end of fetal development the ovary possesses all the elements necessary for its function during the neonatal, prepubertal, and reproductive periods. The follicular components are represented by a multitude of primordial follicles, each consisting of a centrally located oocyte arrested in the diplotene stage of meiotic prophase, a peripheral layer of attenuated follicle cells, and a continuous basement membrane. The interstitial elements are represented by blood and lymphatic vessels, nerves, and interstitial cells. The latter now display features of increased differentiation as compared to the original mesenchymal elements; those situated in the immediate proximity to the basal laminae of individual follicles will, at the time of follicle maturation, differentiate into theca cells.

In spite of the gains made in our knowledge of the mechanisms regulating gonadal development, key aspects continue to elude us: What are the factors that induce the sexually indifferent gonad to differentiate into an ovary rather than a testis or vice versa? What controls the differentiation of a gonocyte into an oogonium rather than a pre-spermatogonium? Is there any relationship between the sexual differentiation of the organ and that of the germinal cells, which is also sexually dimorphic, and, if there is one, how does it operate? Some indirect light on these still unresolved aspects of gonadal development has been shed by recent studies performed in the author's laboratory on germinal cell behavior in ectopic sites, i.e., outside the ovigerous and seminiferous cords (reviewed in 20). Germinal cell ectopism can be distinguished into: intra-, peri-, and extragonadal. The first involves cells that are in the gonads but have not been incorporated in the ovigerous or seminiferous cords and thus reside in extracordal sites such as the stroma, the tunica albuginea, etc. Perigonadal ectopism refers to those germinal cells that are scattered in sites just dorsal to the gonads such as the perigonadal mesenchyme and the vestigia of mesonephric structures, as well as those that are situated within the extragonadal segments of the rete testis and ovarii. The phenomenon of extragonadal ectopism involves, instead, germ cells situated in organs or sites far from the gonads such as the adrenal glands, the retroperitoneal nervous ganglia, the walls of the large vessels (the aorta, the cardinal veins), the erythropoietic mesenchyme surrounding the retroperitoneal organs, the cartilaginous templates of the vertebrae, etc. Several factors are responsible for the ectopic phenomenon; for the scope of this review, suffice it to say that the most important ones are the continuous tissue dynamism typical of embryonal development which is largely responsible for deflecting some germinal cells from their gonadally aimed path and carrying them to extragonadal sites, and the late arrival of some of the germinal cells in the gonads which is responsible for their being excluded from participating in the assembly of the gonadal cords. Be that as it may, the following facts need to be mentioned. In mammals, germ cell ectopism in all of its subvariants is not at all exceptional but, on the contrary, is a frequent and prominent phenomenon; depending upon the species, it may involve most (rodents; 21,22) or all embryos and fetuses (primates; 23), and from a few germinal cells situated only in one or two ectopic sites (rodents; 21,22) to impressive numbers of them distributed over a wide range of extra-, peri-, and intragonadal ectopic locations (primates; 23). In some cases, the number of ectopic germinal cells may exceed that of those that the same embryo has in the gonads (21). Most interesting, however, and most relevant to the topic of this review, is the behavior of the germinal cells in the different ectopic sites. Not only are the ectopic cells able to survive for remarkably long periods of time, up to the end of the third week of postnatal life in rodents (21) and at least up to, and very likely past, the end of intrauterine life in a primate (the *Galago crassicaudatus crassicaudatus*) with a gestation of 133 days (23), but they are also capable of attaining advanced differentiation. Significantly, whereas the ectopic XX germinal cells differentiate just like those inside the ovigerous cords, the XY germinal cells exhibit a dual differentiative behavior. Those in intra- and perigonadal ectopic sites follow patterns of differentiation identical to those of the XY cells inside the seminiferous cords, whereas those in extragonadal locations all differentiate as females, i.e., at first as oogonia and then as oocytes; moreover, they also do so scrupulously following the ovarian germinal cell differentiative timetables typical of the species. For example, the XY germinal cells situated in the adrenal glands of mouse embryos and fetuses differentiate from PGCs into oogonia around day 15 of intrauterine development and enter meiosis at day 17. By day 19, they are all arrested in the diplotene stage of prophase and, henceforth, they behave like follicular oocytes, their functional attitudes including the synthesis and deposition of the zona pellucida and the synthesis of the cortical granules from their Golgi complexes. The fact that all germinal cells, including the XY, differentiate extragonadally as XX germinal cells do inside the ovigerous cords indicates that all germinal cells, irrespective of their genetic sex, are inherently female and that the ovary may not play too significant a role in modulating germinal cell behavior. The observation that the XY germinal cells are deflected from their female differentiative bend only if they are within, or in the immediate proximity of, the testis strongly suggests that the male gonad is instead capable of influencing germ cell differentiation, at least that of the XY. Thus, it would seem that ovaries and testes differ with regard to the existence of a possible relationship between gonadal and germinal cell differentiation.

References

1. Wartenberg H. Germ cell migration induced and guided by somatic cell interaction. Bibl Anat 1983; 24:93-110.
2. Witschi E. Migration of the germ cells of human embryos from the yolk sac to the primitive gonadal folds. Contrib Embryol Carnegie Inst 1948; 32:67-80.
3. Zamboni L, Merchant H. The fine morphology of mouse primordial germ cells in extragonadal locations. Am J Anat 1973; 137:299-336.
4. Eddy EM, Clark JM, Gong D, Fenderson BA. Origin and migration of primordial germ cells in mammals. Gam Res 1981; 4:333-62.

5. Blandau RJ, White BJ, Rumery RE. Observations on the movement of the living primordial germ cells in the mouse. Fertil Steril 1963; 14:482-9.
6. Fujimoto T, Yoshinaga K. The role of fibronectin in the interstitial migration of primordial germ cells in amniotes. Cong Anom 1986; 26:186-96.
7. Donovan PJ, Stott D, Cairns LA, Heasman J, Wylie CC. Migratory and postmigratory mouse primordial germ cells behave differently in culture. Cell 1986; 44:831-8.
8. Merchant H. Rat gonadal and ovarian organogenesis with and without germ cells. An ultrastructural study. Dev Biol 1975; 44:1-21.
9. Yoshinaga K, Hess DL, Hendrickx AG, Zamboni L. The development of the sexually indifferent gonad of the prosimian *Galago crassicaudatus crassicaudatus*. Am J Anat 1988; 181:89-105.
10. Zamboni L, Upadhyay S. Ephemeral, rudimentary glomerular structures in the mesonephros of the mouse. Anat Rec 1981; 201:641-4.
11. Upadhyay S, Luciani JM, Zamboni L. The role of the mesonephros in the development of indifferent gonads and ovaries of the mouse. Ann Biol Anim Biochem Biophys 1979; 19:1179-96.
12. Zamboni L, Bezard J, Mauleon P. The role of the mesonephros in the development of the sheep fetal ovary. Ann Biol Anim Biochem Biophys 1979; 19:1153-78.
13. Zamboni L, Upadhyay S. The contribution of the mesonephros to the development of the sheep fetal testis. Am J Anat 1982; 165:339-56.
14. Butler H. Oogenesis and folliculogenesis. In: Hafez ESE, ed. Comparative reproduction of nonhuman primates. Springfield: CC Thomas, 1971:243-68.
15. Anand Kumar TC. Oogenesis in adult prosimian primates. Contr Primat 1974; 3:82-96.
16. Weakley BS. Light and electron microscopy of developing germ cells and follicle cells in the ovary of the golden hamster: twenty four hours before birth to eight day postpartum. J Anat 1967; 101:435-59.
17. Zamboni L, Gondos B. Intercellular bridges and synchronization of germ cell differentiation during oogenesis in the rabbit. J Cell Biol 1968; 36:276-82.
18. Gondos B, Zamboni L. Ovarian development. The functional importance of germ cell interconnections. Fertil Steril 1969; 20:176-89.
19. Merchant H, Zamboni L. Presence of connections between follicles in juvenile mouse ovaries. Am J Anat 1972; 134:127-32.
20. Zamboni L. Meiosis as a sexual dimorphic character of germinal cell differentiation. Tokai J Exp Clin Med 1986; 11:371-90.
21. Zamboni L, Upadhyay S. Germ cell differentiation in mouse adrenal glands. J Exp Zool 1983; 228:173-93.
22. Francavilla S, Zamboni L. Differentiation of mouse ectopic germinal cells in intra- and perigonadal locations. J Exp Zool 1985; 233:101-9.
23. Yoshinaga K, Hess DL, Hendrickx AG, Zamboni L. Germinal cell ectopism in embryos and fetuses of the prosimian *Galago crassicaudatus crassicaudatus*. Development (submitted).

3

Role of Second Messengers in Early Differentiation of Gonads and Sex Ducts

Anne Grete Byskov, Hanne Tinggaard, and Claus Yding Andersen

Lababoratory of Reproductive Biology II
Department of Obstetrics and Gynecology
Rigshospitalet, 2100 Copenhagen, Denmark

Introduction

The phenotypic sex develops as a result of gonadal differentiation, which again usually reflects the genetic sex. In spite of numerous studies, the mechanisms which control gonadal sex differentiation are still not clear. Neither sex steroids nor gonadotropins direct the process (1). Specific gene products of the Y-chromosome have been proposed to control testicular differentiation, e.g., the HY-antigen (histocompatability Y-antigen) (2) and the TDF (testis determining factor) (3).

Differentiation of the testis is easily disturbed in vitro whereas ovarian differentiation seems to be conservative and difficult to change. In culture, sexually undifferentiated testes can be feminized to such a degree that they are morphologicallly indistinguishable from ovaries: testicular cords do not develop and germ cells enter meiosis (4,5). Feminization of the fetal mouse testis occurs after a few days of culture in media containing the Meiosis Inducing Substance (MIS). MIS activity is present and released from gonads in which meiosis takes place, e.g., in adult testes of different species and in ovarian follicular fluid of preovulatory follicles (6).

It has been suggested that the two events—enclosure of germ cells in testicular cords and premature initiation of meiosis—are correlated events (4). In a study of cultured fetal mouse gonads it was found that testicular cord formation was prevented by adding compounds which interfered with the second messenger system of cyclic nucleotides. However, the germ cells of these testes did not enter meiosis (7). In the rat, differentiation of testicular cords in vitro was prevented by adding fetal calf serum to the culture medium, but meiosis was not induced (8,9). Therefore, the two events are not necessarily correlated.

Previous results show that various components which interfere with the two second messenger systems (cyclic nucleotides and inositol phospholipids) initiate meiosis in fetal male mouse germ cells in vitro (10), some components acting synergistically with MIS (e.g., forskolin) and others antagonistically (e.g., TPA). These interactions strongly suggest that

MIS acts through receptors on the germ cells or associated somatic cells. The purpose of the present study is to see whether second messengers—some of which apparently control regulation of meiosis in our culture system of fetal mouse gonads—simultaneously interfere with gonadal, in particular testicular, differentiation.

Materials and Methods

Cultures of Fetal Gonads

From fetal mice, strain Albino A-Strong, the gonadal ridges with adherent mesonephric tissue which includes the sex ducts, were removed on day 11-1/2 postcoitus (day 1 is the day of plug). One gonad of each fetus served as the control and the other as experiment. The gonads were cultured at 36°C in 100% humidified atmosphere with 5% CO_2 in air for 3 and 6 days. As control medium we used Minimum Essential Medium (MEM), supplemented with 0.2 mM L-glutamine, 100 IU per ml penicillin, 100 µg per ml streptomycin (all from Flow Laboratories) and 10% heat inactivated fetal calf serum. A total of 44 pairs of ovaries and 48 pairs of testes were used. The effect on gonadal differentiation and meiosis of various substances were tested by adding them to the control medium.

Substances Tested

Dibutyric adenosine 3,5 cyclic monophosphate (dbcAMP, Sigma), 0.75 mM; 7 ovaries and 7 testes, cultured for 6 days. Forskolin, (Calbiochem), 0.3, 3, 10, and 100 µM; 17 ovaries and 19 testes, cultured for 6 days. Lithium chloride (Lithium, Merk), 10 mM; 9 ovaries and 9 testes, cultured for 6 days. Lithium, 10 mM; 11 ovaries and 13 testes, cultured for 3 days in lithium followed by 3 days in control medium. All media had a pH of 7.20 in equilibrium with 5% CO_2 in air, and the osmolality was 280 osmol per kg.

Preparation of the Cultured Fetal Gonads

By the end of the culture period, the gonadal tissue was fixed in 50% Karnowsky's fixative, block-stained with uranylacetate and embedded in Epon. Alternating 1 µ and ultrathin sections were prepared.

Results

Cultured Control Gonads

The testis develops testicular cords with numerous Sertoli cells and rather few resting gonocytes (prespermatogonia) (Fig. 1). The delineation of the cords is somewhat irregular, but is often well defined with a basal lamina, at places lined with flattened cells. In the ovary germ cells have entered meiosis, almost all being in zygotene and pachytene stages (Fig. 2).

Gonads Cultured with Various Substances

Forskolin. Addition of forskolin prevents testicular cord formation and induces meiosis in the male in a dose-dependent manner. Thus, male and female gonads cultured in 10 and 100 µM forskolin cannot be distinguished morphologically from each other or from the control ovaries. In all cases, the germ cells have entered meiosis and have often advanced to pachytene stage (Fig. 3). With 3 µM forskolin, meiosis is also induced in the male but the

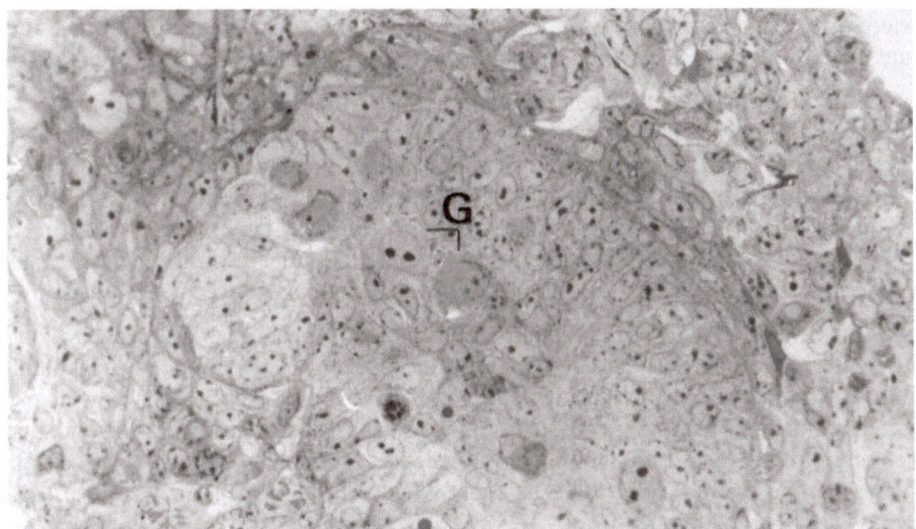

Fig. 1. Testicular cords with many Sertoli cells and some gonocytes (G) of a testis cultured for 6 days. At places, the basal lamina is lined with flattened cells. x 1,890.

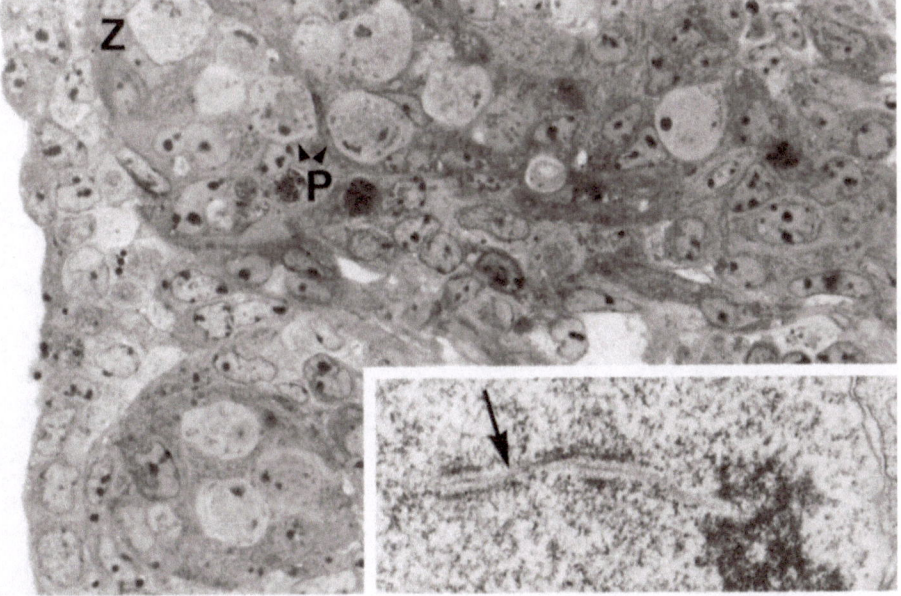

Fig. 2. Cortical part of a control ovary cultured for 6 days showing oocytes in different stages of meiosis, zygotene (Z), pachytene (P). x 2,000. Inset: Synaptonemal complex from an oocyte in pachytene stage with a bivalent twisted 180 degrees (arrow). x 34,000.

structure of the testicular cords is only slightly blurred. Testicular cords are present after culture with 0.3 μM forskolin, a concentration which also leaves the germ cells unaffected.

dbcAMP. The low (0.1 mM) concentration of dbcAMP had no effect, but the high (1.5 mM) concentration was toxic. Concentration of 0.75 mM occasionally caused induction of meiosis to leptotene and zygotene stage in some of the male germ cells but had no inhibitory effect on the differentiation of testicular cords. On the contrary, the delineation of the cords with a distinct basal lamina surrounded by flattened cells was better defined than in the controls (Fig. 4). No effect could be seen in the ovaries except that fewer germ cells seemed to be present than in the controls, an observation which was also noticed in the testes.

Lithium. Addition of 10 mM lithium to cultures for 6 days caused the germ cells of both sexes to enter and remain in leptotene stage (Fig. 5). However, when 3-day cultures in lithium are followed by 3 days in control medium, the germ cells of both sexes proceeded in meiosis to zygotene and pachytene stages (Fig. 6) and the testicular cords became less distinct than in the control. After 6 days in lithium, only fragments of testicular cords were present, the testes resembling ovaries cultured in the same way, with germ cells in leptotene stage scattered in the gonadal tissue.

Influences on the Sex Ducts

The Wolffian duct in all controls, males as well as females, was in degeneration after 6 days of culture (Fig. 7, Fig. 8). However, this degeneration was prevented in cultures with forskolin (3 and 10 μM) (Fig. 9) and to a lesser degree with dbcAMP (Fig. 10). In these cultures many cells of the Wolffian duct epithelium were in mitosis.

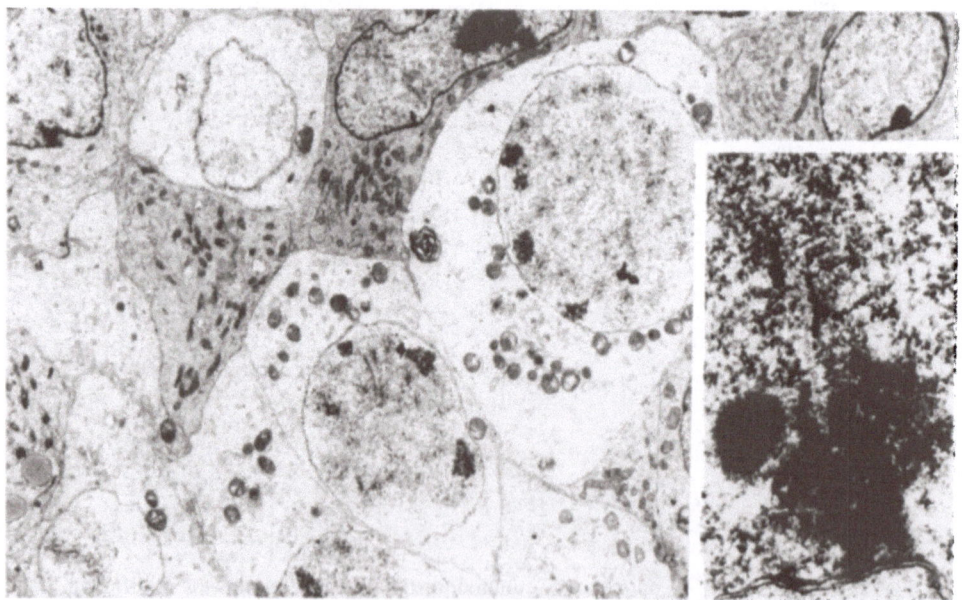

Fig. 3. Testis cultured for 6 days with 3 μM forskolin with germ cells in pachytene stages and no trace of testicular cords. x 4,500. Inset: Synaptonemal complex. x 45,000.

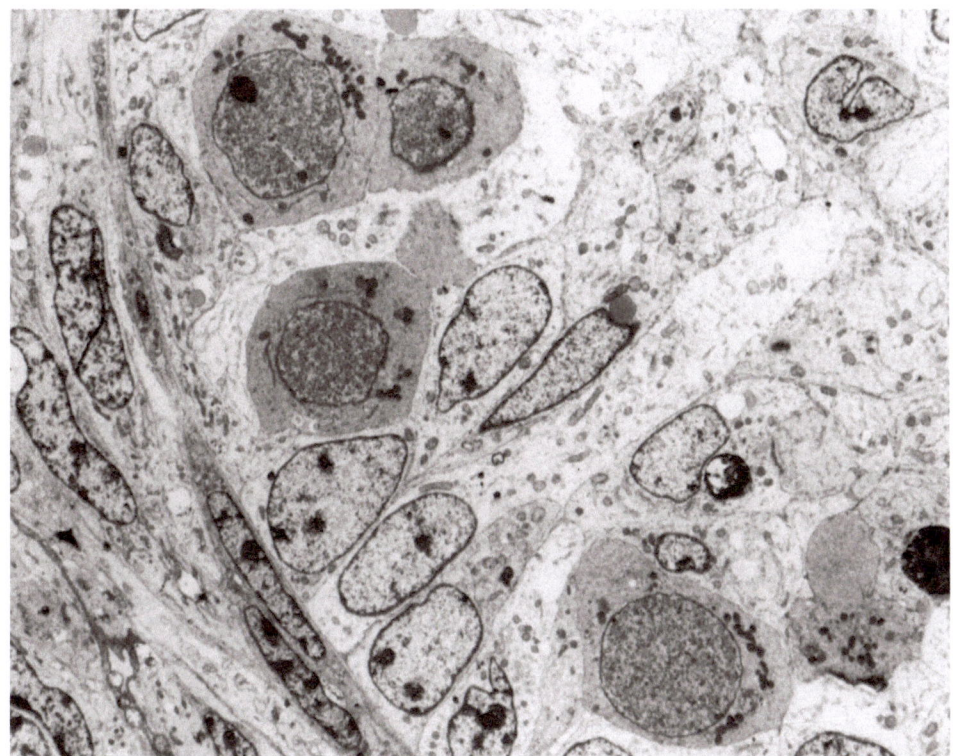

Fig. 4. Well-defined testicular cords with gonocytes of a testis cultured for 6 days with 0.75 mM dbcAMP. x 3,800.

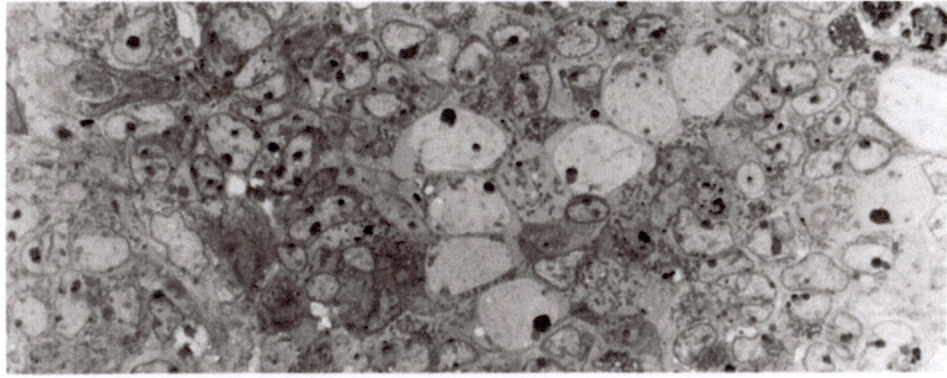

Fig. 5. Ovary cultured with 10 mM lithium for 6 days. The large, clear germ cells are leptotene stages. x 2,000.

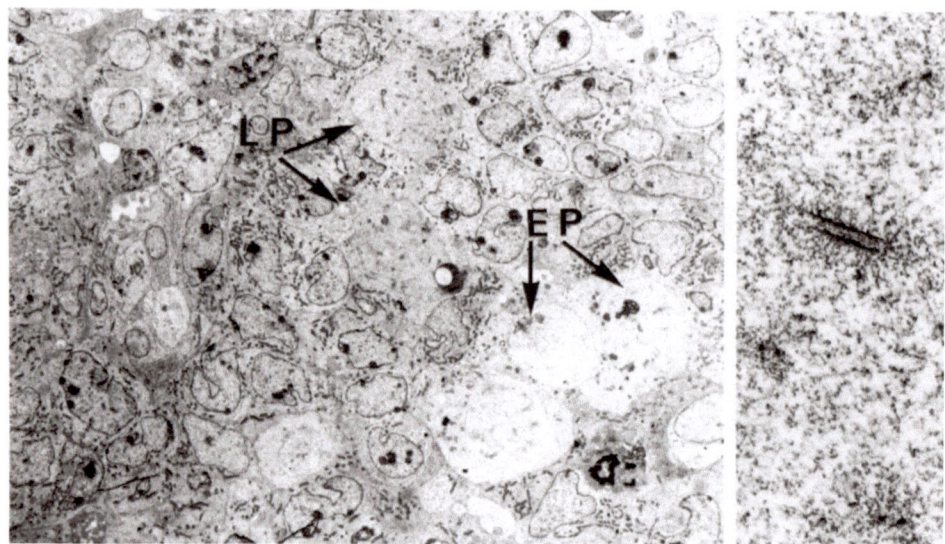

Fig. 6. Testis cultured for 3 days in 10 mM lithium followed by 3 days in control medium with early (EP) and late pachytene (LP) stages. x 2,400. Inset: Four synaptonemal complexes; one is sectioned longitudinally and the others are cross-sectioned. x 30,000.

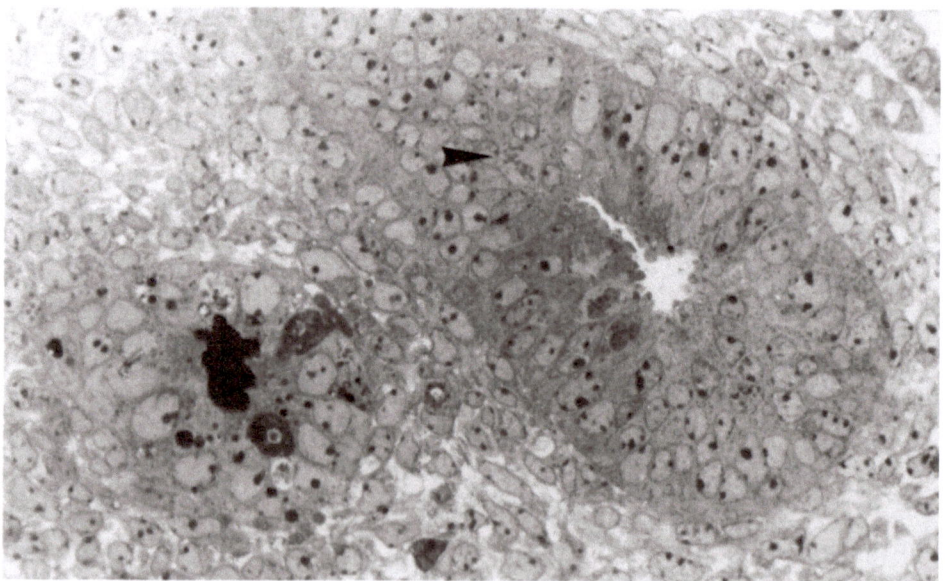

Fig. 7. Female control ducts with a well-developed Mullerian duct with mitosis (arrow) and a degenerating Wolffian duct. x 1,800.

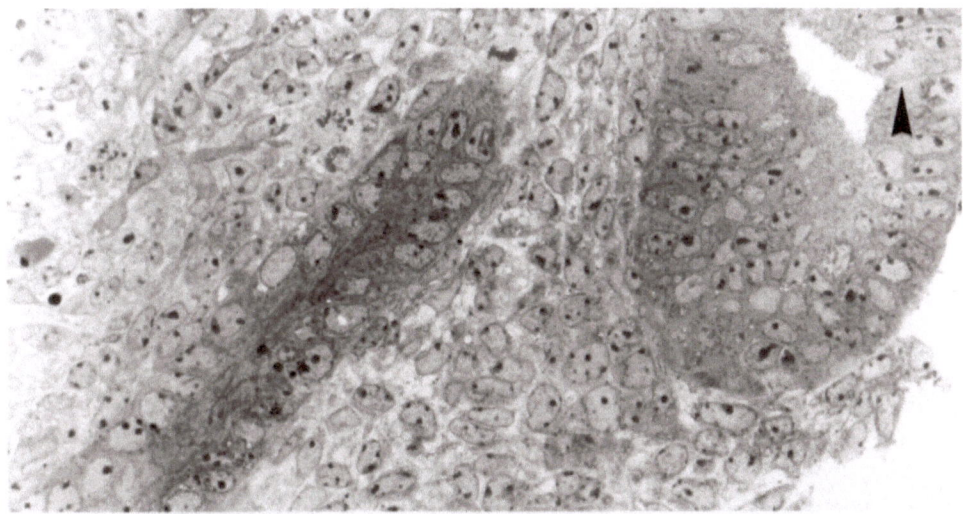

Fig. 8. Male control ducts with a similar appearance as the female of Figure 7. The arrow points at mitosis. x 1,800.

In all cultures, except those with dbcAMP, the Mullerian duct seemed to grow well with many mitotic figures in the epithelium (Fig. 7, Fig. 8). In cultures with dbcAMP, mitotic figures were rare in the Mullerian epithelium although it was not degenerating (Fig. 10).

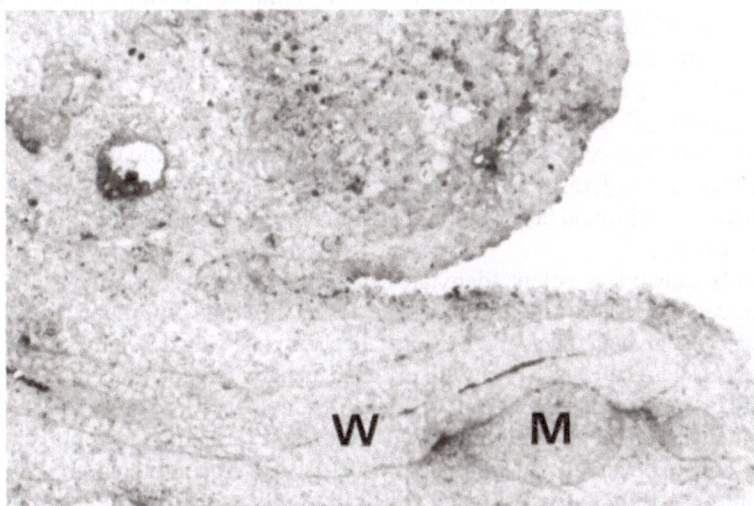

Fig. 9. Male ducts and part of the testis cultured for 6 days in 10 mM forskolin. The Wolffian duct (W) is large with a multilayered epithelium as the Mullerian duct (M). No testicular cords are seen. x 300.

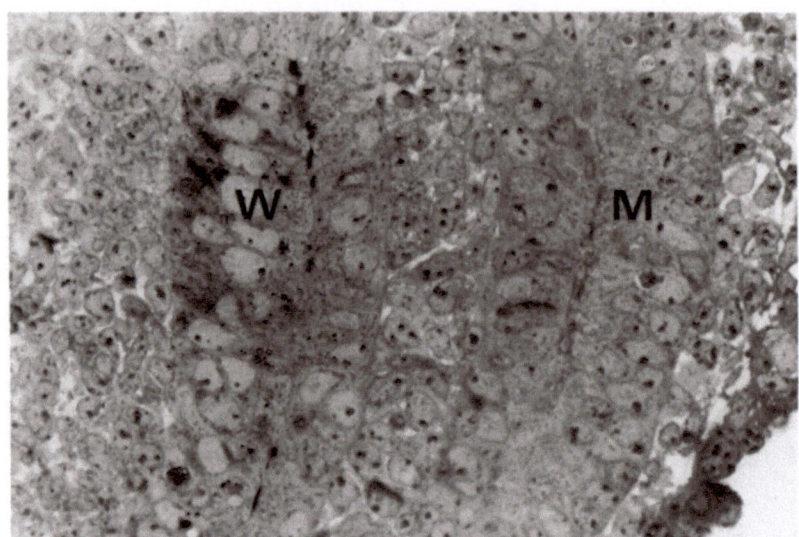

Fig. 10. Female ducts cultured in 0.75 mM dbcAMP for 6 days. The epithelium of the Mullerian duct is low compared with that in Figure 7 and Figure 8, but the epithelium of the Wolffian duct is higher. x 1,800.

Discussion

Our results confirm previous findings that second messengers are involved in initiation of meiosis (10). Moreover, second messengers interfere with the formation of testicular cords and growth of the Wolffian and Mullerian duct. In the lithium experiment it was also shown that premature initiation of meiosis can take place even though the germ cells are enclosed in cords. The results are summarized in Table 1, in which G, L, Z and P are germ cell stages: G - gonocytes; L - leptotene; Z - zygotene; P - pachytene.

Previous studies (7) failed to show an effect of forskolin (20 μM) on the initiation of meiosis in the male germ cells of the mouse. This discrepancy with the present results may be due to the older age of fetuses used in the former study. After gonadal sex differentiation has taken place, we also found no effect by forskolin on germ cells of cultured mouse testes (unpublished results).

Forskolin is known as a potent adenylate cyclase stimulator (11). Since addition of 10 μM forskolin completely prevents formation of testicular cords and induces meiosis and growth of the Wolffian duct, these three events appear, in one way or another, to depend on elevated levels of adenylate cyclase, most likely to result in increased intracellular concentration of cAMP. However, addition of the cAMP analog, dbcAMP, only resulted in a limited induction of meiosis and not in inhibition of testicular cord formation. In contrast, differentiation of the cords appears to be stimulated, which also is in contradiction to a previous report (7). Since exposure to forskolin and dbcAMP results in opposite effects on differentiation of testicular cords, it is possible that the cellular response to the two components differs. While dbcAMP is thought to mimic the effect of cAMP, the stimulation of adenylate cyclase by forskolin may, in addition to increasing cAMP, also activate protein kinase C by

Table 1. Effect of forskolin, dbcAMP and lithium on development of
mouse gonads and ducts in vitro

Compound	Concentration	Inhibition of TC	Meiosis*		Growth of Ducts	
			Testis	Ovary	Wolff	Muller
Forskolin	0.3 µM	0	G	P Z L	0	+++
	3 µM	+	Z G & L	P Z L	+	+++
	10 µM	+++	P Z L	P Z L	++	+++
dbcAMP	0.75 mM	0	G & L	P Z L	+	++
Lithium 3 days	10 mM	0	L	L	0	+++
Lithium (3+3) days	10 mM	(+)	Z L	P Z L	P 0	+++
Lithium 6 days	10 mM	++	L	L	0	+++

*G - gonocytes; L - leptotene; Z - zygotene; P - pachytene.

stimulation of the other second messenger, diacylglycerol. This effect might result in a different cellular response. It is also possible that the two components act on different cell types, resulting in different cellular secretions. This possibility is also supported by the different actions of dbcAMP and forskolin on the growth of the sex ducts.

The well-differentiated testicular cords in the testes cultured with dbcAMP may produce anti-Mullerian hormone (12), thus explaining the growth inhibition of the Mullerian duct. This well-differentiated testicular tissue probably also secretes testosterone as previously reported (7), which would account for stimulation of the Wolffian duct. Lithium is a component which interacts with both the cAMP pathway and the inositol-lipid pathway. Lithium inhibits the degradation of insositol-1,4,5-P3 which induces intracellular release of Ca^{++} ions (13). Lithium also inhibits forskolin-stimulated adenylate cyclase, probably by acting directly on the enzyme (14). Since lithium stimulates DNA synthesis in some cell types (15), we previously proposed that lithium induces the premeiotic DNA synthesis and entrance into leptotene stage in the germ cells, but that further progress is blocked, reversibly, by its inhibition of adenylate cyclase (10). The latter study showed, in fact, that forskolin and lithium acted antagonistically in controlling meiosis.

In conclusion, on the basis of these preliminary results, we propose that early differentiation of the testicular cords depends on a finely controlled elevated level of cAMP. The direct stimulation of adenylate cyclase by forskolin which prevents testicular cord formation may not only raise cAMP to uncontrollable levels but simultaneously act distal to cAMP through diacylglycerol.

References

1. Byskov AG. Differentiation of mammalian embryonic gonad. Physiol Rev 1986; 66:71-117.
2. Wachtel SS. H-Y antigen in gonadal differentiation. In: Austin CR, Edwards RG, eds. Mechanisms of sex differentiation in animals and man. London, New York: Academic Press, 1981:255-99.
3. Page DC, Mosher R, Simpson EM, et al. The sex-determining region of the human Y chromosome encodes a finger protein. Cell 1987; 51:1091-1104.
4. Byskov AG. Regulation of meiosis in mammals. Ann Biol Anim Biochem Biophys 1979; 19:1251-61.
5. Fajer AB, Schneider J, McCall D, Ances IG, Polakis SE. The induction of meiosis by ovaries of newborn hamsters and its relation to the action of the extraovarian structures in the mesovarium (rete ovarii). Ann Biol Anim Biochem Biophys 1979; 19:1273-8.
6. Westergaard LG. Intrafollicular factors regulating human ovarian follicular development and oocyte maturation. Dan Med Bull 1988 (in press).
7. Taketo T, Thau RB, Adeyemo O, Koide SS. Influence of adenosine 3':5'-cyclic monophosphate analogues on testicular organization of fetal mouse gonads in vitro. Biol Reprod 1984; 30:189-98.
8. Magre S, Agelopoulou R, Jost A. Action du serum de veau sur la differenciation in vitro on le maintien des cordon seminiferes du testicule du faetus du rat. C R Acad Sci (Paris) 1981; 292:85-9.
9. Agelopoulou R, Magre S, Patsavoudi E, Jost A. Initial phases of the rat testis differentiation in vitro. J Embryol Exp Morphol 1984; 83:15-31.
10. Byskov AG, Fenger M, Hansen JL, Husum I, Bagger P. Second messengers in control of onset of meiosis in fetal mice. 1988 (submitted).
11. Daly JW. Forskolin, adenylate cyclase, and cell physiology: an overview. In: Greengard P, ed. Advances in cyclic nucleotide and protein phosphorylation research. New York: Raven Press, 1984:81-9.
12. Joso N, Picard J-Y. Anti-Mullerian hormone. Physiol Rev 1986; 66:1038-90.
13. Drummond AH, Joels LA, Hughes PJ. The interaction of lithium ions with lipid signalling systems. Biochem Soc Trans 1987; 15:32-5.
14. Mork A, Geisler A. Mode of action of lithium on the catalytic unit of adenylate cyclase from rat brain. Pharmacol Toxicol 1987; 60:241-8.
15. Tomooka Y, Imagawa W, Nandi S, Bern HA. Growth effect of lithium on mouse mammary epithelial cells in serum-free collagen gel culture. J Cell Physiol 1983; 117:290-6.

4

Ovarian Tumors, Stem Cells and Ontogeny:
Imminentes Cognitiones

Waldemar A. Schmidt

Department of Pathology and Laboratory Medicine
University of Texas Medical School–Houston

Introduction

Two fundamental and inextricably interrelated issues limit understanding of ovarian malignancy. Clinically, we can neither recognize early lesions nor ascertain their potential. Hence, ovarian cancer management depends upon a "recognition/classification" paradigm wherein tumor recognition, classification and therapy depends upon the morphology of advanced lesions. There is a parallel inability to fully describe the participants and processes of early ovarian development, making it impossible to definitively exclude one or more of the three major theories on the ontogeny of ovarian tissues (1,2). Models and methods used to explore these problems have serious limitations. In carcinogenesis the early lesions are yet to be defined, while in ovarian embryology the minuscule size of the tissues involved and the limited numbers of participating cells restrict research opportunities.

Ovarian carcinogenesis and ontogenesis are really two facets of a singular problem, that of ovarian development. Pierce considers cancer a problem of developmental biology (3,4) and tumors tissues where normal developmental and regenerative processes escape control. In fact, for each major event of carcinogenesis (initiation, promotion, progression, invasion and metastasis), a counterpart may be found in normal developmental and reparative processes (5-7).

Hence: if,   the Pierce hypothesis is true,
      and, ovarian ontogeny and carcinogenesis represent dual facets
            of a singular problem,
      and, understanding precedes controlling,

      then, ovarian tumor models are extremely important tools with which
            we may address simultaneously both aspects of the problem.

I present herein studies with a new ovarian tumor system, the Ross Ovarian Tumor Model, which is not plagued by the problems presented by other models (resistance to tumor induction, prolonged time to develop lesions, sparse numbers and undefined nature of lesions produced, and difficulty culturing lesion cells) (8). Data from these studies suggest properties and processes which might be expected of cells involved in early ovarian development.

The Ross Ovarian Tumor Model

Original Studies and Conclusions

Hillier et al. (9) reported a new line of SV40 virus transformed rat granulosa cells, the original purpose of which was to provide numerous cells for functional studies of granulosa cell function. The granulosa cells were obtained from ovaries of estrogen-treated, immature Holtzman variant Sprague-Dawley (HvSD) rats in the NIH colony. After transformation, the cells were maintained in vivo in RPMI until they no longer shed the virus.

The transformed cells were adapted to in vivo growth by serial passage via intraperitoneal (IP) injection into nude mice, total body irradiated HvSD rats and thence to nonirradiated HvSD rats. All of the nude mice and irradiated rats developed tumor (Hillier, personal communication, 1983). IP injection of 10(7) tumor cells resulted, after 6 days, in the development of solid tumors at the injection site or ascites fluid (AF) tumors, or both, in 75% of the nonirradiated 100 g HvSD rats. Tumor growth was linear and resulted in as much as 75 mL of bloody AF with 10(7)-10(8) tumor cells/mL. The term Fran Tumor (FT) was coined.

FT hormonal responsiveness was demonstrated in vivo using ovariectomized, estrogen-treated ovariectomized, ovariectomized and hypophysectomized, and hypophysectomized animals. In oophorectomized animals, the onset of measurable tumor growth was earlier by 2 days and maximum tumor dimensions were 1.5-2.7 times greater than in untreated, adult female hosts; ovariectomy effects were reversed by estrogen replacement therapy or hypophysectomy. Hypophysectomized animals with intact ovaries had a delayed onset of smaller tumors. Hillier et al. (9) suggested that this line of "hormonally responsive, transplantable tumors of isolated follicular cell-types should be of considerable value in future studies of the regulation of folliculogenesis *(sic)* at a cellular level."

Zeleznik et al. (10) studied steroidogenesis using hypoxanthine guanine phosphoribosyltransferase-deficient (HPRT-) FT cells hybridized with nontransformed granulosa cells obtained from diethylstilbestrol-treated, hypophysectomized, immature female HvSD rats (11). The steroidogenic capacity of the nonfused transformed cells, their HPRT (-) derivatives and the hybrids were evaluated by RIA for progesterone and pregnenolone production; neither the original FT cells nor the HPRT (-) mutants produced steroids. The hybrids grew in culture and produced steroids only after stimulation by agents which increase intracellular cAMP in other steroid producing cells (12-14); the agents were dibutyryl-cyclic-AMP (di-B-cAMP), prostaglandin E2 (PGE2), choleratoxin (CT), isoproterenol (I) and 2-chloroadenosine. Further, because the hybrids required 12-24 h of stimulation before steroid production, they appeared similar to normal granulosa cells at an early stage of development (immature follicle) (15). The authors concluded that the "cells obtained by hybridizing transformed ovarian granulosa cells with freshly isolated rat granulosa cells possess the growth properties of the transformed cell and some of the specialized functions of the primary cells. This strategy may be useful in obtaining other cell strains of differentiated endocrine cells in various developmental stages for more detailed study (10)."

Tumor Biology Studies

The FT was examined to determine its usefulness as a model of ovarian neoplasia (15). The intent was to study the early steps of ovarian carcinogenesis to determine the FT cells' differentiation potential. From the former it was desired to obtain a model for studies of early detection and, thereby, early control and from the latter a model for studying late tumor management through differentiation modulation. If the latter approach was successful, it would be possible to use the cell line to probe early ovarian ontogenesis.

FT cells, from an early posttransformation tissue culture, were retrieved after 10 years under liquid nitrogen. These cells were passed to in vivo growth by IP inoculation into nude mice (approximately 10[6] cells/mL/mouse); all 5 developed AF tumors. The (AF) was pooled and was sequentially passed through 4 more sets of 4 nude mice each. In all, 21 nude mice developed tumors and provided enough AF to permit passage into HvSD rats.

Young, adult female HvSD rats were rendered immune incompetent with 600-700 R total body irradiation (TBI) with a ^{137}Cs source providing 461.1 R/min; a total of 39 such rats were inoculated with sequentially passed AF. The first set were inoculated with AF from the last set of nude mice while all subsequent sets received their AF from preceding sets of rats. Thirty-eight irradiated rats developed tumors. There was no evidence of solid or ascites tumor in one animal even though its cohorts developed AF and solid tumors.

Among 47 intact, nonirradiated HvSD rats receiving AF IP, 34 developed tumors; neither solid nor ascites tumors were found in the other 14 animals even though they received inoculations of tumor bearing ascites fluids which produced tumor in their cohorts. A summary of the results of passage of the FT line through these three hosts is shown in Table 1. A summary of the nature of the ascites fluid and solid tumors (omental and abdominal wall masses) produced in the intact HvSD rats is shown in Table 2.

Table 1. Behavior of FT tumor line in three hosts

	Nude Mice	TBI Rats	Intact Rats
No. injected	21	39	47
No. with tumor	21	38	34
% with tumor	100	97.4	72.3
Days to sacrifice			
average	5.4	4.9	5.3
range	12-4	8-4	11-5
AF: obtained (mL)			
average	4.36	16.3	10.9
range	6.5-0.2	35-3	33-1
cells/mL	ND	$3.2 \times 10(8)$	$6.7 \times 10(6)$

TBI = Total body irradiated; ^{137}Cs source, 600-700R; <140 g = 600R, >160 g = 700R. ND = Not done.

Table 2. Nature of the tumors produced in intact HvSD rats

I. Ascites Fluid	
Packed cell volume, average %	14.6
range %	37.7-0.5
T. blue positive cells, average %	2.1
range %	7.7-0
II. Greater omental weights, g	
Animals with tumor (N)	3.64 (34)
range	5.87-1.70
Animals without tumor (N)	0.39 (13)
range	0.62-0.09
Tumor cell size, microns	
Trypan blue negative (N=200)	12.50
Trypan blue positive (N=200)	18.25
Ave., by flow cytometry (N=20,000)	11.78
Cell cycle analysis, by flow cytometry (from pooled fresh ascites fluids)	
Go + G1	45.5 %
S	51.6 %
G2 + M	2.7 %
Total	99.8 %

Development of AF tumor is related to the number of viable tumor cells injected IP and the genetics of the host receiving the inoculum. Seventy to 100% of intact, immune competent, adult female animals of the HvSD type receiving fresh AF which contains at least 10(6) tumor cells/mL with 90% or more tumor cell viability by Trypan blue exclusion testing will develop AF or solid tumors or both. The relationship between the development of AF or solid tumors and inoculum tumor cell concentration is shown in Table 3.

Table 3. Tumor cell concentration in inoculum and
subsequent development of tumors

Cells/mL	Animals with tumor	Animals without tumor	Days to sacrifice
10(7)	6	4	8
10(6)	9	1	9
10(5)	1	9	11
10(4)	0	10	13
10(3)	0	10	13
10(2)	0	10	13

All experiments done with intact, adult female HvSD animals. All animals were injected with fresh pooled ascites fluid with at least 90% tumor cell viability by Trypan blue exclusion.

The genetic nature of the recipient influences the development of tumors after IP passage. Buffalo rats accepted the tumor better than any other while Wistar-Furth animals developed neither ascites fluid nor subcutaneous lesions. The ability of the tumor to persist in the subcutaneous location in the Buffalo, Fisher 344 and ACI strains beyond 14 days is particularly important. After 2 weeks, immune competent animals are capable of mounting an immune response and some will reject well-established subcutaneous tumors. Animals which develop AF tumors do so within 3-4 days and, because they are moribund within 7-8 days, none that do so will survive long enough to benefit from immunologic defenses. The relationship between the genetic strain of recipient and the subsequent development of either ascites fluid or solid tumors is shown in Table 4.

Table 4. Relationship between tumor development and strain of host

Animal Strain	Animals with AF at Day 7	Animals with SQ Tumors				
		Sacrifice		Animals	Average	
		Day	No.	w/ tumor	Weight g	Volume ml
HvSD	10/10	7	2	2	0.36	0.25
		14	2	2	<0.10	<0.10
		21	2	0	–	–
		28	4	0	–	–
Buffalo	10/10	7	2	2	2.49	1 .25
		14	2	2	4.58	4.50
		21	2	2	3.54	3.64
		28	2	2	<0.10	<0.10
		35	2	2	0.74	0.63
Fischer 344	8/10	7	2	2	0.46	0.35
		14	2	2	<0.10	<0.10
		21	2	1	0.30	0.20
		28	4	1	<0.10	<0.10
ACI	5/10	7	2	2	0.10	0.14
		14	2	1	0.20	0.22
		21	2	0	–	–
		28	4	0	–	–
Lewis	2/10	7	2	2	0.10	0.14
		14	2	0	–	–
		21	2	0	–	–
		28	4	0	–	–

Wistar-Furth – – – NEITHER AF NOR SQ TUMORS DEVELOPED – – –

All animals in ascites fluid group injected IP and sacrificed on day 7. All other groups injected subcutaneously (SQ) in one flank. All inocula had >10(6) tumor cells/mL with >90% viability (Trypan blue exclusion).

Hormonal Modulation of In Vivo Tumor Growth

Hormonal responsiveness of FT tumors was demonstrated using nonirradiated, adult female HvSD animals which were: oophorectomized, oophorectomized and estrogen treated, and hypophysectomized. Each set of animals, including the appropriate controls, was inoculated with the same pool of fresh AF with the same number of viable tumor cells. Controls included intact animals injected with viable ascites fluid, intact animals injected with irradiated ascites fluid, and sham hypophysectomized animals.

Results were similar to earlier data (Hillier et al. [9]), again suggesting in vivo tumor growth stimulation by FSH. More of the oophorectomized animals developed AF and solid tumors; the rapid appearance of AF in these animals necessitated earlier sacrifice than was necessary in any of the other groups. Hypophysectomized animals had smaller volumes of AF and solid tumors than the other groups. Both the hypophysectomized and oophorectomized/estrogen-treated animals which developed tumors survived longer than either the oophorectomized or the control groups. These results are summarized in Table 5; notice the sequence of days postinoculation at which the animals with tumor had to be sacrificed: oophorectomy—day 6; controls and sham hypophysectomized—days 7 and 8; hypophysectomized—day 9; and, estrogen treated oophorectomized—day 10.

In Vitro Studies

Initiation of Cultures and the DC3 Clone. FT cells were reestablished in vitro with sterile AF fluid obtained from one immune suppressed but otherwise intact adult female HvSD rat. RPMI washed AF, inoculated at various concentrations (0.15-1.5 x 10(6) cells/25 cm2 flask) in RPMI, DME and JME (spinner culture) media, was cultured under standard conditions (37°C, 95% O_2, 5% CO_2). The RPMI medium was discontinued because the cells therein divided too rapidly; the doubling times in DME and JME stabilized after the first three passes and remained stable thereafter at an average of 16.36 and 25.05 h during the

Table 5. Hormonal modulation of in vivo tumor growth

Recipient type	With tumor (%)	Without tumor	Day of sacrifice
Ovariect.	9 (81.8)	2	6
Sham	8 (80.0)	2	8
Irrad. AF	0	10	11
Ovar. + E2	5 (50.0)	5	10
Sham + E2	4 (40.0)	6	10
Irrad. AF	0	10	11
Hypox.	10 (71.4)	4	9
Sham	6 (60.0)	4	7
Intact	6 (60.0)	4	7
Irrad. AF	0	10	13

Animals inoculated IP 1 mL fresh AF with 10(8) tumor cells/mL, 0% Trypan blue positivity. Irrad. AF = Ascites fluid pool inoculum irradiated (^{137}Cs) with 15,000 R immediately prior to inoculation.

first 6-8 days of culture in DME and JME, respectively. This is similar to the 18-h doubling times recorded by others using these cells (17,18). Seeding efficiencies of FT cells in DME were 81.1-90.6% in the 0.1-0.5 x 10(6)cells/25 cm2 flask range. Large numbers of cells were easily grown; 0.2 x 10(6) cells typically expanded to 40-50 x 10(6) cells in 5 days.

A monoclonal line (DC3) was derived from the morphologically pleocellular FT cultures by limiting dilution. The DC3 cells in vitro had growth characteristics and morphological features similar to the parental FT cell line. After culture for 3 and 6 months respectively, both the monoclonal DC3 and the original FT cell lines had similar in vivo properties when injected IP (Table 6).

Stem Cell Studies. Combined in vivo and in vitro studies quantified the hormonal modulation of in vivo growth and determined the differentiation capabilities of FT-induced tumors. Six groups of at least 10 postpubertal (140-160 g) female HvSD rats were used: intact animals, intact given hCG (Serono Laboratories, Inc., Norwell, Massachusetts), oophorectomized animals, oophorectomized animals given hCG, hypophysectomized animals, and hypophysectomized animals given hCG. Oophorectomy and hypophysectomy was done by the supplier and the animals were observed for 2 weeks to assure health prior to experimentation; only those hypophysectomized rats with stable weights were used. The hCG-treated animals received 250 USP units intramuscularly twice/day from the 4th day postinjection of tumor cells until the day of sacrifice. Each animal received IP 2 mL of pooled AF containing >10(6) tumor cells with >95% viability by Trypan blue exclusion. The ascites fluids from the afflicted animals in the 6 experimental groups were harvested and pooled on the 6th-11th day after injection; various tumor biology parameters were monitored.

RBCs were removed from the pooled AFs with lysing reagent (Ortho Diagnostic Systems, Inc., Raritan, New Jersey) (19), tumor cell clumps were dispersed with 5% collagenase digestion (19), and the resulting single cell suspension was separated into 15 fractions by isopycnic density gradient centrifugation (800 x g, 30 min) on a continuous gradient of 0-100% Percoll (Pharmacia Inc., Laboratory Separation Division, Piscataway, New York) (20,21). The number of cells in each fraction was counted with a hemocytometer and viability was determined by Trypan blue exclusion. Tumor behavior in these 6 groups, the nature of the AF pools, the recovery rates and viability of tumor cells after separation are shown in Table 7.

Table 6. In vivo behavior of FT and DC3 cell lines

| | Cell Line Inoculated Into Host | | | |
| | FT | | DC3 | |
Host	Animals with tumor	Sacrifice day	Animals with tumor	Sacrifice day
TBI	10/10	8–9	10/10	8–9
Intact	2/10	13	8/10	8–9

TBI = Total body irradiated, 600 R; these animals were inoculated 48 h after irradiation. All animals inoculated IP with 1 mL washed cells with <10% Trypan blue positivity. FT cells from pass 25, 7 x 10(6) cells/mL; DC3 cells from pass 19, 3.5 x 10(6) cells/mL.

Table 7. Summary of tumor biology and cell separation data

Exper. Group	Tumor Incid. (%)	Oment Wt. (g)	AF Vol. (mL)	Cells/ mL x10(6)	Total Cells x10(9)	Rate (%)	Viab (%)
	Tumor Biology Data					Recovery Data	
I	80	5.61	37.5	17.8	5.34	71.9	97.8
I + hCG	90	7.15	43.0	10.2	3.94	65.5	96.1
O	90	5.20	23.2	50.1	10.48	46.7	50.1
O + hCG	70	8.69	43.0	31.7	9.53	11.7	94.9
H	39	2.02	6.5	23.6	0.92	44.6	23.6
H + hCG	98	2.37	10.9	30.1	2.95	20.6	30.1

Tumor incid = Tumor incidence. Oment wt = Average omental weight for group. AF vol = Average ascites fluid volume for group. Rate = Average recovery rate. Viab = Average viability of recovered cells. I = Intact animals. O = Oophorectomized animals. H = Hypophysectomized animals. Statistical analysis reveals $P<0.05$ for all comparisons except for the following where $P>0.05$: average omental weights: H vs. H + hCG. Incidence of tumors: I vs. I + hCG; I vs. O; I vs. H + hCG.

Morphologically (normal vs. tumor cell, type of tumor cells [mono- or multinucleated], nuclear location, cell size, shape and surface characteristics), there were no important differences between the fractions and the single cell suspension used for loading the density gradient. The procedure did separate tumor and normal cell types well in each of the experimental groups (Figures 1 and 2). Fractions 1-3 contained dead cells and cell debris.

Distinguishing differences were shown when the degree of tumor cell differentiation (as measured by Oil Red O [ORO] staining of intracytoplasmic neutral lipids) and growth capabilities in culture were examined. AF cells from animals with apparently rapidly growing tumors, such as in the oophorectomized animals, contain little or no lipid which is consistent with the concept that rapidly dividing cells undergo little differentiation. Human CG appeared to modulate the differentiated state of the tumor cells and caused an increase in the amount of intracellular lipid (Fig 3).

Fractions 4-15 and an aliquot of the "load" cell suspension of each animal group were placed into both flask and agar culture. Flasks (25 cm^2) containing 5 mL of DMEM-F12 medium (Dulbecco's modification of Eagle's medium [DMEM]) and modified Ham's F12 (Flow Laboratories, McLean, Virginia) with 15% heat inactivated fetal calf serum (GIBCO Laboratories, Grand Island, New York) were inoculated with 10(5) cells from fractions 4-15 and the preseparation "load" cell suspension. The cultures were maintained at 37°C in a 95% O_2/5% CO_2 humidified atmosphere for 5 days before harvesting. Three replicates of each preparation ("load" suspension and fractions 4-15) were cultured and counted.

Anchorage independent growth was measured according to the procedures described for such cultures of human ovarian carcinoma cells by Buick and MacKillop (22,23). Cells (0.33 x 10[5]) were plated onto 35 mm dishes with enriched DMEM-F12 medium supple-

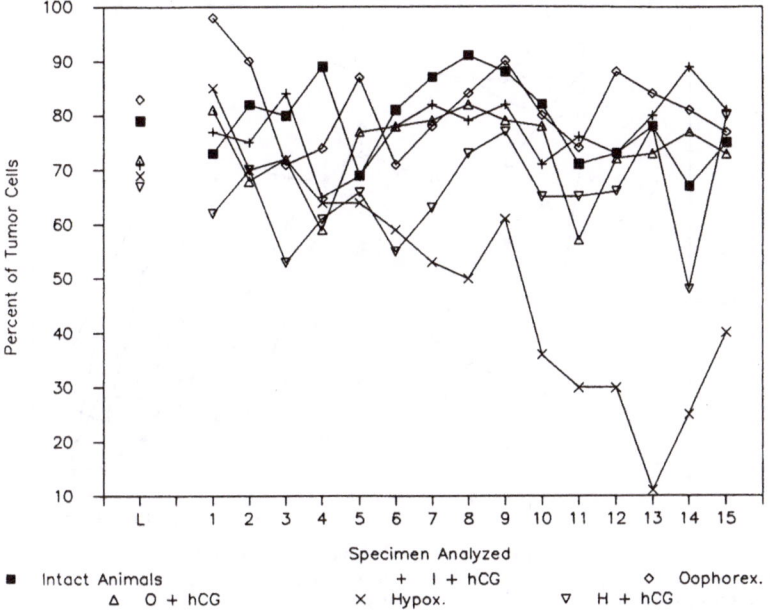

Fig. 1. Percent of tumor cells in the "load" cell suspension and in each fraction.

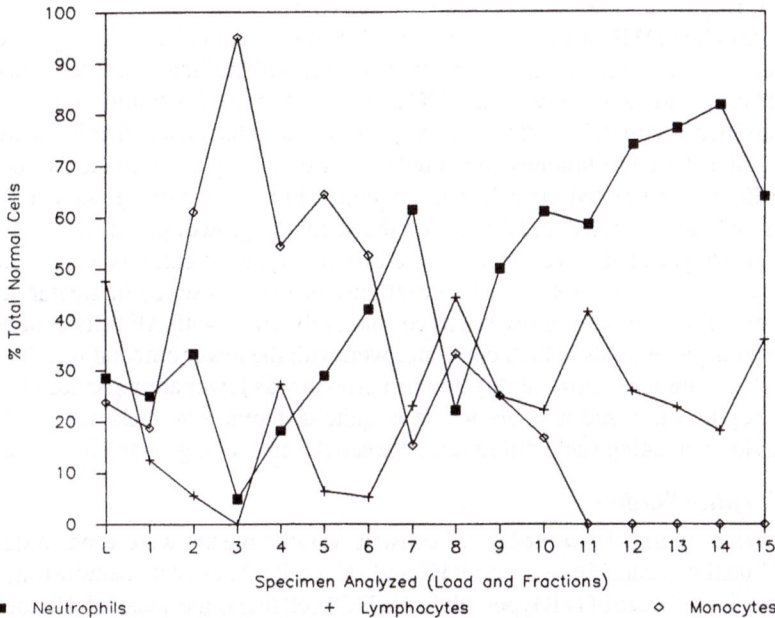

Fig. 2. Differential (%) of normal cells and the "load" cell suspension and in each fraction.

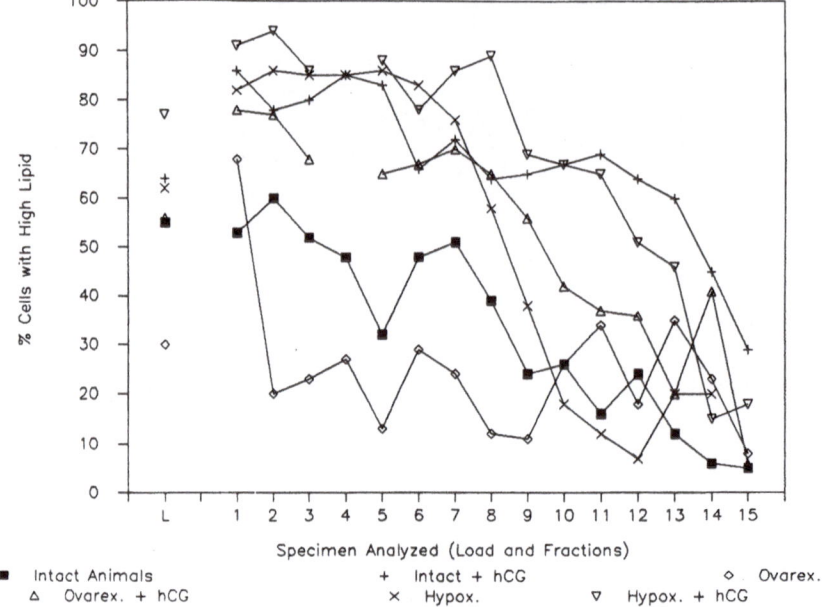

Fig. 3. Percent of tumor cells with >10 ORO intracytoplasmic neutral lipid droplets per cell in the "load" cell suspension and in each fraction.

mented with 15% FCS (final concentration), which contained 0.375% agarose, and covered with 1 mL enriched DMEM-F12 medium with 15% FCS containing 0.6% agarose. Three replicate cultures were made of each of fractions 4-15 and of the "load" cell suspension from each animal group; incubations were at 37°C in a 95% O_2/5% CO_2 humidified atmosphere. Colonies (defined as collections of >50 cells) (23) were counted on day 6 of incubation. The separation and isolation techniques prevented plating of colony-sized clusters of cells.

The techniques separated the cell types, quantified the stationary (or attached) growth capabilities and demonstrated and quantified the stem cell growth properties (24) of these cells. The growth peaks observed in these two different types of cultures occur in identical or adjacent fractions (Figures 4 and 5). In each instance hCG resulted in greater growth in both types of cultures. In vitro growth was considerably lower with AF cells obtained from hypophysectomized animals, which correlates well with the lower omental weights and AF volumes in these animals. Surprisingly, in vitro growth was lower among cultures of tumor cells from oophorectomized animals which is quite different than these animals' in vivo tumor behavior, indicating some difference between AF and solid growth phase tumor cells.

Cellular Identity Studies

Histochemistry and Immunohistochemistry. Various means were used to define the nature and functional capabilities of both FT and DC3 cells. These data demonstrate that the FT cell "line" is a mixture of cell types while the DC3 cell line is monoclonal. Histochemical comparisons of FT tumor nodules and normal tissues are shown in Table 8. Both FT cells in tumor nodules and normal granulosa cells have intracytoplasmic ORO staining droplets (25).

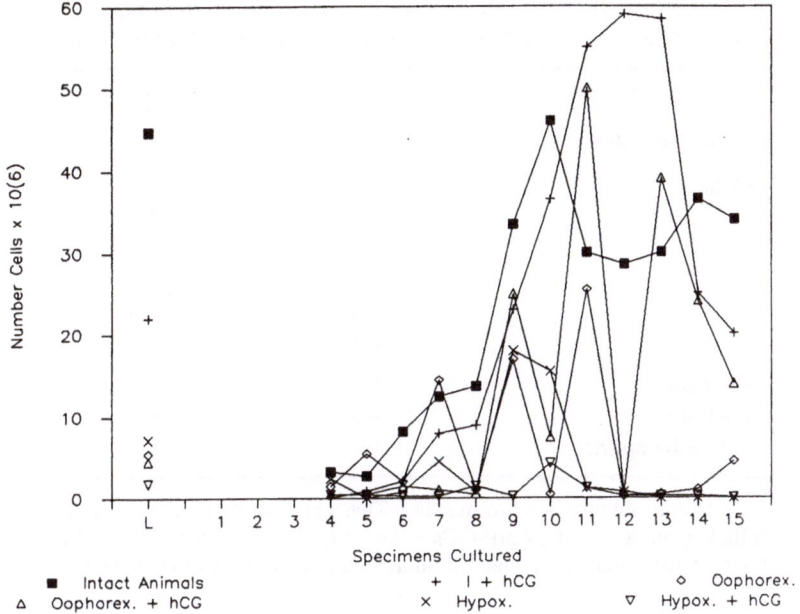

Fig. 4. Number of cells harvested from flask cultures of the "load" cell suspension and fractions 4-15 from each animal group.

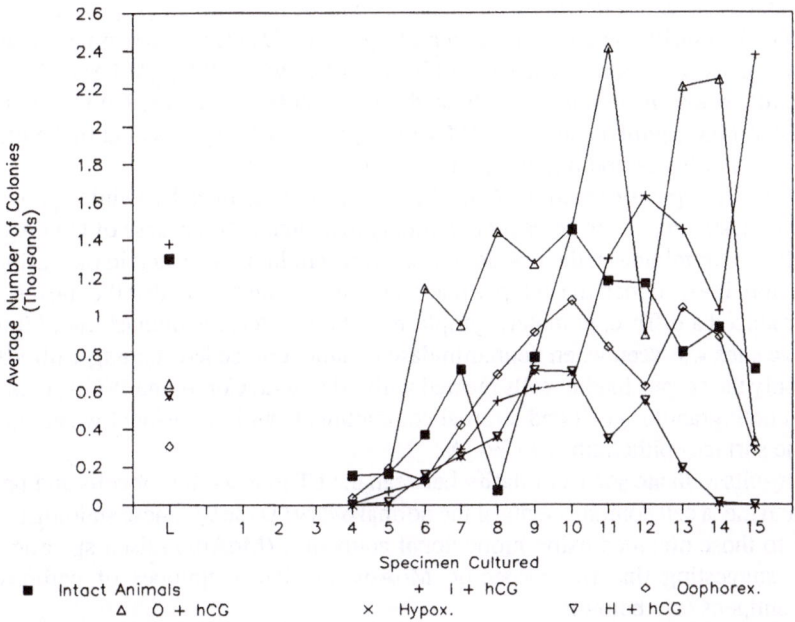

Fig. 5. Number of colonies in agar cultures of the "load" cell suspension and each fractions 4-15 from each animal group.

Table 8. Histochemical analysis of FT-induced tumors.
Oil Red O (ORO) and Gamma-glutamyl Transpeptidase (GGT)

Tissue Examined	ORO	GGT
Tumor nodules	+	–
Ovary	+	+
	CL	CL
	S	
	TI	
	AtrF-GCs	
	AntF-GCs	
Rat testis	NE	+
AAF liver	NE	+
Fall. tube epith.	+/–	+

CL = Corpus luteum. S = Stroma. TI = Theca interna. AtrF-GCs = Atretic
follicle granulosa cells. AntF-GCs = Antral follicle granulosa cells. AAF
liver = GGT control; acetylaminofluorene treated. NE = Not evaluated.

Granulosa cells and FT cells lack gamma-glutamyl transpeptidase (GGT) activity, unlike normal mammalian Sertoli and corpus luteum cells (26).

Lectin histochemical analysis of FT tumor nodules was done using Con A, PNA, WGA, SBA, UEA and DBA with and without pretreatment with neuraminidase (Type V); specificity was determined by using the appropriate inhibitory sugars (27-31). The strongest and most specific reactions were obtained with Con A (200 μg/mL), WGA (100 μg/mL) and SBA (200 μg/mL) lectins, whose reactions were blocked by the inhibitory sugars. No reactivity was seen with DBA (100 μg/mL) and UEA (100 μg/mL) and reactivity was obtained with PNA (500 μg/mL) only after neuraminidase pretreatment.

The lectins with specific reactivity (Con A, WGA and SBA) all had a nodular, geographic reaction pattern, staining some areas more strongly than others. In the case of Con A, WGA and PNA after neuraminidase, the reactions were intracellular and located in the perinuclear or Golgi region. PNA stained the cell periphery and SBA, which provided the most specific reaction, produced a diffuse, granular, cytoplasmic stain. Extensive unmasking of intracellular reactive sites was seen when neuraminidase treatment preceded staining with SBA. In the ovary, only the corpus luteum cells reacted with SBA; with Con A and WGA, there were reactions in both granulosa cell and stromal compartments with occasional weak reactions affecting the surface epithelium with WGA.

These results indicate some similarity between the FT-induced tumor cells and both the granulosa and theca cell compartments of the normal ovary (Table 9). These staining patterns are similar to those obtained using monoclonal antibodies (MoAbs) raised specifically to DC3 cells, suggesting that these specific MoAbs are detect epitopes of carbohydrate containing antigens (see below).

Immunocytochemical analysis of FT tumors and control tissues was done using anti-rat transferrin receptor (TrFeR) antibody (Harlan-Sprague Dawley), anti-fibronectin (Fn) anti-

Table 9. Lectin histochemical analysis of FT-induced tumors

Tissue Examined	Results—without/with neuraminidase					
	Con A	WGA	SBA	PNA	UEA	DBA
Tumor nodules	+/+	+/+	+/+	–/+	–/–	–/+
Ovary	+	+	+	–	–	+
	CL Atr-GCs	FF ZP-GCs	CL			CL
Uterus	+S –LE	+S –LE	+S	+?	+SE	–
Adrenal	+C&ZG	+C	+C	–	–	–
Kidney	+T	+G&T	+CD	?+T	–	+?T
Stomach	+E	+E&M	+E	+E	+E&M	–

Ovary: CL = Corpus luteum. FF = Follicular fluid. Atr-GCs = Atretic follicle granulosa cells. ZP-GCs = Zona pellucida granulosa cells. *Uterus:* S = Serosal surface (mesothelium). SE = Luminal surface epithelium. *Adrenal:* C = Capsule. ZG = Zona glomerulosa. *Kidney:* T = Tubules. G = Glomeruli. CD = Collecting ducts. *Stomach:* E = Epithelium. M = Mucus.

body (Miles Scientific), and antibodies directed against the intermediate filaments cytokeratin (CK—low molecular weight), desmin (D) and vimentin (V) (Labsystems). The results of these studies are shown in Table 10. In the tumor nodules, a very weak, mostly perinuclear, TrFeR reaction was seen. Strong reactions for TrFeR were seen in the red pulp of the spleen, weak reactions in the muscle and stroma of the uterus, the white pulp of the spleen and epithelium and muscle of the stomach, while no reactions were present in the ovary, the uterine epithelium, kidney tissues, the adrenal or the liver.

Table 10. Immuno-histochemical analysis of FT-induced tumors. Transferrin receptor (TrFeR), fibronectin (Fn), and the intermediate filaments cytokeratin (CK), desmin (D) and vimentin (V)

Tissue Examined	TrFeR	Fn	CK	D	V
Tumor nodules	v weak	+	+ & –	+ & –	+ & –
Ovary	–	+	+	+ & –	+
Uterus	+ & –	+	+	+	NS
Kidney	–	+	NS	+	+
Spleen	+ & –	+	+	+	+/–
Adrenal	–	+	NS	+	NS
Liver	–	+	+	+	NS
Stomach	+	+	+	+	+

v weak = very weak. NS = nonspecific staining.

In the tumor nodules, Fn was present in a geographic pattern occupying about 20% of the area of each nodule. In the ovary, strong Fn reactions were found at the basal surface epithelium, in the stroma and between granulosa cells of antral follicles; immature follicles demonstrated little or no Fn. Strong Fn reactions were seen along the muscle cells and the basal surface of uterine epithelium, in renal glomeruli and along tubular basal lamina, with elements of the spleen, adrenal, and liver as well as along the hepatocellular plates and muscle of the stomach.

The reaction for low-molecular weight CK also had a geographic distribution associated with nodular aggregates and randomly distributed tumor cells; about 20% of the cells were reactive. In the ovary, only the surface epithelium demonstrated CKs. Other tissues with prominent reactions for CKs were the uterine serosal surface and luminal epithelium, the surface epithelium of the stomach, the mesothelial surface of the spleen and hepatocytes.

Desmin reactivity was found in very few and scattered cells in tumor nodules; most of this reactivity was in vascular smooth muscle. Contrarily, in the ovary, there was D reactivity in theca interna cells, especially of antral follicles, weakly in the surface epithelium and very weakly among periantral granulosa cells as well as in vascular elements of the corpora lutea. Strong D reactivity was seen in the smooth muscle of all the other tissues, the liver capsule and the nonparenchymal cells of the adrenal zona glomerulosa.

Vimentin reactivity had a geographic pattern in the tumor nodules. All tumor cells had intracellular, often perinuclear, networks of V fibers. Vascular endothelium, granulosa cells of atretic follicles and some corpus luteum cells reacted strongly for V but theca interna cells were uniformly unreactive for V. Strong V reactivity was seen in vascular elements of other tissues as well as in the tubular cells of the kidney.

Monoclonal Antibodies to DC3 Cells. Monoclonal antibodies (MoAbs) were developed using DC3 cells grown in vivo as the immunogen and standard technique (32). Twelve antibodies, 11 IgM and one IgG, were isolated which distinguished subsets of cells among FT and DC3 cells grown in vivo or in vitro (Tables 11 and 12). These MoAbs were grouped according to staining pattern: intracellular fibrils (4), diffuse surface staining (2), punctate surface staining (4) and Golgi region staining (1). A striking lack of substantial antigenic identity between DC3 cells and normal adult ovarian granulosa cells at any stage of follicular development was seen. Most FT and DC cells shared antigenic identity with ovarian stromal cells, particularly those of the theca interna, and stromal/mesenchymal elements in the rat testis (Table 12). As with cytokeratin, a small subset of cells shared antigenic identity with ovarian surface epithelial cells. The MoAb staining patterns with other adult rat tissues (Table 11) demonstrated that the MoAbs were reasonably specific for ovarian tissues.

Receptors and Products

Studies of DC3 cell functional characteristics were done in collaboration with TA Fitz and CA Winkle et al. (TL Walden, RM Wah, and MM Marr at USUHS—Uniformed Services University of the Health Sciences) and with RC Burghardt et al. (IF Greenbaum, RC Kurten and D Gaddy-Kurten—Texas A & M University). These experiments have detailed granulosa cell-like physiologic functions and the properties of DC3 cell gap junctions.

Fitz et al. (33) have shown that DC3 cells in vitro, during logarithmic growth and prior to complete confluence (Iscove's medium with 5% FBS), will bind certain gonadotropins,

Table 11. Immuno-histochemical analysis of FT-induced tumors.
Monoclonal antibodies (MoAbs) specific to DC3 cells

Tissue Examined	MoAb Group			
	A	B	C	D
Tumor nodule	Inter- and intra-cellular fibrils	Diffuse surface stain	Granular surface stain and ectoplasm	Golgi region stain
Ovary	+w TI&S +w, CL Atr-GCs	+ Atr-GCs M-GCs	+ SE, TI, CL Atr-GCs FF	*
Uterus	–	–	+, LE	*
Kidney	+, Gm	–	+, ,PT	
Spleen	–	–	–	*
Adrenal	–	–	+, C +w, ZG +w, ZR	*
Liver	+w, H	+,C	+, H	*
Stomach	+, snE	–	+, dgE	*

+ = positive reaction; +w = weakly positive reaction; * = not yet evaluated. *Ovary:* TI = Theca interna. S = Stroma. Atr-GCs = Granulosa cells of atretic follicles. M-GCs = Mural granulosa cells. SE = Surface epithelium. CL = Corpus luteum. FF = Follicular fluid. *Uterus:* LE = Luminal epithelium. *Kidney:* Gm = Glomerular mesangium. PT = Proximal tubules. *Adrenal:* C = Capsule. ZG = Zona glomerulosa. ZR = Zona reticularis. *Liver:* H = Hepatocellular. *Stomach:* snE = Sub-neck epithelial cells. dgE = Depth of gland epithelial cells, ? paracrine cells.

Table 12. Immuno-histochemical analysis of DC3 cells grown in vitro compared with rat testis. Monoclonal antibodies (MoAbs) specific to DC3 cells

MoAb Group	DC3 Cells In Vitro	Rat Testis
A	Intracellular fibrils	Mesenchymal elements
B	Cell surface	Mesenchymal elements
C	Granular cell surface and ectoplasm	Mesenchymal elements
D	Golgi region	Golgi of epididymal cells spermatids weakly

prostaglandins (PGs) and leukotrienes (LTs) but not murine epidermal growth factor (mEGF). Gonadotropin binding–human luteinizing hormone (hLH), human follicle stimulating hormone (hFSH) has been quantified. Binding of PGs E2 and F-2-alpha and LTs LTC4 and LTE4 has been detected but not quantified; there was no binding of LTD4. In addition, it is possible to modulate hFSH and hLH binding by treating DC3 cells in vitro with pregnant mares serum gonadotropin (PMSG) and human chorionic gonadotropin (hCG) (Table 13).

Using such cultures, Fitz et al. (33) also studied the capacity of DC3 cells to produce PGs and E2 (estradiol) from precursors. After culture with tritiated arachidonic acid, with the calcium ionophore A23187 in the medium, they demonstrated that approximately 8% of the ethyl acetate extractable, tritium labelled metabolites co-migrated in HPLC with authentic PGE2. Using cultures provided with tritiated T (testosterone) as a substrate, they demonstrated that 3% of the tritiated metabolites co-migrated with E2 and that 41% of the metabolites migrated as two substances with a mobility different than that of either T or E2.

From these results, Fitz et al. concluded that "DC3 cells retain several properties of normal rat granulosa cells" and that "DC3 cells may be useful for many experiments in which the luteinization process limits the usefulness of normal granulosa cells (33)."

In other studies, under similar culture conditions, Fitz et al. (34) explored the growth response and steroidogenic capacity of DC3 cells exposed to gonadotropins. Human FSH affected neither the growth rate nor the morphology of the cells but did increase the production of E2 in a dose-dependent manner. Human FSH levels of 0, 20 and 200 ng/mL in the medium resulted in 12, 18 and 27 pg/mL of E2 production. PMSG alone did not influence cell growth rate or E2 production but hCG, with or without PMSG, resulted in a 27% decrease in the number of cells and a 31% decrease in the amount of E2 produced. After correction for steroids in the medium, they were able to detect the production of estrone (96.9 pg/mL), E2 (67.8 pg/mL) and P (progesterone) (46.0 pg/mL) but not pregnenolone, 17-OH-P, androstenedione or testosterone.

The effect of FSH on DC3 cells in vitro is quite limited and different than effects of elevated FSH on in vivo growth. Although DC3 cells will bind hFSH and will increase E2 production, there is no change in cAMP or P in the medium under such conditions. Fitz et al. (35) demonstrated modulation of cAMP and P using other agents known to increase intracellular cAMP levels. With I (isoproterenol), F (forskolin) and 25-OH-C (25-hydroxy-

Table 13. Modulation of hFSH and hLH binding by DC3 cells

Treatment	Extent of Binding	
	hFSH(a)	hLH(b)
None (basal level)	0.28	21.0
PMSG (1.4 IU/mL)	2.19	107.0
PMSG + hCG (1.8 IU/mL)	0.86	11.8

hFSH binding in pmol/mg membrane protein.
hLH binding in fmol/mg membrane protein.

cholesterol) alone and in various combinations, they demonstrated increases in cAMP and P production from DC3 cells in vitro (Table 14). They concluded that DC3 FSH receptors were not coupled to either adenylate cyclase or P production and that P production was related to substrate availability and adenylate cyclase.

These three studies (33-35) and others not detailed here (36,37) suggest that DC3 cells functionally resemble immature granulosa cells in their function, a finding similar to that of Zeleznik et al. (10). The small but detectable FSH binding and the lack of EGF binding resemble properties of granulosa cells from early stages of follicular maturation (38). DC3 cells produce steroids when appropriate conditions are provided and the amount of P produced is directly related to cAMP levels. These authors stated: "On the basis of these data, we conclude that DC3 cells may provide a needed model for the further elucidation of normal granulosa cell function, especially during the early stages of follicular development (36)."

Endocrine Modulation of Gap Junctions

Burghardt et al. (39) demonstrated that DC3 cells in vitro had an undifferentiated morphology and would not spontaneously luteinize as do normal granulosa cells from preantral or older follicles. Using cultures grown on flat surfaces and on collagen beads, they showed that DC3 cell morphology and their gap junctions could be modulated by 8-Br-cAMP (8-Bromo-cyclic AMP) but not FSH (Table 15). DC3 cells grown on collagen beads covered the surface as a sheet and would not retract and round up, as similarly grown normal granulosa cells will do, when exposed to FSH. The DC3 cells would, however, undergo such morphologic changes when 8-Br-cAMP was added to the medium.

Marr et al. (40) demonstrated the functional competence of DC3 cell gap junctions by growing the cells to near confluence in Iscove's medium with 5% FBS. The cultures were loaded with carboxyfluoroscein, selected cells were laser photobleached and fluorescence

Table 14. Modulation of cAMP and P production by DC3 cells

Culture Conditions	cAMP	P (pg/mL)
Control	1.64	24.2
I (1 µg/mL)	24.8	197.0
F (10 µM)	150.4	212.6
25-OH-C 20 pg/mL		56.8
20 ng/mL		66.2
20 µg/mL		143.5
Control		55.5
25-OH-C + I (a)		158.3
25-OH-C + F (b)		6193
25-OH-C + I + F (c)		8835

cAMP expressed as pmol/mL of medium. (a) 20 ng/mL 25-OH-C + 1 µg/mL I. (b) 20 ng/mL 25-OH-C + 10 µM F. (c) 20 ng/mL 25-OH-C + 1 µg/mL I + 10 µM F.

Table 15. Modulation of DC3 morphology and ultrastructure in vitro.
Gap junctions.

Treatment	Number	Size	Internalization
None (a)	Few	Small	None
7.5 h 8-Br-cAMP	More	Small	None
7.5 h 8-Br-cAMP + 24 h (b)	Fewer	Small	Present

(a) = Serum-free DMEM for 48 h after growth to confluence in DMEM + 10% FBS. (b) = Returned to DMEM + 10% FBs. Gap junctions examined by thin section and freeze-fracture techniques.

passage between abutting pairs of cells was monitored. These studies demonstrated gap junctions functional competence and their resistance to modulation by agents which stimulate adenylate cyclase as well as to radiation (Table 16). The irradiation inhibited cellular division and resulted in increased size of the cells and reduced growth (of 40% and 72%) with 5 and 20 Gy at 96 h after irradiation.

Table 16. Function and modulation of DC3 cell gap junctions

Treatment	Cell pairs with transfer/total	Percent pairs with transfer
None (a)	49/130	38
Serum free	6/ 15	40
Bu2-cAMP, 100 µM (b)	8/ 25	32
F, 10 µM (c)	12/ 33	36
CT, 10 ng/mL (d)	14/ 44	32
25-OH-C, 10 µg/mL (e)	13/ 37	35
25-OH-C, 100 ng/mL (f)	3/ 25	12
Co (g), after 4 h	4/ 9	44
Co (h), after 96 h	7/ 18	39
Co (i), after 4 h	1/ 9	11
Co (j), after 96 h	3/ 16	19

(a) = Grown to near confluence; normal granulosa cells under the same conditions demonstrate fluorescence transfer in 19/19 adjoining pairs. (b) Bu2-cAMP = Di-butyryl-cyclic AMP). (c) F = Forskolin. (d) CT = Cholera toxin. (e) 25-OH-C = 25-hydroxy-cholesterol. (f) 25-OH-C = 25-hydroxy-cholesterol. (g) Co = 5 Gy of Co6o irradiation (1 Gy/min). (h) Co = 20 Gy of Co6o irradiation (1 Gy/min). (i) Co = 5 Gy of Co6o irradiation (1 Gy/min). (j) Co = 20 Gy of Co6o irradiation (1 Gy/min).

Conclusions

The FT originates from ovarian-specific cells and seems to be a mixture of at least two transformed cell types, CK+V- surface epithelial and CK-V+ stromal cells. The transformed CK-V+ stromal cells share a number of morphologic and functional characteristics with both theca interna and granulosa cells. The DC3 clone seems to consist of only stromal cells as evidenced by both in vitro and in vivo responses to Gns and other endocrinologically active agents. The ability to bind and respond to Gns and to respond to other agents, such as cAMP, suggests that these are transformed granulosa cells. Histochemical and immunohistochemical studies sustain this contention.

Stem cell growth attributable to FT ascites tumor cells suggests primitive properties and that this model might reveal other properties of cells from early stages of ovarian development. The data presented suggest properties which might be associated with primitive granulosa cells while the cell lines provide the means by which hypotheses may be tested. The FT system, and its monoclonal derivative DC3, also provide a model with which to explore the roots of ovarian carcinogenesis. These options raise the possibility of replacing the recognition/classification paradigm with a new one, the Oncodevelopmental Paradigm, which recognizes cellular origins and potentials and permits modulation of growth and behavior based upon known biochemical control pathways (Table 17).

Table 17. Old and new paradigms of ovarian ontogenesis and oncogenesis compared

	Paradigms	
Process	Old	New
Development	Ontogeny revealed through morphology	ONCO- DEVELOPMENTAL
		PARADIGM:
		Morphology,
Neoplasia	Recognition/ Classification: Cell lineage revealed through morphology and differentiation	Function, Potential and Molecular Identity

Conclusions and Correlations

Stem Cells and Differentiation

The importance of transformed granulosa cells with stem cell properties is revealed by comparing the relationship of stem cells and their progeny to the problem of ovarian ontogenesis/carcinogenesis. Osgood (41,42) presented a unifying concept of the etiology of malignancy, suggesting that: (1) cells of a particular series controlled their own replication through products of the terminally differentiated cells of that line which affected their progenitors; (2) that there were four types of cell division; and, although he did not use the term, (3) that each cell line had stem cell progenitors. The four division types were:

alpha → 2 alpha	stem cell produces two more stem cells.
alpha → alpha, n	stem cell produces one stem cell and one cell destined for terminal differentiation.
alpha → 2n	stem cell produces 2 cells for terminal differentiation; the stem cell pool is depleted.
n → 2n	non-stem cell gives rise to 2 non-stem cells; limited numbers of these divisions are possible.

In this schema, [alpha → 2 alpha] divisions are rare and expand the progenitor pool, [alpha → 2n] divisions would lead inevitably to loss of the line, [alpha → alpha, n] divisions are those which maintain the progenitor pool and provide for development of the line along with [n → 2n] divisions which are limited to expanding the differentiating components of the line. Inhibitors which control these divisions are produced: (1) early in the life of n cells and control [alpha → 2 alpha] divisions; and, (2) later in n cell life and inhibit [alpha → alpha, n] and [n → 2n] divisions.

Zajicek expanded upon these concepts by defining self-controlling proliferation and differentiation compartments in each cell line (43). His concept of the "streaming organism" (44-46) describes tissue development and regeneration of parenchymal elements as composed of 4 compartments: "S"—the stem cells, "P"—the progenitor cells, "Q"—the functioning cells and, lastly, those cells which are dead or dying—by me labelled as "D." The distance from S to D is the "tissue radius," whose length is determined by the duration of the component parts, and which is characteristic for each tissue. The combination of an organ's parenchymal elements with supporting cell populations (connective tissues, blood vessels and nerves) constitute the "proliferon" (47,48). Applying these concepts, he was able to determine the cell migration velocity along the tissue radius in rat incisor teeth inner enamel epithelium (49).

In the human arena, similar concepts have emerged in concepts of growth and differentiation mechanisms in both hematopoietic and ovarian neoplasia. Extensive research into the role of stem cells in the normal hematopoietic process (50), including the understanding of the molecular controls of blood cell development (51), has led to new strategies for control and reversal of hematopoietic malignancies (52). Similar studies in human ovarian neoplasia have detected both stem cell properties and progeny cell differentiation potentials in human ovarian cancer cells (22,23,53-57).

Stem Cells and Ovarian Development

The adult structure and function as well as the ontogenesis of the ovarian follicle also may be explained in the context of these concepts of stem cell proliferation and daughter cell differentiation. The follicle may be considered a cyclic, fast replicating proliferon (Z) (47,58) while the entire organ, at least between puberty and menopause, seems to be a continuous replicator composed of multiple hormonally driven proliferans.

Hirshfield and Schmidt (59), utilizing data from studies of ovarian cellular proliferation, have reexamined follicular development from the standpoint of stem cell proliferation and daughter cell differentiation. They propose that 10 generations are needed for follicles to progress from the primordial to the ovulatory stage. When ovarian follicular development is examined in this fashion, we see, with great dismay, the vast gaps in our knowledge base. Most of what we know (Table 18A/B) has to do with terminally differentiated cells (Zajicek compartments "Q" and "D"), most of that dealing predominantly with granulosa cells. Little is known about participants or processes in early stages of follicular growth (Zajicek compartment "P"), less is known about folliculogenesis and ovarian ontogenesis (Zajicek compartments "S" and "P" remain an enigma). The major limitations to the acquisition of further knowledge in these areas is almost purely technical. That is, it seems impossible to acquire enough cells from primordial follicles or embryonic gonads to permit detailed studies.

Table 18A. Properties of granulosa cells in generations 1-10

Generation	Follicle Cells/ LCS	Diam μm	Extent of Characterization			Differentiation State GCs and Theca
			Morph	Physiol	Bioch	
10	2000	>525	10	8	2-3	Regional specialization of GCs: basal, mural, antral, cumulus; TI w/ steroidogenesis; TE has actin and myosin.
9	1000	360	10	8	2-3	Antral follicle
8	500	250	10	4	0-1	Few in vitro data, GCs have 17-keto steroid reductase, theca cannot make androgens even with cAMP stimulation.
7	256	172	8-10	2	0-1	+/- antrum
6	128	119				"Antral" spaces, full size oocyte, 3-5 GC layers, 1-3 theca cell layers.
5	64-127		6-10	0-1	0	Bilaminar, oocyte growth, independent blood supply.
4	64		6-10	0	0	Unilaminar, spontaneous luteinization TI has 1-3 cells ?
3	20		2-10	0	0	ZP No TI
2	10		2?	0	0	No ZP No TI
1	2-4		1?	0	0	? No TI

Table 18B. Properties of granulosa cells in generations 1-10

Follicle Generation	Duration	Proliferative Rate	Proliferative Potential	Atresia	Notes/Products
(10)	24 h	Slow	Exhausted	Possible	Atresia starts if LH surge is delayed by 8 h; ovulation in 24 h of onset.
(9)	2.5 d	slow	Decreased	Common	Major wave of atresia at metestrus; typical "control" follicles.
(8)	1-1.5 d (>24 h)	Fast	Great; 17 h GT, <7GF	Common	Largest number of atretic follicles from this stage.
(7)	1-1.5 d	Fast	Maximum	Rare	Theca cannot bind LH or hCG.
(6)	3 d	<8GF		Rare	Maximum FSH receptors/GC; P made in infanrs, androgens made.
(5)	4 d	<6GF		Rare	LH receptors on theca cell.
(4)	3-5 d	? = 5GF			FSG receptors on GCs?; aromatase at 7-8 d postpartum.
(3)				Rare	+ 3-beta-hydroxy-steroid reductase.
(2)	GT>14d or 336 h 336 h			None or Rare	Type 3a follicles but includes growing and quiet follicles.
(1)	GF<100%				Quiescent

"Ending Up at the Beginning"

The appropriate ovarian tumor cell lines may, however, provide the quantities and types of cells which will allow hypothesis formulation and testing and data acquisition. With such cell lines, we may explore the roles of known "growth and differentiation" factors on ovarian compartment specific progenitor-type cells (Zajicek compartments "S" and "P," in both pre- and postnatal life). We may use the cell lines to explore the roles played by that new category of inter- and intracellular communication molecules, the so-called oncogene products (60-64).

Chief among these cell lines so qualified lies the Ross Model of SV40 transformed "granulosa" (and other) cells. A similar model, based upon SV40 transformation of human adult keratinocytes, already has demonstrated that those transformed cells acquire multiple features characteristic of embryonal human skin (agar colony growth, decreased growth inhibition from alpha-interferons and 3 low-molecular weight CKs found in fetal epidermis) and loose features which identify fully differentiated epidermal cells (keratinization, expression of involucrin, high molecular weight CKs, and stratified growth in vitro) (65-67). Bernard et al. concluded that their results "strongly suggest that the SV40 Large T antigen may mimic or induce the expression of cellular regulatory protein(s) active only at specific stages of development and reactivated during malignant transformation (67)."

References

1. Byskov AG. Differentiation of the mammalian embryonic gonad. Physiol Rev 1986; 6671-117.
2. Hamilton WJ, Mossman HW, eds. Human embryology; prenatal form and function. 4th ed. Cambridge: Heffer, 1972.
3. Pierce GB, Shikes R, Fink LM. Cancer, a problem of developmental biology. Englewood Cliffs: Prentice Hall, 1978.
4. Pierce GB. Neoplastic stem cells. In: Borek C, Fenoglio CM, King DW, eds. Cancer biology. IV. Differentiation and carcinogenesis. New York: Stratton Intercontinental Medical, 1977.
5. Rubin E, Farber JL. Neoplasia. In: Pathology. Philadelphia: WB Saunders, 1988.
6. Robbins SL, Cotran R, Kumar V. In: Pathology. Philadelphia: WB Saunders, 1984.
7. Meissner WA, Diamandopoulos G-T. Neoplasia. In: Anderson WAD, Kissane JM, eds. Pathology. 7th ed. St. Louis: CV Mosby, 1977.
8. Marchant J. Animal models for tumors of the female genital tract. In: Kurman RJ. Blaustein's pathology of the female genital tract. 3rd ed. New York: Springer-Verlag, 1987:900-8.
9. Hillier SG, Zeleznik AJ, Knazek RA, Legallais FY, Rabson AS, Ross GT. Development of a hormonally-sensitive transplantable granulosa cell tumor. The Endocrine Society, Programs and Abstracts, 1978:344.
10. Zeleznik AJ, Hillier SG, Knazek RA, Ross GT, Coon HG. Production of long term steroid-producing granulosa cell cultures by cell hybridization. Endocrinology 1979; 105:156-62.
11. Hillier SG, Knazek RA, Ross GT. Androgenic stimulation of progesterone production by granulosa cells from pre-antral follicles: further in vitro studies using replicate cell culture. Endocrinology 1977; 100:1539-49.
12. Kolena J, Channing CP. Stimulatory effects of LH, FSH and prostaglandins upon cyclic 3' : 5' AMP levels in porcine granulosa cells. Endocrinology 1972; 90:1543-50.
13. Goff AK, Armstrong OT. Stimulatory action of gonadotropins and prostaglandins on adenosine 3' : 5' monophosphate production by isolated rat granulosa cells. Endocrinology 1977; 101:1461-7.
14. Wolff J, Cook GH. Activation of steroidogenesis and adenylate cyclase by adenosine in adrenal and Leydig tumor cells. J Biol Chem 1977; 252:687-95.

15. Hillier SG, Zeleznik AJ, Ross GT. Independence of steroidogenic capacity and luteinizing hormone receptor induction in developing granulosa cells. Endocrinology 1978; 102:937-46.
16. Schmidt WA, Ross GT. A hormonally responsive transplantable rat granulosa cell tumor. Lab Invest 1985; 52:59A.
17. Burghardt RC, personal communication, 1987.
18. Fitz TA, personal communication, 1987.
19. Pretlow TG, Weir EE, Zettergren JG. Problems connected with the separation of different kinds of cells. In: Richter GW, Epstein MA, eds. Int rev exp path; vol 14. New York: Academic Press, 1975.
20. Hamburger AW, Dunn FE, White CP. Percoll density gradient separation of cells from human malignant effusions. Br J Cancer 1985; 253-8.
21. Pertoft H, Laurent C. Sedimentation of cells in colloidal silica (Percoll). In: Pretlow TG, Pretlow TP, eds. Cell separation: methods and selected applications; vol 1. New York: Academic Press, 1982.
22. Buick RN, MacKillop WJ. Measurement of self-renewal in culture of clonogenic cells from human ovarian carcinoma. Br J Cancer 1981; 44:349-55.
23. MacKillop WJ, Buick RN. Cellular heterogeneity in human ovarian carcinoma studied by density gradient centrifugation. Stem Cells 1981; 1:355-66.
24. Aberts B, Bray D, Lewis J, Raff M, Roberts K, Watson JD. Molecular biology of the cells. New York: Garland Publishing, 1983:911.
25. Guraya SS. Histochemistry of the ovary. In: Motta PM, Hafez ESE, eds. Biology of the ovary. Boston: Martinus Nijhoff, 1980:33-51.
26. Rutenberg AM, Hwakyu K, Fischbein JW, Hanker JS, Wasserkrug HJ, Seligman AM. Histochemical and ultrastructural demonstration of gamma-glutamyl transpeptidase activity. J Histochem Cytochem 1969; 17:517-26.
27. Schulte BA, Poon KC, Rao KPP, Spicer SS. Lectin histochemistry of complex carbohydrates in human cervix. Histochem J 1985; 17:517-26.
28. Schulte BA, Spicer SS. Light microscopic detection of sugar residues in glycoconjugates of salivary glands and the pancreas with lectin-horseradish peroxidase conjugates. I. Mouse. Histochem J 1983; 15:1217-88.
29. Arya M, Vanha-Perttula T. Distribution of lectin binding in rat testis and epididymis. Andrologia 1984; 16:495-508.
30. Arya M, Vanha-Perttula T. Lectin staining of rat testis and epididymis: effect of cyproterone acetate and testosterone. Andrologia 1985; 17:301-10.
31. Teshima S, Hirohashi S, Shimosato Y, et al. Histochemically demonstrable changes in cell surface carbohydrates of human germ cell tumors. Lab Invest 1984; 50:271-7.
32. Galfre G, Milstein C. Preparation of monoclonal antibodies: strategies and procedures. In: Langone JJ, Vunakis HV, eds. Methods in enzymology; vol 73, Part B. New York: Academic Press, 1981:3-46.
33. Fitz TA, Schmidt WA, Walden TL, Winkel CA. Virus transformed rat granulosa cells: a model for the study of granulosa cell function. 6th Biennial Ovarian Workshop, Ithaca, 1986.
34. Fitz TA, Schmidt WA, Winkel CA. Steroidogenic capacity of transformed rat granulosa cells. Biol Reprod 1986; 34:86.
35. Wah RM, Fitz TA, Schmidt WA, Winkel CA. Progesterone synthesis in virus transformed granulosa cells. OB-GYN Armed Forces Meeting, San Diego, 1986.
36. Fitz TA, Wah RM, Schmidt WA, Winkel CA. Physiologic characterization of transformed and cloned granulosa cells. Biol Reprod 1988 (submitted).

37. Winkel CA, Marr MM, Fitz TA, Burghardt RC, Schmidt WA. Morphological and structural-functional characteristics of transformed rat granulosa cells: a model for study of immature granulosa cells. 1988 (in preparation).
38. Amsterdam A, Rotmensch S. Structure-function relationships during granulosa cell differentiation. Endocr Rev 1987; 8:309-37.
39. Burghardt RC, Greenbaum IF, Kurten RC, Gaddy-Kurten D, Schmidt WA. Morphological properties of gap junctions in a transformed granulosa cell line. J Cell Biol 1986; 103:73A.
40. Marr MM, Walden TL, Schmidt WA, Winkel CA, Fitz TA. Gap junctions in transformed rat granulosa cells. Third Annual Contractors Meeting for Biomedical and Materials Science Applications of Free Electron Lasers, Salt Lake City, 1988.
41. Osgood EE. A unifying concept of the etiology of the leukemias, lymphomas and cancers. J Natl Cancer Inst 1957; 18:155-66.
42. Osgood EE. The etiology of leukemias, lymphomas, and cancers. Geriatrics 1964; 19:208-21.
43. Zajicek G, personal communications, 1985.
44. Zajicek G. The histogenesis of glandular neoplasia. Med Hypotheses 1981; 7:1241-51.
45. Zajicek G. Inflammation initiates cancer by depleting stem cells. Med Hypotheses 1985; 18:207-19.
46. Zajicek G. Cancer is a metabolic deficiency. Med Hypotheses 1986; 21:105-15.
47. Zajicek G. Proliferon: the functional unit of rapidly proliferating organs. Med Hypotheses 1979; 5:161-74.
48. Zajicek G. The intestinal proliferon. J Theor Biol 1977; 67:515-21.
49. Zajicek G, Michaeli Y, Regev J. On the progenitor cell migration velocity. Cell Tissue Kinet 1979; 12:453-60.
50. Quesenberry P, Levitt L. Hematopoietic stem cells. New Engl J Med 1979; 301:755-60, 819-23, 868-72.
51. Sachs L. The molecular control of blood development. Science 1987; 238:1374-9.
52. Sachs L. Growth, differentiation and the reversal of malignancy. Sci Am 1986; 254:40-7.
53. MacKillop WJ, Stewart SS, Buick RN. Density/volume analysis in the study of cellular heterogeneity in human ovarian carcinoma. Br J Cancer 1982; 45:812-20.
54. MacKillop WJ, Trent JM, Stewart SS, Buick RN. Tumor progression studied by analysis of cellular features of serial ascitic ovarian tumors. Cancer Res 1983; 43:874-8.
55. Buick RN, Pullano R, Bizzari J-P, MacKillop WJ. The phenotypic heterogeneity of human ovarian tumor cells in relation to cell function. In: Burchiel SW, Rhodes BA, eds. Radioimmunimaging and radioimmunotherapy. New York: Elsevier Science Publishing, 1982:3-12.
56. MacKillop WJ, Ciampi A, Till JE, Buick RN. A stem cell model of human tumor growth: implications for tumor cell clonogenic assays. J Natl Cancer Inst 1983; 70:117-22.
57. Buick RN. Cell heterogeneity in human ovarian carcinoma. J Cell Physiol 1984; 3(suppl):117-22.
58. Zajicek G. The ideal human neoplasm. Med Hypotheses 1979; 5:1133-9.
59. Hirshfield AN, Schmidt WA. Kinetic aspects of follicular development in the rat. In: Mahesh VB, Dhindsa DS, Anderson E, Kalra S, eds. Regulation of ovarian and testicular function. Adv Exp Med Biol; vol 219. New York: Plenum Publishing, 1988.
60. Wheelock FF, Robinson MK. Endogenous control of the neoplastic process. Lab Invest 1983; 48:120-39.

61. Sachs L. Normal regulation, oncogenes and the reversibility of malignancy. Cancer Surveys 1984; 3:220-8.
62. Kaczmarek L. Protooncogene expression during the cell cycle. Lab Invest 1986; 54:365-76.
63. Stiles CD. The biological role of oncogenes—insights from platelet-derived growth factor. Cancer Res 1985; 45:5215-8.
64. Weinberg RA. The action of oncogenes in the cytoplasm and nucleus. Science 1985; 230:770-6.
65. Taylor-Papadimitriou J, Purkis P, Lane EB, McKay I, Chang S. Effects of SV40 transformation on the cytoskeleton and behavioural properties of human keratinocytes. Cell Differ 1982; 11:169-80.
66. Hronis TS, Steinberg ML, Defendi V, Sun T-T. Simple epithelial nature of some simian virus 40-transformed human epidermal keratinocytes. Cancer Res 1984; 44:5797-804.
67. Bernard B, Robinson SM, Semat A, Darmon M. Reexpression of fetal characters in simian virus 40-transformed human keratinocytes. Cancer Res 1985; 45:1707-16.

II. Keynote Speakers

5

Growth Factors, Proto-Oncogenes and the Control of Cell Proliferation: Lessons from the Fibroblast

Judith Campisi

Department of Biochemistry, Boston University School of Medicine
80 East Concord Street, Boston, MA 02118

Introduction

Shortly after fertilization, the rapidly dividing cells of the zygote initiate a multifaceted program of differentiation. Among the earliest changes is a strict regulation of cellular proliferation. Cell proliferation in higher eukaryotes generally depends upon the state of differentiation and the appropriate extracellular factors. For many of the cells that comprise multicellular organisms, extracellular signals control both differentiation and proliferation.

How do signals originating outside the cell alter cellular behavior? This is still largely an unanswered question. However, in recent years, some progress has been made in understanding how certain soluble polypeptide growth factors regulate cell proliferation. Much of this understanding derives from studies of fibroblasts in culture. I will attempt to give a brief, and necessarily incomplete, review of what is known about how some soluble factors modulate the proliferation of fibroblasts. I will then speculate about the applicability of these findings to nonfibroblastic cells in culture.

Polypeptide Growth Modulators, 3T3 Fibroblasts and the Control of Cell Proliferation

The extracellular signals that regulate the proliferation of fibroblasts and other cell types can be grouped into three broad classes. First, most cells are sensitive to both the proximity and identity of their neighbors. Thus, in vivo, cell-cell contacts stimulate or inhibit proliferation, depending upon the cell types of the participants. In many types of adherent cell cultures, cell-cell contact limits or completely inhibits proliferation. Adherent cells are also sensitive to the presence and quality of the substratum to which they are attached. In general, adherent cells will not proliferate unless they are provided with an anchoring substratum. However, the composition of the substratum can either stimulate or inhibit proliferation, in some instances by regulating the state of differentiation. Finally, all cells respond to a variety of soluble factors that can stimulate or inhibit proliferation. Among the soluble factors that control proliferation are polypeptide growth factors and polypeptide growth inhibitors (1).

Polypeptide Growth Modulators

Polypeptide growth factors and inhibitors share several common features. These molecules bind to specific, high affinity receptors present on the cell surface. The occupied receptors convey information to the cell through one or more intracellular signalling mechanisms. Many, but not all, receptors possess an intrinsic protein tyrosine kinase activity that is activated by ligand binding. Ligand binding also triggers the production of small molecular weight, cytoplasmic "second messengers," generally by activating one or more intracellular, membrane-associated enzymes. Second messengers that have been identified include cyclic nucleotides, a transient increase in intracellular free calcium, diacylglycerol and arachidonic acid. Second messenger molecules are presumed to initiate the ultimate cellular response, although how they do so is only incompletely understood (2,3).

One consequence of second messenger production is the activation of one or more intracellular protein kinase. For example, intracellular calcium activates a calmodulin-dependent protein kinase; cyclic AMP (cAMP) activates cAMP-dependent protein kinase (PKA); and diacylglycerol activates protein kinase C (PKC). These protein kinases, each of which phosphorylate several intracellular proteins on serine or threonine, are localized principally in the cytoplasm; however, both cytoplasmic and nuclear substrates have been identified (4-6).

Within a few minutes to hours after binding to their receptors, polypeptide growth factors and inhibitors alter the expression of genes whose protein products are believed necessary or permissive for the proliferative response (1,7). Under some circumstances, the expression of growth factor-inducible genes can be increased by direct activation of a protein kinase (4,8) and protein kinase inhibition can prevent the induction of gene expression by certain growth factors (9,10). Thus, the general paradigm for growth factors is that receptor occupancy activates one or more protein kinases which, directly or indirectly, phosphorylate nuclear proteins that, in turn, interact with DNA sequences responsible for transcriptional regulation.

3T3 Fibroblasts

Much of our understanding about how growth factors and inhibitors alter gene expression and cell proliferation derives from studies of fibroblasts in culture. 3T3 cells are spontaneously immortalized rodent embryo fibroblasts that have been maintained at sub-confluent densities. Most 3T3 cell lines have been established from mass cultures of mouse embryos, but some have been derived by single cell cloning (e.g., A31 cells, derived from a BALB/c mouse embryo). Although immortal, properly maintained 3T3 cells are non-tumorigenic (11,12). The proliferative properties of 3T3 cells are generally shared by non-immortal fibroblasts of many origins, including those from human fetal and adult tissue.

3T3 cells enter a reversible, nonproliferative state, termed quiescence or G0, when cultured in a suboptimal concentration of growth factors (commonly supplied as serum) or when grown to confluence. Quiescent cells reenter the cell cycle and proliferate synchronously when given fresh, serum-containing medium. For fibroblasts, commitment to DNA synthesis is generally tantamount to commitment to cell division. Thus, most of the regulation of cell proliferation is exerted during the G1 phase of the cell cycle. Although this is generally true, there is evidence for control points in other phases of the cell cycle and some mitogens stimulate DNA synthesis without cell division (1,13).

In the 12-h interval between the addition of serum to quiescent cells and the onset of DNA synthesis, four major growth control points have been identified: competence, V, R and W, occurring 12, 6, 2 and 0 h prior to S phase, respectively. These control points were identified by the sequential requirements for three polypeptide growth factors and an optimal rate of protein synthesis.

Growth Factors and the Regulation of Proliferation by 3T3 Cells

Three polypeptide growth factors can replace serum in stimulating quiescent 3T3 cells to initiate DNA synthesis (14,15). These are platelet-derived growth factor (PDGF), epidermal growth factor (EGF) and insulin-like growth factor-I (IGF-I); under some conditions, only EGF and IGF-I is required. PDGF, EGF and IGF-I are not the only growth factors to which 3T3 and other fibroblasts respond. The list of reported fibroblast mitogens is quite long and some 3T3 cell lines (e.g., those derived from Swiss mice) respond to a much broader range of mitogens than others (3). However, a combination of PDGF or EGF and IGF-I stimulates DNA synthesis in most, if not all, fibroblasts.

Confluent BALB/c 3T3 fibroblasts (A31 cells) require the sequential actions of PDGF, EGF and IGF-I in order to initiate DNA synthesis (14-16). A31 cells made quiescent by serum deprivation at subconfluence require only EGF and IGF-I for entry into S phase (17). The timing of these growth factor requirements is summarized by Figure 1.

PDGF establishes a state termed competence, whereby the cells become primed to respond to EGF and IGF-I. Competent cells remain arrested 12 h prior to S phase. EGF enables competent, confluent cells to reach the V point, located 6 h prior to S phase. If the cells are made quiescent by serum deprivation, they do not require PDGF to leave the quiescent state and require only EGF to reach the V point. The transition from G0 to V is accompanied by an increase in the expression of more than 30 genes. As will be discussed below, our data show that although PDGF and EGF act through different intracellular signalling mechanisms in these cells, they can activate the expression of the same set of genes.

The V point is equivalent to the start of G1 during exponential growth. Once cells have reached the V point, they require a rapid rate of protein synthesis to reach the next control point, R. This transition is likely controlled by a labile protein whose synthesis is dependent upon growth factors. In addition, the expression of several genes is induced near or after the V point. IGF-I enables cells in late G1 to initiate DNA synthesis. In the absence of IGF-I, cells arrest at the W point, near the G1/S boundary, from which the cells can return to G0 (1,13,14-17).

Two generalities regarding the control of proliferation by growth factors can be drawn from these studies in 3T3 cells. First, most cells require multiple growth factors for proliferation. Certainly there are reports of cells that grow in growth factor-free media or require only a single factor for proliferation. However, it is generally found that these cells, in fact, produce their own growth factors. Second, the requirements for growth factors appear to be sequential. Unfortunately, very little is known about the molecular events that are responsible for the observed control points. Although it is possible to show that a particular

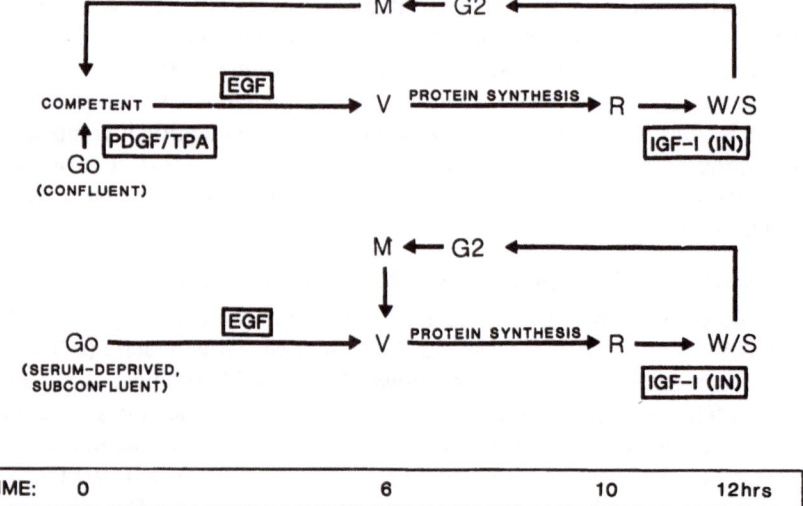

Fig. 1. Control points in the 3T3 cell cycle. Confluent or serum-deprived, sub-confluent 3T3 cells are stimulated to proliferate by the sequential addition of growth factors, as described in the text. Confluent cells undergo one round of cell division, whereas subconfluent cells progress through several rounds, until they reach confluence.

growth factor induces, for example, the activation of specific genes, it is more difficult to identify which of the many effects of a growth factor forms the molecular basis for growth arrest at a single point in the cell cycle.

Growth Inhibitors

In vivo, the positive action of growth factors must be tempered in order to maintain tissue homeostasis and prevent the overgrowth of cells. Several polypeptide growth inhibitors have been identified. Some are produced only under special circumstances, whereas others are produced by signals that initially stimulate proliferation (18). Of particular interest is the recent finding that some polypeptide growth factors induce the expression of interferons (IFNs) that have antiproliferative activity (19,20).

IFNs are multifaceted modulators of cell function (21,22). IFNs were first recognized for their antiviral activity but more recently have been appreciated as inhibitors of cell proliferation. Alpha and beta IFNs retard progress through G0/G1 by growth factor-stimulated fibroblasts. However, in 3T3 and certain other fibroblasts, IFN does not appear to inhibit proliferation by acting at a particular point in the cell cycle (23,24). As will be discussed below, our data suggest that IFN inhibits the expression of a subset of growth factor-inducible genes at the level of translation, as opposed to transcription.

Growth Factor-Inducible Gene Expression

Growth factors, including PDGF, EGF and IGF-I, generally induce the expression of genes by activating transcription, thereby increasing the levels of mRNA in the cytoplasm.

Growth factor-inducible genes include those encoding structural proteins (for example, cytoskeletal and extracellular matrix proteins), metabolic enzymes (for example, ornithinedecarboxylase and ATP:ADP translocase), proteins or enzymes required for DNA synthesis (for example, histones and thymidine kinase) and some members of a small class of genes collectively known as proto-oncogenes (1,7,25). The products of growth factor-inducible genes are presumed necessary or permissive for cell proliferation.

Proto-Oncogenes

When mutated or inappropriately expressed, proto-oncogenes have the ability to contribute to the tumorigenic transformation of certain cells. Genes that have been identified as proto-oncogenes include those encoding growth factors, growth factor receptors, protein kinases and DNA-binding proteins. In 3T3 cells, the mRNAs for at least three proto-oncogenes are induced by growth factors that regulate the proliferation of these cells. These are the c-fos, c-myc and c-ras-Ha proto-oncogenes. Each of these genes has been identified as an (altered) oncogene responsible for the oncogenic properties of acute transforming retroviruses (26).

C-fos encodes a nuclear DNA-binding protein (26). Although c-fos is expressed at high levels in a few differentiated cell types (for example, macrophages), most cells, whether proliferating or quiescent, express little or no mRNA or protein for this gene. However, c-fos mRNA and protein are induced very rapidly, but transiently, by growth factors that stimulate fibroblasts to leave the quiescent state. These growth factors include PDGF and EGF, but not IGF-I (17,27,28). Recent data suggest that the c-fos protein shares properties with nuclear factors that are thought to be general, positive regulators of transcription (29). Thus, in quiescent fibroblasts, c-fos may activate the expression of other genes required for cell proliferation.

C-myc also encodes a nuclear DNA-binding protein, but its function is at present unknown. Unlike c-fos, c-myc is expressed by most, if not all, proliferating cells (26). However, c-myc expression is very low in quiescent cells and transcription, mRNA and protein are generally induced by the same growth factors that activate c-fos expression. The kinetics of c-myc induction are somewhat slower than c-fos induction, occurring within an hour of growth factor stimulation, as opposed to a few minutes (9,17,27,28).

C-ras genes encode a family of proteins localized to the inner surface of the plasma membrane (26) and having homology to the GTP-binding proteins (G proteins) that couple hormone and growth factor receptors to second messenger systems (30). Like G proteins, ras proteins are GTPases, but whether ras proteins do, in fact, function as G proteins is not known. C-ras mRNAs and proteins are expressed by many types of cells, both proliferating and terminally differentiated (31). In quiescent 3T3 cells, the c-ras-Ha mRNA is expressed at a low but detectable level and this level rises a few hours after the cells are stimulated to proliferate by serum (32). In contrast to c-fos and c-myc expression, c-ras-Ha mRNA is induced by IGF-I (Lu, Campisi; unpublished data).

Although growth factors induce the expression of many genes, attention has focused on the proto-oncogenes because of their potential role as critical, intracellular growth regulators. Despite this biased effort, these studies have provided a general framework of knowledge about how growth factors act to induce the expression of growth-related genes.

Regulation of C-fos and C-myc Expression by PDGF and EGF

The transcription, mRNA and protein for the c-fos and c-myc proto-oncogenes increase manyfold beginning 5 (c-fos) to 30 (c-myc) min after quiescent fibroblasts are stimulated to proliferate by fresh serum or purified mitogens. The mitogens that activate the expression of these genes include PDGF, EGF and phorbol ester tumor promoters such as phorbol myristyl acetate (PMA). IGF-I has no effect on the expression of c-fos and c-myc in fibroblasts (9,17,27,28).

Of the mitogens that stimulate c-fos and c-myc expression, PDGF and the phorbol esters share a common mechanism: both mitogens activate PKC. PDGF activates this protein kinase indirectly. Occupancy of the PDGF receptor activates a membrane-associated phospholipase C that specifically hydrolyzes phosphatidyl inositol (PI) (33,34). PI cleavage in turn generates two second messengers: inositol triphosphate, which causes the release of calcium from an intracellular store, and diacylglycerol (DAG), which activates PKC. Phorbol esters activate PKC directly, bypassing the immediate, receptor-mediated events (2,4). By contrast, EGF does not stimulate PI hydrolysis in several types of cells, including A31 fibroblasts (35). There is some evidence that EGF causes an influx of extracellular calcium, but little else is known about the signalling mechanism used by EGF (36).

We have been particularly interested in the intracellular pathways that regulate proto-oncogene expression in fibroblasts (9,17,37). In A31 cells made quiescent by growth to confluence, we found that PMA was a potent inducer of c-fos and c-myc expression, in agreement with the findings of others. However, in subconfluent cells made quiescent by serum deprivation, PMA was a poor inducer of either gene and it was a poor mitogen. This was an unexpected result and we could rule out some trivial explanations for it. First, PKC activity was similar in confluent and subconfluent quiescent cells. Second, PMA could stimulate phosphorylation of the major substrate for PKC (the 80 kDA protein) in both types of quiescent cells. Third, a PDGF-inducible gene of unknown function (JE) was fully inducible by PMA, regardless of the method of growth arrest. Thus, subconfluent, serum-deprived cells contained active PKC that was capable of inducing JE expression but which could not induce appreciable c-fos or c-myc expression. We do not yet understand the basis for this selective block to PKC action. However, the results suggest that cell-cell contacts may selectively influence the action of PMA (17,37), and possibly other mitogens (38).

In contrast to PMA, EGF was a more potent inducer of c-fos and c-myc expression in serum-deprived, subconfluent cells than in confluent cells. From its known inability to stimulate PI hydrolysis in several fibroblasts, it was likely that EGF activated c-fos and c-myc expression by an intracellular pathway that was distinct from that utilized by PDGF or PMA. Indeed, we found that EGF was fully capable of inducing c-fos and c-myc expression in 3T3 cells that had been depleted of PKC activity (9). Thus, EGF clearly utilized a PKC-independent pathway for the induction of c-myc and c-fos expression.

We found that serum-deprived cells contained about twofold higher cAMP levels than confluent cells, raising the possibility that EGF might utilize PKA as part of its intracellular signalling mechanism. Consistent with this view, when the level of cAMP was experimentally elevated in confluent cells (using cholera toxin or isobutylmethylxanthine), EGF was a much more potent inducer of both proto-oncogenes. This induction was blocked by an inhibitor of PKA. In addition, we found that calcium ionophores could mimic the effects of EGF in inducing c-fos and c-myc expression in the presence of elevated cAMP (17,37).

We conclude that there are at least two growth factor-dependent, intracellular pathways for the induction of c-fos and c-myc expression in 3T3 fibroblasts. One pathway is utilized by growth factors that stimulate PI hydrolysis or by phorbol esters. This pathway results in the activation of PKC and is more active in cells that are growth arrested at confluence. A second pathway is utilized by EGF and is more active in serum-deprived cells, which have higher levels of cAMP. This pathway is dependent upon cAMP and PKA; EGF does not stimulate adenylate cyclase. Rather, EGF provides a signal, possibly calcium influx, that cooperates with PKA to induce proto-oncogene expression.

The PKC- and PKA-dependent pathways most likely activate c-fos and c-myc transcription by different ultimate mechanisms. In the 5-regulatory region of the c-fos gene, a phorbol ester response element and a cAMP response element have been identified; these are separable and distinct (39). In the case of c-myc, there are apparently two mechanisms for increasing the level of primary transcripts. The first is an increase in the initiation of new transcripts from the identified promoter sites. The second is a decrease in the frequence of RNA polymerase pausing or premature termination that normally occurs at the boundary of the first exon and first intron. In confluent A31 cells, serum has been shown to increase transcription initiation whereas EGF and cholera toxin decrease pausing or premature termination (40).

Regulation of C-ras-Ha Expression by Insulin and IGF-I

In contrast to c-fos and c-myc expression, we found that serum, but not EGF (regardless of the presence of cholera toxin), induced c-ras-Ha mRNA within about 2 h of addition to quiescent cells. Two purified mitogens could cause this early rise in mRNA: PMA and insulin at hyperphysiological concentrations. Induction by insulin was independent of PKC. Thus, as in the case of c-fos and c-myc, there appears to be two separable pathways for the induction of c-ras-HA.

At hyperphysiological concentrations, insulin binds to and activates its own receptor, as well as that of the IGF-I receptor. The dose response of c-ras-Ha mRNA induction by insulin and IGF-I indicated that both ligands were capable of elevating the levels of this mRNA at nanomolar concentrations. It is, therefore, likely that occupancy of either receptor by the appropriate ligand is capable of inducing the expression of this proto-oncogene.

Unlike the effects of serum, the induction of c-ras-Ha mRNA by insulin and IGF-I was transient. Initially, serum and insulin elevated the mRNA to the same extent and with identical kinetics (within about 2 h of addition). In the presence of serum, the mRNA continued to rise for about 8 h and a maximal level (five- to tenfold over the quiescent level) was maintained as long as the cells continued to proliferate. By contrast, in the presence of insulin alone, the mRNA level began to decline after 4-6 h. Only in the presence of insulin and EGF was the regulation of c-ras-Ha mRNA indistinguishable from the regulation seen in the presence of serum. Indeed, EGF alone did induce this mRNA, but the induction was apparent only after about 6 h. Thus, the early phase of c-ras-Ha mRNA induction was mediated by insulin or IGF-I and the later phase was mediated by EGF (Lu, Campisi; unpublished data).

Like the early induction of c-fos and c-myc expression by PDGF, PMA or EGF, insulin or IGF-I induced c-ras-Ha expression at the level of transcription, and this induction occurred by a mechanism that was independent of new protein synthesis. By contrast, the induction by serum was partially blocked by inhibitors of protein synthesis. This result suggested that the later induction by EGF was dependent upon prior protein synthesis. Unfortunately, we could not test this directly because long exposures to protein synthesis inhibitors are toxic to cells, particularly in the absence of serum.

In summary (Fig. 2), at least three proto-oncogenes are growth factor-inducible in 3T3 cells. For each gene, there is more than one growth factor-linked intracellular pathway. C-fos and c-myc are induced by similar signalling mechanisms, whereas c-ras-Ha is induced by a unique signalling pathway.

Growth Inhibition: Regulation of mRNA Translation by Interferons

In opposition to the actions of growth factors, which stimulate quiescent fibroblasts to progress through G0/G1, interferons retard progress through G0/G1 by growth factor-stimulated fibroblasts (23,24). The finding that PDGF and other growth factors induce IFN expression (19,20) suggests that growth stimulatory factors actually activate a complex, homeostatic program that ensures balanced growth.

The mechanisms by which IFNs inhibit cell proliferation are poorly understood. From studies on the mechanisms of the antiviral activity, it is known that IFNs induce the expression of a ribonuclease, which degrades viral mRNAs, and a protein kinase, which phosphorylates and inactivates a protein synthesis initiation factor (eIF2) (21,22). It is not known whether either of these antiviral mechanisms plays a role in the antiproliferative activity. However, clearly ribonuclease activation or eIF2 inactivation could inhibit cell proliferation if either of these mechanisms acted on cellular mRNAs or proteins that are necessary, positive-acting growth regulators.

However, clearly ribonuclease activation or eIF2 inactivation could inhibit cell proliferation if either of these mechanisms acted on cellular mRNAs or proteins that are necessary, positive-acting growth regulators.

To begin to understand the mechanisms by which IFN negatively regulates cell proliferation, we studied its action on growth factor-inducible gene expression in quiescent and growth factor-stimulated 3T3 cells (Levine, Seshadri, Ng, Hann, Campisi; manuscript submitted for publication). We used for these studies a murine alpha/beta-IFN mixture that

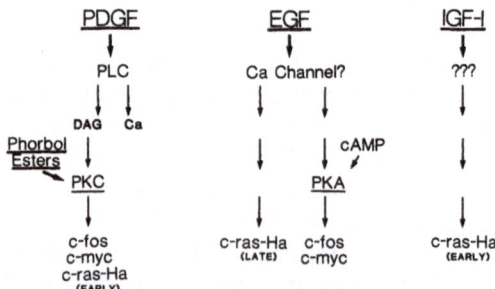

Fig. 2. Regulation of c-fos, c-myc and c-ras-Ha expression by PDGF, EGF and IGF-I in 3T3 cells. See text for complete explanation.

retarded the onset of DNA replication by about 6 h and inhibited the replication of vesicular stomatitis virus, both with nearly identical dose responses.

We found that IFN had no effect on the extent or kinetics of induction of several growth factor-inducible mRNAs, including fibronectin, ornithine decarboxylase and the c-fos and c-myc mRNAs. In fact, IFN prevented the decline in c-myc, ornithine decarboxylase and fibronectin mRNA that normally occurs about 8 h after growth factor stimulation. These results argued against ribonuclease activation as a mechanism for the antiproliferative activity.

In contrast to mRNA levels, we found that IFN selectively inhibited the translation of certain growth factor-inducible genes. This translational inhibition was highly selective: it affected the c-myc, ornithine decarboxylase and fibronectin genes but not the c-fos gene nor the genes encoding most of the cellular proteins resolvable by two-dimensional gel electrophoresis. Thus, IFN substantially inhibited the accumulation of ornithine decarboxylase activity and completely inhibited the induced, but not basal, rate of fibronectin synthesis. In the case of c-myc, IFN delayed the peak of myc protein synthesis, normally apparent 2 h after stimulation, by an interval that was approximately equal to the delay in DNA synthesis.

The IFN-dependent process responsible for the selective, translational inhibition of growth factor-inducible mRNAs is not known. It is unlikely that eIF2 inactivation is entirely responsible because c-myc and fibronectin mRNA were present at high levels on both heavy and light polysomes, not solely in initiation complexes. In addition, IFN stabilized the otherwise labile c-myc mRNA. C-myc mRNA stabilization and accumulation on polysomes is also seen with cycloheximide, an inhibitor of protein synthesis that blocks peptide elongation. It is possible, then, that IFN inhibits the translation of growth factor-inducible mRNAs by inactivating a factor(s) needed for peptide elongation. The basis for the selectivity of the translational inhibition is also not known. It is interesting that translation of c-myc, but not c-fos, mRNA was affected. As discussed above, both mRNAs are induced by the same growth factor signals and both are very labile. Nonetheless, IFN uncoupled the regulation of the c-myc mRNA level from the translation of that mRNA, while having no effect on c-fos mRNA.

Our finding that IFN delays c-myc protein synthesis by an interval coincident with the delay in the onset of DNA synthesis suggests that the myc protein acts or is required several hours prior to the start of S phase. The finding that c-myc protein is required for the initiation of DNA synthesis (41) supports the idea that c-myc is a critical, growth-regulatory target of the antiproliferative action of IFN. However, unlike growth stimulatory polypeptides, which activate transcription, IFN appears to act by inhibiting translation.

Growth Factors, Gene Expression, and the Control of Proliferation in Differentiated Epithelial Cells

In the previous sections, I have described some of the mechanisms by which certain polypeptide growth factors and inhibitors regulate the proliferation of quiescent fibroblasts in culture. These mechanisms include the transcriptional activation of three proto-oncogenes by growth factors and the translational inhibition of at least one of these proto-oncogenes by antiproliferative interferons. We would, of course, like to know whether these findings are applicable to other types of cells in culture and ultimately to cells in vivo.

Some recent data suggest that the mechanisms that regulate fibroblast proliferation may differ from the mechanisms that regulate certain other types of cells in culture, particularly differentiated epithelial cells. In a collaborative effort, we have studied the regulation of proliferation by alveolar type 2 cells from rat lung (Clement, Campisi, Farmer, Brody; manuscript submitted for publication). These cells synthesize and secrete surfactant. In vivo, type 2 cells have the ability to divide and differentiate into type 1 cells, which are terminally differentiated and form the gas transfer barrier, when the need for lung growth or repair arises (42-45).

When isolated from the lungs of adult rats, type 2 cells do not proliferate in culture (46). However, type 2 cells isolated from the lungs of neonatal rats did proliferate in culture, albeit for a limited period of time. Moreover, the proliferation of neonatal type 2 cells was serum dependent: when serum was withdrawn from the medium, proliferation ceased and when serum was resupplied to the cells, proliferation resumed. However, serum stimulated neonatal cells resumed proliferation with little or no lag period that is seen in serum-stimulated fibroblasts. This result suggests that serum deprivation may cause neonatal type 2 cells to arrest growth closer to S phase than fibroblast.

Adult and neonatal type 2 cells in culture provide an opportunity to study the mechanisms that control the proliferation of these differentiated epithelial cells. We studied the expression of four genes whose mRNA levels fluctuate with growth state in fibroblasts and several other cell systems: the c-myc and c-ras-Ha proto-oncogenes and the genes encoding actin and the replication-dependent histine 3.2. These mRNAs were present at identical levels in

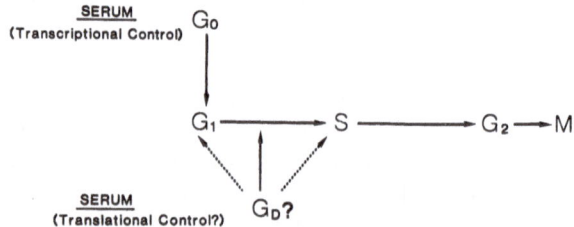

Fig. 3. Control of proliferation by growth factors in fibroblasts or differentiated type 2 epithelial cells. In fibroblasts, cells arrest growth in G0. Growth factors (serum) stimulate progression through G0/G1 and into S phase primarily by increasing the transcription of growth-related genes. The proliferative behavior of serum-deprived neonatal type 2 cells suggest that they may not arrest growth in G0. Rather, these cells appear to arrest growth closer to S phase (GD?). Growth factors may stimulate entry into S phase by increasing the translation of growth-related genes.

proliferating and nonproliferating (serum-deprived) neonatal type 2 cells and in non-proliferating adult type 2 cells. Thus, in contrast to the situation in fibroblasts, the level of mRNA for all four genes was uncoupled from the state of proliferation of the type 2 cells in culture.

Despite constitutively expressed mRNA, we found that replication-dependent histones were synthesized only by proliferating neonatal type 2 cells and not by serum-deprived neonatal cells or by adult cells. Thus, growth factors appear to control the translation, rather than the mRNA abundance of histone 3.2.

Taken together, our results indicate that the control of growth-related gene expression in primary type 2 epithelial cells in culture may differ from the control described for fibroblasts (Fig. 3). The results suggest that in these cells growth factors may control the translation, rather than the transcription, of genes that are growth factor inducible in fibroblasts and that the ability to respond to this translational control may be developmentally regulated.

References

1. Baserga R. The biology of cell reproduction. Cambridge: Harvard University Press, 1985.
2. Hokin LE. Receptors and phosphoinositide-generated second messengers. Annu Rev Biochem 1985; 54:205-35.
3. Rozengurt E. Early signals in the mitogenic response. Science 1986; 234:161-6.
4. Nishizuka Y. The role of protein kinase C in cell surface signal transduction and tumor promotion. Nature 1984; 308:693-8.
5. Hunter T. A thousand and one protein kinases. Cell 1987; 50:823-9.
6. Edelman AM, Blumenthal DK, Krebs EG. Protein serine/threonine kinases. Annu Rev Biochem 1987; 56:567-613.
7. Denhardt DT, Edwards DR, Parfett CLJ. Gene expression during the mammalian cell cycle. Biochim Biophys Acta 1986; 865:83-125.
8. Jetten AM, Ganong BR, Vandenbark GR, Shirley JE, Bell RM. Role of protein kinase C in diacylglycerol-mediated induction of ornithine decarboxylase and reduction of epidermal growth factor binding. Proc Natl Acad Sci USA 1985; 82:1841-945.
9. McCaffrey P, Ran W, Campisi J, Rosner M. Two independent growth factor-generated signals regulate c-fos and c-myc mRNA levels in Swiss 3T3 cells. J Biol Chem 1987; 262:1442-5.
10. Seghal PB, Walther Z, Tamm I. Rapid enhancement of B2-interferon/B cell differentiation factor BSF-2 gene expression in human fibroblasts by diacylglycerols and the calcium ionophore A23187. Proc Natl Acad Sci USA 1987; 84:3663-7.
11. Todaro GJ, Green H. Quantitative studies of the growth of mouse embryo cells in culture and their development into established lines. J Cell Biol 1963; 17:299-313.
12. Ponten J. Relationship between in vitro transformation and tumor formation in vivo. Biochim Biophys Acta 1976; 458:397-422.
13. Pardee AB, Dubrow R, Hamlin JL, Kletzien RF. Animal cell cycle. Annu Rev Biochem 1978; 47:715-50.

14. Scher CD, Shepard RC, Antoniades HN, Stiles CD. Platelet-derived growth factor and the regulation of the fibroblast cell cycle. Biochim Biophys Acta 1979; 560:217-41.
15. Leof EB, Wharton W, Van Wyk JJ, Pledger WJ. Epidermal growth factor and somatomedin C regulate G1 progression of competent Balb/c-3T3 cells. Exp Cell Res 1982; 141:107-15.
16. Campisi J, Pardee AB. Posttranscriptional control of the onset of DNA synthesis by an insulin-like growth factor. Mol Cell Biol 1984; 4:1807-14.
17. Ran W, Dean M, Levine RA, Henkle C, Campisi J. Induction of c-fos and c-myc mRNA by epidermal growth factor or calcium ionophore is cAMP-dependent. Proc Natl Acad Sci USA 1986; 83:8216-20.
18. Keski-Oja J, Moses HL. Growth inhibitory polypeptides in the regulation of cell proliferation. Med Biol 1987; 65:13-20.
19. Zullo JN, Cochran BH, Huang AS, Stiles CD. Platelet-derived growth factor and double-stranded ribonucleic acids stimulate expression of the same genes in 3T3 cells. Cell 1985; 43:793-800.
20. Kohase M, May LT, Tamm I, Vilcek J, Seghal PB. A cytokine network in human diploid fibroblasts: interactions of B-interferons, tumor necrosis factor, platelet-derived growth factor and interleukin 1. Mol Cell Biol 1987; 7:273-80.
21. Lengyel P. Biochemistry of interferons and their actions. Annu Rev Biochem 1982; 51:251-82.
22. Pestka S, Langer JA, Zoon KC, Samuel CE. Interferons and their actions. Annu Rev Biochem 1987; 56:727-77.
23. Taylor-Padimitriou J, Ebsworth N, Rozengurt E. Possible mechanisms of interferon-induced growth and inhibition. In: Ford RJ, Maizel AL, eds. Mediators in cell growth and differentiation. New York: Raven Press, 1985:283-98.
24. Lin SL, Kikuchi T, Pledger WJ, Tamm I. Interferon inhibits the establishment of competence in G0/S-phase transition. Science 1986; 233:356-9.
25. Kaczmarek L. Biology of disease: protooncogene expression during the cell cycle. Lab Invest 1986; 54:365-76.
26. Bishop JM. Cellular oncogenes and retroviruses. Annu Rev Biochem 1983; 52:301-54.
27. Greenberg ME, Ziff EB. Stimulation of 3T3 cells induces transcription of the c-fos protooncogene. Nature 1984; 311:433-7.
28. Muller R, Bravo R, Burckhardt J, Curran T. Induction of c-fos gene and protein by growth factors precedes activation of c-myc. Nature 1984; 312:716-20.
29. Rauscher FJ, Sambucetti LC, Curran T, Distel RJ, Spiegelman BM. Common DNA binding site for fos protein complexes and transcription factor AP-1. Cell 1988; 52:471-80.
30. Hurley JB, Simon MI, Teplow DB, Robisaw JD, Gilman AB. Homologies between signal transducing G proteins and ras gene products. Science 1984; 226:860-2.
31. Barbacid M. Ras genes. Annu Rev Biochem 1987; 56:779-827.
32. Campisi J, Gray HE, Pardee AB, Dean M, Sonenshein GE. Cell cycle control of c-myc but not c-ras expression is lost following chemical transformation. Cell 1984; 36:241-7.
33. Habenicht AJR, Glomset JA, King WC, Nist C, Mitchell CD, Ross R. Early changes in phosphatidylinositol and arachidonic acid metabolism in quiescent Swiss 3T3 cells stimulated to divide by platelet-derived growth factor. J Biol Chem 1981; 23:12329-35.
34. Chu SW, Hoban CJ, Owen AJ, Geyer RP. Platelet-derived growth factor stimulates rapid phosphoinositide breakdown in fetal human fibroblasts. J Cell Physiol 1985; 124:391-6.

35. Besterman JM, Watson SP, Cuatrecasas P. Lack of association of epidermal growth factor-, insulin- and serum-induced mitogenesis with stimulation of phosphatidylinositide degradation in BALB/c 3T3 fibroblasts. J Biol Chem 1986; 261:723-7.

36. Hesketh TR, Moore JP, Morris JDH, Taylor MV, Rogers J, Smith GA, Metcalfe JC. A common sequence of calcium and pH signals in the mitogenic stimulation of eucaryotic cells. Nature 1985; 313:481-4.

37. Ran W, Dean M, Levine RA, Campisi J. Activation of protooncogene expression by growth regulatory signals. Curr Top Microbiol and Immunol 1986; 132:313-9.

38. Dean M, Levine RA, Ran W, Kindy MS, Sonenshein GS, Campisi J. Regulation of c-myc transcription and mRNA abundance by serum growth factors and cell contact. J Biol Chem 1986; 261:9161-6.

39. Sheng M, Dougan ST, McFadden G, Greenberg ME. Calcium and growth factor pathways of c-fos transcriptional activation require distinct upstream regulatory sequences. Mol Cell Biol 1988; 8:2787-96.

40. Nepveu A, Levine RA, Campisi J, Greenberg ME, Ziff EB, Marcu KB. Alternative modes of c-myc regulation in growth factor-stimulated and differentiating cells. Oncogene 1987; 1:243-50.

41. Heikkila R, Schwab G, Wickstrom E, Loke SL, Pluznik DH, Watt R, Neckers LM. A c-myc antisense oligonucleotide inhibits entry into S phase but not progress from G0 to G1. Nature 1987; 328:445-9.

42. Crapo JD, Barry BE, Gehr P, Bachofen M, Weibel ER. Cell number and cell characteristics of the normal human lung. Am Rev Respir Dis 1982; 125:740-5.

43. Adamson IYR, Bowden DH. The type 2 cell as a progenitor of alveolar epithelial regeneration: a cytodynamic study in mice after exposure to oxygen. Lab Invest 1974; 30:35-41.

44. Evans MJ, Cabral LJ, Stephens RJ, Freeman G. Transformation of alveolar type 2 cells to type 1 cells following exposure to NO2. Amer Rev Respir Dis 1978; 17:307-26.

45. Smith LJ, Brody JS. Influence of methylprednisolone on mouse alveolar type 2 cell response to acute lung injury. Amer Rev Respir Dis 1981; 123:459-64.

46. Leslie CC, McCormick-Shannon K, Robinson PC, Mason RJ. Stimulation of DNA synthesis in cultured rat alveolar type 2 cells. Exp Lung Res 1985; 8:53-66.

6

Molecular Characterization of Fibroblast Growth Factor and Possible Role in Early and Late Embryonic Development

Denis Gospodarowicz

Cancer Research Institute M-1282, University of California
Medical Center, San Francisco, CA 94143

Introduction

In recent years growth factors have been shown to influence the in vitro proliferation and differentiation of endocrine cells (1). It has been postulated that they could play an important in vivo role in local control mechanisms involving either autocrine or paracrine regulation of endocrine cell proliferation and/or differentiation (1). Through their ability to modulate each other's activity, they are well suited to control the complex morphogenetic events taking place in various organs during embryonic development or in specialized endocrine organs such as ovaries or testis during the adult phase (2,3).

Among the growth factors which could be relevant to the development and functions of endocrine organs are the fibroblast growth factor(s) and their modulator, transforming growth factor (4). Fibroblast growth factor exists under two closely related forms: basic and acidic FGF, which interact with common cell surface receptors (5). The ability to share receptors enable aFGF and bFGF to exert similar biological effects on a wide range of mesoderm and neuroectoderm cells controlling both their proliferation and differentiation (6). The wide range of FGF-responsive cells is best explained by the possibility that FGF could be the vegetalizing factor responsible in early embryos for mesenchyme induction (4,7). One would, therefore, expect that during the ontogeny of development, FGF would control the proliferation and differentiation of all tissues derived from the primary and secondary mesenchyme. The bioactivity of both basic and acidic FGF can be positively or negatively regulated, depending on the cell type, by transforming growth factor-β (4). Therefore, depending on the relative concentrations of these growth factors in the microenvironment, cell proliferation and differentiation could be selectively enhanced or repressed.

In this review we concentrate on the role of FGF in early embryonic development and in the development and functional regulation of the pituitary gland and gonads. These organs have been shown to contain predominantly the basic form of FGF.

Molecular Characterization of the FGF Genes, Their mRNA and Protein Products

The high degree of structural homology (55%) between aFGF and bFGF suggests that they are derived from a common ancestral gene (8,9). The FGF genes have been cloned and complementary DNA sequences of both bFGF and aFGF have been synthesized. The organization of the genes encoding bFGF and aFGF has been described (10-13). The bFGF gene is localized on human chromosome 4, while that of aFGF is on chromosome 5 (10,14). This suggests that bFGF and aFGF have become separate gene products through a process of gene duplication and evolutionary divergence. The basic FGF gene has a size greater than 38 kbp. It encodes 3 exons widely separated by 2 large introns: the first one separates codons 60 and 61, and the second separates codons 94 and 95 (11). The aFGF gene has a similar organization, with 2 large introns located in identical positions in the coding sequence once basic and aFGF are properly aligned (13). Southern blot analysis of human genomic DNA has shown that there is only one bFGF and one aFGF gene. Therefore, all of the characterized or uncharacterized heparin-binding endothelial cell mitogens related to bFGF or aFGF are the products of a single bFGF or aFGF gene (10-12). In various cultured cells and tissues, the bFGF gene gives rise to 2 polyadenylated mRNAs of approximately 3.7 and 7.0 kb (15,16). The aFGF gene appears to encode a single mRNA species of approximately 4.1 kb (17).

The primary translation product for either bFGF or aFGF is composed of 155 amino acids (12,17). Proteolytic cleavage from the precursor molecule of the first 9 or 15 residues (aFGF) results in the generation of the mature proteins which can then be cleaved further in homologous positions to give the NH2-truncated form of bFGF (des.1-15) or aFGF (des.1-6) (6,9,18).

Comparison of the primary structure of bFGF and aFGF have shown that 55% of their amino acid sequences are identical (8,18). Up to 64% of the remaining sequences may involve nucleotide substitutions, where a single base change could result in amino acid replacement and concomitant homology (8). A distant sequence homology exists between bFGF or aFGF and Interleukin-1b (25 and 27%, respectively) (8,9). A distant homology has also been reported between residues 102 to 111 of aFGF and several neuropeptides (9). These homologies are of little functional consequence, since neither Interleukin-1b nor the various neuropeptides which include bombesin, substances P and K, neuromedin C, physalaemin, and eledoisin compete with basic or aFGF for binding to their common cell surface receptor (Neufeld G and Thomas K, private communication).

Three oncogenes have been shown to be structurally related to FGF. These oncogenes are a diverse group and have been identified in Kaposi's sarcoma, human stomach and bladder cancers, and mouse mammary cancer. The oncogene derived from Kaposi's carcinoma appears to be the same as the hst oncogene, which was previously isolated from human stomach cancers and also from normal stomach tissue (19). The proteins encoded by the hst and Kaposi's sarcoma oncogenes both contain 206 amino acids. Once properly aligned, the sequences of the oncogenes are about 45% identical with the sequence of bFGF and show less resemblance to the sequence of aFGF (20).

The protein product of Int-2, an oncogene that was originally detected in mouse mammary cancers caused by the mouse mammary tumor virus (MMTV) (21), also belongs to the FGF family. Although one substantial gap has to be introduced to maximize the alignment, it, too, resembles (46% homology) bFGF more closely than aFGF (22). The third oncogene found to encode an FGF-like protein was isolated from human bladder cancer cells and named FGF-3 (23). Its protein product has a 45% degree of homology with bFGF, with a lesser degree of homology with aFGF (23).

These results are intriguing in view of findings that the FGFs not only stimulate the division of mesoderm and neuroectoderm-derived cells (4), but are also potent angiogenic agents that foster the growth of new blood vessels (4,24). Such new blood vessel formation is essential if solid tumors are to develop to a significant size (25). Production of the FGFs or related proteins might, therefore, contribute to the development of solid cancers both because of the proteins' effects on cell division and on angiogenesis. Although there is evidence implicating Int-2 as a developmental control gene (26), the precise functions of the genes that gave rise to the FGF-related oncogenes are currently unknown.

Basic FGF seems to have been extremely well conserved through evolution. For example, bovine and human bFGF differ in only 2 of their 146 amino acids, giving an overall amino acid sequence homology of 98.7% (11). Avian and bovine bFGF have the same amino acid composition and avian bFGF cross-reacts on an equimolar basis with bovine bFGF in an RIA using rabbit anti-bFGF polyclonal antibodies. Thus, homologous epitopes are well conserved (4). The deduced amino acid sequence from cDNA coding for the first and last exon of *Xenopus laevis* bFGF show 70% and 90% identity, respectively, to the coding sequence for the first and last exons of bovine bFGF (Kimelman D and Abrahams J, private communication). Acidic FGF seems to be less well conserved, and the bovine form differs from the human by 11 amino acids out of a total of 140 (27,28).

FGF and Mesodermal Induction in Early Embryos

In early embryonic development, the basic body plan arises because cells in different regions of the egg become programmed to follow different pathways (29). During oogenesis, differences arise between the animal and vegetal halves of the eggs. Fertilization results in a subdivision of the vegetal half into a dorsal vegetal and a ventral vegetal region. Mesoderm is then induced from the animal hemisphere by signal(s) originating from the vegetal region of the egg (29-31). This induction is an instructive phenomenon that suppresses epidermal differentiation of cells from the animal pole, and directs them instead to differentiate into mesodermal cells. Signal(s) originating from the dorsal vegetal region lead to the formation of dorsal-type mesoderm, mostly consisting of notochord and somites, while signal(s) originating from the ventrovegetal region lead to the formation of ventral-type mesoderm, consisting primarily of blood cells, mesenchyme, and mesothelium. It has been proposed that this process of regional specification arises from the action of inducing factors, or morphogens. Until recently their chemical natures were unknown since only minute amounts of the substances that cause mesodermal induction can be isolated from early stage embryo. However, agents that cause induction have been isolated from more abundant sources such as late-stage chick embryo or guinea pig bone marrow, and have been characterized as 13000 Mr polypeptides with basic pI (32,33).

In recent studies, Slack and his colleagues (7) have investigated the possibility of bFGF mimicking the effect of the ventrovegetal signal(s) responsible for the formation of ventral-type mesoderm. When explants of ectoderm cut from animal pole of stage 8 Xenopus blastulae were exposed to bFGF, cells, instead of differentiating into epidermis or remaining undifferentiated, differentiated into mesodermal structures. Between 2 to 30 ng bFGF/ml, the induction closely resembled ventral-type mesoderms formed by explants where ventrovegetal regions were combined with animal poles. They consisted of concentric arrangements of loose mesenchyme, mesothelium, and blood cells within an epidermal jacket. At higher bFGF concentrations (30 to 120 ng/ml), most of the explants contained significant amounts of muscle blocks. The inducing effect of bFGF seems to be highly specific since it could not be mimicked by other growth factors such as TGFβ or TGFα, TNF, IFNγ and -α, insulin, Interleukin-1α and -β, G-CSF and GM-CSF (colony-stimulating factors).

These results have recently been confirmed and expanded by Kimelman and Kirschner (34), who reported the presence in Xenopus embryo of an mRNA encoding a protein highly homologous to bFGF. FGF mRNA levels were described as high in the oocyte and dropped by twenty-fivefold during oocyte maturation with an abrupt increase at the midblastula transition, a stage during which vegetalizing factor expression would be expected. It was also reported that the relatively weak effect of bFGF on muscle formation observed earlier by Slack et al. (7) could be potentiated by TGFβ (34). Interestingly, Weeks and Melton have also recently reported (35) that a maternal mRNA called Vg1 localized to the vegetal hemisphere of frog eggs encodes a member of the TGFβ family. These results suggest, then, that the prelocalized maternal messages for FGF and the analog of TGFβ (Vg1) are the mesoderm inducers. While induction of ventral mesoderm tissue may be caused by bFGF alone, induction of dorsal mesoderm (including muscle tissue) may require the participation of both bFGF and TGFβ, with TGFβ having no effect of its own but rather serving to potentiate FGF's bioactivity. Differences in the concentration of the Vg1 peptide across the dorsal ventral axis of blastulae could explain how dorsal (notochord) versus ventral (blood) mesodermal tissues are specified (35).

Recent studies have compared the effect of the two subclasses of TGFβ: TGFβ-1 and -β-2 on muscle formation. They show that TGFβ-2 is active in inducing somites while TGFβ-1 is not (35a). Since the inducing activity present in conditioned medium from XTC cells (a cell line derived from Xenopus and shown in earlier studies to induce animal caps to form various mesodermal derivatives) (35b) can be abolished by neutralizing anti-TGFβ-2 antibodies, but not by anti-TGFβ-1, this suggests that TGFβ-2 could be the dorsal vegetalizing factor present in early blastula. FGF, which induced preferentially ventral mesoderm, would be the ventro-vegetalizing factor.

The FGF levels in whole embryo and limb bud during chick development have also been analyzed. First detected in the yolk and white of unfertilized chick eggs, the level of FGF in the embryonic chick body is fairly constant before days 2 to 6. Thereafter, the levels increase so that by day 13 the increase is sevenfold. In contrast, the FGF level in limb bud is higher than in the rest of the body until day 5, and undergoes a transient decrease between days 6 and 7 (36). It is tempting to speculate that there may be a correlation between the decrease in the FGF level observed during days 5 to 9 in the limb and the extensive myotube formation which occurred during this period (37). Consistent with previous studies (38) that demonstrate that FGF stimulates the proliferation of myoblasts and delays their differentiation, FGF delays the onset of differentiation of days 4-12 embryonic chick wing bud myoblasts (39). However, at an earlier stage (days 4-5), FGF seems to be required for the myogenic differentiation of myoblasts (39). The limited period during which FGF-dependent myoblasts are found in the limb bud suggests that they may play a role in early muscle morphogenesis, and also suggests that FGF may affect muscle development differently during various phases of embryogenesis (39).

FGF could also be involved in early embryonic brain development (reviewed in reference 40), as reflected in its ability to stimulate the proliferation of embryonic neuroblasts which later expressed a cholinergic differentiation (41). It has also been shown to stimulate the proliferation and differentiation of oligodendrocytes and astroglial cells (40), and recent studies have suggested that endogenous brain FGF produced by astroglial cells could be involved in neuronal differentiation (42).

Although the tissues named above (animal pole, muscle and central nervous system) have been the focus of most of the in vivo studies done with FGF, due to the wide range of cell types which are known to be affected by FGF (4), it is likely that FGF will be shown to play a complex role during embryogenesis. Its function and/or availability to target cells is likely to be intimately linked to the changing extracellular matrix which contains several components known to affect FGF activity (4), and which has been shown to be involved in the control of morphogenetic events (43,44).

Expression of FGF in Pituitary Tissues and Cultured Pituitary Cells: Possible In Vivo Function

Of all organs tested, pituitary glands have the highest concentrations of bFGF (45) and, despite a recent report, have no detectable levels of its closely related counterpart, aFGF (46). What has been mistaken in the pituitary for aFGF is the long form [155AA] of bFGF, which on heparin Sepharose elutes earlier than the shorter form [146AA], and which does not cross-react with polyclonal antibodies directed against the NH_2 terminal region of the shorter form of bFGF (unpublished observations). Recent studies have shown that the main cellular source of bFGF in pituitary glands are follicular cells, which can contain as many as 5×10^5 bFGF molecules per cell (47). Previous studies (48) have suggested that follicular cells may play an important role in the restoration of degenerated pituitary glandular tissues during the early stage of transplantation. This is in agreement with the suggestion by Farquhar et al. (49) that follicular cells play the role of nurse cells in the pituitary gland, similar to that of the Sertoli cells in the testes. Follicular cells are also involved in extracellular matrix (ECM) synthesis (50), and there is a large amount of experimental evidence that indicates that ECM plays an important role in cell growth and differentiation (51,52). Previous studies (51,53) have shown that FGF controls the production of ECM components and could become an integral part of such structures (54), thereby further supporting the growth and differentiation of cells becoming associated with newly produced ECM. The ability of follicular cells to support the restoration of pituitary granular cells (48) could reflect their ability to synthesize and release heparan sulfate proteoglycan-FGF complexes which would become an integral part of their ECM. It has also been suggested that follicular cells, which are mainly concentrated in the pars tuberalis, would provide support for its microvascularization (55). The presence of an angiogenic factor such as bFGF in follicular cells could relate to the development and maintenance of the differentiated states of the pars tuberalis microvasculature (55). Follicular cells are known to be the predominant cellular element in the Rathke pouch, the anlagen from which the adenohypophysis will later differentiate (56). The presence of bFGF in that cell type could, therefore, be relevant to the embryonic development of the pituitary gland.

The cyclic behavior of the pituitary intermediate lobe, which is mostly composed of follicular cells, provides one possible explanation for the release of bFGF by these cells in vivo. This lobe exhibits three phases of cellular activity: (1) resting; (2) degeneration and autolysis; and, (3) regeneration. During the second phase, cells increase in size and autolyze, giving rise through a holocrine mechanism of secretion to an intraglandular lumen full of colloid, the breakdown product of marginal intermediate lobe cells (57). As the intermediate lobe reestablishes itself by direct division of its remaining cells, the colloid is expelled from the intraglandular lumen into the venous cavernous sinuses by way of well-defined capsular clefts (57). Since follicular cells have a high bFGF content, one would expect that colloid breakdown products would contain high concentrations of bFGF. This is, in fact, what could have been concluded from the early studies of Boyd who reported in 1970 that pituitary-derived colloid is mitogenic in vivo for cells of mesodermal origin, which are known to respond to FGF (4,58). These included glomerular capillary endothelial cells (59), reticulo-endothelial cells from the liver (60), and microglial cells in the gray and white matter of the brain (61). Recent studies have shown that heparin-Sepharose affinity-purified colloid extracts contained high concentrations of bFGF (Ferrara N, in preparation). This does, indeed, conclusively demonstrate that bFGF could be responsible for the previously reported growth-promoting activity of pituitary-derived colloid (59,61), and provides evidence for a holocrine release of bFGF by follicular cells.

Besides stimulating pituitary cell proliferation and differentiation, bFGF could also have other regulatory functions, in particular, acting as a paracrine regulator of pituitary hormone secretion. Basic FGF has been shown to increase the release of prolactin and decrease basal growth hormone release in established pituitary-derived cell lines such as Ch_4C_1 cells (62). It also modifies the response of primary cultures of rat anterior pituitary cells to TRH, thus increasing both the sensitivity of the cells to TRH and the amount of prolactin and TSH released (63). Within that context, it is interesting to point out that pituitary follicular cells which are the main source of pituitary FGF (47) can exert a complex regulatory role in pituitary hormone release through paracrine mechanisms (64). It is, therefore, tempting to speculate that some of the modulator effects of FGF on pituitary hormone release observed in vitro could also occur in vivo.

Expression of FGF in Gonads and Possible Role In Vivo

Ovaries

Basic FGF is present in ovarian tissue and has been purified to homogeneity from bovine corpus luteum extract, where it is present in a truncated form (65). As in the case of pituitary, extracts from the corpus luteum do not contain detectable levels of aFGF (65). Recent studies have shown that granulosa cells (66) and possibly luteal cells are among the cell types producing bFGF in ovarian tissue. Theca cells, which have recently been shown to produce both EGF and TGFβ (67,68), could also be a source of ovarian bFGF since nonluteinized ovarian tissue contains FGF-like activity (69).

The activities that are required for follicular development and selection include angiogenesis, the release of plasminogen activator and the growth of granulosa cells (70,71). Each of these biological activities are also characteristic of the effects of FGF (65,72-74). The ability of granulosa cells to express the bFGF gene and produce bioactive bFGF suggests that this factor could act as an autocrine growth factor (66) for that cell type, as well as a paracrine regulator of the differentiation of granulosa cells.

The ovarian follicle is one of the most rapidly proliferating normal tissues in vivo, and granulosa cell growth accounts for the majority of follicular cell expression (75). Previous studies have shown that bFGF is mitogenic for granulosa cells maintained in vitro (76) and delays their terminal differentiation (77). This is likely to reflect the ability of bFGF to keep granulosa cells actively cycling (77), thereby preventing them from entering a G0 phase. BFGF could, therefore, play a role in the initiation of follicular morphogenesis by controlling the growth of granulosa cells in ovarian follicles prior to their preantral stage where hormonal control would take over (3). At the same time that FGF acts as an autocrine growth factor for granulosa cells, it could also regulate metabolic activity by controlling the release of cellular products into the liquor folliculi and the delivery of nutrients to oocytes (78). The ability of FGF to act as an autocrine growth factor and as a morphogen for granulosa cells could be influenced by TGFβ. This factor is known to be produced by theca cells (68) and can positively or negatively modulate the biological activity of FGF, depending on the situation. This interplay between FGF and TGFβ could explain, in part, the developmental coordination of the various tissues present within preantral follicles.

In addition to affecting granulosa cell proliferation and differentiation, bFGF also influences their hormonal response. Although bFGF does not increase the proliferation of rat granulosa cells, it inhibits the FSH-mediated induction of LH receptor (43,79), reversibly attenuates the FSH-induced cell aromatase activity (80,81) and stimulates progesterone biosynthesis (81). This tends to suggest that FGF may play an inhibitory cytodifferentiative role in the ontogeny of granulosa cells. The capacity of FGF to interrupt a specific steroidogenic pathway (i.e., estrogen formation) in the granulosa cells and promote another (i.e., progesterone formation) might then be linked to the hormonal events that precede corpus luteum formation and follicular development. Each of these processes are highly dependent on the transitory presence of progesterone without estrogen or vice versa. Therefore, a molecule like FGF could deliver multifunctional signals in the intraovarian milieu to promote cell growth on one hand and predetermine the pattern of the steroidogenic response to FSH, in concert with other growth promoting and growth inhibiting substances, on the other. As such, bFGF may be added to the growing list of growth factors shown to regulate the acquisition of aromatase activity by granulosa cells. These include IGF-1 (82), insulin (82), EGF/TGFα (83,84), and TGFβ (80).

TGFβ is known to act on FSH-induced cell aromatase activity (85) in a mode diametrically opposed to bFGF. It has also been reported to regulate the expression of LH receptors in granulosa cells (86). Thus the presence of TGFβ, produced by theca cells (68), in the microenvironment of granulosa cells could lead to a modulation of the events controlled by FGF. During follicular development stage, a fine tuning in steroid production could, therefore, result from the control of the ratio at which theca versus granulosa cells could express TGFβ versus FGF.

In order for the ovum to escape from the graafian follicle at the time of ovulation, extensive degradation of the follicular wall is necessary. Although several theories have been proposed to explain this phenomenon, its biochemical basis is not firmly established. Schochet, in 1916, suggested that the process has an enzymatic rather than mechanical basis and gave evidence that a proteolytic enzyme is associated with preovulatory follicles (87). Other investigators have also proposed that changes in the amount of lytic enzymes might be involved in ovulation (88,89).

Recently, a specific biochemical mechanism for ovulation has been proposed (90). According to this hypothesis, plasminogen activator (PA) is responsible for the disruption of the follicle. This proposal is based on the fact that rat ovarian granulosa cells produce PA in a manner which is closely correlated with ovulation. The substrate for this enzyme, plasminogen, is present in follicular fluid, and the product of the reaction catalyzed by the action of PA on plasminogen, plasmin, has been shown to weaken follicular wall strips in vitro (91). In addition, in vitro exposure of granulosa cell cultures to preparations of bovine luteinizing hormone and cAMP results in increased amounts of extracellular PA. Taken together, these findings suggest a role for plasminogen activator in ovulation.

Basic FGF is among the growth factors known to stimulate protease and collagenase activity in responsive cells. Although these activities have not yet been studied using granulosa cell cultures with vascular endothelial cells or various tumor cells, FGF stimulates production of PA, as well as collagenase, and further acts to decrease the production of a PA inhibitor (74,92-94). TGFβ influences PA expression induced by bFGF and can inhibit the production of secreted proteases as well as increase the production of a protease inhibitor (95,96). Since both TGFβ and bFGF are present in ovarian follicles, one could speculate that these factors could ultimately play a role in modulating PA activity as well as that of other proteolytic enzymes and collagenase, which plays an important role in the extensive degradation of the follicular wall at the time of ovulation.

Basic FGF, through its angiogenic properties, could also play an important role in the early phase of corpus luteum development when angiogenic events play a critical role. Basic FGF has been shown to be a potent angiogenic factor in vivo in assays as different as the rabbit cornea, the chick chorioallantoic membrane (CAM), or the hamster cheek pouch (65,73,97). The presence of bFGF as the main mitogen in corpus luteum (65) and its presence in granulosa cells (66), the precursor of luteal cells, could be of significance in the angiogenic events, taking place during the early phases of the luteinization process. This is reflected by the extremely rapid and radical vascular changes that take place in the capillary wreath surrounding the follicle at the time of ovulation, and the invasion of the previously avascular granulosa cell layers by numerous and rapidly proliferating capillaries. Previous studies have shown that rabbit luteinizing granulosa and luteal cells produce a diffusible substance that triggers the early vascular changes which occur during development of the corpus luteum and elicit a strong angiogenic response on the part of the host (98). Similar activities have been described by Jakob et al. (99) who demonstrated that bovine corpus luteum grafted on the CAM, the ventral subcutaneous pouch of the mouse, or the hamster cheek pouch elicit a strong angiogenic response. Similarly, Koos and LeMaire (100) have described gonadotropin responsive angiogenesis in rat follicles and corpus luteum. Frederik et al. (101), using human follicular fluid, also established the presence of an angiogenic factor that they associated with the perifollicular neovascularization that occurs during folliculogenesis.

Taken together, these results suggested that granulosa and luteal cells could produce angiogenic factors that trigger capillary invasion in the avascular granulosa cell layer. Basic FGF, which is present in granulosa cells (66), accounts for the full mitogenic potential of corpus luteum crude extract (65) and is mitogenic for corpus luteum-derived capillary endothelial cells (102). Therefore, bFGF could be responsible for the angiogenic activity observed in the developing corpus luteum. Here again, TGFβ could play a significant role in modulating the angiogenic activity of FGF, since it is a potent growth inhibitor of bFGF (in the case of vascular endothelial cells) (103,104), and blocks FGF-induced angiogenesis in vitro (105).

Testes

Basic FGF is present in testicular tissue and has been purified to homogeneity (106). Both mature and truncated forms of bFGF have been shown to coexist (106). Acidic FGF is apparently not expressed in testicular tissues (106) despite a previous report by Feig et al. (107) of a factor called seminiferous growth factor (SGF), which has molecular weight and isoelectric point similar to that of aFGF. The cellular source of bFGF is presently unknown, but by analogy with ovarian tissue, Leydig and/or Sertoli cells could express and synthesize bioactive bFGF.

It is likely that through its ability to stimulate proliferation and differentiation of responsive testicular cells, as well as to modulate their hormonal response and trigger/control ongoing angiogenesis, bFGF could have in the testes most of the effects it has been assigned in ovarian tissue. Sertoli cells are somatic cells that form the seminiferous epithelium within which spermatogenic cells differentiate. Sertoli cells may serve many functions in spermatogenesis, including (i) creating a microenvironment necessary for germ-cell differentiation; (ii) acting as target cells through which follicle-stimulating hormone and testosterone influence spermatogenesis; and, (iii) selectively translocating germ cells from the peripheral to the central compartment of the seminiferous epithelium (108). It is tempting to speculate that the Sertoli cell-derived bFGF could play a role in the regulation of spermatogenesis. An exciting possibility is that this factor mediates the active proliferation of spermatogonia. Other potential target cells include preleptotene spermatocytes and interstitial cells.

Cells of the interstitial compartment represent another possible target for bFGF. These cells rarely divide in normal adult animals (109,110), and yet hyperplasia occurs in response to certain experimental perturbations. Interstitial cell hyperplasia occurs in the cryptorchid testes even in hypophysectomized rats in which gonadotropins are absent (111). Similarly, the inhibition of spermatogenesis by testicular implants of androgen antagonists results in localized hyperplasia of Leydig cells (112). In both cases, the ensuing cell proliferation could be due to the local release of the Sertoli cell-derived growth factor.

One would expect that in testis, and by analogy, with what we know of ovarian tissue, bFGF could modulate the hormonal response of Sertoli cells to FSH through several possible mechanisms. BFGF could inhibit FSH-mediated induction of LH receptor on Sertoli cells. BFGF could also attenuate the FSH-mediated cell aromatase activity and stimulate testosterone synthesis. These events are likely to occur since Sertoli cells, the counterpart of granulosa cells, are known to be both FSH and LH responsive and are capable of synthesizing estrogen (113). In the case of Leydig cells, which are predominantly LH responsive and synthesize mostly androgens, the possible modulation of their hormonal response by bFGF cannot be speculated upon at this time.

Through its angiogenic properties, bFGF could also control the development of the testis microvasculature. The major vessels of the testis are already determined at birth in the rat, but have no special relationship with the seminiferous tubules. At around 15-20 days of age, which corresponds to the onset of intragonadal hormonal activity (114), the microvasculature organizes into two different capillary networks, one confined to the interstitial tissue between the seminiferous tubules, the other connecting the intertubular networks and lying in close contact with the walls of the seminiferous tubules. In the rat, most of the peritubular network appears at about 25-35 days of age, at the time of spermatid formation and consequent tubular enlargement (115).

There is evidence (116,117) that organization of the microvasculature is under endocrine control. Whether this is due to the direct action of hormones such as steroids, or results from hormone-induced differentiation of the interstitial and tubular tissues to produce angiogenic factors, has not been established. An evaluation of the relative importance of bFGF in controlling the organization of the testes microvasculature could, therefore, shed some light on the nature of the testicular angiogenic factors.

Ovarian and Testicular Neoplasms

Much less is known of the causes of ovarian cancer than those of the other major gynecologic neoplasms. Since cancer of the ovary will strike 1 to 2% of women during their lifetime, and will be responsible for the death of most women who develop this cancer, the lack of knowledge is particularly unfortunate (118). Malignant tumors originating in cells derived from coelomic epithelium constitute the large majority (60%) of ovarian cancers (119). They are followed in frequency by sex cord stromal tumors, and over 90% of these malignancies are granulosa cell tumors (119). The presence of bFGF in ovarian tissue could be a contributing factor to tumor formation. Although its presence in coelomic epithelium has not yet been demonstrated, it is expressed in granulosa cells (66). Previous studies have shown that in BHK-21 cells transfected with plasmids carrying the bFGF gene, inappropriate expression of the bFGF gene results in autonomous cell growth and in the expression of the transformed phenotype (120). Similar results have been reported when Swiss 3T3 cells are transfected with an aFGF expression vector (121). Inappropriate expression of the bFGF gene in granulosa cells could, therefore, have similar consequences. In testis, the most frequent tumors derived from endocrine cells are those derived from Sertoli cells, which are the counterpart of the granulosa cells and which could also express the bFGF gene. The possibility, therefore, exists that, like in granulosa cells, aberrant expression of bFGF could be a contributing factor in the biogenesis of tumors derived from Sertoli cells, and possibly Leydig cells.

The various loci at which bFGF acts could make it an important agent in tumor progression. It could act as an autocrine growth factor, responsible for the aberrant growth of ovarian or testicular tumor cells. In the case of ovarian or testicular cells depending only on FGF, uncontrolled expression of the bFGF gene during neoplastic transformation could make them divide in an aberrant manner. In the case of cells responding to multiple exogenous growth factors, uncontrolled expression of endogenous bFGF could make them independent for further growth of an exogenous growth factor supply. By increasing capillary endothelial cell proliferation, bFGF could be responsible for the increased vascular supply which delivers O_2 and nutrients and removes waste products in actively growing ovarian and testicular tumors. Finally, by increasing tumor PA level (92,95,122), as well as by increasing the secreted levels of various protease (122) and collagenase (123), bFGF would facilitate the metastatic process and tumor invasion.

Conclusion

Although a number of growth factors have recently been isolated and characterized, their roles in vivo as well as their physiological relevance is still largely conjectural. In most cases [TGFβ, TGFα, EGF, PDGF], identification rests on the correlation between their respective mRNA expression in various tissues at various stages of development, rather than on a direct causality between growth factor expression and morphogenetic events. Until recently, of all the growth factors characterized to date, only NGF had a well-established physiological role, based on its ability to control the development of both peripheric and central nervous systems. The recent studies, conducted primarily at an early embryonic stage, have helped to establish a physiological role for FGF and its modulator, TGFβ. The demonstration that bFGF can act as a primordial morphogen at one of the earliest embryonic stages by instructing cells destined to form ectodermal structure to shift and form mesodermal structure instead will, in all likelihood, have a profound impact in the field of embryology and provide for the first time a clue as to the nature of the early embryonic inducers. It is also worth noting that those observations are in close agreement with previous in vitro studies which have shown that FGF had a transforming activity and could act as a morphogen as well as a mitogen on practically all mesoderm- and neuroectoderm-derived cells studied to date (4). Nevertheless, one cannot conclude that FGF will act to induce only the proliferation and differentiation of mesodermal and neuroectodermal cells, since a few cell types shown to be sensitive to FGF can also be of ectodermal origin (such as corneal epithelial, lens and glial cells) (72), and ectodermal cells such as pituitary-derived follicular cells are known to contain bFGF.

The role of the microenvironment in the regulation of the development and function of endocrine organs such as pituitary and gonads has recently been the subject of renewed interest. Among the factors which could be involved in such regulation are growth factors which, through their ability to act in an autocrine or paracrine manner, can mediate the short-range interactions between the various tissues and cell types present in complex organs during development.

Growth factors such as FGF and its modulator, TGFβ, could play an important role in pituitary development/regeneration and ovarian follicular morphogenesis. They could also play a role in the development of complex structures such as the seminiferous tubules where cell proliferation and differentiation are ongoing and intensive processes throughout the life of the individual.

The role of growth factors in complementing and modulating the control offered by long-range effectors such as hormones can no longer be ignored. In the case of ovarian tissue, for example, FGF as well as TGFβ could be involved in preparing follicles either for the luteinization process or atresia. In the case of FGF, this could be achieved by shifting steroidogenic pathways toward progestogen production, as a consequence of FGF's ability to inhibit aromatase activity. By inducing capillaries to invade the follicular structure, FGF would further favor ovulation. TGFβ, by inhibiting FGF to act either at the level of granulosa cells or capillary endothelial cells, would lead the follicles toward atresia. What functional role FGF and TGFβ would have in testicular tissue is presently unknown, but is likely to be the object of increased interest in the future.

Finally, the role of growth factors in the development of ovarian and testicular neoplasms, the etiology of which is too often unknown, could be an important area of research in the future. Recent evidence links inappropriate expression of growth factors or their cell surface receptors to malignancies. Strong evidence also indicates a similar linkage between oncogenes and growth factors or their receptors. Together, this experimental evidence points toward the increasing importance of growth factors in neoplastic etiology (122).

References

1. Schomberg DW, May JV, Mondschein JS. Interaction between hormones and growth factors in the regulation of granulosa cells differentiation in vitro. J Steroid Biochem 1983; 19:291-5.
2. Gospodarowicz D, Vlodavsky I, Bialecki H, Brown K. The control of proliferation of ovarian cells by the epidermal and fibroblast growth factors. In: Spilman CH, Wilkes J, eds. Fifth Brook Lodge Meeting on Novel Aspects of Reproductive Biology. New York: SP Medical and Scientific Books, Spectrum Publ Inc., J. Wiley and Sons, 1978:107-8.
3. Gospodarowicz D. Growth and differentiation factors for cell populations in the normal ovaries. In: Murphy ED, Beamer WG, eds. Ovarian neoplasia—Workshops on the biology of human cancer. Report No. 11, Technical Report Series, Int Union Against Cancer, vol 50; 1980:2-21.
4. Gospodarowicz D, Ferrara N, Schweigerer L, Neufeld G. Structural characterization and biological functions of fibroblast growth factor. Endocr Rev 1987; 8:95-114.
5. Neufeld G, Gospodarowicz D. Basic and acidic fibroblast growth factor interacts with the same cell surface receptor. J Biol Chem 1987; 261:5631-7.
6. Gospodarowicz D. Purification of brain and pituitary FGF. In: Barnes D, Sirbasku D, eds. Methods in enzymology: peptide growth factors; vol 147B. Orlando, Florida: Academic Press, 1987:106-19.
7. Slack JM, Darlington B, Heath H, Godsave S. Heparin binding growth factors as agents of mesoderm induction in early Xenopus embryo. Nature 1987; 326:197-200.
8. Esch F, Ueno N, Baird A, et al. Primary structure of bovine brain acidic fibroblast growth factor (FGF). Biochem Biophys Res Commun 1985; 133:554-62.
9. Gimenez-Gallego G, Rodkey C, Bennett C, Rios-Candelore M, Disalvo J, Thomas K. Brain-derived acidic fibroblast growth factor: complete amino acid sequence and homologies. Science 1985; 230:1385-8.
10. Abraham JA, Whang L, Tumolo A, Mergia A, Fiddes JC. Human basic fibroblast growth factor: nucleotides sequence, genomic organization, and expression in mammalian cells. In: Molecular biology of homo sapiens; vol 51. New York: Cold Spring Harbor, 1987:657-68.
11. Abraham JA, Whang JL, Tumolo A, et al. Human basic fibroblast growth factor: nucleotide sequence and genomic organization. EMBO J 1986; 5:2523-8.

12. Abraham JA, Mergia A, Whang JL, et al. Nucleotide sequence of a bovine clone encoding the angiogenic protein, basic fibroblast growth factor. Science 1986; 233:545-8.
13. Mergia A, Tumolo A, Haaparanta T, et al. Isolation and characterization of the human gene for acidic FGF. DNA 1988 (in press).
14. Mergia A, Eddy R, Abraham JA, Fiddes JC, Shows TB. The genes for basic and acidic fibroblast growth factors are on different human chromosomes. Biochem Biophys Res Commun 1986; 138:644-51.
15. Schweigerer L, Neufeld G, Friedman J, Abraham JA, Fiddes JC, Gospodarowicz D. Capillary endothelial cells express basic fibroblast growth factor, a mitogen that stimulates their own growth. Nature 1987; 325:257-9.
16. Schweigerer L, Neufeld G, Mergia A, Abraham JA, Fiddes JC, Gospodarowicz D. Basic fibroblast growth factor in human rhabdomyosarcoma cells: implications for the proliferation and neovascularization of myoblast-derived tumors. Proc Natl Acad Sci USA 1986; 84:842-6.
17. Jaye M, Howk R, Burgess W, et al. Human endothelial cell growth factor: cloning, nucleotide sequence, and chromosome localization. Science 1986; 233:541-4.
18. Esch F, Baird A, Ling N, et al. Primary structure of bovine pituitary basic fibroblast growth factor (FGF) and comparison with the amino terminal sequence of bovine brain acidic FGF. Proc Natl Acad Sci USA 1985; 6507-11.
19. Sakamoto H, Mori M, Taira M, et al. Transforming gene from human stomach cancers and a noncancerous portion of stomach mucous. Proc Natl Acad Sci USA 1986; 83:3997-4001.
20. Taira M, Yoshida T, Miyagawa K, Sakamoto H, Terada M, Sugimura T. cDNA sequence of human transforming gene hst and identification of the coding sequence required for transforming activities. Proc Natl Acad Sci USA 1987; 84:2980-4.
21. Dickson C, Smith R, Brookes S, Peters G. Tumorogenesis by mouse mammary tumor virus: proviral activation of a cellular gene in the common integration region, Int-2. Cell 1984; 37:529-36.
22. Dickson C, Peters G. Potential oncogene product related to growth factors. Nature 1987; 326:833.
23. Marx JL. Oncogene action probed. Science 1987; 237:602.
24. Gospodarowicz D, Neufeld G, Schweigerer L. Molecular and biological charac-terization of fibroblast growth factor: an angiogenic factor which also controls the proliferation and differentiation of mesoderm and neuroectoderm derived cells. Cell Differ 1986; 19:1-17.
25. Folkman J. How is blood vessel growth regulated in normal and neoplastic tissue? Cancer Res 1986; 46:467-73.
26. Jakobovits A, Shackleford GM, Varmus HE, Martin GR. Two proto-oncogenes implicated in mammary carcinogenesis, Int-1 and Int-2, are independently regulated during mouse development. Proc Natl Acad Sci USA 1986; 83:7806-10.
27. Gimenez-Gallego G, Conn G, Hatcher VB, Thomas K. The complete amino acid sequence of human brain derived acidic fibroblast growth factor. Biochem Biophys Res Commun 1986; 138:611-7.
28. Gautschi-Sova P, Muller T, Bohlen P. Amino acid sequence of human acidic fibroblast growth factor. Biochem Biophys Res Commun 1986; 140:874-80.
29. Slack JMW. From egg to embryo: determinative events in early development. Cambridge and London: Cambridge University Press, 1983.

30. Nieuwkoop PD. The formation of mesoderm in Urodelean amphibians. I. Induction by the endoderm, Wilhelm Roux' Arch Entw Mech Org 1969; 162:341-73.
31. Smith JC, Dale L, Slack JMW. Cell lineage and region-specific markers in the analysis of inductive interactions. J Embryol Exp Morphol 1985; 89(supp):317-27.
32. Tiedemann H, Jaenicke L, eds. In: Biochemistry of differentiation and morphogenesis. 23rd Colloquium Ges Biol Chem, Springer, Berlin, 1982:275-8.
33. Born J, Geithe HP, Tiedemann H, Tiedemann HP, Kocher-Becker U. Isolation of a vegetalizing inducing factor, Hoppe-Seylers. Z Physiol Chem 1972; 353:1075-87.
34. Kimelman D, Kirschner M. Synergistic induction of mesoderm by FGF and TGFb and the identification of an mRNA coding for FGF in early Xenopus embryo. Cell 1987; 51:869-77.
35. Weeks DL, Melton DA. A maternal mRNA localized to the vegetal hemisphere in Xenopus eggs codes for a growth factor related to TGFb. Cell 1987; 51:861-6.
35a Rosa F, Roberts AB, Danielpour D, Dart LL, Sporn MB, David IB. Mesoderm induction in amphibians: the role of $TGF\beta_2$-like factors. Science 1988; 239:783-5.
35b Smith JC. A mesoderm-inducing factor is produced by a Xenopus cell line. Dev Biol 1987; 99:3-14.
36. Seed J, Olwin BB, Hauschka SD. Fibroblast growth factor level in whole embryo and limb bud during chick development. Dev Biol 1988; 128:50-7.
37. Marchok AC, Herrmann H. Studies of muscle development. I. Changes in cell proliferation. Dev Biol 1967; 15:129-55.
38. Gospodarowicz D, Weseman J, Moran JS, Lindstrom J. Effect of fibroblast growth factor on the division and fusion of bovine myoblasts. J Cell Biol 1976; 70:395-405.
39. Seed J, Hauschka SD. Clonal analysis of vertebrate myogenesis VIII FGF dependent and independent muscle colony types during chick wing development. Dev Biol 1988; 128:40-9.
40. Gospodarowicz D. Fibroblast growth factor. In: Critical reviews in oncogenesis. 1988 (in press).
41. Gensburger C, Labourdette G, Sensenbrenner M. Brain basic FGF stimulates the proliferation of rat neuronal precursor cells in vitro. FEBS Lett 1987; 217:1-5.
42. Hatten ME, Lynch M, Rydel RE, et al. Dev Biol 1988; 125:280-9.
43. Bernfield M, Banerjee SK, Koda JE, Rapraeger AC. Remodeling of the basement membrane as a mechanism of morphogenetic tissue interaction. In: The role of extracellular matrix in development. New York: A. R. Liss, 1984:548-72.
44. Eckblom P. Basement membrane protein and growth factors in kidney differentiation. In: Tolstad RL, ed. The role of extracellular matrix in development. 42nd Symposium of the Soc for Dev Biol. New York: A. R. Liss, 1984:173-206.
45. Gospodarowicz D. Localization of a fibroblast growth factor and its effect alone and with hydrocortisone on 3T3 cell growth. Nature 1974; 249:123-7.
46. Biswas SB, Hammond RW, Anderson LD. Fibroblast growth factors from bovine pituitary and human placenta and their functions in the maturation of porcine granulosa cells in vitro. Endocrinology 1988; 123:559-66.
47. Ferrara N, Schweigerer L, Neufeld G, Mitchell R, Gospodarowicz D. Pituitary follicular cells produce basic fibroblast growth factor. Proc Natl Acad Sci USA 1987; 84:5773-7.
48. Gon G, Shirasawa N, Ishikawa H. Appearance of the cyst or ductile like structures and their role in the restoration of the rat pituitary autograft. Anat Rec 1987; 217:371-8.

49. Farquhar MG, Stutelsky EH, Hopkins CR. Structure and function of the anterior pituitary and dispersed pituitary cells, in vitro studies. In: Tixer-Vidal A, Farquhar MG, eds. The anterior pituitary gland. New York: Academic Press, 1975:82-135.

50. Vila-Porcile E, Olivier L. The problem of the folliculo-stellate cells in the pituitary gland. In: Motta PM, ed. Ultrastructure of endocrine cells and tissues. Boston: Martinus Nijihoff Publishers, 1984:64-76.

51. Gospodarowicz D. The control of mammalian cell proliferation by growth factors, extracellular matrix, and lipoproteins. J Invest Dermatol 1983; 81:41-50.

52. Gospodarowicz D. Extracellular matrix and the control of proliferation and differentiation of endothelial cells. In: Vogel HJ, Nossel HL, eds. Pathobiology of the endothelial cell. New York: Academic Press, 1982:19-61.

53. Gospodarowicz D, Cohen DC, Fujii DK. Regulation of cell growth by the basal lamina and plasma factors: relevance to embryonic control of cell proliferation. In: Sato G, Pardee A, Sirbasku D, eds. Cold Spring Harbor Conferences on Cell Proliferation. Growth of cells in hormonally deficient media; vol 9. New York: Cold Spring Harbor, 1982:95-124.

54. Vlodavsky I, Folkman J, Sullivan R, et al. Endothelial cell-derived basic fibroblast growth factor: synthesis and deposition into subendothelial extracellular matrix. Proc Natl Acad Sci USA 1987; 84:2292-6.

55. Harris GW. Function of the pituitary stalk. Bull Johns Hopkins Hosp 1955; 97:359-72.

56. Halmi NS, Moriarity GC. The hypophysis. In: Weiss L, Greep RO, eds. Histology. 4th ed. New York: McGraw-Hill, 1974:1039.

57. Boyd WH. Morphological feature of the hypophyseal intermediate lobe directly related to its activity. Arch Histol Jpn 1972; 34:1-17.

58. Gospodarowicz D. Biological activity in vivo and in vitro of pituitary and brain fibroblast growth factor. In: Ford RJ, Maizel AL, eds. Mediators in cell growth and differentiation. New York: Raven Press, 1985:109-34.

59. Boyd WH. Proliferation of glomerular capillary endothelial cells under the influence of hypophyseal intermediate lobe materials. Z Anat Entwick Gesch 1970; 130:306-15.

60. Boyd WH. Influence of hypophyseal intermediate lobe tissue and colloid on reticuloendothelial cells of the liver. Experientia 1970; 26:72-4.

61. Boyd WH. The effect of bovine hypophyseal intermediate lobe tissue and colloid on microglia. J of Neuro Visc Relat 1970; 31:382-6.

62. Schonbrunn A, Krasnoff M, Westerdorf JM, Tashjian AH. EGF and TRH act similarly on a clonal pituitary cell strain. J Cell Biol 1980; 85:786-97.

63. Baird A, Mormede P, Ying S, et al. A non-mitogenic pituitary function of fibroblast growth factor: regulation of thyrotropin and prolactin secretion. Proc Natl Acad Sci USA 1985; 82:5545-9.

64. Allaerts W, Denef C. Modulation of hormone secretion by folliculo-stellate cells in rat anterior pituitary cell aggregates [Abstract]. Program of the First International Congress of Neuroendocrinology, San Francisco, CA, 1986; 83:2.

65. Gospodarowicz D, Cheng J, Lui G-M, Baird A, Bohlen P. Corpus luteum angiogenic factor is related to fibroblast growth factor. Endocrinology 1985; 17:201-13.

66. Neufeld G, Ferrara N, Mitchell R, Schweigerer L, Gospodarowicz D. Granulosa cells produce basic fibroblast growth factor. Endocrinology 1987; 121:597-603.

67. Skinner MK, Lobb D, Dorrington JH. Ovarian theca/interstitial cells produce an epidermal growth factor like substance. Endocrinology 1987; 121:1892-9.

68. Skinner MK, Keski-Oja J, Osteen KG, Moses HL. Ovarian theca cells produce transforming growth factor-b which can regulate granulosa cell growth. Endocrinology 1986; 121:786-92.
69. Makris A, Ryan KJ, Yasumisu T, Hill CL, Zetter BR. The nonluteal porcine ovary as a source of angiogenic activity. Endocrinology 1984; 115:1672-8.
70. Hsueh AJW, Adashi EY, Jones PBC, Welsh TH. Hormonal regulation of the differentiation of cultured ovarian granulosa cells. Endocr Rev 1984; 5:76-127.
71. Ny T, Bjersing L, Hsueh AJW, Loskutoff DJ. Cultured granulosa cells produce two plasminogen activators and an antiactivator, each regulated differently by gonadotropins. Endocrinology 1985; 116:1666-8.
72. Gospodarowicz D, Greenburg G, Bialecki H. Factors involved in the modulation of cell proliferation in vivo and in vitro: the role of fibroblast and epidermal growth factors in the proliferative response of mammalian cells. In Vitro 1978; 14:85-118.
73. Gospodarowicz D, Bialecki H, Thakral TK. The angiogenic activity of the fibroblast and epidermal growth factor. Exp Eye Res 1979; 28:501-14.
74. Montesano R, Vassalli JD, Baird A, Guillemin R, Orci L. Basic fibroblast growth factor induces angiogenesis in vitro. Proc Natl Acad Sci USA 1986; 83:7297-301.
75. Gougeon A. Rate of follicular growth in the human ovary. In: Rolland R, Van Hall EV, Hillier SG, McNatty KP, Shoemaker J, eds. Follicular maturation and ovulation. North Holland, Amsterdam: Elsevier, 1982:155.
76. Gospodarowicz D, Ill CR, Birdwell CR. Effects of fibroblast and epidermal growth factors on ovarian cell proliferation in vitro: I. Characterization of the response of granulosa cells to FGF and EGF. Endocrinology 1977; 100:1108-20.
77. Gospodarowicz D, Bialecki H. The effects of the epidermal and fibroblast growth factor on the replicative life span of bovine granulosa cells in culture. Endocrinology 1978; 103:854-8.
78. Savion N, Gospodarowicz D. Patterns of cellular peptide synthesis by cultured bovine granulosa cells. Endocrinology 1980; 107:1798-807.
79. Mondschein JS, Schomberg DW. Growth factors modulate gonadotropin receptors induction in granulosa cell cultures. Science 1981; 211:1179-80.
80. Adashi EY, Resnick CE, Bergeman CS, Gospodarowicz D. Fibroblast growth factor as a regulator of ovarian granulosa cell differentiation: a novel non-mitogenic role. Mol Cell Endocrinol 1987 (in press).
81. Baird A, Hsueh AJW. Fibroblast growth factor as an intraovarian hormone: differential regulation of steriodogenesis by an angiogenic factor. Regul Pept 1986; 16:243-50.
82. Hsueh AJW, Welsh TH, Jones PBC. Inhibition of ovarian and testicular steroidogenesis by EGF. Endocrinology 1981; 108:2002-4.
83. Adashi EY, Resnick CE, D'Ercole J, Svoboda ME, Van Wyk JJ. Insulin-like growth factors as intraovarian regulators of granulosa cell growth and function. Endocr Rev 1985; 6:400-20.
84. Schomberg DW, May JV, Mondschein JS. Interaction between hormones and growth factors in the regulation of granulosa cell differentiation in vitro. J Steroid Biochem 1983; 19:291-5.
85. Adashi EY, Resnick CE. Antagonistic interactions of transforming growth factors in the regulation of granulosa cell differentiation. Endocrinology 1986; 119:1979-84.
86. Kneckt M, Peng P, Catt KJ. Transforming growth factor-beta regulates the expression of luteinizing hormone receptors in ovarian granulosa cells. Biochem Biophys Res Commun 1986; 139:800-8.

87. Schochet SS. A suggestion as to the process of ovulation and ovarian cyst formation. Anat Rec 1916; 10:447-57.
88. Espey LL. Ovarian proteolytic enzymes and ovulation. Biol Reprod 1974; 10:216-35.
89. Rondell P. Role of steroid synthesis in the process of ovulation. Biol Reprod 1974; 10:199-215.
90. Beers WH, Strickland S, Reich E. Ovarian plasminogen activator: relationship to ovulation and hormonal regulation. Cell 1975; 6:387-94.
91. Beers WH. Follicular patterns in plasminogen and plasminogen activator and the effect of plasmin on ovarian follicle wall. Cell 1975; 6:379-86.
92. Presta M, Moscatelli D, Silverstein JJ, Rifkin DB. Purification from a human hepatoma cell line of a basic FGF like molecule that stimulates capillary endothelial cell plasminogen activator production, DNA synthesis and migration. Mol Cell Biol 1986; 6:4060-6.
93. Mira Y, Lopez R, Joseph-Silverstein J, Rifkin DB, Ossowski L. Identification of a pituitary factor responsible for enhancement of plasminogen activator activity in breast tumor cells. Proc Natl Acad Sci USA 1986; 83:7780-4.
94. Moscatelli D, Presta M, Rifkin DB. Purification of a factor from human placenta that stimulates capillary endothelial cell protease production, DNA synthesis and cell migration. Proc Natl Acad Sci USA 1986; 83:2091-5.
95. Saskela O, Moscatelli D, Rifkin DB. The opposing effects of basic fibroblast growth factor and transforming growth factor beta on the regulation of plasminogen activator activity in capillary endothelial cells. J Cell Biol 1987; 105:957-63.
96. Thalacker FW, Nilsen-Hamilton M. Specific induction of secreted proteins by TGFb and TPA. Relationship with an inhibitor of plasminogen activator. J Biol Chem 1987 (in press).
97. Gospodarowicz D, Cheng J, Lui G-M, Baird A, Bohlen P. Isolation by heparin-Sepharose affinity chromatography of brain fibroblast growth factor: identity with pituitary fibroblast growth factor. Proc Natl Acad Sci USA 1984; 81:6963-7.
98. Bassett DL. The changes in the vascular pattern of the ovary of the albino rat during the estrous cycle. Am J Anat 1943; 73:251-91.
99. Jakob W, Jentzsch JW, Mauersberger B, Oehme P. Demonstration of angiogenesis in activity in the corpus luteum of cattle. Exp Pathol 1977; 13:231-6.
100. Koos R, LeMaire W. Evidence for an angiogenic factor from rat follicles. In: Greenwald GE, Terranova PF, eds. Factors regulating ovarian functions. New York: Raven Press, 1983:191.
101. Frederik JL, Shimanuki T, DiZerega GS. Initiation of angiogenesis by human follicular fluid. Science 1984; 224:389-90.
102. Gospodarowicz D, Massoglia S, Cheng J, Fujii DK. Effect of fibroblast growth factor and lipoproteins on the proliferation of endothelial cells derived from bovine adrenal cortex, brain cortex and corpus luteum capillaries. J Cell Physiol 1986; 127:121-36.
103. Frater-Schroeder M, Muller G, Burchmeier W, Bohlen P. Transforming growth factor-b inhibits endothelial cell proliferation. Biochem Biophys Res Commun 1986; 137:295-302.
104. Baird A, Durkin T. Inhibition of endothelial cell proliferation by type-b transforming growth factor: interactions with acidic and basic fibroblast growth factors. Biochem Biophys Res Commun 1986; 183:476-82.
105. Muller G, Behrens J, Nussbaumer U, Bohlen P, Birchmeier W. Inhibitory action of transforming growth factor-b on endothelial cells. Proc Natl Acad Sci USA 1987; 84:5600-4.

106. Ueno N, Baird A, Esch F, Ling N, Guillemin R. Isolation and partial characterization of basic fibroblast growth factor from bovine testis. Mol Cell Endocrinol 1987; 49:189-94.

107. Feig LA, Klagsbrun M, Bellve AR. Mitogenic polypeptide of the mammalian seminiferous epithelium: biochemical characterization and partial purification. J Cell Biol 1983; 97:1435-43.

108. Fawcett DW. Frontiers in reproduction and fertility control. Part 2. In: Greep RO, Koblinsky MA, eds. Cambridge, MA: M.I.T. Press, 302-20.

109. Baillie AH. Observations on the growth and histochemistry of the Leydig tissue in the postnatal prepubertal mouse testis. J Anat 1961; 95:357-70.

110. Reddy KJ, Svoboda DJ. Alterations in rat testes due to an antispermatogenic agent. Arch Pathol 1967; 84:376-92.

111. Iturriza FC, Irusta O. Hyperplasia of the interstitial cells of the testis in experimental cryptorchidism. Acta Physiol Lat Am 1979; 19:236-42.

112. Aoki A, Fawcett DW. Is there a local feedback from the seminiferous tubules affecting activity of the Leydig cells? Biol Reprod 1978; 19:144-58.

113. Dorrington JH, Armstrong DT. Effect of FSH on gonadal functions. Recent Prog Horm Res 1979; 35:301-33.

114. Setchell BP. Testicular blood supply, lymphatic drainage and secretion of fluid. In: Johnson AD, Gomes WR, VanDenmark NL, eds. The testis; vol 5. New York: Academic Press, 101-239.

115. Kormano M. An angiographic study of the testicular vasculature in the postnatal rat. Z Anatomie und Entwicklungsgeschichte 1967; 126:138-53.

116. Williams RF. Some responses of living blood vessels and connective tissue to testicular grafts in rabbits. Anat Rec 1949; 104:147-61.

117. Gunn SA, Gould TC. Vasculature of the testes and adnexa. In: Hamilton DW, Greep RO, eds. Handbook of physiology, Section 7: Endocrinology; vol V. Washington: American Physiological Society; 117-42.

118. Weiss NS. Epidemiology of ovarian cancer. In: Murphy ED, Beamer NG, eds. Biology of ovarian neoplasia; vol 50. Geneva: UICC, 1980:34-9.

119. Cutler SJ, Young JL, eds. Third national cancer survey: incidence data. National Cancer Institute Monograph 1975; 41:1-27.

120. Neufeld G, Mitchell R, Ponte P, Gospodarowicz D. Expression of human basic fibroblast growth factor cDNA in baby hamster kidney-derived cells results in autonomous cell growth. J Cell Biol 1988; 106:1385-94.

121. Jaye M, Lyall RM, Mudd R, Schlessinger J, Sarver N. Expression of aFGF cDNA confers growth advantage and tumorigenesis to Swiss 3T3 cells. EMBO J 1988; 7:965-9.

122. Moscatelli D, Presta M, Joseph-Silverstein J, Rifkin DB. Both normal and tumor cells produce basic fibroblast growth factor. J Cell Physiol 1986; 129:273-6.

123. Denhardt DT, Hamilton RT, Parfett CL, et al. Close relationship of the major excreted protein of transformed murine fibroblasts to thiol dependent cathepsin. Cancer Res 1986; 66:4590-6.

124. Sporn MB, Roberts AB. Autocrine growth factors and cancer. Nature 1985; 313:745-7.

III. Growth Factors and the Ovary

7

Rodent Studies on the Potential Relevance of Insulin-Like Growth Factor (IGF-I) to Ovarian Physiology

Eli Y. Adashi,[1] Carol Resnick,[1] Eleuterio R. Hernandez,[1] Marjorie E. Svoboda,[2] E. Hoyt,[3] David R. Clemmons,[4] Pauline K. Lund,[3] and Judson J. Van Wyk[2]

[1]Division of Reproductive Endocrinology, Department of Obstetrics and Gynecology, University School of Medicine, Baltimore, Maryland 21201 and Departments of [2]Pediatrics and [3]Physiology, and Medicine. [4]University of North Carolina at Chapel Hill, Chapel Hill, North Carolina 27514

Introduction

The recurring process of ovarian follicular growth is an exponential rather than a linear process characterized by substantial dramatic proliferation and differentiation of the granulosa cell. Although the pivotal role(s) of gonadotropins and of gonadal steroids in this explosive agenda is well recognized, the variable fate of follicles subject to comparable gonadotropic support suggests the existence of additional intraovarian regulatory mechanism(s). Among potential novel intraovarian regulators, insulin-like growth factor I (IGF-I) has been receiving increasingly intense scrutiny (1-2). Taken together these studies strongly suggest the existence of an *intraovarian autocrine* control mechanism, wherein *IGF-I may serve as the central signal*, and the *granulosa cell its site of production, reception, and action*. Viewed in this light, IGF-I may promote the growth and/or differentiation of the granulosa cell, acting for the most part as an amplifier of gonadotropin action. Granulosa cell-derived IGF-I may also provide paracrine input to the nearby theca-interstitial cell compartment in the interest of coordinated follicular function.

The Granulosa Cell as a Site of IGF-I Production

Significantly, of all adult *rat* organs tested (3), *the ovary (O) displays the third highest level of IGF-I gene expression*, the uterus (U) and liver (Li) being the most active in this regard (Fig. 1). Although the *rat* ovarian content of IGF-I appears to be growth hormone dependent (4), a direct effect of growth hormone at the level of the rat granulosa cell remains to be demonstrated. Extending the investigation to the transcriptional level, we have recently shown that the adult and immature *rat* ovary (as well as the isolated, granulosa cell) is a site of IGF-I gene expression (5) and that it may be subject to gonadotropic regulation.

Ovarian IGF-I Gene Expression in the Rat. To evaluate the possibility of ovarian IGF-I gene expression, polyadenylated RNA from the ovaries of immature (21-23 days old; DES treated) or randomly cycling adult (70-80 days old; non-DES treated) rats was hybridized with a 32_p-labelled rat IGF-I complementary DNA probe (Fig. 2). As in liver, northern blot analysis revealed at least three major RNA species sized at 1.7, 4.7 and 7.5 kb. Significantly, however, comparison of the hybridization signals indicates enhanced abundance of Pre Pro IGF-I RNAs (mostly 7.5 and 1.7 kb) in ovaries of immature DES-treated (Lane 2) as compared with adult (Lane 1) rats. As such, these findings suggest measurable IGF-I gene expression at the level of the ovarian granulosa cell since the ovaries of immature DES-treated rats are comprised largely (>90%) of granulosa cells.

Reprobing of the blots with a ubiquitin cDNA probe revealed similar abundance of ubiquitin mRNA in all samples (not shown), indicating that the observed differences are not due to differences in the polyadenylated message load. The significance and the translational competence of the multiple relatively high molecular weight RNA transcripts (the smallest of which is of sufficient size to encode Pre Pro IGF-I) remains uncertain. However, it is likely that these RNA transcripts represent processing variants since Pre Pro IGF-I is encoded by a single gene. Importantly, these studies support the suggestion that the ovary is a site of IGF-I gene expression and that locally produced rather than circulatory-derived IGF-I may play a role in ovarian physiology. Further studies will be necessary to determine whether the differences observed between immature and adult rats are, in effect, age dependent or whether DES (applied to immature but not adult rats) may be the culprit.

Ovarian IGF-I Gene Expression: Effect of FSH. Given the central role of FSH in supporting granulosa cell differentiation, the possibility of FSH-regulated IGF-I gene expression appears worthy of study. To this end, increasing amounts of total RNA from the ovaries of FSH-treated (0, 5, or 10 µg/rat/day; bid), immature hypophysectomized rats were dotted onto Genescreen and hybridized with a 32_p-labelled rat Pre Pro IGF-I$_A$ cDNA probe. The results (shown in Figure 3) suggest that the treatment with increasing concentrations of FSH results in dose-dependent increments in ovarian IGF-I (but not ubiquitin; not shown)

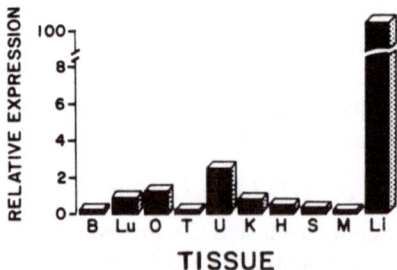

Fig. 1. Relative expression of IGF-I gene in various tissues. Li = liver; U = uterus; 0 = ovary. (Reprinted with permission from Murphy et al., Endocrinology 1987; 120:1279.)

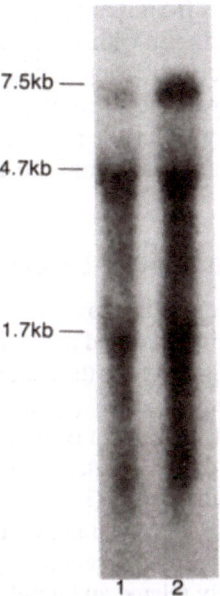

Fig. 2. Polyadenylated RNA (20 µg/lane) samples are from (1) immature (21-23 days old), DES-treated, or (2) randomly cycling adult (70-80 days old) rats.

gene expression. While these observations do not conclusively pinpoint the granulosa cell as a site of IGF-I gene expression, the very fact that the granulosa cell (rather than the theca-interstitial cell) is a site of FSH reception and action supports such a possibility.

Granulosa Cell IGF-I Gene Expression. To determine whether the granulosa cell is a site of IGF-I gene expression, use was made of cytoplasmic RNA from increasing concentra-

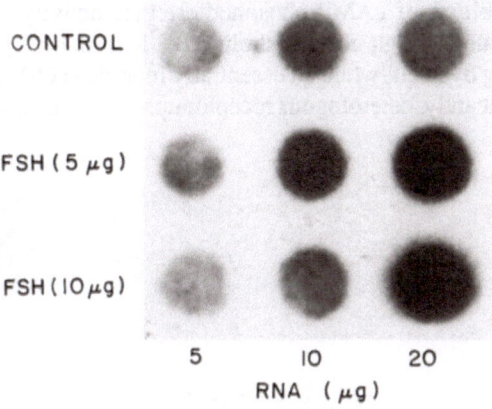

Fig. 3. Ovarian IGF-I gene expression: effect of FSH.

tions ($0.5\text{-}5.0 \times 10^6$) of granulosa cells from immature, DES-primed rats. Extracted RNA was dotted onto Genescreen, and hybridized with a 32_p-labelled rat Pre Pro IGF-I_A cDNA probe. As shown (Fig. 4), provision of increasing concentrations losa cells yielded dose-dependent increments in the intensity of the hybridization signal given 3 h of exposure. Whereas these findings indicate readily detectable presence of Pre Pro IGF-I message in the granulosa cell, the occurrence of similar transcripts in theca-interstitial cells cannot be excluded at this time.

The Granulosa Cell as a Site of IGF-I Reception

Binding to FSH-primed rat granulosa cells proved time-, temperature-, and pH-dependent, optimal steady state conditions being achieved following an 8-h incubation at 15°C and a pH of 8.0 (6). Although subject to regulation by the cellular density of plating, the binding of [^{125}I] IGF-I to its receptor proved saturable (apparent Kd 3.3×10^{-9}M) as well as reversible, complete or partial tracer displacement being effected by competitive inhibition and dilution, respectively (6). Scatchard and Hill analyses yielded linear plots consistent with a single class of nonintereacting binding sites (Fig. 5). Specificity studies revealed the competition for [^{125}I] IGF-I binding to follow a rank order of potency of IGF-I > MSA > insulin, a pattern compatible with a Type I IGF receptor (Fig. 6). Limited or no displacement was observed for a series of chemically related and unrelated polypeptides as well as by a human insulin receptor antiserum (6). Using affinity cross-linking, we have also been able to observe that whole ovarian membranes of untreated (or FSH-treated) immature hypophysectomized DES-treated rats are endowed with specific Type I IGF receptors (2). Similar results have later been obtained with isolated granulosa cells from the same experimental model.

We have recently reported (7,8) FSH and LH to be capable of upregulating granulosa cell IGF-I binding, an effect further augmented by growth hormone but not prolactin. Specifically, we were able to show that FSH is capable of upregulating IGF-I binding in a time- and dose-dependent fashion and that cAMP, its purported intracellular second messenger, may play an intermediary role in this regard (7). Indeed, granulosa cell IGF-I binding was enhanced following elevation of the intracellular cAMP content by a series of cAMP-generating agonists, inhibition of cAMP-phosphodiesterase activity, or the provision of nondegradable cAMP analogs. High dose forskolin (10^{-5}M), like FSH, proved capable of augmenting IGF-I binding by itself, while an essentially inert dose (10^{-7}M) synergized with FSH in this regard. Significantly, heterologous receptor upregulation was not limited to FSH,

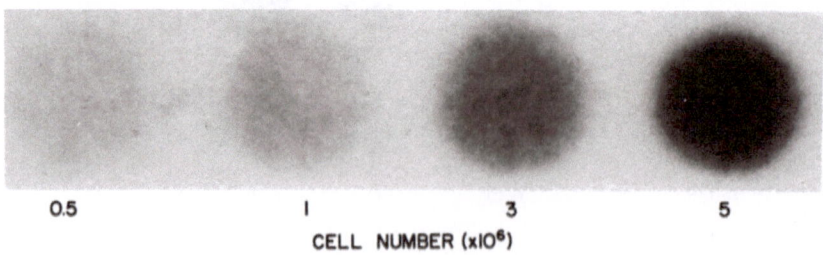

Fig. 4. Rat granulosa cell IGF-I gene expression.

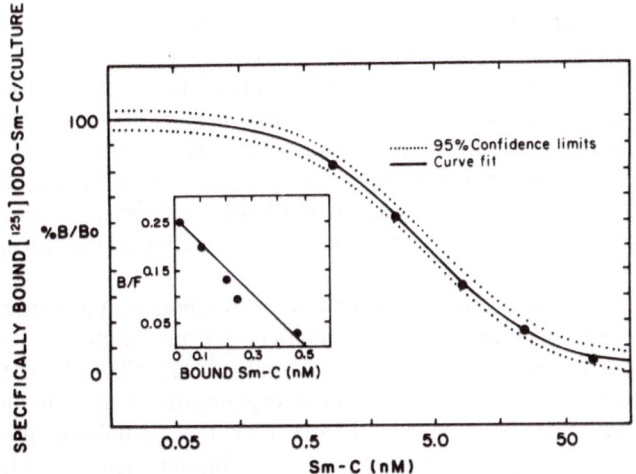

Fig. 5. IGF-I binding to whole granulosa cells: Scatchard analysis.

similar increments being observed for luteotropic, β_2-adrenergic, but not lactogenic granulosa cell agonists (6). Related in vivo studies using immature, hypophysectomized, DES-treated rats revealed that the ability of FSH to upregulated granulosa cell IGF-I binding: (a) is not strictly an in vivo phenomenon and that it can be fully reproduced in vivo; (b) is due to enhancement of IGF-I binding capacity rather than affinity; (c) may be subject to diametrically opposed modulation by somatogenic and GnRH-like granulosa cell agonists (up- and downregulation, respectively); and, (d) is best maintained by gonadotropins but not

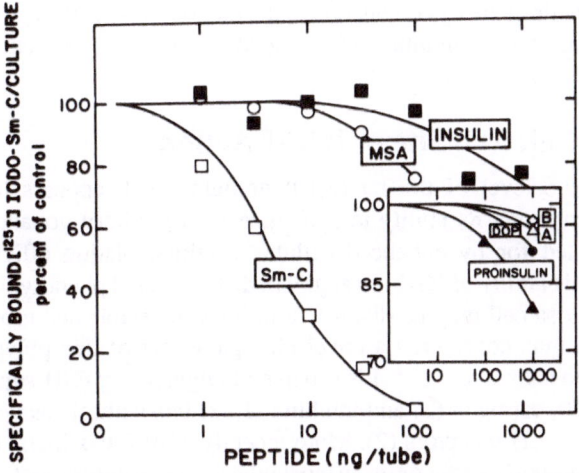

Fig. 6. IGF-I binding to whole ovarian granulosa cells: competition analysis.

prolactin (8). Inasmuch as gonadotropin dependence constitutes a unique attribute of the ovarian granulosa cell, our findings further suggest that the granulosa cell IGF-I receptor may have thoroughly adapted to its unique environment, providing the first example of a cell type for which the complement of IGF-I receptors may be cAMP dependent. Given the pivotal role of FSH in the induction of granulosa cell receptors for luteotropic and lactogenic ligands, this finding strongly suggests that the acquisition of IGF-I responsiveness may be part and parcel of granulosa cell ontogeny. Accordingly, gonadotropins may condition the cell to respond optimally to IGF-I, thereby conferring selective advantage upon follicles so endowed.

Both IGF-I and IGF-II synergize with FSH in the promotion of granulosa cell differentiation (9). However, the identity of the IGF receptor type(s) mediating the cytodifferentiative action of the IGFs remains uncertain. Whereas the role of the rat Type I IGF receptor cannot be evaluated at this time due to the lack of specific reagents, the recent availability of a unique antiserum to the rat Type II receptor (R-II-PAB1) has made studies of this receptor type possible for the first time. That R-II-PAB1 antiserum immunoneutralizes the Type II IGF receptor at the level of the rat granulosa cell was validated by its ability to inhibit $[^{125}I]$ IGF-II but not $[^{125}I]$ IGF-I binding or cross-linking to granulosa cell preparations. Moreover, R-II-PAB1 proved capable of immunoprecipitating $[^{125}I]$ IGF-II cross-linked to rat granulosa cell membranes. To assess the functional roles of the Type II IGF receptor in IGF-I and IGF-II hormonal action, FSH (20 ng/ml)-primed granulosa cells were cultured for 72 h in the absence or presence of IGF-I or IGF-II (both at 50 ng/ml), with or without increasing (receptor-active) concentrations of R-II-PAB1 (0.1-100 μg/ml). Control incubations were carried out with an ammonium-sulphate precipitate of nonimmune rabbit serum dialyzed against phosphate-buffered saline. Significantly, both IGF-I and IGF-II enhanced the FSH-stimulated accumulation of progesterone. However, R-II-PAB1 was without effect on the cytodifferentiative action of either IGF-I or IGF-II, suggesting that IGF-I and IGF-II hormonal action may be exerted largely, if not exclusively, by the Type I IGF receptor. As such, these findings are in keeping with the notion that inasmuch as cytodifferentiation (i.e., progesterone biosynthetic capacity) is concerned, the rat granulosa cell Type II receptor does not appear to participate in transmembrane IGF signalling and that its functional role, if any, remains to be determined.

The Granulosa Cell as a Site of IGF-I Action

IGF-I action at the level of the rat (2,10) granulosa cell appears largely, but not exclusively, contingent upon its ability to synergize with pituitary gonadotropins. These effects are unaccounted for by enhanced cellular viability, plating efficiency or DNA synthesis (2). Thus, this ability of IGF-I to augment differentiated phenotypic expression of the developing granulosa cell may be distinct from its well established growth-promoting property (2) and was thus considered a novel biologic effect of this polypeptide. In this connection, it has been shown that IGF-I is capable of augmenting FSH-supported (but not basal) progesterone (2), estrogen (2) and inhibin (11,12) biosynthesis as well as the FSH-mediated acquisition of LH receptors (2). More recently, IGF-I was found to augment the basal as well as FSH-supported proteoglycan biosynthesis (2). In this respect, IGF-I appeared to exert its classic "sulfation factor" activity at the level of the granulosa cell, the very chondrotropic effect which led to its discovery. Fractionation of the major extracellular proteoglycan species revealed FSH to favor the exclusive production of dermatan sulfate, whereas IGF-I supported the simultaneous biosynthesis of both heparan and dermatan sulfate. These findings suggest that IGF-I may effect marked quantitative as well as qualitative alterations in proteoglycan economy. Given the possible role of proteoglycans in follicular antrum formation and follicular atresia, these findings raised the possibility that IGF-I of granulosa cell origin may partake into the growth as well as demise of the developing ovarian follicle.

Specifically, IGF-I proved capable of amplifying the FSH transduction sequence at multiple cellular site(s) both proximal (13) and distal (13) to cAMP generation. Although without effect on cAMP breakdown (13), IGF-I appeared to exert a complex in the face of *unaltered* FSH receptor content (13). However, additional studies will be required to distinguish between direct effect(s) of this peptide on the stimulatory ($G_s=N_s$) or inhibitory ($G_i=N_i$) regulatory membrane proteins, the catalytic (C) cyclase protein, or combinations thereof. In addition, IGF-I was observed to exert a potent stimulatory effect on cAMP action as reflected in cAMP-supported progesterone biosynthesis (13). However, additional studies will be required to determine which of the post-cAMP events may be involved. The above notwithstanding, there is reason to believe that the ability of IGF-I to enhance FSH hormonal action may not be limited to perturbation of intracellular signalling but may also involve enhanced intercellular communication, e.g., granulosa cell clumping and intercellular gap junction formation (14).

Recent studies have clearly established that granulosa cells are a site of growth hormone reception and action. However, the cellular mechanism(s) underlying this phenomenon remain uncertain. On the one hand, it is possible that growth hormone may activate a series of receptor-mediated events independent of IGF-I generation. Alternatively, the transduction of the growth hormone signal might require the intermediary generation of IGF-I which in turn could act as the ultimate mediator of growth hormone action. Given that IGF-I, like growth hormone, is capable of augmenting FSH hormonal action, it is tempting to speculate that the growth hormone-FSH synergy may be due, if only in part, to the ability of growth hormone to enhance IGF-I generation, and hence FSH action. To test this possibility, FSH-supported (20 ng/ml) granulosa cells (8 x 10^5 viable cells/dish) from immature, DES-primed rats were cultured for 72 h in the absence or presence of ovine growth hormone (200 ng/ml), with or without 1:1000 dilution of sml.2 (a monoclonal antibody to IGF-I). Significantly, the utility of the sml.2 monoclone in the detection (and neutralization) or biologically active and endogenously produced IGF-I has previously been demonstrated. Accordingly, an sml.2-induced attenuation of abolition (i.e., immunoneutralization) of growth hormone action may be construed as evidence supporting the intermediacy of endogenously produced and released IGF-I, whereas the lack of sml.2 effect would render such possibility unlikely. As shown (Fig. 7), concurrent treatment with growth hormone (GH) resulted in a 2.6-fold increase in the FSH-stimulated accumulation of progesterone. However, provision of the sml.2 monoclone produced a significant ($P<0.05$) inhibition (60%) of the growth hormone effect. As such, these findings suggest that growth hormone action at the level of the granulosa cell may involve, if only in part, the intermediacy of the locally generated IGF-I. In this respect, these findings are in keeping with an extended somatomedin hypothesis wherein locally (rather than distantly) generated IGF-I may be acting as a mediator of growth hormone action. However, to the extent that sml.2 is incapable of complete neutralization of the growth hormone effect, our findings are also consistent with the possibility that growth hormone may act, at least in part, through IGF-I independent mechanism(s). Above and beyond these considerations, these findings may account, if only in part, for the putative puberty-promoting effect of growth hormone in that local generation of IGF-I may well potentiate gonadotropic hormonal action.

The Granulosa Cell as a Generator of a Functional IGF-I Binding Protein

Preliminary studies now suggest the existence of gonadotropin- and cAMP-dependent IGF-I binding activity in media conditioned by luteinizing human granulosa cell monolayers. Unaccounted for by possible follicular fluid or serum contamination, the granulosa cell-derived IGF-I binding protein (BP) appears immunologically related to a comparable human amniotic fluid protein previously purified to homogeneity (5). Although only partially purified at this time, preliminary studies suggest the existence of a comparable protein in human follicular fluid as well. Significantly, once secreted, IGF-I-BP is thought to adhere to the cell surface (by, as yet, uncertain nonreceptor mechanisms) thereupon amplifying IGF-I binding and hormonal action (16-18). Significantly, IGF-I-BP may well be identical to the so-called placental protein 12 (PP 12), the N-terminal amino acid sequence of which proved identical (19). Localized immunohistochemically to luteinized human granulosa cells (20), iPP12 is found in abundance in human follicular fluid (20). This exciting development introduces a new and potentially important regulatory element concerned with the amplification of IGF-I and, hence, gonadotropin hormonal action. Using a polyclonal antibody raised

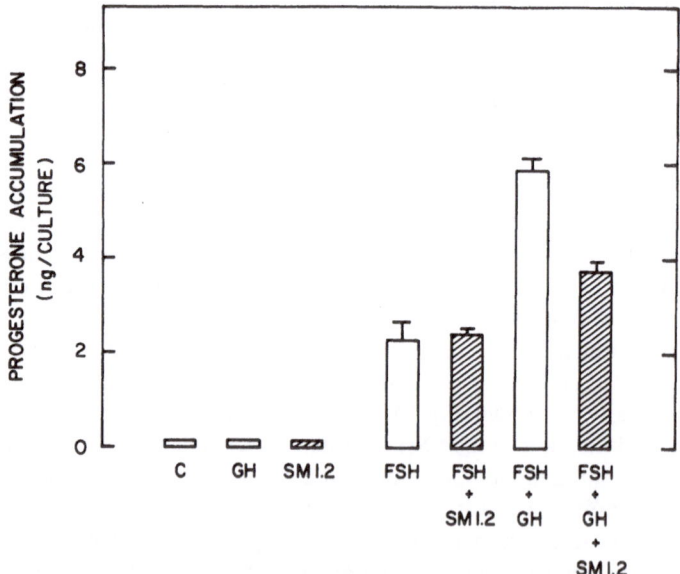

Fig. 7. Role of locally generated IGF-I in growth hormone action.

against highly purified IGF-I-BP from human amniotic fluid, we were able to detect substantial immunoreactivity (up to 70 ng/ml) in follicular fluid samples obtained from women undergoing ovum retrieval for in vitro fertilization and embryo transfer. To determine the cellular source of this immunoreactivity, identically derived, serum-weaned luteinizing human granulosa cell monolayers (0.75×10^5 cells/dish) were cultured for 24 h. Conditioned media exhibited significant activity in both radioimmune (Fig. 8) and binding (not shown) assays for IGF-I-BP, displaying dose-dependent displacement parallel to a highly purified human amniotic fluid standard. Significantly, both assay methods yielded comparable quantitative data thereby highlighting the utility of the RIA and its ability to reflect IGF-I binding activity.

To study the potential hormonal dependence of iIGF-I-BP, serum-weaned luteinizing human granulosa cell monolayers were cultured for 24 h in the absence or presence of hCG (500 mIU/ml). Significantly, basal iIGF-I-BP release (2.9 ± 0.6 ng/10 µg cellular protein) was increased 1.8-fold to 5.2 ± 0.6 ng/10 µg cellular protein. Similarly, treatment with 8-bromo-cAMP (1.5 mM) for 6 h resulted in substantial enhancement (2.8-fold increase) of iIGF-I-BP release. These findings suggest that granulosa cell IGF-I-BP release may be gonadotropin dependent and that cAMP may play an intermediary role in this regard. It is thus tempting to speculate the gonadotropins may not only enhance granulosa cell IGF-I production and reception, but that they may also concurrently modulate IGF-I hormonal action by means of its locally generated binding protein.

Summary

We have observed that the theca-interstitial cell, like the granulosa cell, may be a site of IGF-I reception and action and that physiological concentrations of IGF-I may also participate in the regulation of ovarian androgen biosynthesis (21). As such, these observations

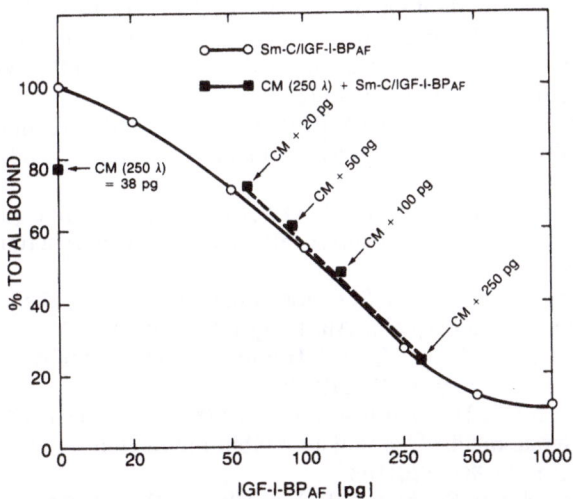

Fig. 8. CM = conditioned media. IGF-I-BP$_{AF}$ = human amniotic fluid IGF-I binding protein standard.

are in keeping with the view that IGF-I of granulosa cell origin may not only play an *autocrine* role but may also serve as one of several signals through which the granulosa cell may communicate in a *paracrine* fashion with the adjacent theca-interstitial cell compartment. In doing so, the granulosa cell may exert some control over its own destiny by enhancing ovarian androgen provision to suit its aromatizing capabilities and the estrogen requirements of the developing follicle as a whole. This line of reasoning introduces a level of complexity not previously envisioned implicating IGF-I in the orchestration of the coupling of androgen to estrogen biosynthesis, thereby promoting coordinated follicular development.

Acknowledgments

Supported in part by NIH Research Grant HD-19998 (EYA) and USPHS Research Career Development Award 1-K04-HD-00697 from the NICHHD, NIH.

References

1. Hammond JM. Peptide regulators in the ovarian follicle. Aust J Biol Sci 1981; 34:491.
2. Adashi EY, Resnick CE, D'Ercole AJ, Svoboda ME, Van Wyk JJ. Insulin-like growth factors as intraovarian regulators of granulosa cell growth and function. Endocr Rev 1985; 6:400.
3. Murphy LJ, Bell GI, Friesen HG. Tissue distribution of insulin-like growth factor I and II messenger ribonucleic acid in the adult rat. Endocrinology 1987; 120:1279.
4. Davoren JB, Hsueh AJW. Growth hormone increases ovarian levels of immunoreactive somatomedin-C/insulin-like growth factor I in vivo. Endocrinology 1986; 118:888.
5. Hernandez ER, Hoyt E, Van Wyk JJ, Adashi EY. The somatomedin-C/insulin-like growth factor I (Sm-C/IGF-I) gene is expressed in the rat ovary. [Abstract]. Abstract 821, 69th Annual Meeting of the Endocrine Society, Indianapolis, IN, 1987.
6. Adashi EY, Resnick CE, Hernandez ER, Svoboda ME, Van Wyk JJ. Characterization and regulation of a specific cell membrane receptor for somatomedin-C/insulin-like growth factor I in cultured rat granulosa cells. Endocrinology 1988; 122:194-201.
7. Adashi EY, Resnick CE, Svoboda ME, Van Wyk JJ. Follicle-stimulating hormone enhances somatomedin-C binding to cultured rat granulosa cells: evidence for cAMP dependence. J Biol Chem 1986; 261:3923.
8. Adashi EY, Resnick CE, Svoboda ME, Van Wyk JJ. In vivo regulation of granulosa cell somatomedin-C/insulin-like growth factor I receptors. Endocrinology 1988; 122:383-1390.
9. Davoren JB, Kasson BG, Li CH, Hsueh AJW. Specific insulin-like growth factor (IGF) I- and II-binding sites on rat granulosa cells: relations to IGF action. Endocrinology 1986; 119:2155.
10. Davoren JB, Hsueh AJW, Li CH. Somatomedin C augments FSH-induced differentiation of cultured rat granulosa cells. Am J Physiol 1985; 249:E26.
11. Bicsak TA, Tucker EM, Cappel S, et al. Hormonal regulation of granulosa cell inhibin biosynthesis. Endocrinology 1986; 119:2711.
12. Zhiwen Z, Carson RS, Herington AC, Lee VWK, Burger HG. Follicle-stimulating hormone and somatomedin-C stimulate inhibin production by rat granulosa cells in vitro. Endocrinology 1987; 120:1633.
13. Adashi EY, Resnick CE, Svoboda ME, Van Wyk JJ. Somatomedin-C as an amplifier of follicle-stimulating hormone action: enhanced accumulation of adenosine 3′,5′-monophosphate. Endocrinology 1986; 118:149.

14. May JV, Schomberg DW, Grodon S, Amsterdam A. Synergistic effect of insulin and follicle-stimulating hormone on biochemical and morphological differentiation of porcine granulosa cells. Bio Reprod 1985; 32(suppl):53.
15. Busby WH, Klapper DL, Clemmons DR. Purification of a 34,000 dalton somatomedin-C binding protein from human amniotic fluid. Isolation of two forms with different biologic actions. J Biol Chem 1987.
16. Clemmons DR, Elgin RG, Han VKM, Casella SJ, D'Ercole AJ, Van Wyk JJ. Cultured fibroblast monolayers secrete a protein that alters the cellular binding of somatomedin-C/insulin-like growth factor I. J Clin Invest 1986; 77:1548.
17. DeVroede MA, Tseng L-YH, Katsoyannis PG, Nissley SP, Rechler MM. Modulation of insulin-like growth factor I binding to human fibroblast monolayer cultured by insulin-like growth factor carrier proteins released to the incubation media. J Clin Invest 1986; 77:602.
18. Elgin RG, Busby WH, Clemmons DR. An insulin-like growth factor (IGF) binding protein enhances the biologic response to IGF-I. Proc Natl Acad Sci USA 1987; 84:3254.
19. Koistinen R, Kalkkinen N, Huhtala M-L, Seppala M, Bohn H, Butanen EM. Placental protein 12 is a decidual protein that binds somatomedin and has an identical N-terminal amino acid sequence with somatomedin-binding protein from human amniotic fluid. Endocrinology 1986; 118:1375.
20. Seppala M, Koskimies AI, Tenhunen A, et al. Pregnancy proteins in seminal plasma, seminal vesicles, preovulatory follicular fluid and ovary. Ann NY Acad Sci 212.
21. Hernandez ER, Resnick CE, Svoboda ME, Van Wyk JJ, Payne DW, Adashi EY. Somatomedin-C/insulin-like growth factor I as an enhancer of androgen biosynthesis by cultured rat ovarian cells. Endocrinology 1988; 122:1603-13.

8

Insulin-Like Growth Factors (IGFs) as Autocrine/Paracrine Regulators in the Porcine Ovarian Follicle

J. M. Hammond, J. S. Mondschein, and S. F. Canning

Department of Medicine, The Milton S. Hershey Medical Center
The Pennsylvania State University, P.O. Box 850, Hershey, PA 17033

Introduction

Our laboratory was attracted to ovarian growth factors as a potential mechanism for regulating the growth and development of the ovarian follicle. At the time we began our studies, it was known that peptide growth factors were potent mitogens for granulosa cells of the pig and other species (1,2). In addition, insulin at high concentrations was known to influence granulosa cell growth and differentiation (3), but effects of IGFs on ovarian cells had not been shown. In the process of investigating the hormonal regulation of the growth-related enzyme ornithine decarboxylase, we discovered that the IGF multiplication stimulating activity (MSA, rat IGF-II) was an extremely potent stimulator of this activity in porcine granulosa cells and was considerably more potent than insulin (4,5). As reviewed below, the characterization of IGF effects on granulosa cell replication and the interaction of the insulin-like factors with other growth factors on these responses has continued to be an interest of our laboratory. In addition, studies from our group (6), as well as more numerous data from others represented at this symposium, indicated that the IGFs had stimulatory effects on the cytodifferentiation of ovarian cells. Accordingly recent studies have focused on the relative importance of the growth-promoting and steroidogenic effects of insulin-like factors on porcine granulosa cells.

To understand the manner in which the ovarian effects of IGFs might be mediated, it became crucial to determine local concentrations of these factors in the ovary, and to evaluate the possibility of ovarian secretion. Initially, the IGFs or somatomedins were regarded principally as circulating factors of hepatic origin which mediated the effects of growth hormone (reviewed in 7). However, it has become clear that these factors are secreted in a number of additional tissues where they can serve as local regulators of organ-specific growth and differentiated function (reviewed in 7). To establish these mechanisms in the ovary, we examined the levels and regulation of the IGFs in porcine follicular fluid (8-10) and granulosa cell-conditioned medium (9,11-14). More recently, other laboratories have also demonstrated that the ovary contains high levels of IGFs and/or their mRNAs (15-18) and that granulosa cells have the capacity to synthesize and secrete such factors (17,19). IGF secretion and/or mRNA levels can be stimulated by gonadotropins (10,11,16,17,19), gonadal steroids (11,16), and other growth factors (13,14). As reviewed below, IGFs, in turn, can dramatically enhance the effects of such agents on granulosa cell replication or steroidogenesis. Thus, the stage is set for a mutually amplifying autocrine/paracrine system which could materially enhance the possibility of an ovarian follicle reaching maturity.

IGF Actions on Porcine Granulosa Cells

Since porcine granulosa cells actively replicate in vitro, the control of this process, and the interplay between replication and cytodifferentiation, can be studied in detail. We found that all three insulin-like peptides, IGF-I, IGF-II, and insulin, were potent mitogenic agents in cultured granulosa cells (6). Insulin or the IGFs were essential for sustained replication in serum-free medium (20), and they stimulated thymidine incorporation in a time- and dose-dependent fashion (6,21) (Figures 1 and 2). These studies indicated that IGF-I was

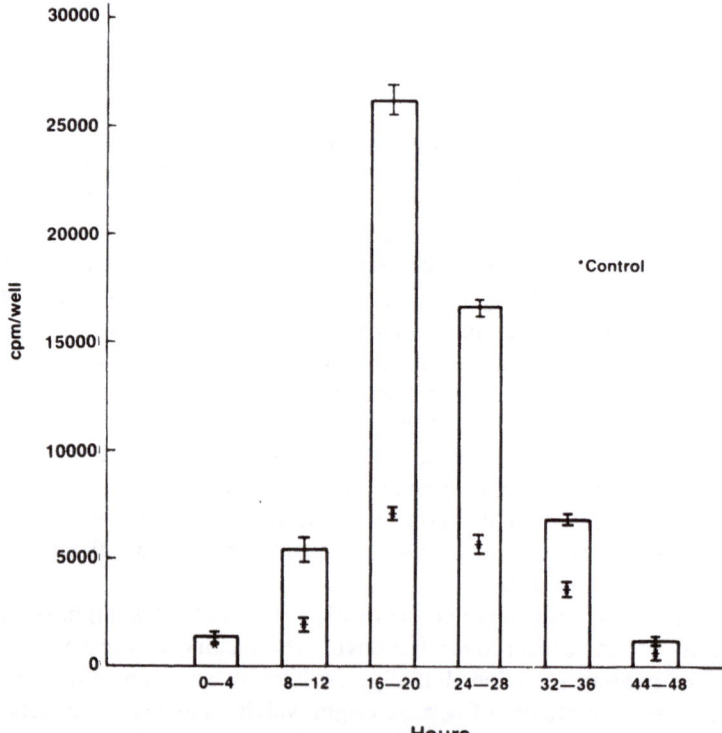

Hours

Fig. 1. Time course of IGF-dependent DNA synthesis in cultured porcine granulosa cells. Granulosa cells from immature follicles were cultured in 10% serum for 3 days, serum-deprived for 24 h, and then treated with MSA (rat IGF-II), 1 μg/ml. ^{3}H-methyl thymidine was added to replicate cultures at the times indicated, 4 h before the cultures were harvested. From Hammond and English (21).

slightly more potent in this mitogenic assay (see also Figure 4, below). The insulin-like peptides were not additive at maximally effective concentrations, suggesting a common, saturable mechanism of action (6,21). For this reason insulin has been used as a surrogate for the IGFs in some studies. The IGFs and insulin are particularly potent mitogenic agents when combined with other growth factors such as epidermal growth factor (EGF), transforming growth factor alpha (TGFα), fibroblast growth factors (FGFs) or platelet-derived growth factor (PDGF) (Fig. 3). In the aggregate these data suggest that PDGF, the insulin-like peptides, FGF, and the EGF-like peptides (EGF and TGFα) have mutually reinforcing discrete mechanisms of action. Since peptides resembling FGF as well as EGF and/or TGFα are present in the ovary (reviewed in 22), these stimulatory interactions could take place in vivo.

In contrast to the positive interaction among the several growth factors, there is a negative interation between the IGFs and hormonal stimulators of cytodifferentiation with regard to granulosa cell replication (21). For example, when cells are maintained with estradiol (E_2) and FSH for 3 days prior to treatment with insulin and the IGFs, the mitogenic response is reduced (Fig. 4). This antagonism does not result from a loss of the responsivity of these cells to the IGFs or to gonadotropins. In fact, IGFs and FSH interact in a synergistic

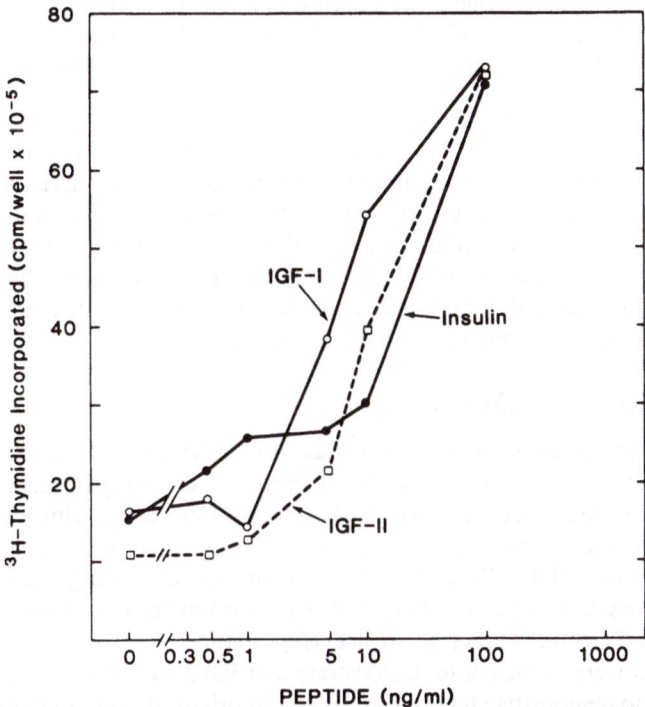

Fig. 2. Dose-dependent stimulation of DNA synthesis by insulin-like peptides. Cells were cultured as described in Figure 1 and treated with growth factors and ^{3}H-methyl thymidine for 36 h beginning 24 h after serum deprivation. From Baranao and Hammond (6).

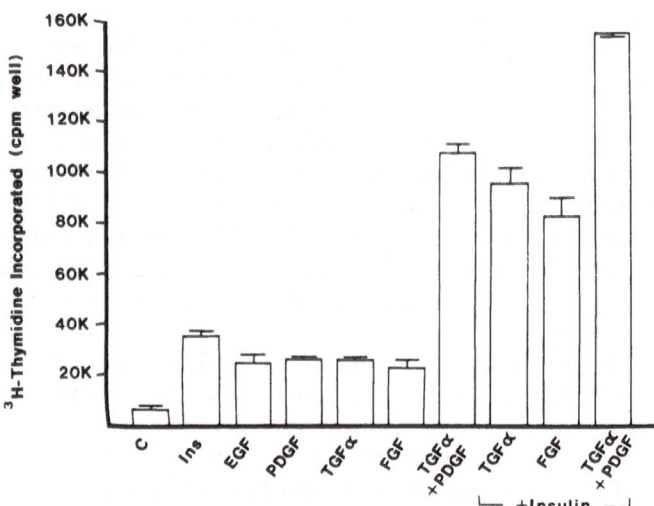

Fig. 3. Interactions of insulin and other growth factors on DNA synthesis by cultured granulosa cells. Cells were cultured as described in Figure 2 and treated with insulin (1 μg/ml), EGF (10 ng/ml), PDGF (5 ng/ml), TGFα (10 ng/ml, EGF equivalents), basic FGF (100 ng/ml), alone and in combination.

stimulatory fashion on differentiation of the steroidogenic pathway (Fig. 5) (6). The biochemical mechanisms involved in the steroidogenic actions of the IGFs will be presented in greater depth by other laboratories represented at this symposium. In summary, the IGFs can promote either replication or cytodifferentiation of granulosa cells. The dominant action of these peptides depends on their interaction with other paracrine or hormonal regulators such as ovarian growth factors and pituitary and gonadal hormones. Under conditions optimal for differentiation of granulosa cells such as gonadotropin treatment in vitro, the cytodifferentiative actions of the IGFs appear to predominate.

IGF Secretion in the Ovary

To establish the plausibility of the IGFs as intrafollicular regulators in vivo, it was necessary to demonstrate that these factors were present in the ovary in quantities sufficient to mediate the physiological effects discovered in culture. Our studies with ovarian follicular fluid indicate that such concentrations occurred in the porcine ovarian follicle (5,9). In addition to authentic IGFs, follicular fluid was found to contain high molecular weight IGF-binding proteins which could be recognized by direct binding of IGF tracer and resolved from IGFs by gel filtration in molar acetic acid (Fig. 6) (8,9).

These studies were sufficient to demonstrate that IGFs were present in the ovary but were inadequate to demonstrate their nature or cell of origin. A point of particular interest was the relative abundance of basic IGF-I and neutral IGF-II in the porcine ovary. Our initial studies with a relatively specific IGF-II receptor assay and a more specific IGF-I immunoassay (RIA) suggested that both peptides might be present in pig ovary (9). More recently,

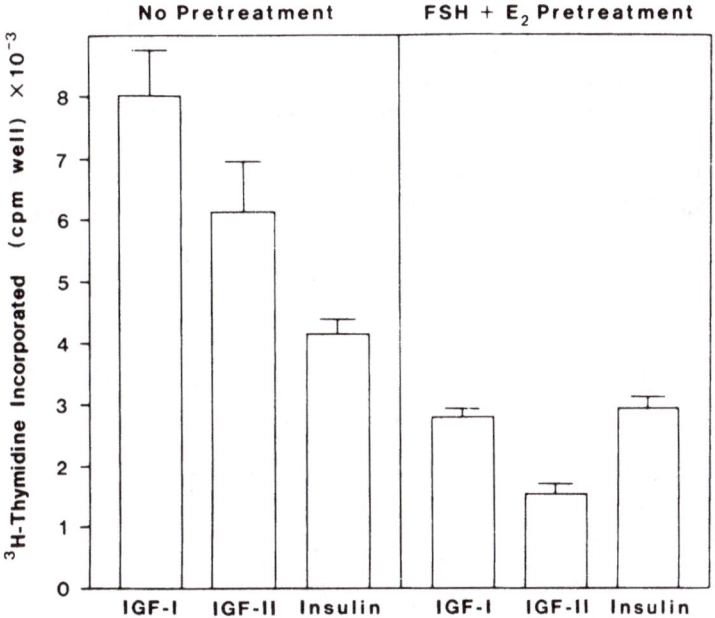

Fig. 4. Effect of granulosa cell differentiation on the mitogenic response to insulin-like peptides. Cultures were maintained and assessed as described in Figure 2 except that serum-free medium (20) was used during the initial culture period to optimize hormone responsiveness, and half the cultures were treated with FSH (200 ng/ml) and E_2 (1 µg/ml) for the duration of the experiment. The dose of insulin-like peptides during the 36 h labeling period was 100 ng/ml.

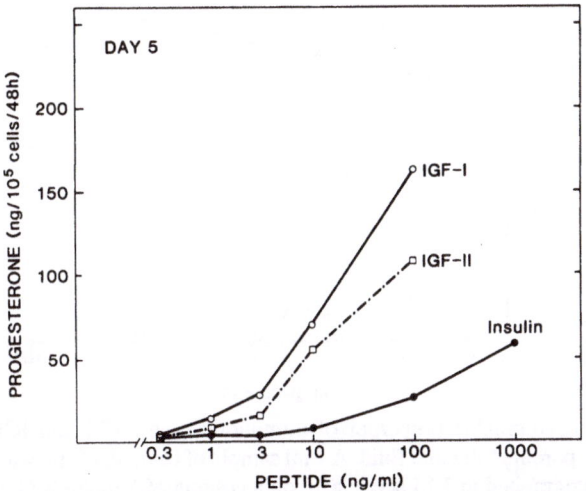

Fig. 5. Synergistic interaction of FSH and insulin-like peptides on steroidogenesis. Granulosa cells were cultured for 5 days in serum-free medium containing FSH, 200 ng/ml, and the doses of insulin-like peptides indicated. In the absence of FSH, the steroidogenic response to the IGFs was not demonstrable (data not shown). From Baranao and Hammond (6).

hybridization analysis and/or RIA performed in other laboratories have suggested that IGF-I is the dominant IGF in rat ovary (16,23), whereas IGF-II predominates in the human (17-19).

In our most recent studies, we have used a variety of techniques to reexamine these issues in the porcine ovary. The binding protein in follicular fluid cross reacted in radioreceptor assays (RRA) as well as radioimmunoassays (RIA) for IGFs, presumably by binding radioligand in competition with antibodies or receptors (Fig. 6, ref. 9), and resulted in erroneously high estimates for ovarian IGF levels. In our hands, this has proved to be a

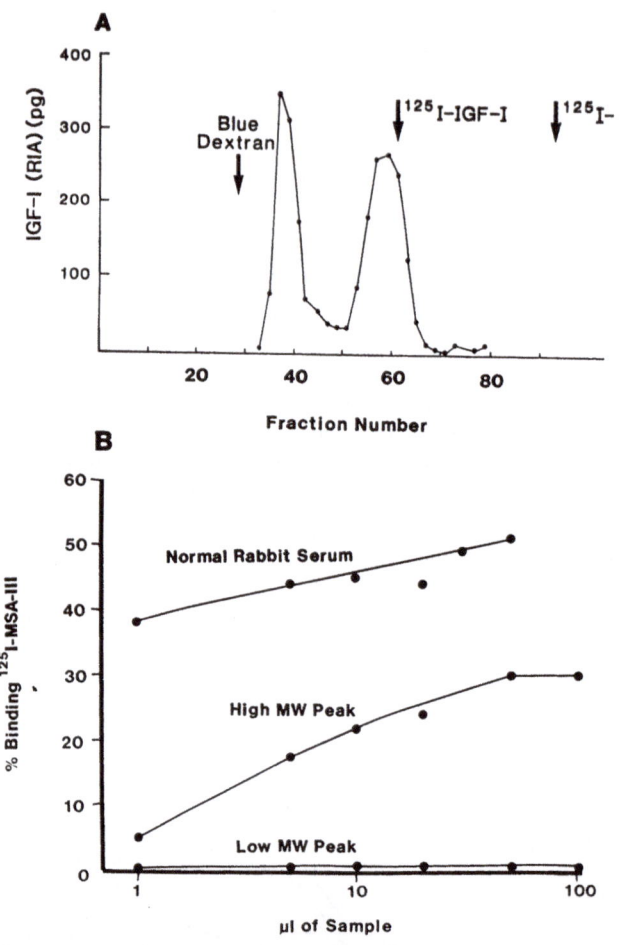

Fig. 6. Chromatographic properties of immunoreactive IGF-I and IGF-binding protein(s) in porcine follicular fluid. A 1 ml sample of follicular fluid was acidified and chromatographed in 1 M acetic acid on a column of Sephadex G-75 (43 x 3 cm). The fractions indicated were assayed for IGF-I immunoreactivity (A). For analysis of direct binding of ^{125}I-MSA-III (B), fractions contained in the high and low molecular weight peaks were pooled, lyophilized and resuspended in 2.0 ml assay buffer. From Hammond et al. (9).

particularly severe problem for IGF-II assays. Using selective IGF-I and II RIAs, coupled with gel filtration and chromatofocusing to separate IGF-I, II and binding protein activity, we have found that both IGF-I and II are present in abundance in porcine follicular fluid (24) (Fig. 7).

To establish the ovarian origin of at least part of the IGFs in follicular fluid, we have employed cultures of porcine granulosa cells maintained in highly supplemented serum-free medium (20). In these circumstances, the secretion of IGF-I can be demonstrated for more than 10 days in culture (9,11). To date, secretion of IGF-II has not been comparably demonstrated when binding protein has been rigorously eliminated. Thus, culture studies in the pig provide little support for IGF-II secretion by granulosa cells. On the other hand, IGF-II mRNA as well as mRNA for IGF-I is easily detected in porcine ovarian extracts (Hammond et al., unpublished). Finally, immunohistochemical studies (Lin CT, et al., manuscript in preparation) with a monoclonal antibody (which recognizes both IGF-I and IGF-II [25]) have shown that IGF immunoreactivity is present in theca and luteal cells in addition to granulosa cells, raising the possibility of additional secretory sites for IGF-I and/or IGF-II. Collectively, these observations have led to the working hypothesis that IGF-I and II are both synthesized in the porcine ovary. Further studies will be required to conclusively demonstrate their cells of origin and respective physiological roles. As shown above, IGF-I appears to be the more potent ovarian stimulator in several assays, but IGF-II

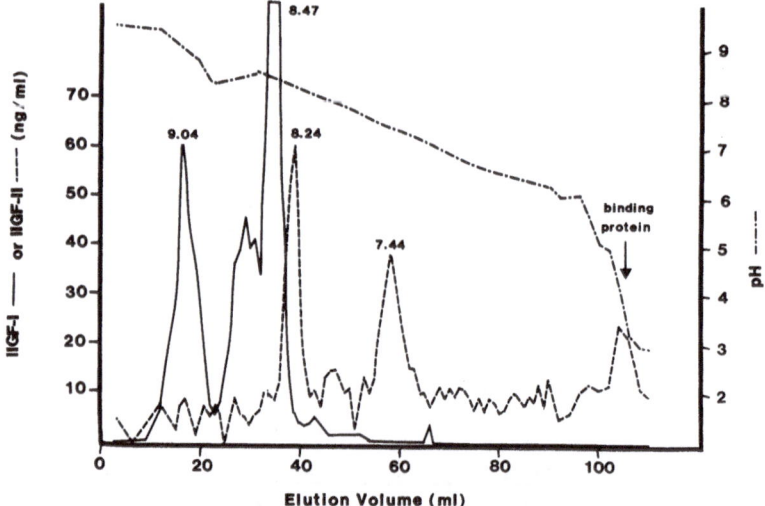

Fig. 7. Resolution of IGF-I and IGF-II in follicular fluid. The low molecular weight (IGF-containing) fractions from gel filtration (see Figure 6) were lyophilized and chromatographed on a chromatofocusing column to resolve the IGFs based on their isoelectric point (31). The eluted fractions were analyzed by RIA for IGF-I using a previously published assay (9) and for IGF-II with antibodies from the Amano Corp. and chemically synthesized IGF-II (19) as radioligand and standards. The apparent PI of the dominant IGF-I and IGF-II peaks and the elution position of residual-binding protein activity are indicated.

is also active in the porcine ovary. In the light of recent structural comparisons of the IGF-I and IGF-II receptors (26,27), the cellular processes entrained to IGF-II receptors (if any) may be quite different from those controlled by IGF-I binding sites.

Using immunoassays specific for IGF-I and a variety of techniques to eliminate or minimize the influence of IGF-binding proteins, we have studied physiological regulation of ovarian IGF-I levels and/or secretion in vivo and in vitro. Initial studies suggested that the levels of immunoreactive IGF-I in follicular fluid correlated with follicle size (9). More recently, we showed that treatment of immature pigs with gonadotropins caused a coordinated increase in follicular size, intrafollicular steroids, and follicular IGF-I (Fig. 8) (10). Similarly, treatment of pigs with growth hormone increases ovarian IGF-I levels (28).

The regulation of IGF-I secretion has been examined in greater detail in cultured porcine granulosa cells. In culture, the secretion of IGF-I was shown to be regulated by a number of hormones and growth factors. Perhaps the most physiologically interesting are the gonadotropins and the gonadal steroid, E_2 (Figures 9 and 10) (11). Of these classic ovarian regulators, FSH was found to be the most effective. CAMP derivatives were also found to be potent stimuli of IGF-I secretion (11). In addition to these established regulators of ovarian function, growth hormone (GH) (12) and a number of growth factors (13,14) were found to modulate IGF-I secretion in vitro. The GH stimulation was roughly equivalent to that of FSH and estradiol combined (Fig. 11). Among the growth factors, EGF was found to be the most

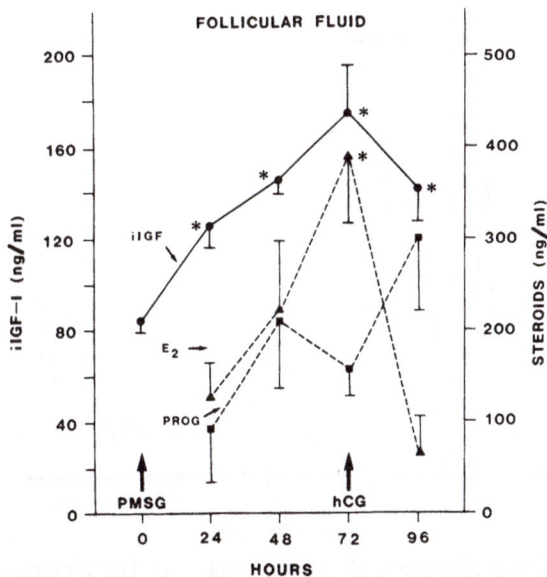

Fig. 8. Gonadotropin-induced changes in steroids and immunoreactive insulin-like growth factor-I (iIGF-I) in follicular fluid. Animals were treated with pregnant mare's serum gonadotropin (PMSG) at Time 0 and human chorionic gonadotropin (hCG) at 72 h. Follicular fluid was harvested at the times indicated and assayed for E_2, progesterone (prog), and iIGF-I. Values depicted represent mean and SEM for 5 animals at each time point. *Different from first time point, P<0.01. From Hammond et al. (10).

potent stimulator of IGF-I secretion while TGFβ inhibited IGF-I secretion (Fig. 12) (13). More recent studies (14) have shown a modest stimulatory effect of TGFβ at very low concentrations as well as the dramatic inhibitory action at higher levels. In the aggregate, these studies indicate that IGF-I is produced by granulosa cells and that its secretion is regulated by a number of factors which are currently felt to impinge on follicular growth and development. Taken together with the facilitatory effects of these hormones and growth factors on IGF action described above, these data suggest a complex intrafollicular network of growth factors and hormones which could influence ovarian cell function through several mechanisms.

Linkage between IGF Secretion and Follicular Cell Function

The evidence presented above concerning the concomitant action and secretion of IGFs in the ovary suggests, but does not prove, an important local modulatory role for the IGFs in follicular growth and development. Our data with gonadotropin-treated pigs (10) (see Figure 8, above) are consistent with a local effect of ovarian IGFs as amplifiers of gonadotropin-dependent steroidogenesis in vivo. In contrast, when we increased intrafollicular and systemic IGF levels by the administration of porcine growth hormone (28), we were unable to demonstrate an increase in intraovarian steroids or of granulosa cell differentiation when cells from GH-treated pigs were cultured. In fact, a significant inhibitory effect of GH on several reproductive parameters was encountered (28). These data suggest that a

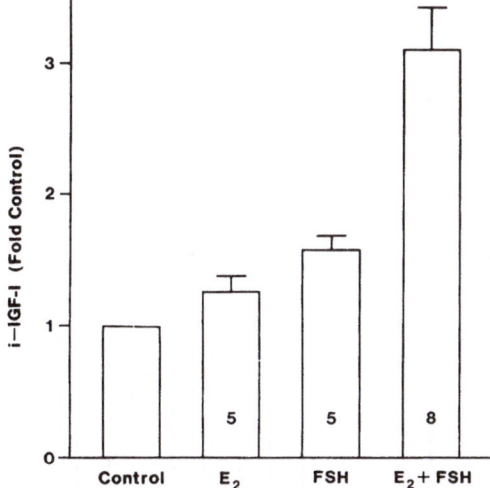

Fig. 9. Effects of E_2 and FSH on immunoreactive iIGF-I secretion by cultured granulosa cells. Cells were maintained in serum-free medium for 7 days and treated with E_2 (1 µg/ml) and/or FSH (200 ng/ml) from day 3 through 7. iIGF-I in medium conditioned from days 5-7 was determined by RIA after C-18 chromatography to minimize interference by binding protein. The values depicted are the average of N experiments (see numbers in bars) normalized by cell counts and as fold control. Each value depicted is different from the others (P<.05). Redrawn from Hsu and Hammond (11).

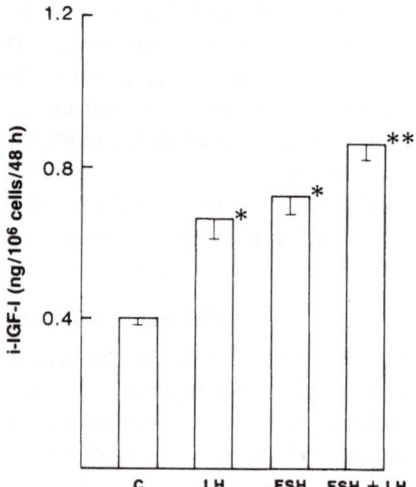

Fig. 10. Effects of FSH and LH on secretion of iIGF-I by cultured granulosa cells. Experimental conditions were the same as depicted in Figure 8 except for hormone treatments comprising FSH (200 ng/ml) and/or LH (200 ng/l). *P<.05; **P<.01 vs. control. From Hsu and Hammond (11).

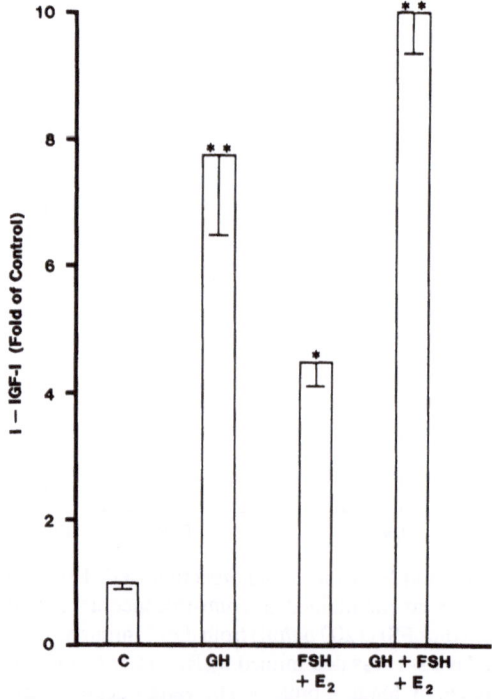

Fig. 11. Comparative effects of growth hormone (GH) and FSH/E$_2$ on iIGF-I secretion. Granulosa cells were cultured as described in Figure 8 except that some cultures received GH (300 ng/ml). *P<.05 and **P<.01 vs. control. From Hsu and Hammond (12).

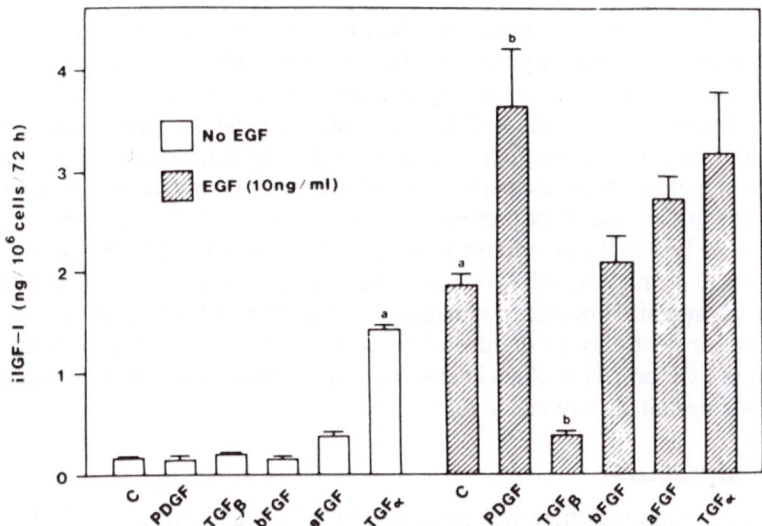

Fig. 12. Effects of growth factors on secretion of iIGF-I by cultured granulosa cells. Cells were cultured for 3 days in serum-free medium from which exogenous growth factors were eliminated except for those shown: PDGF, TGFβ, and EGF (10 ng/ml); basic (b) and acidic (a) FGF (100 ng/ml); and TGFα (10 ng/ml, EGF equivalents). (a) Different from no EGF control, (b) different from EGF control, $P<.05$. From Mondschein and Hammond (13).

rise in intrafollicular IGFs, in and of itself, is insufficient to promote enhanced follicular growth or steroidogenesis. Apparently support by pituitary gonadotropins and/or other follicular factors was lacking in the GH-treated animals.

Recently (Mondschein et al., this workshop), we have attempted more direct assessment of the role of IGF in these processes than afforded by these correlative studies. These experiments have relied on the neutralizing properties of the monoclonal antibody to IGF-I used for immunohistochemistry as described above. Two experimental paradigms have been employed. First, the antibody was added to cultured granulosa cells deprived of exogenous insulin or IGFs and treated with E_2 and/or FSH; under these circumstances, E_2 and FSH individually stimulate progesterone secretion and cause a synergistic stimulatory interaction which is dependent on insulin-like peptides (29). Second, the antibody was added to granulosa cell cultures treated with follicular fluid from highly differentiated (preovulatory) porcine follicles; such follicular fluid causes a brisk stimulation of progesterone secretion (30) and a substantial increase in granulosa cell replication (5,21). In both experimental paradigms the antibody inhibited progesterone secretion by greater than 50%. In contrast, it had modest effects on granulosa cell replication.

Summary and Conclusions

The accumulated data from numerous laboratories and multiple approaches has provided strong circumstantial evidence for IGFs as important modulators of ovarian function. Studies in the porcine ovarian follicle have been particularly informative and coherent since they have addressed IGF action, levels, and secretion and the manner in which these phenomena are interfaced with other pituitary and gonadal regulators. While the evidence in hand falls short of compelling proof of an obligatory role for these peptides as mediators of follicular growth and development, studies with neutralizing antibodies in vitro and ex vivo (with follicular fluid) attest to the importance of these peptides as hormonal amplifiers. Although the IGFs are important mitogenic peptides for immature or poorly differentiated granulosa cells, their principal actions in the presence of gonadotropins and in the preovulatory follicle would appear to be cytodifferentiative rather than growth promoting. Since it is in these follicles in which the highest IGF levels are to be found, these actions of the IGFs seem the most secure at present. However, it remains plausible, indeed likely, that earlier stages of follicular development may be dominated by interactions between the IGFs and growth factors such as EGF or TGFα. Such interactions would function to enhance granulosa cell replication and restrain differentiated function.

Acknowledgments

The research presented here was supported by NIH grants HD16952, HD10122, and K04 336 (to JMH). Several of the studies presented were conducted with collaborating laboratories including those of B. K. Tsang and B. R. Downey in Canada, D. R. Hagen, University Park, PA, and M. M. Rechler, NIH. In addition, we have received critical antibodies, growth factors, or probes from J. J. Van Wyk, Rene Humbel, M. M. Rechler, C. H. Li, K. Ramasharma, Genentech, and F. A. Simmen. Further, we acknowledge the contribution of previous postdoctoral fellows, J. D. Veldhuis, J. L. S. Baranao, and C. J. Hsu, to the evolution of this project. Finally, the technical expertise of Ms. Sheila Herman and the secretarial skills of Mrs. Sheila Barley and Mrs. Sandra Christian have been essential.

References

1. Gospodarowicz D, Ill CR, Birdwell CR. Effects of fibroblast and epidermal growth factors on ovarian cell proliferation in vitro. I. Characterization of the response of granulosa cells to FGF and EGF. Endocrinology 1977; 100:1108-20.
2. Gospodarowicz D, Bialecki H. Fibroblast and epidermal growth factors are mitogenic agents for cultured granulosa cells of rodent, porcine, and human origin. Endocrinology 1979; 104:757-64.
3. Channing CP, Tsai V, Sachs D. Role of insulin, thyroxine and cortisol in luteinization of porcine granulosa cells grown in chemically defined media. Biol Reprod 1976; 15:235-47.
4. Veldhuis JD, Hammond JM. Multiplication stimulating activity regulates ornithine decarboxylase in isolated porcine granulosa cells in vitro. Endocr Res Commun 1979; 6:299-309.
5. Hammond JM, Yoshida K, Veldhuis JD, Rechler MM, Knight AB. Intrafollicular role of somatomedins: comparison with effects of insulin. In: Greenwald GS, Terranova P, eds. Factors regulating ovarian function. New York: Raven Press, 1983:197-201.
6. Baranao JLS, Hammond JM. Comparative effects of insulin and insulin-like growth factors on DNA synthesis and differentiation of porcine granulosa cells. Biochem Biophys Res Commun 1984; 124:484-90.
7. Tissue growth factors. Daughaday WH, ed. Clinics in endocrinology and metabolism; vol 13, no 1. Philadelphia: WB Saunders Company, 1984.

8. Hammond JM, Veldhuis JD, Seale TW, Rechler MM. Intraovarian regulation of granulosa-cell replication. In: Channing CP, Segal, eds. Intraovarian control mechanisms. New York: Plenum Publishing Company, 1982:341-56.

9. Hammond JM, Baranao JLS, Skaleris D, Knight AB, Romanus JA, Rechler MM. Production of insulin-like growth factors by ovarian granulosa cells. Endocrinology 1985; 117:2553-5.

10. Hammond JM, Hsu C-J, Klindt J, Tsang BK, Downey BR. Gonadotropins increase concentrations of immunoreactive insulin-like growth factor-I in porcine follicular fluid in vivo. Biol Reprod 1988; 38:304-8.

11. Hsu C-J, Hammond JM. Gonadotropins and estradiol stimulate immunoreactive insulin-like growth factor-I production by porcine granulosa cells in vitro. Endocrinology 1987; 120:198-207.

12. Hsu C-J, Hammond JM. Concomitant effects of growth hormone on secretion of insulin-like growth factor-I and progesterone by cultured porcine granulosa cells. Endocrinology 1987; 121:1343-8.

13. Mondschein JS, Hammond JM. Growth factors regulate immunoreactive insulin-like growth factor-I production by cultured porcine granulosa cells. Endocrinology 1988, 123:463-8.

14. Mondschein JS, Canning SF, Hammond JM. Effects of transforming growth factor beta on the production of immunoreactive insulin-like growth factor-I and progesterone and on ^{3}H-thymidine incorporation in porcine granulosa cell cultures. Endocrinology 1988 (in press).

15. Davoren JB, Hsueh AJW. Growth hormone increases ovarian levels of immunoreactive somatomedin C/insulin-like growth factor I in vivo. Endocrinology 1986; 118:888-90.

16. Hernandez ER, Hoyt E, Van Wyk JJ, Adashi EY. The somatomedin-C/insulin-like growth factor-I (Sm-C/IGF-I) gene is expressed in the rat ovary. Annual Meeting of the Endocrine Society, 1987.

17. Voutilainen R, Miller WL. Coordinate tropic hormone regulation of mRNAs for insulin-like growth factor II and the cholesterol side-chain-cleavage enzyme, P450scc, in human steroidogenic tissues. Proc Natl Acad Sci USA 1987; 84:1590-4.

18. Ramasharma K, Cabrera CM, Li CH. Identification of insulin-like growth factor-II in human seminal and follicular fluids. Biochem Biophys Res Commun 1986; 140:536-42.

19. Ramasharma K, Li CH. Human pituitary and placental hormones control human insulin-like growth factor II secretion in human granulosa cells. Proc Natl Acad Sci USA 1987; 84:2643-7.

20. Baranao JLS, Hammond JM. Serum-free medium enhances growth and differentiation of cultured pig granulosa cells. Endocrinology 1985; 116:51-8.

21. Hammond JM, English HF. Regulation of deoxyribonucleic acid synthesis in cultured porcine granulosa cells by growth factors and hormones. Endocrinology 1987; 120:1309-46.

22. Hammond JM, Hsu C-J, Mondschein JS, Canning SF. Paracrine and autocrine functions of growth factors in the ovarian follicle. J Anim Sci 1988; 66:21-31.

23. Murphy LJ, Bell GI, Friesen HG. Tissue distribution of insulin-like growth factor I and II messenger ribonucleic acid in the adult rat. Endocrinology 1987; 120:1279-82.

24. Mondschein JS, Canning SF, Hammond JM. Profiles of immunoreactive (i) insulin-like growth factors (IGFs) -I and -II in porcine follicular fluid (FF) and granulosa cell conditioned medium (GCCM) [Abstract]. Biol Reprod 1988; 38(suppl 1):191.

25. Han VKM, Hill DJ, Strain AJ, et al. Identification of somatomedin/insulin-like growth factor immunoreactive cells in the human fetus. Pediatr Res 1987; 22:245-9.

26. Morgan DO, Edman JC, Standring DN, et al. Insulin-like growth factor II receptor as a multifunctional binding protein. Nature 1987; 329:301-7.
27. MacDonald RG, Pfeffer SR, Coussens L, et al. A single receptor binds both insulin-like growth factor II and mannose-6-phosphate. Science 1988; 239:1134-7.
28. Bryan KA, Hammond JM, Canning S, et al. Reproductive and growth responses of gilts to exogenous porcine pituitary growth hormone. J Anim Sci 1988 (in press).
29. Baranao JLS, Hammond JM. Multihormone regulation of steroidogenesis in cultured porcine granulosa cells: studies in serum-free medium. Endocrinology 1985; 116:2143-51.
30. Ledwitz-Rigby F, Petito SH, Tyner JK, Rigby BW. Follicular fluid effects on progesterone secretion are not due to follicle-stimulating hormone or steroids. Biol Reprod 1985; 33:277-85.
31. Zumstein PP, Humbel RE. Purification of human insulin-like growth factors I and II. Methods Enzymol 1985; 109:782-8.

9

Regulatory Actions of the Insulin-Like Growth Factor, IGF-I (Somatomedin-C), on Sterol Metabolism by Ovarian Cells

Johannes D. Veldhuis

Box 202, Department of Internal Medicine, University of Virginia
School of Medicine, Charlottesville, VA 22908

Introduction

Steroidogenic cells require large quantities of sterol substrate for utilization in the biosynthesis and secretion of relevant steroid hormones (1,2). Although the regulation of cholesterol's economy in ovarian (granulosa and luteal) cells has been characterized extensively for gonadotropic hormones (particularly LH and HCG), fewer studies are available that delineate the nature of trophic growth factor control of sterol delivery to, and utilization by, the steroidogenic apparatus. To examine the mechanisms subserving the actions of differentiating growth factors, we have employed an in vitro serum-free culture system of swine granulosa cells that is highly responsive to the insulin-like growth factor, IGF-I (Somatomedin-C) (3,4).

General Methods

Using pure human IGF-I synthesized by recombinant DNA technology, we have probed the specific nature of growth factor action on the following four loci of sterol metabolism in serum-free cultures of porcine granulosa cells: (1) the binding, uptake, degradation, and utilization of lipoprotein-borne sterol (low-density lipoprotein, LDL, and high-density lipoprotein, HDL); (2) the turnover of intracellular cholesteryl ester stores (by the enzymes acyl coenzyme A cholesterol acyltransferase, ACAT, and cholesteryl ester hydrolase, CEH); (3) the de novo synthesis of cholesterol by the rate-limiting enzyme, HMG CoA reductase; and, (4) the effective delivery of sterol to and its utilization in the cholesterol side-chain cleavage apparatus, assessed by monitoring the conversion of radiolabeled sterol to chromatographically isolated progestins and by examining the ability of IGF-I to induce specific immunoprecipitable protein constituents of the cholesterol side-chain enzyme reaction system. Figure 1 schematically summarizes these four major regulatory loci in sterol metabolism. These questions were addressed using the classical experimental tools pioneered by Goldstein and Brown in studies of LDL metabolism in the human fibroblast (5).

Results and Discussion

The specificity of the stimulation of granulosa cell steroidogenesis by human IGF-I was examined by the use of a monoclonal antibody to the trophic hormone, which in dilutions of 1/1000-1/250 reduced IGF-I action by 63-95%. This is illustrated in Figure 2A for IGF-I stimulated progesterone production by porcine granulosa cells in serum-free monolayer cultures. Moreover, the relevance of IGF-I action to intrafollicular function was suggested by the ability of IGF-I antibody to significantly (60-75%) suppress the stimulation of progesterone accumulation by swine granulosa cells exposed to homologous follicular fluid: Figure 2B.

In addition, the stimulatory effects of human plasma with or without added estradiol can also be inhibited significantly by specific IGF-I antiserum: Figure 2C. Thus, an important plasma-derived trophic factor may be IGF-I. More importantly, since the ability of swine follicular fluid to enhance basal rates of progesterone accumulation is significantly antagonized by a monoclonal antibody to human IGF-I, we can infer that one significant trophic constituent of follicular fluid is IGF-I or IGF-I-like peptide(s). This inference has been further supported by IGF-I sequence-specific immunoassay of porcine follicular fluid, which contains concentrations of immunoreactive IGF-I commensurate with those attained in circulating plasma and similar to those which exert near-maximal stimulatory effects in vitro (6,7). Thus, overall, we can conclude that granulosa cells are targets for the trophic actions of IGF-I and that the follicular fluid milieu contains plasma and/or locally derived IGF-I peptide(s). The latter inference is suggested by the ability of cultured pig granulosa cells to accumulate immunoreactive and radioreceptor-active IGF-I material (8).

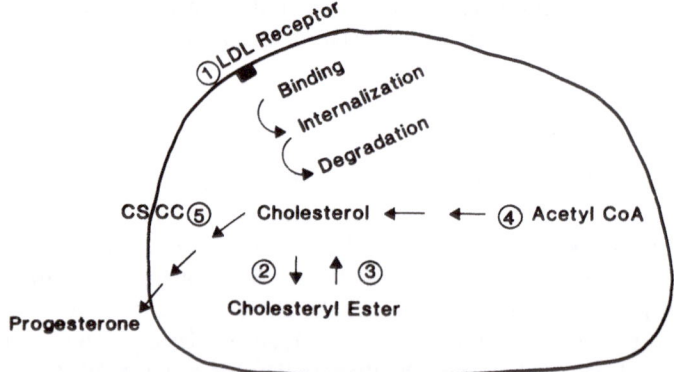

Fig. 1. Schematized depiction of key regulatory sites in cellular sterol metabolism and steroidogenesis that are stimulated by the trophic actions of IGF-I. IGF-I enhances: (1) lipoprotein (LDL and HDL) processing; (2,3) cholesteryl ester turnover (ACAT and CEH reactions); (4) *de novo* biosynthesis of cholesterol (HMG CoA reductase); and, (5) cholesterol side-chain cleavage activity (cytochrome P-450$_{scc}$ and adrenodoxin). Evidence has been presented that each of these steps is significantly regulated by IGF-I (see Discussion).

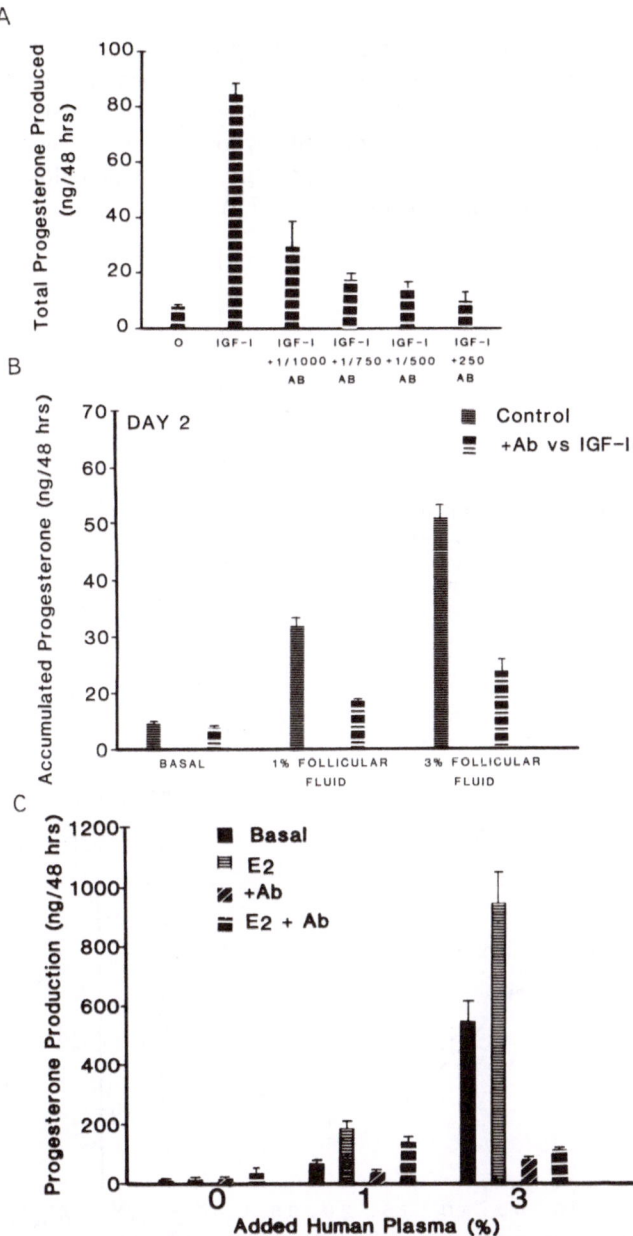

Fig. 2. *Panel A*. Dose-dependent inhibitory effect of monoclonal antiserum to human IGF-I peptide on IGF-I stimulated progesterone accumulation by swine granulosa cells cultured in serum-free medium (Veldhuis JD and Van Wyck J, unpublished). *Panel B*. Ability of a monoclonal antibody to IGF-I peptide to impede the stimulatory effect of swine follicular fluid on progesterone production by porcine granulosa cells (Veldhuis JD and Van Wyck J, unpublished). *Panel C*. Monoclonal antibody to IGF-I inhibits progesterone accumulation stimulated by human plasma alone or combined with estradiol (E_2, 1 mcg/ml) (Veldhuis JD and Van Wyck J, unpublished).

Initial studies demonstrated that intact swine granulosa cells exhibit high-affinity, low-capacity specific receptors for radiolabeled IGF-I, whose binding could be antagonized by unlabeled IGF-I (0.48-0.68 nM) and by monoclonal antibody directed to the human IGF-I receptor, but sparingly by insulin, MSA, or antibody to the insulin receptor (3); see Figure 3A through D. Similar observations have been confirmed in rat granulosa cells which also express specific and high-affinity IGF-I receptors (7,9).

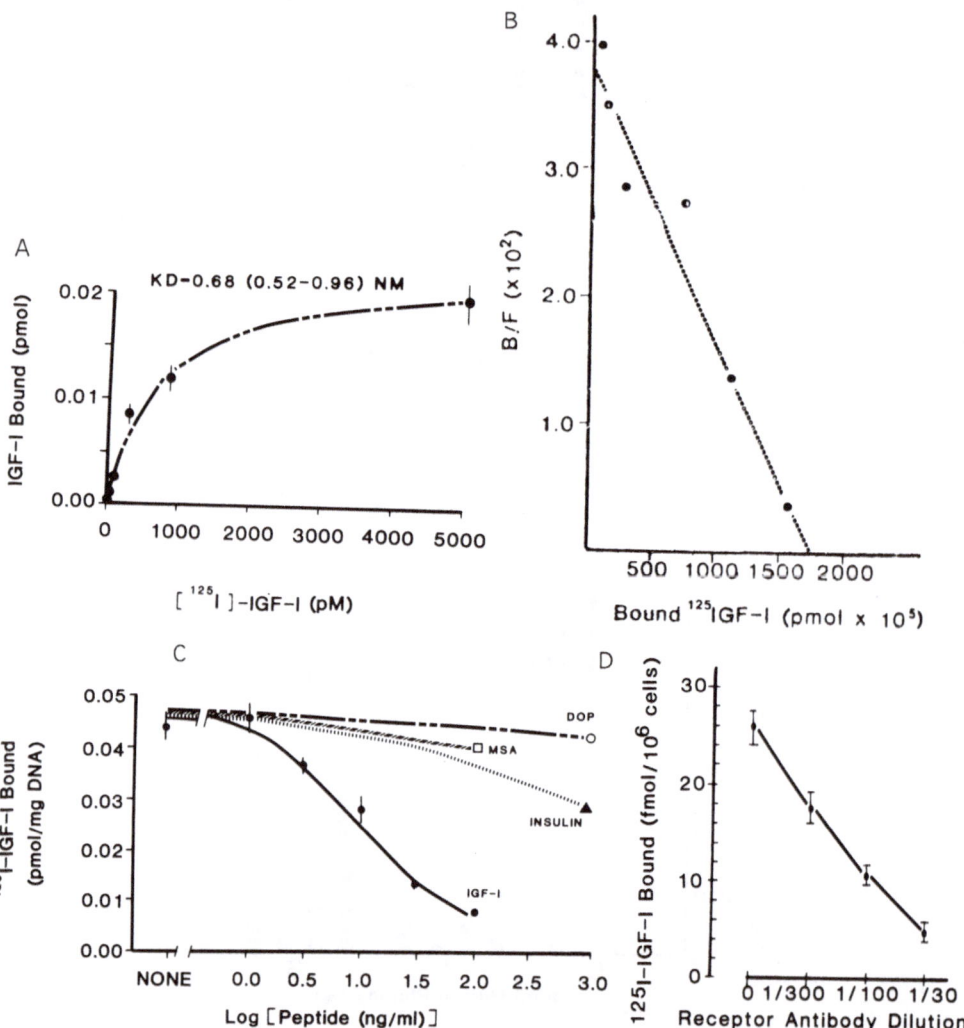

Fig. 3. *Panel A*. High-affinity binding of [^{125}I]-Somatomedin-C by swine granulosa cells. Serum-free cultures of pig granulosa cells were incubated with increasing concentrations of [^{125}I]-Somatomedin-C/IGF-I as indicated for 2 h at 4°C. The total binding curve was analyzed by nonlinear curve fitting and the nonspecific component (designated NS) and the specific high-affinity component resolved. The specific binding reaction exhibited an apparent K_d of 0.68 nM. *Panel B*. Data are plotted according to the method of Scatchard and analyzed by linear least-squares *(continued on next page)*

The trophic actions of IGF-I on steroidogenesis can be explained in part by effective stimulation of lipoprotein-borne sterol metabolism. Thus, IGF-I synergistically amplified the stimulatory effect of LDL on progesterone biosynthesis. This synergism was associated with a decrease in the mean half-maximally stimulatory concentration of LDL from 20 to 3.5 mcg/ml, which accompanied a three- to sixfold increase in the *number* of specific high-affinity LDL receptors assessed with [^{125}I]-iodo-LDL on swine granulosa cells, with no change in their apparent binding affinity (Kd = 4.4 mcg/ml) (10). IGF-I also augmented by three- and eighteenfold, respectively, the maximal rates of radioiodinated LDL internalization and degradation, without altering the half-maximally effective concentrations of LDL supporting these processes. These trophic effects of IGF-I on LDL processing are depicted in Figure 4.

The stimulatory effects of IGF-I on LDL metabolism were accompanied by a two- to 2.5-fold increase in the total mass of free and esterified cholesterol measured by microfluorometric assay of sonicated granulosa cells (10). Such measurements strongly support the inferences made using iodinated LDL particles, in which the fate of the iodotyrosines of apoprotein B, but not the sterol (cholesterol) moiety per se, is monitored. In addition, IGF-I stimulated the intracellular accumulation of free ^{3}H-cholesterol and ^{3}H-cholesteryl ester from exogenous ^{3}H-cholesteryl linoleate-labeled LDL, and amplified ^{3}H-progesterone secretion by granulosa cells exposed to the source of lipoprotein-borne sterol (10). The latter use of sterol-labeled reconstituted LDL particles allows one to assess more explicitly the processing of lipoprotein-borne cholesterol per se. Thus, we have been able to demonstrate that IGF-I enhances the metabolism of LDL-associated radio-iodinated apoprotein B ([^{125}I]-iodo-LDL binding, internalization and degradation), accelerates the uptake and utilization of LDL-carried cholesterol (^{3}H-cholesteryl-linoleate-labeled LDL), and increases the total cellular mass of sterol. Estradiol and FSH also alone stimulate LDL metabolism (11-13). Notably, the trophic actions of IGF-I on LDL metabolism were demonstrated at thirty- to one hundredfold lower concentrations of IGF-I than insulin. IGF-I also significantly increased the specific high-affinity binding of radiolabeled high-density lipoprotein (HDL), and enhanced the formation of ^{3}H progesterone (separated by two-dimensional thin-layer chromatography) from ^{3}H-cholesteryl-linoleate reconstituted human HDL (Veldhuis JD, Gwynne JT, unpublished). Thus, the metabolism of both LDL and HDL occurs in swine granulosa cells and is regulated in a stimulatory (trophic) fashion by IGF-I.

To assess the ability of IGF-I to stimulate cholesteryl ester formation in granulosa cells, cultures were exposed to ^{3}H-oleic acid complexed to albumin, and the rate of formation of ^{3}H-cholesteryl ester assessed. IGF-I significantly increased the maximal rate of cholesteryl

---

(Fig. 3 continued) curve fitting, which yielded an estimated K_d of 0.48 (± 0.11) nM and an X-axis intercept of 0.0181 (± 0.0021 pmol). *Panel C.* Typical equilibrium competition curve, in which increasing concentrations of unlabeled Somatomedin-C/IGF-I were incubated in the presence of 20 pM [^{125}I]-Somatomedin-C/IGF-I at 4°C for 4 h. In certain cultures, MSA, insulin, or desoctapeptide (DOP) insulin were added at the indicated concentrations. Data are means ± SEM (three to five cultures) from four experiments. *Panel D.* Ability of a monoclonal (mouse) antibody to the human IGF-I receptor provided by Dr. Steven Jacobson (Burroughs-Wellcome Co., Research Triangle Park, NC) to inhibit the binding of [^{125}I]-iodo-IGF-I to intact swine granulosa cells. The binding of IGF-I was assessed as described above. (Data in A-C are from reference 3 with permission.)

ester formation in intact cells. Moreover, IGF-I also enhanced the enzymatic activity of ACAT as assessed in microsomal preparations of granulosa cells previously treated with this growth factor. The effect of IGF-I was to increase the maximal velocity of the ACAT reaction from 3.83 ± 0.64 pmol/min/mg protein to 8.4 ± 0.85 pmol/min/ng protein (P<0.01), without changing the apparent Km of the reaction; *viz.* 37 (32-43) mcM control vs. 35 (31-41) mcM in IGF-I treated cultures (means with 67% confidence limits). When cells were prelabeled with oleic acid under equilibrium conditions, the hydrolysis of cholesteryl oleate was signif-

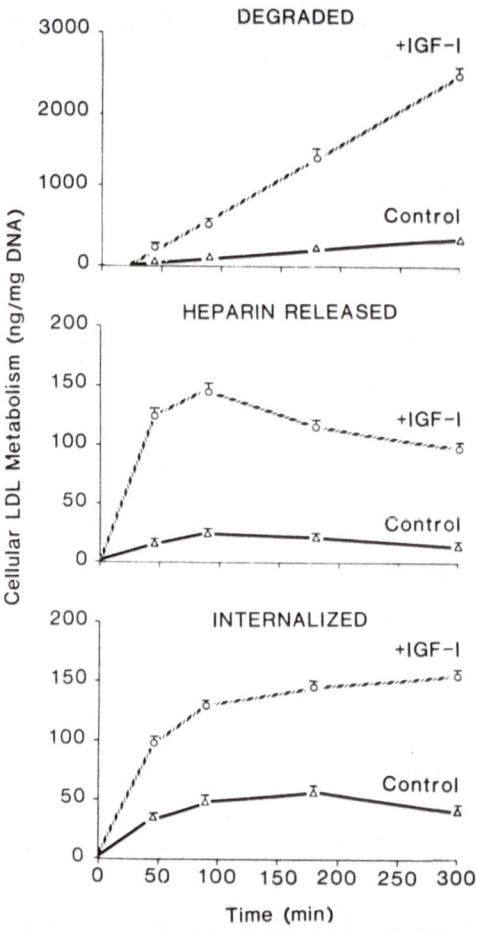

Fig. 4. Time-dependent influence of IGF-I on LDL metabolism by swine granulosa cells. Granulosa cells were maintained in the serum-free culture in the presence of [^{125}I]-iodohuman LDL (1.5 mcg/ml) for the indicated time intervals. Granulosa cells were permitted to metabolize LDL, and that portion degraded (upper panel), releasable by heparin (middle panel), or retained by the heparin-treated cells (internalized, bottom panel) was determined. Each data point represents the mean. SEM (n=3 replications) from two independent experiments. (Data are from reference 10 with permission.)

icantly accelerated by treatment with IGF-I. Accordingly, IGF-I accelerates both the formation and degradation of cholesteryl esters, i.e., it stimulates cholesteryl ester turnover and
exchange between free sterol and cholesteryl ester stores. The relevance of such actions has
been suggested in studies using an experimental inhibitor of the ACAT reaction; *viz.*
compound 58-035 (14). Chemical blockade of cellular ACAT activity resulted in enhanced
trophic actions of insulin on steroidogenesis: Figure 5. Such results can be interpreted to
indicate that the relative partitioning of cholesterol between its free and ester stores can
participate in controlling overall rates of steroid biosynthesis at least under conditions of
restricted substrate availability.

   To assess the impact of IGF-I on *de novo* cholesterol synthesis, granulosa cells were
cultured with [^{14}C]-acetate in the presence or absence of this growth factor (50 ng/ml). IGF-I
significantly increased the formation of [^{14}C] labeled free cholesterol with a corresponding
increase in the mass of free cholesterol assayed by microfluorimetry from 12 ± 0.83 to $15 \pm$
0.85 mcg/10^7 cells. The mass of cholesteryl ester stores was unchanged (7.0 ± 0.3 control,
vs. 6.7 ± 0.3 mcg/10^7 cells in IGF-I treated. The stimulatory effect of IGF-II on [^{14}C]-acetate
conversion to cholesterol was corroborated by the direct demonstration that IGF-I enhanced
^{3}H-cholesterol formation from ^{3}H water by 1.5-fold, and increased the activity of the
rate-limiting microsomal enzyme, HMG CoA reductase, by twofold (15). Thus, as determined by ^{3}H- water or ^{14}C-acetate incorporation and by mass measurements, i.e., by three

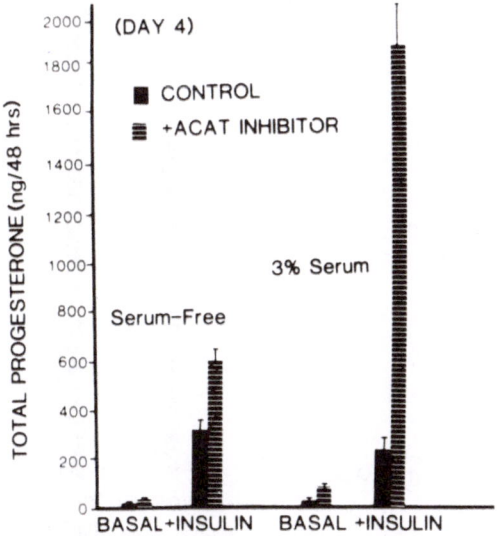

Fig. 5. Swine granulosa cells were cultured for 4 days in the presence or absence
of 3% serum under basal conditions or with a maximally stimulating concentration
of insulin. Cultures were treated with control solvent or Compound 58-035 (3
mcg/ml), an experimental inhibitor of the ACAT reaction. Data are the mean $\pm$
SEM (n=4 separate cultures), expressed as nanograms of total progesterone per 48
h/3×10^6 cells. The ability of the ACAT inhibitor to amplify insulin's stimulatory
action was confirmed in two other independent experiments. (Data are from
reference 14 with permission.)

independent techniques, IGF-I accelerates the *de novo* biosynthesis of cholesterol in ovarian cells. The relevance of this source of intracellular sterol is suggested by the ability of compactin (ML-236B), a competitive inhibitor of HMG COA reductase to suppress to a significant degree the stimulatory effect of IGF-I (alone or combined with FSH) on progesterone biosynthesis (16): Figure 6. This suppressive effect of compactin could be overcome to a significant degree by provision of mevalonolactone, the product of the HMG CoA reductase reaction.

The relevance of increased available sterol substrate to the cholesterol side-chain cleavage enzyme was assessed by monitoring the conversion of 25-hydroxycholesterol to progestin in control and IGF-I treated cells. IGF-I enhanced by two- to sixfold the synthesis of pregnenolone, progesterone, and 20-alpha-hydroxypregn-4-en-3-one (15,16). This evidence of increased functional cholesterol side-chain cleavage activity was accompanied by enhanced incorporation of [^{35}S]-methionine into specific immunoisolated components of the cholesterol side-chain cleavage apparatus, namely, cytochrome P-450$_{scc}$ and adrenodoxin (15,16). Moreover, in conjunction with FSH or estradiol, IGF-I served as a biological amplifier of hormonally stimulated steroidogenesis by synergistically activating side-chain cleavage activity and the cellular uptake delivery and utilization of lipoprotein-carried sterol substrate (16).

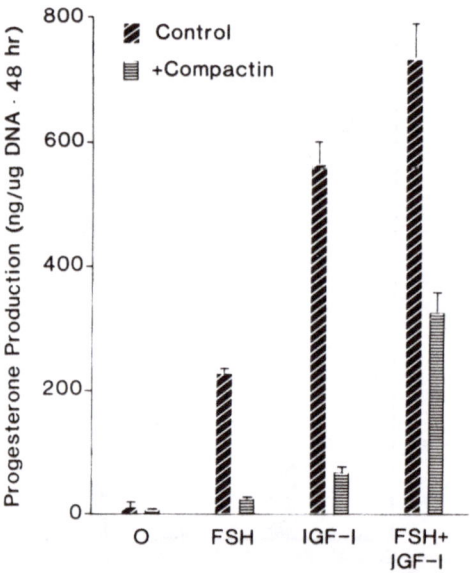

Fig. 6. Influence of compactin, a competitive inhibitor of *de novo* cholesterol synthesis, on the synergistic stimulation by FSH and IGF-I of progesterone production by swine granulosa cells. Ovarian cells were cultured in the absence or presence of compactin (25 mcM), with or without FSH (200 ng/ml), IGF-I (20 ng/ml), or both hormones. Data are expressed on a culture-by-culture basis as progesterone production per mcg of DNA per 48 h. Data are means ± S.E., n=4 determinations in each of two experiments. (Data are from reference 15 with permission.)

Conclusion

The trophic growth factor and differentiating hormone, IGF-I, can augment absolute rates of progestin biosynthesis by ovarian cells by activating four complementary mechanisms summarized schematically in Figure 1: (1) stimulating the binding, cellular uptake, and effective utilization of low- and high-density lipoprotein-borne sterol substrate (LDL and HDL); (2) increasing *de novo* synthesis of cholesterol; (3) facilitating cholesteryl ester turnover; and, (4) enhancing functional cholesterol side-chain cleavage activity and stimulating synthesis of cholesterol side-chain cleavage proteins. These specific potent trophic actions of IGF-I on each of the key regulatory loci in sterol homeostasis in granulosa cells indicate that IGF-I can play a critical role in the steroidogenic differentiation of granulosa-luteal cells during preovulatory follicular development. The future application of molecular biology probes should allow additional elucidation of the biochemical mechanisms subserving these trophic actions of IGF-I on sterol economy in the ovary.

Acknowledgments

This work was supported in part by RCDA KO4 HD 00634, and NIH Grants HD 16806 and HD 16393. The studies of cholesterol side-chain cleavage were performed in collaboration with Dr. R. J. Rodgers (Dallas, TX); those with reconstituted LDL with Dr. J. F. Strauss, III (Philadelphia, PA); and those with reconstituted HDL with Dr. J. T. Gwynne (Chapel Hill, NC).

References

1. Strauss JF III, Schuler LA, Rosenblum MF, Tanaka T. Cholesterol metabolism by ovarian tissue. Adv Lipid Res 1981; 18:99-127.
2. Gwynne JT, Strauss JF III. The role of lipoproteins in steroidogenesis and cholesterol metabolism in steroidogenic cells. Endocr Rev 1982; 3:299-321.
3. Veldhuis JD, Furlanetto RW. Trophic actions of human somatomedin C/insulin-like growth factor I (IGF-I) on ovarian cells: in vitro studies using swine granulosa cells. Endocrinology 1985; 116:1235-42.
4. Veldhuis JD, Demers LM. A role for somatomedin C as a differentiating hormone and amplifier of hormone action on ovarian cells: studies with synthetically pure somatomedin C and swine granulosa cells. Biochem Biophys Res Commun 1985; 130:234-40.
5. Goldstein JL, Brown MS. The low-density lipoprotein pathway and its relation to atherosclerosis. Annu Rev Biochem 1977; 46:897-930.
6. Veldhuis JD, Rodgers RJ, Furlanetto RW. Synergistic actions of estradiol and the insulin-like growth factor, somatomedin C, on swine ovarian (granulosa) cells. Endocrinology 1986; 119:530-8.
7. Barano JLS, Hammond JM. Comparative effects of insulin and insulin-like growth factors on DNA synthesis and differentiation of porcine granulosa cells. Biochem Biophys Res Commun 1985; 124:484-91.
8. Hammond JM, Baranao LS, Skleris D, Knight AB, Romanus JA, Rechler MM. Production of insulin-like growth factors by ovarian granulosa cells. Endocrinology 1985; 117:2553-7.

9. Hsueh AJW, Adashi EY, Jones PBC, Welsh TH Jr. Hormonal regulation of the differentiation of cultured ovarian granulosa cells. Endocr Rev 1984; 5:76.

10. Veldhuis JD, Nestler JE, Strauss JF III. The insulin-like growth factor, IGF-I (somatomedin c), modulates low-density lipoprotein metabolism by swine granulosa cells. Endocrinology 1987; 121:340-6.

11. Veldhuis JD, Gwynne JT. Properties of low-density lipoprotein binding by cultured swine granulosa cells. Endocrinology 1985; 117:1067-74.

12. Veldhuis JD, Gwynne JT. Estrogen regulates low-density lipoprotein metabolism by cultured swine granulosa cells. Endocrinology 1985; 117:1321-7.

13. Veldhuis JD. Follicle-stimulating hormone replaces low-density lipoprotein metabolism by swine granulosa cells. Endocrinology 1988 (in press).

14. Veldhuis JD, Strauss JF III, Silavin SL, Kolp LA. The role of cholesterol esterification in ovarian steroidogenesis: studies in cultured swine granulosa cells using a novel inhibitor of acyl coenzyme A: cholesterol acyltransferase. Endocrinology 1985; 116:25-30.

15. Veldhuis JD, Rodgers RJ. Mechanisms subserving the steroidogenic synergism between FSH and the insulin-like growth factor, IGF-I (somatomedin C): alterations in cellular sterol metabolism in swine granulosa cells. J Biol Chem 1987; 262:7658-64.

16. Veldhuis JD, Rodgers RJ, Dee A, Simpson ER. The insulin-like growth factor, somatomedin C, induces the synthesis of cholesterol side-chain cleavage cytochrome P-450 and adrenodoxin in ovarian cells. J Biol Chem 1986; 261:2499-502.

10

Growth Factor–Gonadotropin Interactions in Ovarian Cells

David W. Schomberg

Departments of Obstetrics and Gynecology and Cell Biology
Duke University Medical Center, Durham, NC 27710

Introduction

The literature now contains several publications demonstrating that classical reproductive hormones and growth factors interact to modulate ovarian cellular function (see reviews 1-3). Examples on a general level are: (1) regulation by reproductive hormones of growth factor production; (2) modulation of growth factor receptor expression/function by reproductive hormones; or conversely, (3) modulation of the production of reproductive hormones by growth factors; and, (4) growth factor involvement in regulating the expression/function of receptors for reproductive hormones. However, detailed biochemical knowledge in terms of the intracellular mechanisms by which these various effectors interact to regulate growth or differentiation is not yet available for any cell type. Also, at this level, there is no information to indicate whether growth factor-initiated mechanisms are the same in reproductive hormone-responsive vs. nonresponsive cells.

In this chapter, results from our laboratory will be discussed which address, to a limited extent, some of the more general aspects mentioned above. Interactions of follicle-stimulating hormone (FSH) with platelet-derived growth factor (PDGF) preparations, transforming growth factor-beta (TGF-β), and epidermal growth factor (EGF) will be highlighted. Other contributors to this symposium will address the role(s) of insulin-like growth factor-I (IGF-I) and fibroblast growth factor (FGF).

FSH-PDGF Interactions

We initially reported that PDGF potentiated FSH-mediated LH receptor induction in the rat granulosa cell culture system and postulated that PDGF may play a physiological role in the terminal differentiation of granulosa cells into luteal cells during the corpus hemorrhagicum stage following follicle rupture (4). We later observed that different and successively more highly purified preparations diverged widely in terms of mitogenic activity in Balb/c-3T3 cells and differentiating activity (LH receptor induction) in granulosa cells (5).

Further work in our laboratory shows that the active differentiation-inducing material from platelet extracts purified essentially according to Heldin et al. (6) is TGF-β rather than PDGF (7). Figure 1 shows that the active material from Bio-gel P-60 column eluates migrates as a Mr 25,000 species on SDS polyacrylamide gel electrophoresis under nonreducing conditions. The biological activity of this electro-eluted material was neutralized by anti-TGF-β IgG (7). These results indicate that the previously reported effects of highly purified PDGF upon granulosa cell LH/hCG receptor induction and cAMP production are not due to PDGF itself (8). PDGF prepared in our laboratory from the "PDGF only" region of Bio-gel P-60 eluates which were very potent in stimulating ^{3}H-thymidine incorporation in Balb/c-3T3 fibroblasts did not potentiate FSH-dependent LH receptor induction in rat granulosa cell cultures (2,7). Thus, granulosa cells obtained from the DES-treated immature rat are not responsive to very highly purified PDGF. Perhaps this result can be generalized to rat cells from other developmental stages and to cells from other species as well, but these aspects await further work. As an example, PDGF (obtained from commercial sources) participates with other growth factors in enhancing the mitotic activity of porcine granulosa cells maintained in platelet-poor, plasma-derived serum (9).

There is as yet no information to indicate that PDGF is present in follicular fluid or whether it is synthesized anywhere in the follicle. There is a precedent for production of PDGF by steroidogenic cells, however. Cytotrophoblastic cells produce PDGF in a temporally circumscribed manner, strongly suggesting the possibility of hormonal regulation in this tissue (10).

FSH-TGF-β Interactions

TGF-β is a 25 kilodalton (kD) homodimeric peptide produced by a wide variety of cell types including the ovarian thecal component (11). Structurally, TGF-β possesses a significant degree of amino acid sequence homology with inhibin, activin or follicle-stimulating hormone releasing protein (FRP), and Mullerian inhibiting substance (MIS), all of which are produced by the ovarian follicle (2). Depending upon conditions, granulosa cells may produce small or large quantities of TGF-β in culture (11; our unpublished observations). Freshly harvested granulosa cells at the stages of follicle development investigated did not express TGF-β mRNA although thecal preparations did (Skinner, this symposium). In a preliminary study, TGF-β mRNA was detected in extracts of whole rat ovaries (12). High concentrations of TGF-β-like material were found in human follicular fluid in another preliminary study (13). TGF-β may actually be secreted (at least in vitro) in a high molecular weight precursor form which is biologically inactive, requiring chemical or enzymatic action to achieve the mature, biologically active 25 kD form (14-15). In other cell culture systems, i.e., established cell lines, the regulation of TGF-β production has been shown to vary. In several cell lines, TGF-β itself has been shown to increase TGF-β mRNA expression and cellular secretion of the translated product (16). In malignant cell lines (MCF-7 breast and PC-3 prostatic adenocarcinoma), however, TGF-β, or TGF-β$_2$ production is increased by the antiestrogen tamoxifen. A mechanism(s) other than increased mRNA expression is involved, suggesting that the processing of inactive to active or mature TGF-β can be more important in some circumstances (17-19).

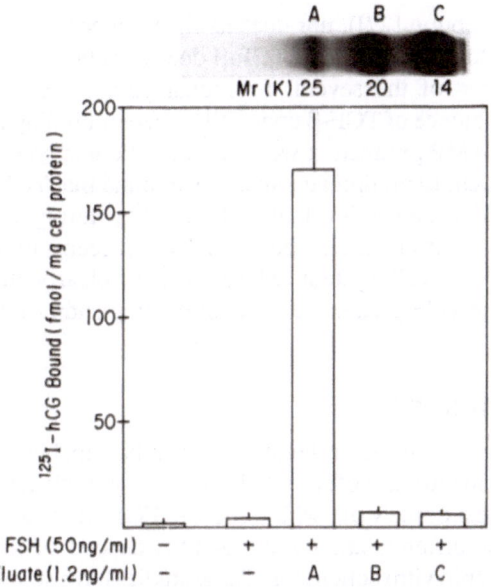

Fig. 1. SDS polyacrylamide gel electrophoresis of the active p-60 column chromatography region potentiating granulosa cell differentiation. Only the Mr 25,000 region contained activity. From (7) with permission.

TGF-β has been described as a bifunctional regulator since it elicits disparate effects upon several cell parameters in vitro depending upon the cell type investigated and/or the presence of other growth factor components in the culture milieu (20). Similarly, in combination with FSH, TGF-β stimulates ^{3}H-thymidine incorporation and cell number of rat granulosa cells during the first week of culture (21) although it inhibits these responses in EGF-stimulated bovine (11) and porcine granulosa cells (9). With respect to FSH-dependent LH receptor induction in rat granulosa cell cultures, the response to FSH plus TGF-β appears to be bifunctional, but can be more accurately described as a left-shift in the FSH dose-response curve with TGF-β potentiating both the stimulatory and the "downregulatory" responses (22). TGF-β alone does not have significant stimulating or inhibitory effects upon LH receptor induction, steroidogenesis, or cAMP production in this system (7,23). The steroidogenic response to TGF-β plus FSH in the rat granulosa cell system is more uniform; both progesterone and estrogen production are potentiated (23-25). The situation is quite complicated, however, for current work in our laboratory indicates that in the porcine granulosa cell system TGF-β attenuates the FSH-stimulated responses of LH receptor induction and progesterone secretion (unpublished observations).

How can these disparate responses be understood at the cellular level? At the present time this is a tremendously difficult question to answer, especially since the signal transduction mechanism(s) mediating TGF-β action are not known. Three different membrane species which bind to TGF-β with high-affinity have been demonstrated in fibroblasts (26). Yet by itself, TGF-β does not stimulate adenylyl cyclase activity or protein kinase C activity (with one reported exception [27]), nor does its ligand-receptor complex possess tyrosine kinase activity (28). On the other hand, TGF-β does significantly modulate FSH receptor responsiveness in terms of the several functional parameters mentioned above. Thus, investigation of the influence of TGF-β upon FSH receptor binding and function in terms of hormone-stimulated cAMP production would seem to be one potential pathway amenable to more detailed research. In preliminary studies we found that TGF-β plus FSH relative to FSH alone maintained a higher level of FSH binding during long-term culture of rat granulosa cells (29). In current studies, however, TGF-β seems to have the opposite effect in the porcine granulosa cell system. More work is clearly needed to delineate the mechanism(s) by which TGF-β alters the level of binding and/or function of this important receptor.

FSH-EGF Interactions

EGF was the first growth factor demonstrated to be capable of stimulating granulosa cell mitogenic activity in vitro and of stimulating ovarian growth in vivo (30,31). Since these initial observations, most of the work with respect to EGF and ovarian cellular function has involved endpoints of differentiation such as FSH-dependent steroidogenesis and LH receptor induction under in vitro conditions. These studies have supported the generalization that the processes of growth and differentiation are largely mutually exclusive, especially in cells which remain mitotically competent under culture conditions. Thus, the general effect of EGF has been to antagonize the effectiveness of FSH in vitro. In studies in vivo utilizing the sheep, systemically administered EGF also decreased circulating steroid concentrations and gonadotropin responsiveness (32,33).

Although the extent of EGF production by ovarian cells is not known, prepro EGF mRNA has been detected in the mouse ovary (34). Porcine follicular fluid contains EGF-like activity (35); the radioreceptor assay employed in these studies did not distinguish between EGF and transforming growth factor-alpha (TGF-α). The source of EGF/TGF-α activity in the ovarian follicle seems to be the theca interna compartment (36,37). Work is proceeding in various laboratories to isolate and sequence the active component (36,38). Based upon the biochemical evidence currently available, the consensus view of investigators in this field is that the active component will be TGF-α, or will more closely resemble TGF-α than EGF. In any event, since EGF and TGF-α interact with the same receptor, the biological response in terms of cell-cell paracrine interactions is likely to be the same although certain theoretical issues could be raised which might argue for differential responses.

Very little is known about the hormonal regulation of EGF or TGF-α production or of their receptor populations. Several studies have identified specific, high-affinity, low capacity EGF receptor-binding sites on granulosa cells (39-41). The regulation of these sites by FSH seems to be different in the pig and the rat (40-41). In porcine granulosa cells, Scatchard analysis demonstrated the presence of a single class of receptors for EGF. FSH treatment in vitro lowered slightly the binding capacity, but did not change receptor-binding affinity (41). This is shown in more detail in Figure 2, indicating that cAMP-generating effectors but not steroids, alone or in combination with FSH, were able to modulate EGF-binding capacity. Conversely, and in contrast to its general mode of action to decrease differentiated function, EGF is able to increase the FSH-binding capacity of porcine granulosa cells in vitro (42). Figure 3 demonstrates the increase in FSH receptor binding in insulin plus EGF-treated cultures over that of insulin-treated controls. Chronic FSH treatment at saturating levels markedly decreased both total monolayer [^{125}I]iodo-FSH binding and binding per unit protein in insulin controls and insulin plus EGF-treated cells. The demonstration of increased FSH binding by EGF treatment has potentially important physiological implications. EGF or TGF-α, acting locally at appropriate developmental stages, could increase follicle responsiveness to FSH, especially at early preantral stages where growth factor-gonadotropin interactions could facilitate follicle growth. Also, as pointed out previously (42), the actions of EGF or TGF-α on granulosa cell proliferation and FSH receptor expression are consistent with a role during early follicle development, perhaps during the gonadotropin-independent phase. Lastly, the decrease in FSH receptor binding affinity and inhibitory actions of EGF or TGF-α on FSH-stimulated processes could be viewed as positive effects if they prevent premature granulosa cell differentiation. These aspects could be true at any stage of follicle development.

Results similar to those shown above were obtained in separate experiments when the effects of 100 ng/ml FSH plus 10 μg/ml EGF upon ^{3}H-thymidine incorporation and cell numbers were measured (Fig. 4), in that saturating levels of FSH decreased both [^{125}I]iodo-EGF binding and mitotic responsiveness. Since this level of FSH maximizes differentiation in this system, it is of interest to know the effects of lower concentrations of FSH on EGF receptor binding and mitotic responsiveness to exogenous EGF. Preliminary results obtained indicate that FSH dose dependently decreased mitotic responsiveness but only decreased [^{125}I]iodo-EGF binding at the highest level. Thus, at this stage of development there appears to be no correlation between EGF receptor binding and EGF responsiveness in the context of FSH-directed mitotic activity. Results such as these may be relevant to growth inhibition/atresia of some follicles inappropriately synchronized with surge levels of FSH, and to the decreased rate of growth in antral vs. preantral follicles. A decreased rate of growth in antral follicles has been noted previously in rat and hamster follicles using ^{3}H-thymidine uptake methodology (43,44). Since FSH is necessary to maintain the development of early to late preantral follicles in the hypophysectomized animal, more work is needed to understand how FSH-dependent mechanisms stimulate cell division at these early stages of development.

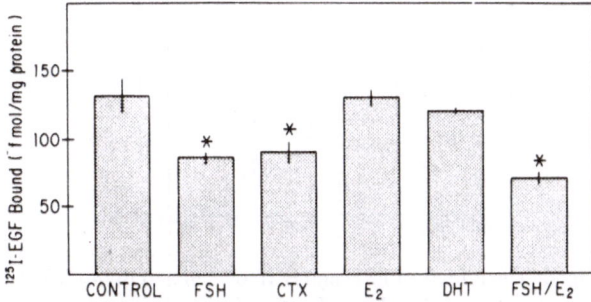

Fig. 2. The effects of reproductive hormones on the [^{125}I]iodo-EGF binding capacity of porcine granulosa cells from 1-3 mm follicles. From (41) with permission.

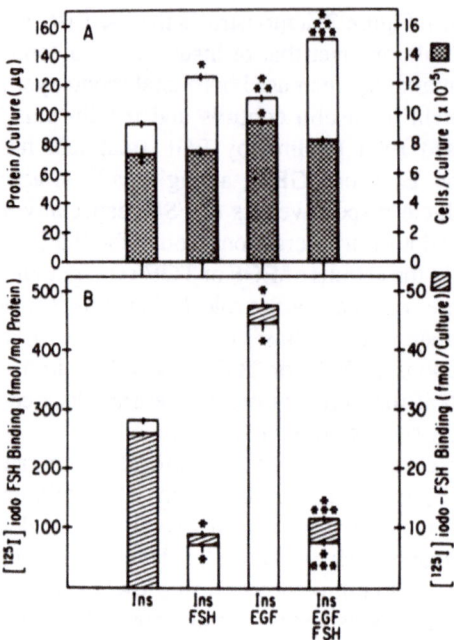

Fig. 3. The interactions between EGF and FSH on [^{125}I]iodo-FSH binding and monolayer cell and protein contents. From (42) with permission.

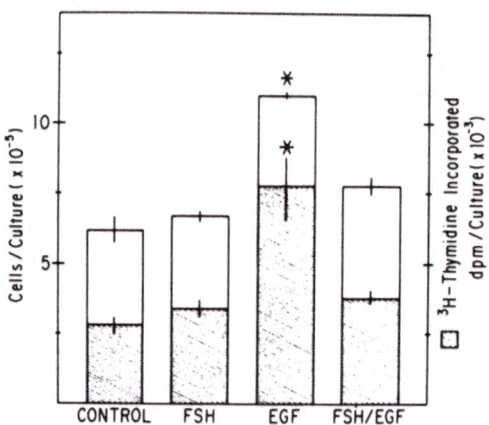

Fig. 4. The effects of FSH and EGF on tritiated thymidine incorporation and cell proliferation in porcine granulosa cell cultures. Cells were obtained from 1-3 mm follicles. From (41) with permission.

Conclusion

These results and those of others presented at this symposium continue to support the concept that growth factor-gonadotropin interactions are important in ovarian cellular function. Much more work is needed, however, to establish the precise nature of these interrelationships. Important issues such as the nature and extent of the regulation by reproductive hormones of growth factor production and the issue of paracrine regulation between putative growth factor-producing and growth factor-responsive cellular subpopulations remain to be addressed. And, as pointed out in the introduction, detailed biochemical knowledge in terms of the intracellular signalling mechanisms by which these various effectors interact is not yet available.

Acknowledgments

Supported in part by Grants HD 11827 and HD 21261 from the NICHD, NIH. I also want to acknowledge the expert secretarial assistance of Ms. Donna Camp.

References

1. Adashi EY, Resnick CE, D'Ercole AJ, Svoboda ME, Van Wyk JJ. Insulin-like growth factors as intraovarian regulators of granulosa cell growth and function. Endocr Rev 1985; 6:400.
2. Schomberg DW. Regulation of follicle development by gonadotropins and growth factors. In: Stouffer RL, ed. The Primate Ovary. New York: Plenum Press, 1987:25-33.
3. Schomberg DW. The role of growth factors in the regulation of ovarian growth and function. In: Parvinen M, Huhtaniemi I, Pelliniem LJ, eds. Rome: Ares-Serono Symposia, 1988:127-38.
4. Mondschein JS, Schomberg DW. Growth factors modulate gonadotropin receptor induction in granulosa cell cultures. Science 1981; 211:1179-80.
5. Mondschein JS, Schomberg DW. Effects of partially and more highly purified platelet-derived growth factor preparations on luteinizing hormone receptor induction in granulosa cell cultures. Biol Reprod 1984; 30:603-8.
6. Heldin CH, Westermark B, Wasteson A. Platelet-derived growth factor: purification and partial characterization. PNAS (USA) 1979; 76:3722-6.
7. Blair EI, Kim I-C, Estes JE, Keski-Oja J, Schomberg DW. Human PDGF preparations contain a separate activity which potentiates FSH-mediated induction of LH receptor in cultured rat granulosa cells: evidence for transforming growth factor beta. Endocrinology (in press).
8. Knecht M, Catt KJ. Modulation of cAMP-mediated differentiation in ovarian granulosa cells by epidermal growth factor and platelet-derived growth factor. J Biol Chem 1983; 258:2789-94.
9. May JV, Frost JP, Schomberg DW. Differential effects of epidermal growth factor, somatomedin-C/insulin-like growth factor I, and transforming growth factor-β on porcine granulosa cell deoxyribonucleic acid synthesis and cell proliferation. Endocrinology 1988; 123:168-79.
10. Goustin AS, Betsholz C, Pfeifer-Ohlsson S, et al. Coexpression of the sis and myc protooncogenes in developing human placenta suggests autocrine control of trophoblastic growth. Cell 1985; 41:301.

11. Skinner MK, Keski-Oja J, Osteen KG, Moses HL. Ovarian thecal cells produce transforming growth factor-beta which can regulate granulosa cell growth. Endocrinology 1987; 121:786-92.

12. Hernandez ER, Twardzik DR, Purchio A, Adashi EY. Gonadotropin-dependent ovarian transforming growth factor-beta gene expression. Biol Reprod 1987; 36(suppl 1):58.

13. Ruegseggar Veit C, Assoian RK. Identification of transforming growth factor-beta in human ovarian follicular fluid [Abstract]. Abstract No. 1225, Proc 70th Ann Meeting of The Endocrine Society, New Orleans, 1988.

14. Miyazono K, Hellman U, Wernstedt C, Heldin C-H. Latent high molecular weight complex of transforming growth factor B1. J Biol Chem 1988; 263:6407-15.

15. Wakefield LM, Smith DM, Flanders KC, Sporn MB. Latent transforming growth factor-β from human platelets. J Biol Chem 1988; 263:7646-54.

16. Van Obberghen-Schilling E, Roche N, Flanders KC, Sporn MB, Roberts AB. Transforming growth factor B1 positively regulates its own expression in normal and transformed cells. J Biol Chem 1988; 263:7741-6.

17. Knabbe C, Lippman ME, Wakefield LM, et al. Evidence that transforming growth factor-beta is a hormonally regulated negative growth factor in human breast cancer cells. Cell 1987; 48:417-28.

18. Ikeda T, Lioubin MN, Marquardt H. Human transforming growth factor type B2: production by a prostatic adenocarcinoma cell line, purification, and initial characterization. Biochemistry 1988; 26:2406-10.

19. Lawrence DA, Pircher R, Jullien P. Conversion of a high molecular weight latent β-TGF from chicken embryo fibroblasts into a low molecular weight active β-TGF under acidic conditions. Biochem Biophys Res Commun 1985; 133:1026-34.

20. Sporn MB, Roberts AB, Wakefield LM, Assoian RK. Transforming growth factor-β: biological function and chemical structure. Science 1986; 233:532-4.

21. Dorrington JA, Chuma V, Bendell JJ. Transforming growth factor β and follicle-stimulating hormone promote rat granulosa cell proliferation. Endocrinology 1988; 123:353-9.

22. Knecht M, Feng P, Catt KJ. Transforming growth factor-beta regulates the expression of luteinizing hormone receptors in ovarian granulosa cells. Biochem Biophys Res Commun 1986; 139:800-7.

23. Dodson WC, Schomberg DW. The effect of transforming growth factor-β on follicle-stimulating hormone-induced differentiation of cultured rat granulosa cells. Endocrinology 1987; 120:512-6.

24. Adashi EY, Resnick CE. Antagonistic interactions of transforming growth factors in the regulation of granulosa cell differentiation. Endocrinology 1986; 119:1879-81.

25. Knecht M, Feng P, Catt KJ. Bifunctional role of transforming growth factor-β during granulosa cell development. Endocrinology 1987; 120:1243-9.

26. Cheifetz S, Weatherbee JA, Tsang M L-S, et al. The transforming growth factor-β system, a complex pattern of cross-reactive ligands and receptors. Cell 1987; 48:409-15.

27. Markovac J, Goldstein GW. Transforming growth factor beta activates protein kinase C in microvessels isolated from immature rat brain. Biochem Biophys Res Commun 1988; 150:575-82.

28. Libby J, Martinez R, Weber MJ. Tyrosine phosphorylation in cells treated with transforming growth factor-β. J Cell Physiol 1986; 129:159-66.

29. Kim I-C, May JV, Schomberg DW. The potential mechanism by which human transforming growth factor-β (hTGF-β) modulates FSH-induced differentiation of

cultured rat granulosa cells (GC) [Abstract No. 237]. Biol Reprod 1987; 36(suppl 1):125.

30. Gospodarowicz D, Ill CR, Birdwell CR. Effects of fibroblast and epidermal growth factors on ovarian cell proliferation in vitro. I. Characterization of the response of granulosa cells to FGF and EGF. Endocrinology 1977; 100:1108-20.

31. Gospodarowicz D, Mescher AL, Birdwell CR. Control of cellular proliferation by the fibroblast and epidermal growth factors. In: Third decennial review conference: cell, tissue, and organ culture. National Cancer Institute Monograph 48. Bethesda: USPHS, NIH 1978:109-30.

32. Shaw G, Jorgenson GI, Tweendale R, Tennison M, Waters MJ. Effect of epidermal growth factor on reproductive function of ewes. J Endocrinol 1985; 107:429-36.

33. Radford HM, Panaretto BA, Avenell JA, Turnbull KE. Effect of mouse epidermal growth factor on plasma concentrations of FSH, LH, and progesterone and on oestrus, ovulation and ovulation rate in merino ewes. J Reprod Fertil 1987; 80:383-8.

34. Rall LB, Scott J, Bell GI. Mouse preproepidermal growth factor synthesis by the kidney and other tissues. Nature 1985; 313:228-30.

35. Hsu C-J, Holmes SD, Hammond JM. Ovarian epidermal growth factor-like activity. Concentrations in porcine follicular fluid during follicular development. Biochem Biophys Res Commun 1987; 147:242-7.

36. Skinner MK, Lobb D, Dorrington JH. Ovarian thecal/interstitial cells produce an epidermal growth factor-like substance. Endocrinology 1987; 121:1892-9.

37. Kudlow JE, Kobrin MS, Purchio AF, et al. Ovarian transforming growth factor-alpha gene expression: immunohistochemical localization to the theca-interstitial cells. Endocrinology 1987; 121:1577-9.

38. Lobb DK, Skinner MK, Dorrington JH. Rat thecal/interstitial cells produce a mitogenic activity that promotes the growth of granulosa cells. Mol Cell Endocrinol 1988; 55:209-17.

39. Jones PBC, Welsh TH Jr, Hsueh AJW. Regulation of ovarian progestin production by epidermal growth factor in cultured rat granulosa cells. J Biol Chem 1982; 257:11268-73.

40. Feng P, Knecht M, Catt KJ. Hormonal control of epidermal growth factor receptors by gonadotropins during granulosa cell differentiation. Endocrinology 1987; 120:1121-6.

41. Buck PA, Schomberg DW. [^{125}I]iodo-epidermal growth factor binding and mitotic responsiveness of porcine granulosa cells are modulated by differentiation and follicle-stimulating hormone. Endocrinology 1988; 122:28-33.

42. May JV, Buck PA, Schomberg DW. Epidermal growth factor enhances [^{125}I]iodo-follicle stimulating hormone binding by cultured porcine granulosa cells. Endocrinology 1987; 120:2413-20.

43. Roy SK, Greenwald GS. Quantitative analysis of in vitro incorporation of [^{3}H]thymidine into hamster follicles during the oestrous cycle. J Reprod Fert 1986; 77:143-52.

44. Hirshfield AN, Schmidt WA. Kinetic aspects of follicular development in the rat. In: Mahesh VB, Dhindsa DS, Anderson E, Kalia SP, eds. Regulation of ovarian and testicular function. New York: Plenum, 1987:211-36.

11

Transforming Growth Factor Production and Action in the Ovarian Follicle: Theca Cell–Granulosa Cell Interactions

Michael K. Skinner

Department of Pharmacology, Vanderbilt University
School of Medicine, Nashville, TN 37232

Introduction

Cell-cell interactions have an important role in the physiology of an individual cell and a whole organ. Interactions between cells result in the maintenance or alteration of several parameters, including growth, function and differentiation. It is unlikely that any individual interaction could maintain and regulate all cellular processes. Therefore, a number of different types of cell-cell interactions are required. The types of specific cellular interactions possible have previously been categorized into environmental, nutritional and regulatory cell-cell interactions (1). The current manuscript will review the interactions between different cell types in the ovarian follicle which regulate cell growth.

Cell proliferation within the ovarian follicle is required for both the maintenance of ovarian function and the endocrine status of the female. The progression of a primordial follicle to become an ovulatory follicle is a process that involves a rapid rate of somatic cell proliferation. The two primary somatic cell types in the ovarian follicle are granulosa cells and theca cells. Granulosa cells help form the follicle and provide the cytoarchitectural support for the developing oocyte. Theca cells surround the follicle and provide structural support. A combination of granulosa cell growth, theca cell growth and antrum formation result in the expansion of the ovarian follicle. Although stimulation of cell growth is required for the ovulatory follicle to develop, the vast majority of follicles undergo atresia in which cell growth is arrested at various stages of follicle development. Therefore, in addition to the need for a growth stimulator, a growth inhibitor may also be required. The regulation of ovarian cell proliferation is an important and complex process that will require an array of externally and locally derived regulatory agents.

Investigations into the regulation of ovarian cell growth have primarily focused on the factors which regulate granulosa cell proliferation (2). Several growth factors have been shown to stimulate granulosa cell proliferation including fibroblast growth factor (FGF)

(3,4), insulin-like growth factor (IGF) (5), and epidermal growth factor (EGF) (3,4). Granulosa cells contain high affinity EGF receptors (6) and respond in vitro to EGF through an increase in cell proliferation (3,4). In addition, EGF has been shown to alter the hormonal regulation of granulosa cell function (2) by having an inhibitory effect on the ability of FSH to stimulate estrogen biosynthesis (6). These observations have led to the proposal that EGF may have an important role in regulating ovarian cell growth and differentiation (2). Because circulating levels of EGF are negligible (7), the local production of an EGF-like substance in the ovarian follicle would appear to be needed. Studies to determine the potential local production of an EGF-like substance in the ovary will be reviewed.

Transforming growth factor-alpha (TGF-alpha) is a protein that has structural homology with EGF (8), binds to the EGF receptor (9), and has similar biological activities as EGF (10). TGF-alpha is a unique gene product that is produced as a precursor integral membrane protein which is processed into a soluble extracellular protein (11). TGF-alpha was initially isolated from the conditioned medium of virally transformed fibroblasts (12) and has subsequently been shown to be produced by a large number of neoplastic cells (13). Cells of embryonic origin have also been shown to produce TGF-alpha (14). These observations have led investigators to propose that TGF-alpha may function during transformation as an autocrine growth factor (10). Reports have recently demonstrated that TGF-alpha is produced by normal adult cell types, including bovine pituitary cells (15) and human keratinocytes (16). These observations imply that TGF-alpha may also be a growth regulator in normal adult tissue. Therefore, TGF-alpha is a candidate for an EGF-like growth regulator in the ovarian follicle.

Since the majority of developing follicles undergo atresia and growth arrest, the potential presence of a growth inhibitor needs to be considered. Transforming growth factor-beta (TGF-beta) is a protein that has both stimulatory and inhibitory effects on cell proliferation (17). TGF-beta generally inhibits the growth of epithelial cell types, particularly if they are responsive to EGF (18). Although TGF-beta was initially isolated from the conditioned medium from virally transformed fibroblasts (19), it has subsequently been shown to be produced by a large number of neoplastic and normal cell types (20). This highly conserved protein is produced by a number of different species and acts via unique cell surface receptors (21). TGF-beta has also been shown to influence the differentiation and functions of a number of cell types (20). Granulosa cells are an epithelial cell type that respond to EGF; therefore, it was postulated that TGF-beta may influence granulosa cell growth. Recent observations that TGF-beta can regulate granulosa cell steroidogenesis (22,23) support this hypothesis.

Evidence for the local production of transforming growth factors in the ovary and data regarding the regulation of ovarian cell growth will be reviewed. Discussion of the proposed physiological significance of transforming growth factors in the ovary and their relationship to other growth regulators will also be presented.

Methodology

The experimental design used to determine the local production of growth factors in the ovary utilized the isolation and culture of individual cell types. The use of a purified cell population provides a direct means to determine both the sites of synthesis and action of locally produced growth factors. Results obtained with impure cell populations must be qualified because of the potential presence of cell-cell interactions between the different cell types. Although purified populations of granulosa cells can be isolated from rat ovaries (24), homogeneous populations of theca cells are not easily obtained. Because of this fact and the observation that rat granulosa cells do not readily proliferate in vitro, an alternate animal model was utilized. The bovine is a mono-ovulator and the size of the ovary allows for the isolation of homogeneous populations of both granulosa cells and theca cells. These bovine cell types proliferate in vitro and can be cultured under serum-free conditions (3,4,25). Serum-free conditioned medium can be obtained from these cell cultures and used as a potential source for locally produced growth factors. Alternatively, these cell cultures can also be used to determine potential sites of action of specific growth regulators.

Quantitation of the presence of an EGF-like substance can be accomplished with an EGF radioreceptor assay and a bioassay that relies on the growth of an EGF-dependent cell line (7). TGF-alpha can also be analyzed with these same EGF assays. TGF-beta is analyzed with radioreceptor and radioimmunoassays, as well as a bioassay that relies on colony formation on soft agar (25). Confirmation of the presence of a growth factor with a bioassay demonstrates the biological activity of the components detected.

Transforming Growth Factors

Initial observations utilized a rat theca/interstitial cell culture which was a mixed population of cells depleted of granulosa cells. Serum-free conditioned medium from this culture system contained growth-promoting activity for a number of cell types, including bovine granulosa cells (26). The growth-promoting activity from this rat theca/interstitial cell conditioned medium was found to be a heat-stable protein of approximately 20 kDa by size exclusion chromatography (26). These observations demonstrated the local production of a growth factor in the ovary by a theca/interstitial cell population in culture. This growth-promoting activity was subsequently identified as an EGF-like substance with an EGF radioreceptor assay (27). It was found that rat granulosa cell-secreted proteins, obtained from serum-free conditioned medium, did not contain detectable EGF activity with an EGF radioreceptor assay. Secreted proteins from theca/interstitial cell cultures, however, did contain a component that specifically bound to the EGF receptor (27). Theca/interstitial cell-secreted proteins also stimulated the growth of an EGF-dependent cell line (27). The EGF-like substance was isolated by reverse phase hydrophobic chromatography and found to be a single molecular species by both the EGF radioreceptor assay and EGF growth assay (27). These observations indicated that a population of rat theca/interstitial cells, but not rat granulosa cells, produce an EGF-like substance that can promote the growth of granulosa cells and other EGF responsive cells (26,27).

To determine more precisely the site of synthesis of the EGF-like substance, bovine theca cells and granulosa cells were isolated and cultured (25). Theca cell and granulosa cell-secreted proteins were prepared from serum-free conditioned medium that was concentrated by ultrafiltration. Theca cell-secreted proteins were found to contain a component that specifically bound to the EGF receptor as determined by an EGF radioreceptor assay (28). As was found with rat granulosa cell-secreted proteins, bovine granulosa cell-secreted protein preparations were not found to contain an EGF-like substance (28). To confirm these observations, a bioassay for EGF was utilized that is dependent on the growth of an

EGF-sensitive cell type (7). Theca cell-, but not granulosa cell-secreted protein preparations were found to contain EGF-like bioactivity with this EGF growth assay. These combined observations demonstrate that theca cells are the site of synthesis for an EGF-like substance produced locally in the ovarian follicle.

Several biochemical characteristics of the EGF-like substance produced by theca cells were found to be different from those of authentic EGF. The molecular weight of the EGF-like substance was between 20-30 kDa under both denaturing and physiological conditions (27). The molecular weight of authentic EGF is approximately 6,000 (29). The hydrophobicity of the EGF-like substance was also found to be greater than that of authentic murine EGF (27). Therefore, either a large molecular weight form of EGF was produced, as has previously been identified in several physiological fluids (29), or a different EGF-like protein is present. To determine whether a different EGF-like protein is produced, a TGF-alpha molecular probe was obtained. This probe was a complimentary RNA (cRNA) previously described (16). Polyadenylated RNA was prepared from bovine theca cells and granulosa cells and analyzed by Northern analysis. Theca cells, but not granulosa cells, were found to express the TGF-alpha gene with a 4.5 kb RNA species being detected (28). This observation demonstrated that theca cells can produce TGF-alpha and imply that the EGF-like substance detected in theca cell-secreted protein preparations is TGF-alpha. Similar analysis with a human EGF cDNA probe indicated the absence of EGF gene expression in theca cells or granulosa cells (28). Since granulosa cells do not appear to produce TGF-alpha, EGF or any detectable EGF-like substance, the TGF-alpha produced by theca cells may have a paracrine role in regulating granulosa cell growth (28).

During the analysis of the presence of the EGF-like substance in theca cell-secreted protein preparations, it was found that a component was also present which could inhibit the ability of EGF to promote cell growth. The presence of an apparent growth inhibitor indicates that the growth assay may not provide an accurate estimate of the amount of EGF-like material present (27). The growth inhibitory substance was found to be separated from the EGF-like substance by reverse phase chromatography (27). These observations indicated that an EGF growth inhibitory substance was present in theca cell-secreted protein preparations that was distinct from the EGF-like substance or TGF-alpha. A protein that has previously been shown to inhibit the ability of EGF to promote cell growth is TGF-beta (17,20). Therefore, the possible presence of TGF-beta production by theca cells was examined. TGF-beta was detected in theca cell-secreted protein preparations using both radioimmunoassays and radioreceptor assays. TGF-beta biological activity was also detected with an assay based on colony formation on soft agar (25). Granulosa cell-secreted protein preparations did not contain any detectable TGF-beta (25). To demonstrate active synthesis and secretion of TGF-beta by theca cells, a TGF-beta antisera was used to immunoprecipitate radiolabeled theca cell-secreted proteins. A 25 kDa radiolabeled protein that co-migrated with authentic TGF-beta was specifically immunoprecipitated with the antisera (25). These observations demonstrated that theca cells, but not apparently granulosa cells, produce TGF-beta as a potential growth inhibitor for granulosa cell growth.

Growth Regulation

To examine the physiological significance of TGF-alpha and TGF-beta production by theca cells, the effects of transforming growth factors on bovine follicle cell growth were examined. TGF-alpha was found to stimulate granulosa cell growth (28) which confirms previous observations made on the effects of EGF on granulosa cell growth (2-4). Since the circulating levels of EGF are negligible (7), the local production of TGF-alpha by theca cells provides a source of an EGF-like substance in the ovarian follicle. TGF-alpha may have an important role in promoting and maintaining follicle cell growth during the growth phase of the ovary when a primordial follicle develops into an ovulatory follicle. Although TGF-beta alone had no effect on granulosa cell growth, TGF-beta does inhibit the ability of TGF-alpha and EGF to promote bovine granulosa cell growth (25). Demonstration of TGF-beta production by theca cells provides a source for a locally produced growth inhibitor (25). TGF-beta may be required to inhibit cell growth in the atretic follicle and also to prevent premature cell growth in the primordial follicle. Therefore, both TGF-alpha and TGF-beta can influence granulosa cell growth which provides a physiological function for the transforming growth factors produced by theca cells. Previous observations have also indicated that EGF can influence theca/interstitial cell steroidogenesis (30); therefore, the transforming growth factors may also influence theca cells. Theca cells were found to contain high-affinity EGF receptors using a Scatchard analysis (28). This data correlates with the need during follicle development for both granulosa cell and theca cell growth. TGF-alpha and TGF-beta production by theca cells may, therefore, have both an autocrine role in influencing theca cell growth and a paracrine role in regulating granulosa cell growth. The inverse actions of TGF-alpha and TGF-beta provide an efficient mechanism to control the rapid growth stimulation and inhibition required in the ovarian follicle.

In addition to the cell proliferation-related effects, growth factors have also been shown to influence the differentiation of granulosa cells. EGF has previously been shown to have inhibitory effects on the ability of FSH to promote estrogen biosynthesis (2,6). Subsequently these observations have been confirmed with TGF-alpha (31). Therefore, EGF-like substances that promote granulosa cell growth have inhibitory effects on the ability of agents to stimulate a functional parameter such as estrogen biosynthesis. It is not known whether the EGF-like substances directly inhibit granulosa cell steroidogenesis or indirectly inhibit steroidogenesis by altering the rate of granulosa cell proliferation. It is speculated that the reduced ability of regulatory agents to stimulate a differentiated function such as steroidogenesis in the presence of a growth factor may be due to the ability of the growth factor to promote cell proliferation. Promoting granulosa cell proliferation puts the cell into the growth phase of the cell cycle in which differentiated functions such as steroidogenesis may not be readily stimulated. This is supported by the actions of TGF-beta on the ability of FSH to stimulate granulosa cell steroidogenesis. TGF-beta augments the actions of FSH to stimulate granulosa cell estrogen production (22). TGF-beta inhibits cell growth and puts the cell into a nonproliferative differentiated state. Due to the cell being in this stage of the cell cycle, regulatory agents have an enhanced ability to stimulate granulosa cell-differentiated functions such as steroidogenesis. Therefore, it is speculated that the inhibitory and stimulatory effects of TGF-alpha and TGF-beta, respectively, on granulosa cell steroidogenesis are an indirect effect of the growth-promoting ability of these growth factors.

Any agent which could inhibit growth and thus promote a more differentiated state of the cells will likely have a stimulatory effect on granulosa cell functions. Alternatively, any agent which promotes the growth of granulosa cells will likely reduce the differentiated state of the cell and have inhibitory effects. This type of separation of differentiated functions and the growth of granulosa cells has previously been postulated (32). The physiological significance of the effects of transforming growth factors on granulosa cell hormonal regulation are currently unknown.

A number of different growth factors have been shown to influence granulosa cell growth (2-4) which may cooperate in the control of follicle cell expansion (Table 1). Insulin like-growth factor (IGF) has previously been shown to be produced by granulosa cells (33) and influence the growth (34) and functions of granulosa cells (5). Due to the local production of IGF, it has been proposed that IGF may have an important role in regulating granulosa cell growth and differentiation (5). IGF has been shown to be produced by the majority of cell types examined and is involved in the regulation and maintenance of cellular differentiation for many cell types. Therefore, it is likely that IGF will also play an integral role in the control of ovarian cell function, differentiation and hormonal regulation. Examination of cell growth has shown that IGF is a progression factor that regulates the DNA synthesis phase of cell proliferation (35). It is the combined actions of a growth initiator such as EGF and a progression factor such as IGF that maintain optimal cell growth within a tissue (35). From these observations it is speculated that the synergistic actions of TGF-alpha and IGF will be required to maintain optimal follicle cell proliferation. Fibroblast growth factor (FGF) has also been shown to promote granulosa cell growth (3,4). FGF has a number of functions which include being an angiogenic factor (36). Whether FGF will be a physiologically important growth factor for follicle cells such as granulosa cells or theca cells remains to be elucidated. However, the high degree of vascularization of the ovarian follicle, particularly in the corpus luteum, suggests that FGF may have an important role as an angiogenic factor for the follicle (36). Although it is possible that different growth factors have similar functions in the ovary, it is proposed that the primary roles for the different growth factors will be distinct. Therefore, TGF-alpha may function as a growth initiator and through the synergistic actions of IGF maintain optimal follicle cell growth. FGF may primarily function as an angiogenic factor to promote vascularization of the follicle and TGF-beta may function to inhibit cell growth when growth arrest is required. Although a number of growth factors have been identified to be involved in ovarian cell growth, investigations are now required to determine the physiological functions of these different growth factors.

Theca Cell-Granulosa Cell Interactions

The types of cellular interactions possible between theca cells and granulosa cells are numerous. These interactions will be divided into three general categories of environmental, nutritional and regulatory cell-cell interactions (1). The first category deals with the extracellular environment of the cell. Interactions mediated by an extracellular matrix and specific proteins such as cell adhesion molecules make up the environmental category. This type of interaction has an important role in providing the proper structural support and surroundings for the cell to maintain a normal morphology and differentiated state. This interaction is also very important during development and morphogenesis. The second category, called nutri-

Table 1. Ovarian growth regulators

Growth Factor	Site of Synthesis	Site of Action	Response/Function
TGFα	Theca	Theca/granulosa	Growth stimulator
EGF	—	Theca/granulosa	Growth stimulator
TGFβ	Theca	Theca/granulosa	Growth inhibitor
IGF	Granulosa/theca?	Granulosa/theca?	Cell differentiation and growth stimulator
FGF	—	Granulosa/ vasculature	Angiogenic factor and growth stimulator

tional, deals with a cell obtaining essential components needed for survival. The maintenance of normal cellular functions requires many externally derived components such as energy metabolites. When an essential component such as a sugar metabolite, vitamin, or metal is derived from one cell type and delivered to a different cell type, a nutritional type of cell-cell interaction has occurred. The third category of cell-cell interaction deals with a component that is produced by one cell type that acts on a second cell type to cause a signal transduction event. This action induces a cellular response on the molecular level associated with the differentiation, function, or growth of the cell. This type of interaction is called regulatory. Interactions of this type are important in the control and maintenance of many cellular parameters. Regulatory agents involved in this type of interaction are paracrine factors. This interaction generally requires a receptor-mediated event to induce a second messenger that alters cellular parameters on the molecular level.

Examples of several theca cell-granulosa cell interactions are shown in Table 2. Environmental interactions are mediated by an extracellular matrix between the outer layer of mural granulosa cells and inner layer of theca interna. This extracellular matrix is speculated to be produced cooperatively by both cell types as has been shown in other tissues like the testis (1). One of the primary functions of this extracellular matrix is to provide structural support to the follicle. Additional effects of environmental cellular interactions on cell morphology and function have not been thoroughly investigated (38). A nutritional interaction between theca cells and granulosa cells that has been established is mediated through the production of androgens by theca cells. Testosterone produced by theca cells can be utilized by granulosa cells for the biosynthesis of estrogen (24). This interaction is a classic example of a nutritional interaction where a substrate, testosterone, is provided to an enzyme, aromatase. This interaction is critical for the maintenance of ovarian function and the endocrine status of the female. Regulatory interactions require a receptor-mediated signal transduction event on the molecular level. A recently identified regulatory interaction between theca cells and granulosa cells involves progestin production by granulosa cells. Progestins produced by granulosa cells can act on theca cells to influence cellular differentiation and function (39). Evidence has also been provided that estrogens may also influence theca cell functions (39). These steroid-mediated interactions may have an important role in mediating cellular differentiation in the follicle.

Table 2. Theca cell-granulosa cell interactions

Cell-Cell Interaction Category	Mediator	Ovarian Site of Synthesis	Response/Function
Environmental	Extracellular matrix	Granulosa/theca	Structural support for follicle
Nutritional	Androgen	Theca	Estrogen biosynthesis by granulosa
Regulatory	Progestin	Granulosa/theca	Theca cell differentiation
	TGFα	Theca	Growth stimulator for granulosa/theca
	TGFβ	Theca	Growth inhibitor for granulosa/ theca

The production of transforming growth factors by theca cells also provide mediators of cell-cell interactions in the follicle. TGF-alpha and TGF-beta produced by theca cells have a paracrine role in the regulation of granulosa cell growth and a possible autocrine role in the regulation of theca cell growth (Fig. 1). Growth factor-mediated paracrine interactions within a tissue provide an efficient mechanism for different cell types to form a functional unit to control tissue growth. The evolution of this process indicates the importance of cell-cell interactions between different cell types within a tissue and implies that few cell types will be autonomous in the regulation of growth and differentiation. Theca-granulosa cell interactions provide an example of mesenchymal-epithelial cell interactions. The importance of mesenchymal-epithelial cell interactions have been demonstrated during development (37), but remain to be elucidated in adult tissue. TGF-alpha and TGF-beta production by theca cells and subsequent actions on granulosa cells are examples of growth factor-mediated mesenchymal-epithelial cell interactions. The synthesis of TGF-alpha by theca cells also provides an example of TGF-alpha production by a normal adult mesenchymal cell type. Previous studies have implicated TGF-alpha as an important growth regulator during transformation (10,13) and embryonic development (14). Recently the demonstration of TGF-alpha by normal epithelial cell types has led to the proposal that TGF-alpha may also have an important role as a growth regulator in normal adult tissue (15,16). The observation that TGF-alpha is produced by theca cells supports this proposal and indicates that TGF-alpha may be an important growth regulator in EGF responsive tissues requiring rapid cell proliferation (28).

The observations reviewed indicate that theca cells produce both TGF-alpha and TGF-beta which may function as a growth stimulator and growth inhibitor, respectively, in the ovarian follicle (Fig. 1). The speculation is made that TGF-alpha production by theca cells would be predominate during the growth phase of the follicles and TGF-beta production would be predominate in the atretic and primordial follicle when growth is inhibited. These inverse actions of TGF-alpha and TGF-beta provide an efficient mechanism to control the

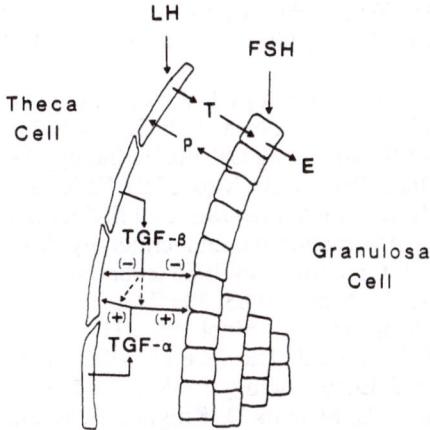

Fig. 1. Schematic of theca cell-granulosa cell
interactions mediated by TGF-alpha, TGF-beta,
testosterone (T), progestin (P) and estrogen (E).

rapid stimulation and inhibition of cell growth required in the ovarian follicle. Therefore,
the local production of transforming growth factors will have an important role in the
regulation of ovarian cell growth.

References

1. Skinner MK. Ann NY Acad Sci 1987; 513:158.
2. Hsueh AJW, Adashi EY, Jones PBC, Walsh TH. Endocr Rev 1984; 5:76.
3. Gospodarowicz D, Ill CR, Birdwell CR. Endocrinology 1977; 100:1108.
4. Gospodarowicz D, Bialecki H. Endocrinology 1979; 104:757.
5. Adashi EY, Resnick CE, D'Ercole AJ, Svoboda ME, Van Wyk JJ. Endocr Rev 1985;
   6:400.
6. Jones PB, Welsh TH, Hsueh AJ. J Biol Chem 1982; 257:11268.
7. Carpenter G, Zendegui J. Anal Biochem 1986; 153:279.
8. Marquardt H, Hunkapillar MW, Hood LE, Todaro GJ. Science 1984; 223:1079.
9. Todaro GJ, Fryling C, Delarco JE. Proc Natl Acad Sci USA 1980; 77:5258.
10. Derynck R. J Cell Biochem 1986; 32:293.
11. Bringman TS, Lindquist PB, Derynck R. Cell 1987; 48:429.
12. DeLarco JE, Todaro GJ. Proc Natl Acad Sci USA 1978; 75:4001.
13. Derynck R, Goeddel DV, Ullrich A, et al. Cancer Res 1987; 47:707.
14. Lee DC, Rochford RM, Todaro GJ, Willareal LP. Mol Cell Biol 1985; 5:3644.
15. Samsoonder J, Kobrin MS, Kudlow JE. J Biol Chem 1986; 261:14408.
16. Coffey RJ, Derynck R, Wilcox JN, et al. Nature 1987; 328:817.
17. Keski-Oja J, Leof EB, Lyons RM, Coffey RJ, Moses HL. J Cell Biochem 1987; 33:95.
18. Moses HL, Tucker RF, Leof EB, Coffey RJ, Halper J, Shipley GD. In: Feramisco J,
    Ozanne B, Stiles C, eds. Cancer cell; vol 3. New York: Cold Spring Harbor Press,
    1984:65-71.
19. Roberts AB, Arzano MA, Lamb LC, Smith JM, Sporn MB. Proc Natl Acad Sci USA
    1981; 78:53359.

20. Sporn MB, Roberts AB, Wakefield LM, Assoian RK. Science 1986; 233:532.
21. Tucker RF, Branum EC, Shipley GD, Ryon RJ, Moses HL. Proc Natl Acad Sci USA 1984; 81:6757.
22. Adashi EY, Resnick CE. Endocrinology 1986; 119:1879.
23. Feng P, Catt KJ, Knecht M. J Biol Chem 1986; 261:14167.
24. Dorrington JH, Moon YS, Armstrong DT. Endocrinology 1975; 97:1328.
25. Skinner MK, Keski-Oja J, Osteen KG, Moses HL. Endocrinology 1987; 121:786.
26. Lobb DK, Skinner MK, Dorrington JH. Mol Cell Endocrinol 1988; 55:209.
27. Skinner MK, Lobb DK, Dorrington JH. Endocrinology 1987; 121:1892.
28. Skinner MK, Coffey RJ. Endocrinology 1988 (submitted).
29. Gray A, Dull TJ, Ullrich A. Nature 1983; 303:722.
30. Erickson GF, Case E. Mol Cell Endocrinol 1983; 31:71.
31. Adashi EY, Resnick CE, Twardzik DR. J Cell Biochem 1987; 33:1.
32. Epstein-Almog R, Orly J. Endocrinology 1985; 116:2103.
33. Hammond JM, Baranao JL, Skaleris D, Knight AB, Romanus JA, Rechler M. Endocrinology 1985; 117:2553.
34. Savion N, Lui GM, Laherty R, Gospodarowicz D. Endocrinology 1981; 109:409.
35. O'Keefe EJ, Pledger WJ. Mol Cell Endocrinol 1983; 31:167.
36. Gospodarowicz D, Ferrara N, Schweigrer L, Neufeld G. Endocr Rev 1987; 8:95.
37. Cunha GR, Chung LWK, Shannen JM, Taguchi O, Fujii H. Recent Prog Horm Res 1983; 39:595.
38. Carnegie JA, Byard R, Dardick I, Tsang BK. Biol Reprod 1988; 38:881.
39. Fortune JE. Biol Reprod 1986; 35:292.

12

Fibroblast Growth Factors as Local Mediators of Gonadal Function

Andrew Baird, Naoya Emoto, Shunichi Shimasaki, Ana Maria Gonzalez, Bart Fauser* and Aaron J. W. Hsueh*

Laboratories for Neuroendocrinology, The Salk Institute
10010 N. Torrey Pines Road, La Jolla, California 92037
*Department of Reproductive Medicine, University of California
at San Diego, San Diego, California 92038

Although the presence and effects of many growth factors in gonadal tissues has been established by several investigators (1-4), their physiological function remains, to a large extent, speculative. The main reason behind this problem is the fact that in in vitro assays, growth factors have a tremendous number of biological activities. A case in point is basic fibroblast growth factor, basic FGF (3,4). This mitogen is characterized by its ability to elicit a neovascular response in in vivo assays of angiogenesis (5) and is thought to participate in these processes in the reproductive system (3). Yet these growth factors are also characterized by their capacity to modulate the growth and function of a wide number of cells (6,7). These include granulosa, adrenocortical, endothelial and smooth muscle cells, chondrocytes and fibroblasts, just to name a few. In some instances, basic FGF has no effect on cell proliferation, but only affects differentiated function (8-10). In other cases, its mitogenic activity appears to be the predominant activity (6,7). With the structural characterization of basic FGF, it has become of paramount importance to establish its possible physiological function(s) in tissues where it has been identified. At first glance, its pleiotropic activities might seem to preclude determining a specific function for this molecule; however, the discovery that it is widely distributed and found in almost all tissues suggests that its biological activities are local and thus potentially highly specific for any given environment. On this basis, it seems unlikely that an adrenal-derived FGF plays the function of a wound healing and/or angiogenic factor. More likely it is involved in adrenocortical homeostasis, an activity of the molecule in vitro (11).

The present research was initiated with the primary goal of establishing the presence of basic FGF in gonadal tissues and examining its possible function and regulation in these tissues. Because the ovary is a tissue that undergoes regular and highly regulated angiogenesis, it is also an attractive model to investigate the mechanisms responsible for regulating the bioavailability of basic FGF and its role in angiogenesis.

Materials and Methods

Isolation of FGFs

Basic FGF was isolated from ovary and testes as described by Gospodarowicz et al. (3) and Ueno et al. (4). In each instance, a combination of ammonium sulfate precipitation, cation exchange chromatography and heparin-Sepharose affinity chromatography and reverse phase HPLC achieved homogeneity as assessed by amino acid analysis and amino terminal sequencing. In biological studies, human recombinant basic FGF has been used and possesses all of the biological activities of the native molecule (12).

Cell Culture

Vascular and capillary endothelial cells and Swiss 3T3 cells were cultured and used in proliferation and mitogenesis assays as described (3,4,6). Granulosa cell assays and neonatal testes were grown as described by Jones et al. (13) and Fauser et al. (14), respectively. Human dermal fibroblasts were cultured as described by Emoto and Baird (15).

FGFs in Follicular Fluid

A total of 500 ml of porcine follicular fluid was centrifuged and diluted threefold with Tris-buffered (10 mM) saline (TBS). The solution was loaded onto a 10-ml heparin-Sepharose gel column by gravity and the bound proteins were eluted with a step gradient of 0.15, 0.6, 1.1, 2.0 and 3.0 M NaCl in TBS. Aliquots of the column fractions were tested for FGF activity in proliferation and mitogenic assays and in a RIA for basic FGF.

Angiogenesis Assays

The effects of basic FGF on the rabbit cornea were performed with recombinant basic FGF obtained from Chiron Corp., Emeryville, CA (12). Elvax pellets were prepared containing 200 ng of basic FGF and were implanted into a rabbit corneal pouch. Angiogenesis was assessed 12 to 18 days after surgery.

Aromatase and Steroid Assays

The capacity of rat granulosa cells in vitro to form estrogens was measured by RIA as described (9,13). The effects of basic FGF on aromatase activity in peripheral fibroblasts were assessed using a radiometric assay measuring the capacity of these cells to release water from the metabolism of radiolabelled androstenedione (15). The effects of basic FGF on testosterone production were measured by RIA (14).

Identification of Rat Ovarian FGF

A library was prepared from PMSG-stimulated rat ovaries and screened for the presence of basic FGF. Positive clones were isolated and sequenced as described by Shimasaki et al. (in preparation), and used to predict an amino acid sequence for rat ovarian basic FGF.

Receptor Studies

Basic FGF was radioiodinated using lactoperoxidase (16) and used in binding studies as described by Moscatelli (17). Cross-linking basic FGF to its receptor on granulosa cells was accomplished using DSS as described by Neufeld and Gospodarowicz (18).

Results and Discussion

Activities of Basic FGF in Gonadal Tissues In Vitro

The presence of many growth factors has been established in the ovary (1,2). Among these is basic FGF, a potent angiogenic, growth and differentiation factor. Like many growth factors, basic FGF has the capacity to inhibit aromatase activity in cultured rat granulosa cells (Fig. 1A).

Like its effect on cell proliferation, the potency of its effect on aromatase activity is well within a range to suggest a physiological importance. In contrast, the effects of basic FGF on testicular function require a considerably higher concentration of basic FGF (Fig. 1B). The significance of this finding is not known. The affinity and specificity of the receptor are similar to those reported for other cell types (see below), making it unclear why the testes cells require higher concentrations of basic FGF to detect a response. Whether basic FGF is acting through the acidic FGF receptor or whether neonatal testes cells are refractory to basic FGF and possibly producing an inhibitory factor remains to be investigated. This latter possibility is supported by the identification of TGF beta (transforming growth factor beta) as a potent inhibitor of basic FGF activity in endothelial cells (19,20).

Local Presence of Basic FGF in Gonadal Tissues

Heparin-Sepharose affinity chromatography of porcine follicular fluid reveals the presence of basic FGF-like activities (Fig. 2). The major peak of endothelial cell-stimulating activity elutes with 2 M NaCl, a characteristic of basic FGF. This material also contains immunoreactive basic FGF as measured by RIA (not shown). A small peak of activity is detected in the 1.1 M eluate which may correspond to acidic FGF. No immunoassays were

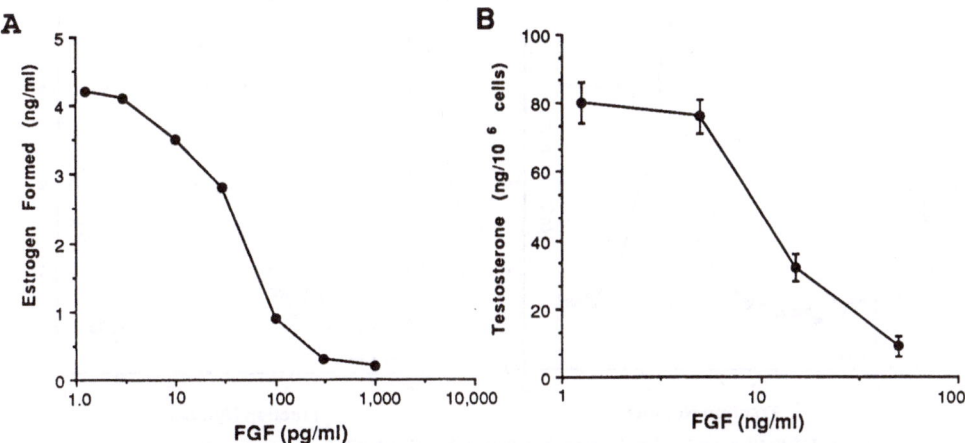

Fig. 1. Effect of basic FGF on estrogen and testosterone formation by (A) rat granulosa cells, and (B) neonatal rat testes cells in vitro. Cells were challenged with luteinizing hormone (10 ng/ml) and various concentrations of basic FGF. The conditioned media was collected and estrogens *(Panel A)* or testosterone *(Panel B)* formation was measured by RIA.

performed to test this hypothesis. The quantities of basic FGF in porcine follicular fluid are small. The batch processing of 500 ml of porcine follicular fluid failed to yield sufficient quantities for further chemical analysis.

The presence of basic FGF in porcine follicular fluid does not necessarily establish a gonadal origin for the mitogen. To investigate this possibility, we examined the immunohistological staining of basic FGF in the ovary and testes. Using a monoclonal antibody raised against recombinant basic FGF, we were able to detect staining in granulosa and Leydig cells, respectively, but not exclusively (not shown). Thus, there is an intragonadal source of the mitogen. It remains to be established whether granulosa and Leydig cells are the sole source of basic FGF in the gonads. The recent demonstration that basic FGF can be cloned from libraries prepared from PMSG-treated rat ovaries establishes the fact that basic FGF is locally synthesized in the ovary. An analysis of its primary structure (Table 1) shows it to be highly homologous to bovine and human basic FGF with only four conservative changes and one amino acid deletion.

Characterization of the FGF Receptor in Gonadal Tissues

We have also examined the receptor for basic FGF on cultured rat testes cells and on granulosa cells (Fig. 3). An analysis of both cell types reveals the presence of saturable binding that, when translated by Scatchard analyses, identifies high affinity receptors (Ka $\sim 10^{-12}$ M). With an estimated number of binding sites at $\sim 2000\text{-}3500$/cell, there is good evidence that the binding reflects a cell-specific receptor. Accordingly, it was established that the binding of basic FGF is specific. Although other growth factors like NGF (nerve growth factor), PDGF (platelet-derived growth factor), IGF (insulin-like growth factor), TGF alpha, TGF beta and insulin have no effect on basic FGF binding, acidic FGF can

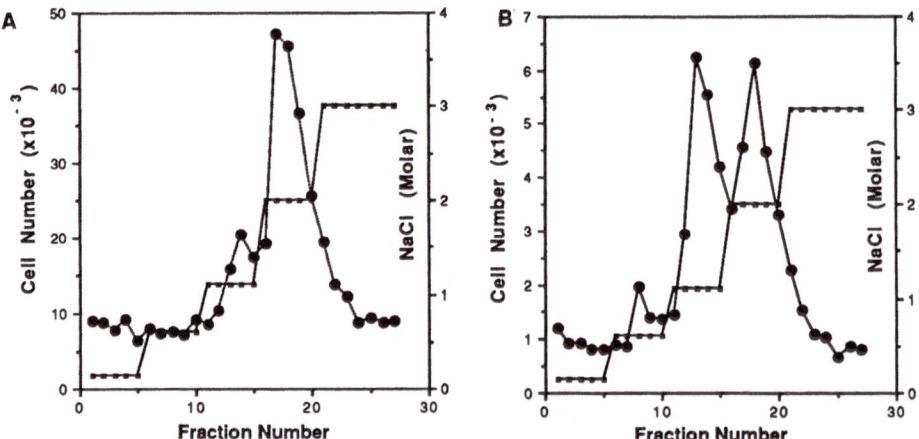

Fig. 2. FGF-like activities in porcine follicular fluid. Column fractions obtained after passing 500 ml of porcine follicular fluid through a heparin-Sepharose column were tested for their capacity to stimulate the proliferation of adrenocortical capillary endothelial cells *(Panel A)* or thymidine incorporation into Swiss 3T3 cells *(Panel B)*. The proteins were eluted with a step gradient of NaCl in Tris buffer as described in the text.

Table 1. Predicted primary structure of rat ovarian basic FGF

---

maagsitsl PALPE DGG * GA FPPGH FKDPK RLYCK NGGFF LRIHP
DGRVD GVREK SDPHV KLQLQ AEERG VVSIK GVCAN RYLAM
KEDGR LLASK CVTEE CFFFE RLESN NYNTY RSRKY SSWYV
ALKRT GQYKL GSKTG PGQKA ILFLP MSAKS

---

*Indicates the deletion of serine at residue 9 compared to the bovine sequence (6).
Substitutions include S for T at position -2, V for I at position 51, E for D at position 80,
and S for P at position 126, compared to the sequence of bovine pituitary basic FGF (6).

displace the labelled mitogen on both cell types. Thus, it is reasonable to suggest that these
two ligands cross-talk on a similar receptor. Binding studies with acidic FGF will address
this question.

The molecular nature of the binding protein on rat granulosa cells was investigated by
cross-linking the growth factor to its receptor. As shown in Figure 5, these experiments
identified a 130,000-dalton protein. This is in marked contradistinction to the two molecular
weight species that bind basic FGF on baby hamster kidney cells (135 and 160 Kd) and the
protein (160 Kd) identified on 3T3 cells (21-23).

Effects of Basic FGF on Extragonadal Aromatase

The capacity of basic FGF to modify aromatase activity in granulosa cells is not unique
to granulosa cells. The addition of basic FGF and other growth factors to cultured fibroblasts
reveals the ability of each of these factors to inhibit the formation of estrogens from
radiolabelled androstenedione. Thus, there exists a common inhibitory effect of growth
factors on the aromatase activity found in gonadal and in peripheral tissues. In view of the
paracrine nature of basic FGF activity, it is likely that the mitogen plays a local role in each

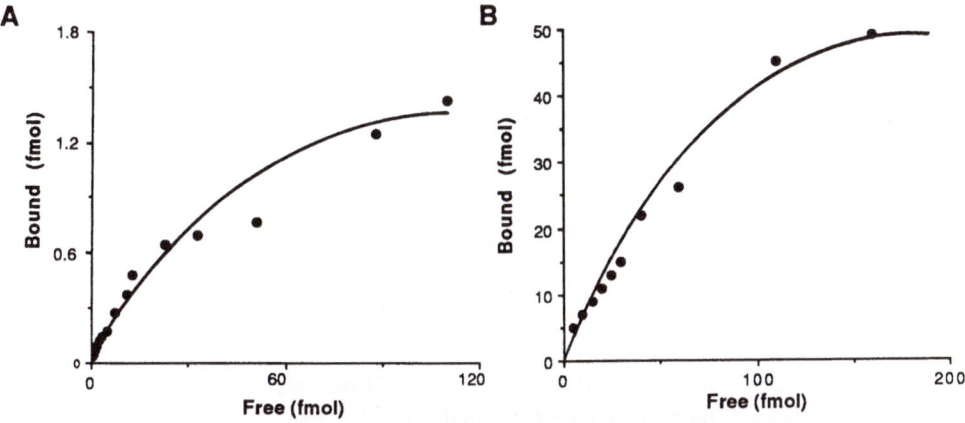

Fig. 3. Saturation of FGF binding to granulosa and neonatal testes cells. Rat
granulosa *(Panel A)* or rat neonatal testes cells *(Panel B)* were incubated with
various concentrations of radiolabelled basic FGF and examined for saturation of
receptor binding.

of these tissues. By inference then, dysfunction in the aromatization of androgens in the periphery need not reflect similar problems in the ovary. Thus, it will become of paramount importance to understand the molecular mechanisms that regulate the local production of basic FGF in tissues and establish the identity of factors that modulate its bioavailability.

There is a wealth of information to suggest that FGFs are important components in maintaining normal gonadal function. These data come primarily from in vitro studies, but are also beginning to develop from in vivo work. Consistent with their proposed role as ovarian angiogenic factors, FGFs have been implicated in the neovascular events associated with normal ovarian function. Yet it is important to consider the fact that FGFs possess a wide range of activities in vitro that extend to delaying cell senescence and maintaining differentiated function. Because these factors appear to be present in the local hormonal milieu, they are in a good position to modulate gonadal function. It is in view of this observation that it will be particularly important to establish which biological activities of basic FGF in vitro correspond to physiological functions in the gonads in vivo. Furthermore, the observation that FGFs are locally present in the gonads raises the important necessity of understanding the mechanisms that are responsible for regulating their bioavailability.

The reagents necessary to investigate the in vivo functions of basic FGF in tissues have only been available in the last 3 years. In all of the instances so far, the in vitro activities of basic FGF have been translated into effective in vivo activities. As an example, the effects

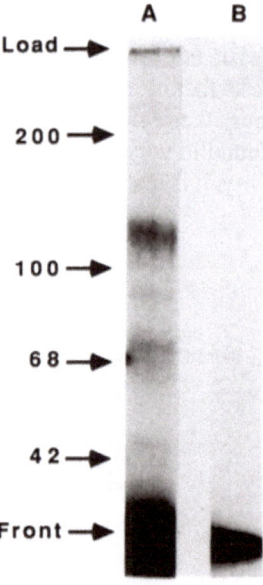

Fig. 4. Identification of the basic FGF receptor on rat granulosa cells. Radioiodinated basic FGF was incubated with cells and covalently cross-linked to its receptor using DSS. The cells were extracted and the binding visualized after SDS-PAGE by autoradiography.

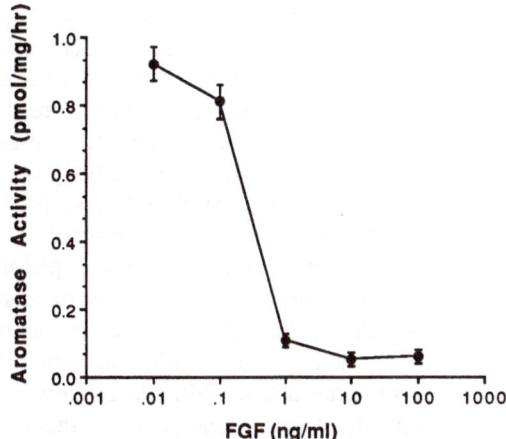

Fig. 5. Effects of basic FGF on peripheral aromatase activity. Human-derived fibroblasts were tested for their capacity to convert radiolabelled androstenedione to estrogens as described in the text. Basal aromatase activity was stimulated with 1 mM dbcAMP and various concentrations of basic FGF were added to the cells. Basic FGF has no effect in the absence of dbcAMP.

of basic FGF on endothelial cell growth in vitro have led to the identification of basic FGF as an angiogenic factor capable of stimulating new blood vessel growth in the cornea (see Figure 6).

The angiogenic activity for basic FGF is also observed on the vasa vasorum (in preparation), and in regenerating nerves (24) and when injected into the brain (25). Its effects

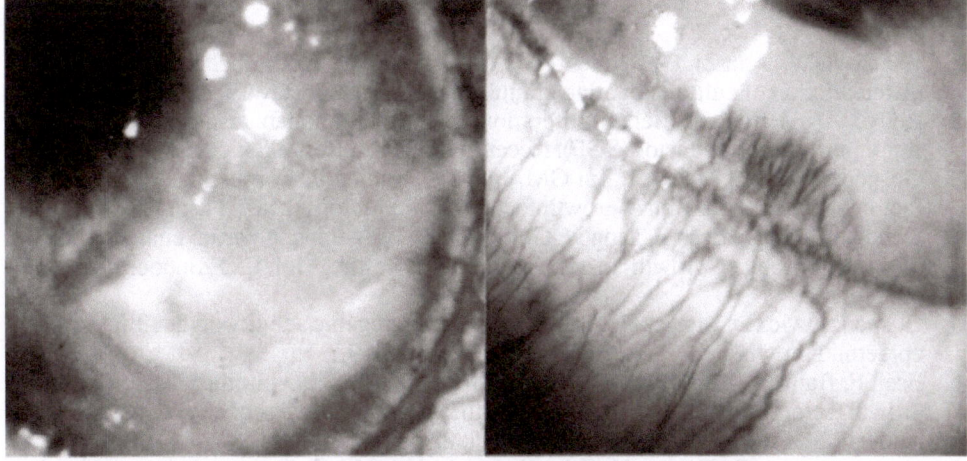

Fig. 6. Angiogenesis stimulated by basic FGF. Elvax pellets without *(Panel A)* or with *(Panel B)* basic FGF were implanted into rabbit corneal pouches and the angiogenesis observed 12 days after surgery (magnification x 40).

on chondrocyte proliferation gives it the capacity to induce cartilage repair in vivo (26), and its effects as a morphogen in vitro have been confirmed by Nicoll's laboratory who have used antisera to basic FGF to establish a function for this growth factor in mammalian embryonic development (27). On this basis, in the near future there should be a wealth of information made available from ongoing research in reproductive biology. Because the ovary provides one of the few physiological models for studying neovascularization, the results obtained in this area of growth factor research will have profound effects on our understanding of the pathophysiological effects of growth factors in other tissues.

Finally, it is important to emphasize that, just as basic FGF is pleiotropic in vitro and in vivo, so are many other growth factors. Thus, it is not reasonable to conclude that basic FGF is necessarily *the* ovarian angiogenic factor. Many molecules possess the capacity to stimulate neovascularization. These include EGF (epidermal growth factor), TGF alpha, TGF beta, and acidic FGF, just to name a few (29). More likely is the possibility that angiogenesis in the ovary is dependent on a multitude of factors that are present in the local hormonal environment. The time- and concentration-dependent effects of each of these factors combined with their interactions with each other will determine cellular responsiveness. From in vitro studies in defined media, where their activities were first described, it is now necessary to study their interactions in vitro and in vivo to understand how, together, they modulate gonadal function in their native milieu.

Acknowledgments

We are grateful for the expert technical assistance of Emelie Amburn, Jim Farris and Mike Ong, and for the skillful secretarial work of Denise Higgins. This research was supported by grants from the National Institutes of Health (HD-09690 and DK-18811), from the Robert J. Kleberg and Helen C. Kleberg Foundation, and from the G. Harold and Leila Y. Mathers Charitable Foundation.

References

1. Hsueh AJW, Adashi EY, Jones PBC, Welsh TH Jr. Hormonal regulation of the differentiation of cultured ovarian granulosa cells. Endocr Rev 1984; 5:76-127.
2. Bellve AR, Feig LA. Cell proliferation in the mammalian testis: biology of the seminiferous growth factor (SGF). Recent Prog Horm Res 1984; 40:531-67.
3. Gospodarowicz D, Cheng J, Lui GM, Baird A, Bohlen P. Corpus luteum angiogenic factor is related to fibroblast growth factor. Endocrinology 1985; 117:2383-91.
4. Ueno N, Baird A, Esch F, Ling N, Guillemin R. Isolation and partial characterization of basic fibroblast growth factor from bovine testis. Mol Cell Endocrinol 1987; 49:189-94.
5. Gospodarowicz D, Bialecki H, Takral TK. The angiogenic activity of the fibroblast and epidermal growth factor. Exp Eye Res 1979; 28:501-9.
6. Esch F, Baird A, Ling N, et al. Primary structure of bovine pituitary basic fibroblast growth factor (FGF) and comparison with the amino-terminal sequence of bovine brain acidic FGF. Proc Natl Acad Sci USA 1985; 82:6507-11.
7. Gospodarowicz D, Ferrara N, Schweigerer L, Neufeld G. Structural characterization and biological functions of fibroblast growth factor. Endocr Rev 1987; 8:95-114.

8. Baird A, Mormede P, Ying S-Y, et al. A nonmitogenic function of fibroblast growth factor: regulation of thyrotropin and prolactin secretion. Proc Natl Acad Sci USA 1985; 82:5545-59.

9. Baird A, Hsueh AJW. Fibroblast growth factor as an intraovarian hormone: differential regulation of steroidogenesis by an angiogenic factor. Regul Pept 1986; 16:243-50.

10. Mormede P, Baird A. Estrogens, cyclic adenosine 3', 3'-monophosphate, and phorbol esters modulate the prolactin response of GH_3 cells to basic fibroblast growth factor. Endocrinology 1988; 122:2765-71.

11. Hornsby PJ, Gill GN. Characterization of adult bovine adrenocortical cells throughout their life span in tissue culture. Endocrinology 1978; 102:926-36.

12. Barr PJ, Cousens LS, Lee-Ng CT, et al. Expression and processing of biologically active fibroblast growth factors in the yeast *Saccharomyces cerevisiae*. J Biol Chem 1988 (in press).

13. Jones PBC, Hsueh AJW. Direct effects of gonadotropin-releasing hormone and its antagonist upon ovarian function stimulated by FSH. Biol Reprod 1981; 24:747-54.

14. Fauser BCJM, Baird A, Hsueh AJW. Fibroblast growth factor inhibits luteinizing hormone-stimulated androgen production by cultured rat testicular cells. J Clin Endocrinol Metab 1988 (in press).

15. Emoto N, Baird A. The regulation of aromatase activity in cultured human skin fibroblasts [Abstract]. Abstract 15, Endocr Soc Mtg, Indianapolis, 1987.

16. Baird A, Schubert D, Ling N, Guillemin R. Receptor- and heparin-binding domains of basic fibroblast growth factor. Proc Natl Acad Sci USA 1988; 85:2324-8.

17. Moscatelli D. High and low affinity binding sites for basic fibroblast growth on cultured cells: absence of a role for low affinity binding in the stimulation of plasminogen activator production by bovine capillary endothelial cells. J Cell Physiol 1987; 131:123-30.

18. Neufeld G, Gospodarowicz D. The identification and partial characterization of the fibroblast growth factor receptor of baby hamster kidney cells. J Biol Chem 1985; 260:13860-8.

19. Baird A, Durkin T. Inhibition of endothelial cell proliferation by type beta-transforming growth factor: interactions with acidic and basic fibroblast growth factors. Biochem Biophys Res Commun 1986; 138:476-82.

20. Frater-Schroder M, Muller G, Burchmeir W, Bohlen P. Transforming growth factor beta inhibits endothelial cell proliferation. Biochem Biophys Res Commun 1986; 137:295-302.

21. Moenner M, Chevallier B, Badet J, Barritault D. Evidence and characterization of the receptor to eye-derived growth factor I, the retinal form of basic fibroblast growth factor, on bovine epithelial lens cells. Proc Natl Acad Sci USA 1986; 83:5024-8.

22. Neufeld G, Gospodarowicz D. Basic and acidic fibroblast growth factors interact with the same cell surface receptors. J Biol Chem 186; 262:5631-7.

23. Olwin BB, Hauschka SD. Identification of the fibroblast growth factor receptor Swiss 3T3 cells and mouse skeletal muscle myoblasts. Biochemistry 1986; 25:3487-92.

24. Cuevas P, Carceller F, Baird A, Guillemin R. Basic fibroblast growth factor (bFGF) increases peripheral nerve regeneration rate. 7th Gen Mtg Europ Soc Neurochem, Goteborg, 1988.

25. Cuevas P, Baird A, Guillemin R. Angiogenic response to fibroblast growth factor in the rat brain in vivo. 8th Int Symp Microsur Anas Cerbr Ischem, Florence, Italy, 1986.

26. Cuevas P, Burgos J, Cuevas B, Baird A, Guillemin R. Basic fibroblast growth factor (bFGF) stimulates cartilage regeneration. XXVI World Congr Int Coll Surg, Milan, Italy, 1988.
27. Liu L, Nicoll CS. Evidence for a role of basic fibroblast growth factor in rat embryonic growth and differentiation. Endocrinology 1988 (in press).
28. Folkman J, Klagsbrun M. Angiogenic factors. Science 1987; 235:442-6.

IV. Poster Presentation Manuscripts

13

Analysis of Binding Sites for IGF-I on Membranes from Granulosa Cells of Small, Medium, and Large Porcine Follicles

Vincent W. Hylka, Brigitte Caubo, and Sharon A. Tonetta

Livingston Reproductive Biology Laboratory
University of Southern California School of Medicine
1321 N. Mission Road, Los Angeles, California 90033

Abstract. We examined binding of IGF-I to granulosal membranes from small (<3 mm), medium (3-6 mm) and large (>8 mm) porcine follicles. Granulosa cells were aspirated and membranes prepared by dounce homogenization. Membranes from each group were incubated for 16 h at 4°C (optimal conditions) with ^{125}I-IGF-I in the absence or presence of unlabeled IGF-I (0.01-1 µg/ml), IGF-II (0.5-5 µg/ml), or insulin (0.1-20 µg/ml). Scatchard analysis of the data demonstrated a curvilinear plot for all three groups. The high-affinity sites had the following Ka values (mean ± SEM; nM): small = 6.50 ± O.09; medium = 6.45 ± 0.44; large = 6.48 ± 0.44. The binding capacities of the high-affinity sites for each group were (pmol/mg protein): small = 1.51 ± 0.17; medium = 1.15 ± 0.14; large = 1.40 ± 0.15. The low-affinity sites had the following Ka values (nM): small = 0.053 ± 0.008; medium = 0.077 ± 0.019; large = 0.077 ± 0.007. The low-affinity sites had the following binding capacities (pmol/mg protein): small = 20.40 ± 3.10; medium = 13.76 ± 0.78; large = 12.99 ± 0.55. Preferential binding for the high-affinity sites was IGF-I > IGF-II > insulin. These data show that although IGF-I plays a role in granulosal differentiation, the affinity and number of high-affinity binding sites do not change during follicular maturation. However, the number of low-affinity binding sites appears to be greater in granulosa cells from small follicles, suggesting a possible role for IGF-II and/or insulin in early follicular maturation.

Introduction

Insulin-like growth factor-I (IGF-I) acts as a regulator of ovarian function. In the pig, IGF-I is produced by granulosa cells (1) and is found in high concentrations in follicular fluid (2). Additionally, IGF-I receptors are present on both granulosa (3) and theca (4) from porcine follicles, and IGF-I can modulate both basal and gonadotropin-induced secretion of steroids in granulosa (5) and theca cells (6).

In granulosa cells, IGF-I enhances basal secretion of progesterone [P] (7), as well as FSH-induced increases in P (8), estradiol [E2] (7,9), cyclic AMP [cAMP] (10), and receptors for luteinizing hormone [LH] (11). Conversely, secretion of IGF-I can be augmented in porcine granulosa cells by gonadotropins, E2, and cAMP (12).

Several changes that occur in porcine granulosa cells as the follicle matures (enhanced sensitivity to FSH, increase in LH receptors, etc.) can also be enhanced by IGF-I. Therefore, modulation of granulosa cells by IGF-I during follicular maturation may be a function of: (a) an increased amount of IGF-I available to the cells; or, (b) a change in the number and/or affinity of IGF-I receptors. The present study examined the number and affinities of IGF-I binding sites on granulosa cells from small, medium, and large porcine follicles.

Methods

Fresh porcine ovaries were obtained from a local abattoir. Follicles were separated into 3 groups: small (<3 mm), medium (3-6 mm), and large (>8 mm). Granulosa cells and follicular fluid were removed by slow aspiration and gentle scraping with a 5 ml syringe fitted with a 25-gauge needle. Granulosa cells were separated from follicular fluid by centrifugation at 800 x g for 8 min. (After this point, procedures were done on ice.) Cells were then washed 3x with 0.025 M tris, 1 µg/ml aprotinin, pH 7.5. Cells were then diluted in receptor buffer (0.025 M tris, 1% sodium azide, 1 µg aprotinin/ml, pH 7.4; = RB), homogenized in a ground glass homogenizer, then dounce homogenized and centrifuged at 5,000 x g for 20 min. The resulting crude membrane pellet was diluted into RB, sonicated for 5 seconds, and then aliquoted and frozen at -70°C until used. There were no differences between frozen and fresh tissue. Protein content of the membrane homogenates was estimated using the method of Lowry et al. (13), with BSA used as standard. Maximum binding curves and optimal conditions were determined. Membranes from each maturational group were incubated for 16 h at 4°C with ^{125}I-IGF-I (Amersham, Arlington Heights, IL) in the absence or presence of unlabeled IGF-I (Collaborative Research, Bedford, MA; 0.1-1 µg/ml), IGF-II (MSA from Collaborative Research; 0.5-5 µg/ml), or porcine insulin (Eli Lilly Co., Indianapolis, IN; 0.1-20 µg/ml) in a total incubation volume of 150 µl, containing 1% BSA. After incubation, tubes were spun at 5,000 x g (4°C) for 15 min.. Pellets were washed 2 more times using 2 ml of RB + 1% BSA as resuspension buffer. Final pellets were counted in a gamma counter. Data were analyzed using a curvilinear Scatchard analysis computer program, ISIS-59. Each Scatchard binding analysis experiment was repeated 3 times. Significant differences were determined using analysis of variance followed by Duncan's multiple comparison test. P<0.05 was considered significant.

Results

Maximum binding capacity of membranes from granulosa cells of all three groups is shown in Figure 1. Granulosa from small and medium-sized follicles had maximum binding of about 36% of total counts added, whereas cells from large follicles reached a maximum of 47% of total counts. In order to perform Scatchard analysis of IGF-I binding sites, we used 3-5 µg membrane protein/tube (14-22% specific binding).

The displacement of ^{125}I-IGF-I from granulosa membranes of small and large follicles by IGF-I, IGF-II, or insulin is shown in Figure 2. The rank order of displacement potency

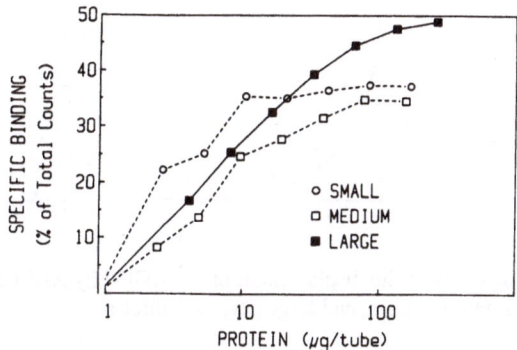

Fig. 1. Binding of ^{125}I-IGF-I to increasing membrane protein from granulosa cells of small, medium, and large porcine follicles.

was IGF-I > IGF-II > insulin. Curves were similar for membranes from granulosa of small or large follicles.

Characterization of IGF-I binding sites by Scatchard analysis is illustrated in Figure 3. Membranes from all three sizes of follicles gave curvilinear plots. Statistical analysis of binding sites is given in Table 1. Membranes from all three groups of granulosa cells had both high-affinity/low capacity and low-affinity/high capacity sites. During follicular maturation, there was no significant difference in the affinity and/or number of the high-affinity sites. Although there was no significant difference in the binding or affinity of the low-affinity receptors between the three groups, granulosal membranes from small follicles had slightly elevated levels of binding sites (P=0.06) of the low-affinity receptors compared with the other groups.

Discussion

The present study demonstrated that granulosa cells from small, medium, and large follicles have specific receptors for IGF-I. Cells from all three maturational groups also

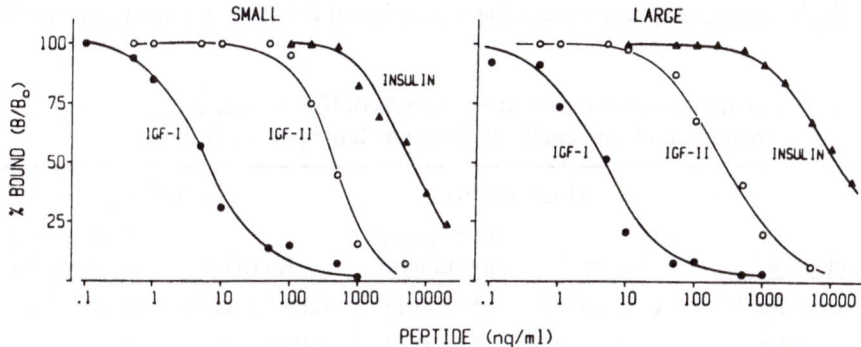

Fig 2. Displacement of ^{125}I-IGF-I by IGF-I, IGF-II, and insulin using granulosa membranes from small and large porcine follicles.

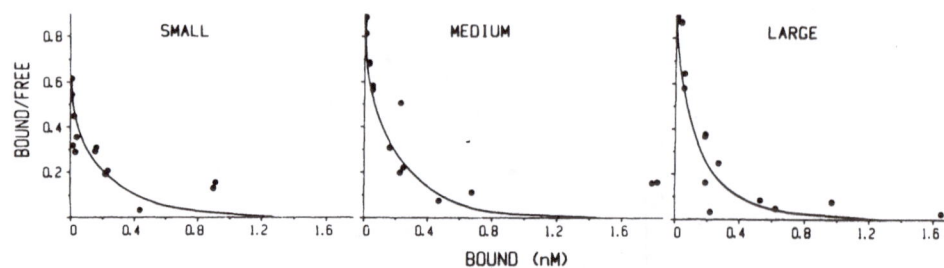

Fig. 3. Scatchard analysis of the displacement of ^{125}I-IGF-I by IGF-I from granulosa membranes from small, medium, and large porcine follicles.

demonstrated curvilinear Scatchard plots, indicating the presence of additional receptors with low affinity for IGF-I. These low-affinity receptors might be explained by (a) the possible existence of receptors for insulin and/or IGF-II (which have a low affinity for IGF-I); or, (b) negative cooperativity that might be exhibited by the type I receptor (14). Although specific receptors for insulin have been characterized on porcine and rat granulosa cells (5), type II receptors have only been identified in the rat (15). With high levels of insulin (20 μg/ml), a substantial amount of labeled IGF-I (>25%) remained bound to membranes (Fig. 2). However, lower levels of IGF-II (1 μg) displaced almost all of the labeled IGF-I from granulosal membranes. Thus, it seems highly likely that porcine granulosa cells possess type II receptors. Characterization of IGF-II receptors on porcine granulosa cells remains to be determined.

We also found some evidence that the low-affinity receptors for IGF-I on granulosa cells might change during follicular maturation. Granulosa cells from small follicles demonstrated slightly elevated levels of binding sites for the low-affinity receptor when compared with cells from medium and large follicles (Table 1). Since previous studies have shown no change in the number of receptors for insulin during follicular maturation (16), the possibility exists that type II receptors might be elevated in granulosa in the immature follicle.

Although mechanisms regulated by IGF-I are enhanced as the follicle matures, the present study rules out a change in type I receptor number and/or affinity as a cause. Since local production of IGF-I by granulosa cells can play a major part in the differentiation of these cells (8), another explanation of enhanced action of IGF-I during maturation could be

Table 1. Summary data of Scatchard analysis of IGF-I binding to granulosa membranes from small, medium, and large porcine follicles

	High Affinity		Low Affinity	
Follicle size	Ka (nM)	Sites (pmol/ mg protein)	Ka (nM)	Sites (pmol/ mg protein)
Small (<3 mm)	6.50 ± 0.09	1.51 ± 0.17	0.053 ± 0.008	20.40 ± 3.10
Medium (3-6 mm)	6.45 ± 0.44	1.15 ± 0.14	0.077 ± 0.019	13.76 ± 0.78
Large (>8 mm)	6.48 ± 0.44	1.40 ± 0.15	0.077 ± 0.007	12.99 ± 0.55

that granulosal secretion of IGF-I increases as the follicle matures. Hammond et al. (2) have shown that concentrations of IGF-I in porcine follicular fluid appear to increase as the follicle develops. Whether these follicular fluid levels are due to secretion by granulosa or theca remains to be determined.

Data from the present study, together with the fact that porcine theca cells contain specific receptors for IGF-I (4), suggest that modulation of follicular function by insulin and insulin-like growth factors is a complex process.

References

1. Hsu C-J, Hammond JM. Gonadotropins and estradiol stimulate immunoreactive insulin-like growth factor-I production by porcine granulosa cells in vitro. Endocrinology 1987; 120:198-207.
2. Hammond JM, Yoshida K, Veldhuis JD, Rechler M, Knight AP. Intrafollicular role of somatomedins: comparison with effects of insulin. In: Greenwald GS, Terranova PF, eds. Factors regulating ovarian function. New York: Raven Press, 1983:197-205.
3. Baranco JLS, Hammond JM. Comparative effects of insulin and insulin-like growth factors on DNA synthesis and differentiation of porcine granulosa cells. Biochem Biophys Res Commun 1984; 124:484-90.
4. Caubo B, Tonetta SA. Binding sites for IGF-I identified on theca cells from large porcine follicles. In: Hirshfield A, ed. Paracrine communication in the ovary—oncogenesis and growth factors. New York: Plenum Press (in press).
5. Adashi EY, Resnick CE, D'Ercole AJ, Svoboda ME, Van Wyk JJ. Insulin-like growth factors as intraovarian regulators of granulosa cell growth and function. Endocr Rev 1985; 6:400-20.
6. Caubo B, Tonetta SA. Growth factors modulate steroidogenesis in porcine theca cells [Abstract]. Society for the Study of Reproduction, Seattle, WA, 1988; 44.
7. Hammond JM, Baranao LS, Skaleris D, Knight AB, Romanus JA, Rechler MM. Production of insulin-like growth factors by ovarian granulosa cells. Endocrinology 1985; 117:2553-5.
8. Adashi EY, Resnick CE, Svoboda ME, Van Wyk JJ. A novel role for somatomedin-C in the cytodifferentiation of the ovarian granulosa cell. Endocrinology 1984; 115:1227-9.
9. Adashi EY, Resnick CE, Brodie AMH, Svoboda ME, Van Wyk JJ. Somatomedin-C mediated potentiation of follicle-stimulating hormone-induced aromatase activity of cultured rat granulosa cells. Endocrinology 1985; 117:2313-20.
10. Adashi EY, Resnick CE, Hernandez ER, et al. Insulin-like growth factor I as an amplifier of follicle stimulating hormone action: studies on mechanism(s) and site(s) of action in cultured rat granulosa cells. Endocrinology 1988; 122:1583-91.
11. Adashi EY, Resnick CE, Svoboda ME, Van Wyk JJ. Somatomedin-C enhances induction of luteinizing hormone receptor by follicle-stimulating hormone in cultured rat granulosa cells. Endocrinology 1984; 116:2369-75.
12. Hammond JM, Hsu C-J, Klindt J, Tsang BK, Downey BR. Gonadotropins increase concentrations of immunoreactive insulin like growth factor-I in porcine follicular fluid in vivo. Biol Reprod 1988; 38:304-8.
13. Lowry OH, Rosebrough NJ, Farr AL, Randall RJ. Protein measurement with the Folin phenol reagent. J Biol Chem 1951; 193:265-75.

14. De Meyts P, Roth J, Neville DM, Gavin JR, Lesniak MA. Insulin interaction with its receptor: experimental evidence for negative cooperativity. Bichem Biophys Res Commun 1973; 55:154-61.
15. Davoren JB, Kasson BG, Li CH, Hsueh AJW. Specific insulin-like growth factor (IGF) I- and II- binding sites on rat granulosa cells: relation to IGF action. Endocrinology 1986; 119:2155-62.
16. Otani T, Maruo T, Yukimura N, Mochizuki M. Effect of insulin on porcine granulosa cells: implications of a possible receptor mediated action. Acta Endocrinol (Copenh) 1985; 108:104-10.

14

Binding Sites for IGF-I Identified on Theca Cells from Large Porcine Follicles

Brigitte Caubo and Sharon A. Tonetta

Livingston Reproductive Biology Lab, University of Southern California Medical Center, Los Angeles, CA 90033

Abstract. Theca from large porcine follicles (>8mm) were examined for specific IGF-I binding sites. Thecal membranes were prepared and then incubated overnight at 4°C with ^{125}I-IGF-I with or without increasing concentrations of IGF-I, IGF-II and insulin. Specific high-affinity IGF-I binding sites were demonstrated. Scatchard analysis gave a curvilinear plot with a Ka for the high affinity sites of 1.97 ± 0.35 nM (binding capacity, 305.7 ± 37.2 fmol/mg protein). Preferential binding was IGF-I>IGF-II>insulin. Interestingly, IGFs modulate steroidogenesis in porcine theca cells with a similar order of potency. These data demonstrate high affinity, low capacity binding of IGF-I to porcine thecal membranes and suggest that IGF-I and related peptides act on thecal steroidogenesis through IGF-I receptors.

Introduction

Growth factors play an important role in the paracrine and/or autocrine regulation of follicular development (1). Insulin-like growth factors (IGFs) constitute a family of insulin-related polypeptide growth factors (IGF-I, IGF-II/MSA). IGF-I is secreted by granulosa cells (2,3). Estradiol and gonadotropins enhance secretion of IGF-I from porcine granulosa cells in vitro (4). Recently, the secretion of IGF-I by ovarian homogenates was increased by growth hormone (5). IGF-I in follicular fluid from porcine preovulatory follicles was significantly greater than levels in either follicular fluid of immature follicles or serum (6). Therefore, there appears to exist an autocrine loop for IGFs in the ovary since various aspects of granulosal function, including proliferation, are modulated by these factors (3). IGF-I can increase gonadotropin-induced synthesis of estrogen and progestin, and enhance FSH induction of granulosal LH/hCG receptors in the rat (7,8).

In addition to granulosa cells, theca cells play a major role in follicular steroidogenesis, and thecal steroidogenesis in large porcine follicles is altered by IGFs and insulin (9). Although this suggests that theca cells contain a type I receptor, the presence of receptors for IGF-I on porcine theca cells has not been demonstrated. In the present study, the binding of IGF-I to porcine thecal membranes from large follicles was examined.

Materials and Methods

Fresh porcine ovaries were obtained from a local abattoir. Follicular fluid was aspirated from large follicles (>8 mm) and the thecal layer was removed stereomicroscopically. Tissue was washed 3 times in buffer (Tris-HCl 0.025M, 1 µg/ml of Aprotinin, pH 7.4), minced with scissors, then gently digested with 0.2% type I collagenase (Sigma) for 1 h to remove any adhering granulosa cells (10). All subsequent experiments were performed on ice unless noted otherwise. After 3 more washes in buffer, tissue was homogenized in a glass tissue grinder and centrifuged at 5000 x g for 15 min. The pellet was weighed and suspended in buffer (Tris-HCl 0.025 M, 1 µg/ml Aprotinin, 1% BSA, pH 7.4). The protein content of the membrane homogenates was estimated using the method of Lowry et al. (11) with BSA as standard.

Binding experiments were conducted by incubating thecal membranes with ^{125}I-IGF-I (Amersham, Arlington Heights, IL; specific activity: 1938 Ci/mMol, 15000 cpm/tube) and increasing concentrations of IGF-I (0.1 ng/ml-1 µg/ml; Collaborative Research, Bedford, MA) in a final volume of 150 µl. The incubation was stopped by addition of 2 ml of ice cold buffer. The pellet was washed several times and radioactivity measured in a gamma counter. To assess specific binding, nonspecific binding (excess unlabeled hormone) was subtracted from total binding. Optimal conditions were determined and used for the rest of the assays.

For Scatchard analysis, the experiment was repeated 3 times and the binding competition data were analyzed using a curvilinear Scatchard analysis computer program: ISIS-59. To determine the binding specificity of the receptors, ^{125}I-IGF-I (15000 cpm/tube) was incubated with increasing amounts of IGF-I, IGF-II (MSA; Collaborative Research), or porcine insulin (Eli Lilly, Indianapolis, IN). The assay was performed as described above.

Results

Specific binding of ^{125}I-IGF-I on thecal membranes was assessed for time and temperature dependence. These data are summarized in Figure 1. Specific binding was significant at both 4°C and 24°C (25% and 22%, respectively) and appeared to reach a plateau at 8 h (24°C) and 4 h (4°C) of incubation. Nonspecific binding ranged from 20% at 4°C to 50% at 37°C (Figure 1A). Thus, optimal conditions (overnight incubation at 4°C) were used in subsequent experiments. The maximum binding capacity of the tissue was then examined (Figure 1B). Maximum specific binding was 32% for 285 µg of protein per tube. In further experiments, we incubated 17.7 µg protein/tube (10% specific binding).

Thecal membrane homogenates were incubated with ^{125}I-IGF-I and increasing concentrations of IGF-I (0.1 ng/ml-1 µg/ml), IGF-II (0.5 ng/ml-5 µg/ml), and insulin (100 ng/ml-33 µg/ml) (Figure 2). Insulin-related hormones competed for the binding sites on thecal membranes. The rank order of potency was IGF-I>IGF-II>insulin and the ED_{50}s were 10 ng/ml, 300 ng/ml, 10 µg/ml, respectively. Scatchard analysis gave a curvilinear plot (Figure 2, inset); the Ka of the high affinity site was 1.97 ± 0.35 nM with a binding capacity of 305.7 ± 37.2 fmol/mg protein (values for the low affinity site(s) were Ka = 0.042 ± 0.007 nM, binding capacity = 1594 ± 264.8 fmol/mg protein).

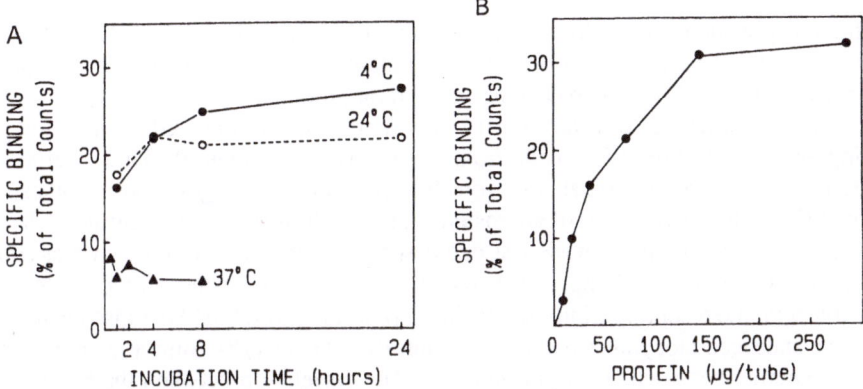

Fig. 1. (A) Time and temperature dependence of ^{125}I-IGF-I binding. (B) Maximum binding of ^{125}I-IGF-I on thecal membranes.

Discussion

The data reported here demonstrate the existence of specific IGF-I receptors on porcine theca cells from large follicles. IGF-II and insulin competed for the binding sites, but only at much higher concentrations than IGF-I (ED$_{50}$ for IGF-I = 300 ng/ml, for insulin = 10 µg/ml). The Scatchard analysis of the IGF-I binding data gave a curvilinear plot which can be explained by either the coexistence of IGF-II and/or insulin receptors or by negative cooperativity given the similarity between insulin and IGF-I receptors (12,13). Indeed, the presence of insulin receptors has been demonstrated on thecal/interstitial cells from human ovaries (14). Moreover, in our experiment, insulin at doses up to 33 µg/ml was unable to displace more than 70% of the ^{125}I-IGF-I from its binding sites. Since insulin does not bind to IGF-II receptors, these data strongly suggest the presence of IGF-II receptors on theca cells. Similarly, specific binding sites for IGF-I have been demonstrated on granulosa cells

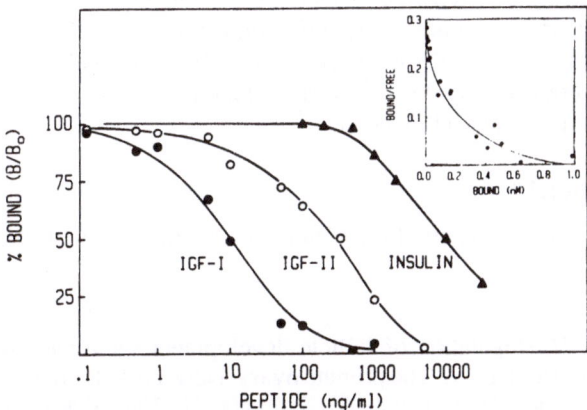

Fig. 2. Displacement of ^{125}I-IGF-I by IGF-I, IGF-II, and insulin on thecal membranes. Inset: Representation of a Scatchard analysis.

in the human, pig and rat, exhibiting the same rank order of affinities IGF-I>IGF-II>insulin (15-17); the order of potency of the peptides on granulosal function was similar (2). Specific binding sites for IGF-II have also been reported in rat granulosa cells (16).

In separate studies, our laboratory has also shown that IGFs can modulate steroidogenesis in cultured theca cells from large porcine follicles (9). Under serum-free conditions, IGFs increased basal and gonadotropin-induced progesterone synthesis. In addition, hCG-induced synthesis of androstenedione and testosterone was further enhanced by IGFs, whereas estradiol synthesis was decreased. The rank order of potency was similar to that found for receptor binding: IGF-I>IGF-II>insulin and the concentrations used were compatible with the receptor affinity shown in the present report. IGF-I has also been shown to enhance androgen biosynthesis in rat theca/interstitial cells (18). Similar data have been found on porcine theca cells using insulin (19). The correlation between the binding data and the biological activity of IGF-I on theca cells strongly suggests that the actions of IGF-I are mediated through a type I receptor. Thus, it appears that in addition to its autocrine activities on granulosa cells, IGF-I can act on theca cells to modulate ovarian steroidogenesis. Whether or not theca cells can themselves produce IGF-I is not yet known.

The IGF-I receptors on theca cells may play a role in polycystic ovary disease (PCO). In women, PCO is often associated with insulin resistance. Affected patients present hyperandrogenism, anovulation, and acanthosis nigricans. Interestingly, the postulated mechanisms for insulin resistance reside at the insulin receptor level, i.e., defect in insulin receptor binding or postreceptor binding events, or anti-insulin receptor autoantibodies (20,21). Because of their insulin resistance, these patients are often hyperinsulinemic. Since in this case the insulin receptor is not functional and insulin can bind to the IGF-I receptor, it is tempting to suggest that the high levels of insulin found in these patients may play a pathological role on ovarian steroidogenesis via binding to the thecal IGF-I receptor. Thus, insulin would synergize with LH to hyperstimulate theca cells to synthesize more androgens and then induce the secondary pathological findings of PCO. As proposed by Poretsky et al. (22), the androgen excess would induce follicular atresia with loss of estrogen-producing cells. Thus, androgen-producing cells would become predominant and could perpetuate the cycle by producing more androgens in response to insulin and LH.

In conclusion, the presence of specific high-affinity IGF-I receptors on thecal membranes was demonstrated. These data, together with recent evidence of IGF-I regulation of basal- and gonadotropin-induced thecal steroidogenesis (16), suggest that IGF-I modulates thecal as well as granulosal function.

Acknowledgments

B. Caubo supported by a grant from Communaute Francaise de Belgique.

References

1. Schomberg DW. Regulation of follicle development by gonadotropins and growth factors. In: Stouffer RL, ed. The primate ovary. New York: Plenum Press, 1988:25-34.
2. Adashi EY, Resnick CE, D'Ercole AJ, Svoboda ME, Van Wyk JJ. Insulin-like growth factors as intraovarian regulators of granulosa cells growth and function. Endocr Rev 1985; 6:400-20.

3. Hammond JM, Baranao JLS, Skaleris D, Knight AB, Romanus JA, Rechler MM. Production of insulin-like growth factors by ovarian granulosa cells. Endocrinology 1985; 117:2553-5.

4. Hsu CJ, Hammond JM. Gonadotropins and estradiol stimulate immunoreactive insulin-like growth factor-I production by porcine granulosa cells in vitro. Endocrinology 1987; 120:198-207.

5. Davoren JB, Hsueh JW. Growth hormone increases ovarian levels of immunoreactive somatomedin C/insulin-like growth factor I in vivo. Endocrinology 1986; 118:888-90.

6. Hammond JM, Hsu CJ, Klindt J, Tsang BK, Downey BR. Gonadotropins increase concentrations of immunoreactive insulin-like growth factor-I in porcine follicular fluid in vivo. Biol Reprod 1988; 38:304-8.

7. Adashi EY, Resnick CE, Hernandez ER, et al. Insulin-like growth factor I as an amplifier of follicle-stimulating hormone action; studies on mechanism(s) and site(s) of action in cultured rat granulosa cells. Endocrinology 1988; 122:1583-91.

8. Veldhuis JD, Rodgers RJ, Furlanetto RW, Azimi P, Juchter D, Garmey J. Synergistic actions of estradiol and the insulin-like growth factor somatomedin C on swine ovarian (granulosa) cells. Endocrinology 1986; 119:530-8.

9. Caubo B, Tonetta SA. Growth factors modulate steroidogenesis in porcine theca cells [Abstract]. Society for the Study of Reproduction, 1988:44.

10. Tonetta SA, De Vinna RS, diZerega GS. Modulation of porcine thecal cell aromatase activity by human chorionic gonadotropin, progesterone, estradiol-17B, and dihydrotestosterone. Biol Reprod 1986; 35:785-91.

11. Lowry OH, Rosebrough NJ, Farr AL, Randall RJ. Protein measurement with the folin-phenol reagent. J Biol Chem 1951; 193:265-75.

12. Nissley PS, Haskell JF, Sasaki N, De Vroede M, Rechler MM. Insulin-like growth factor receptors. J Cell Sci 1985; 3(suppl):39-51.

13. De Meyts P, Roth J, Neville DM, Gavin JR, Lesniak MA. Insulin interaction with its receptor: experimental evidence for negative cooperativity. Biochem Biophys Res Commun 1973; 55:154-61.

14. Poretsky L, Grigorescu F, Seibel M, Moses AC, Flier JS. Distribution and characterization of insulin and insulin-like growth factor I receptors in normal human ovary. Endocrinology 1985; 61:728-34.

15. Gates GS, Bayer S, Seibel M, Poretsky L, Flier JS, Moses AC. Characterization of insulin-like growth factor binding to human granulosa cells obtained during in vitro fertilization. J Recept Res 1987; 7:885-902.

16. Davoren BJ, Kasson BG, Li CH, Hsueh AJW. Specific insulin-like growth factors (IGF) I- and II-binding sites on rat granulosa cells: relation to IGF action. Endocrinology 1986; 2155-62.

17. Hylka VW, Caubo B, Tonetta SA. Analysis of binding sites for IGF-I on membranes of granulosa cells of small, medium and large porcine follicles. In: Hirshfield A, ed. Paracrine communication in the ovary—oncogenesis and growth factors. New York: Plenum Press (in press).

18. Hernandez ER, Resnick CE, Svoboda ME, Van Wyk JJ, Payne DW, Adashi EY. Somatomedin C/insulin-like growth factor I as an enhancer of androgen biosynthesis by cultured rat ovarian cells. Endocrinology 1988; 122:1603-12.

19. Barbieri RL, Makris A, Ryan KJ. Effects of insulin on steroidogenesis in cultured porcine ovarian theca. Fertil Steril 1983; 40:237-41.

20. Kahn CR, Flier JS, Bar RS, et al. The syndromes of insulin resistance and acanthosis nigricans. N Engl J Med 1976; 294:739-51.

21. Taylor SI, Dons RF, Hernandez E, Roth J, Gorden P. Insulin resistance associated with androgen excess in women with autoantibodies to the insulin receptor. Ann Intern Med 1982; 851-7.
22. Poretsky L, Kalin MF. The gonadotropic function of insulin. Endocr Rev 1987; 8:132-41.

15

The Role of Insulin-Like Growth Factors in Granulosa Cell Steroidogenesis: Studies with a Neutralizing Antibody to IGF-I

J. S. Mondschein, S. F. Canning, and J. M. Hammond

Department of Medicine, The Milton S. Hershey Medical Center
The Pennsylvania State University, Hershey, PA 17033

Summary

Evidence that granulosa cells secrete and respond to insulin-like growth factors (IGFs) suggests, but does not prove, the importance of IGFs as intraovarian regulators. To further assess the role of these peptides in ovarian function, we have employed a neutralizing monoclonal antibody to IGF-I to block the actions of IGFs in porcine follicular fluid and in granulosa cell-conditioned medium. Granulosa cells from immature porcine follicles were cultured in medium containing follicular fluid from large (6-10 mm) porcine follicles which had been charcoal stripped to remove steroids. Granulosa cells cultured with follicular fluid produced five- to twentyfold more progesterone than did those cultured with charcoal-treated porcine serum. However, for granulosa cells treated with the blocking antibody, follicular fluid-stimulated progesterone production was inhibited 67%. Granulosa cells were also cultured without exogenous growth factors; the effects of FSH, estradiol, GH, and combinations thereof on progesterone production were inhibited by 45-76% by the antibody. The stimulatory effect of follicular fluid on ^{3H}-thymidine incorporation in granulosa cell cultures was reduced by only 12% by the antibody. These results suggest that the stimulatory effects of follicular fluid and hormones on progesterone production are mediated, at least in part, by IGFs. Under these culture conditions, ovarian IGFs appear to be more important to cytodifferentiation than to replication.

Introduction

Evidence from a number of laboratories suggests that IGFs are important autocrine/paracrine regulators in the ovary (reviewed in 1). Granulosa cells of several species possess receptors for IGFs and respond to IGFs with stimulation of many growth and differentiation-related endpoints. Ovarian follicular fluid (FF) contains abundant quantities of IGFs. In addition, we have recently shown that granulosa cells produce IGF-I in culture and that the production of IGF-I can be regulated by gonadotropins, estradiol (E_2, 2), growth hormone (GH, 3) and growth factors (4,5). More definitive proof for an autocrine/paracrine role of IGFs in the ovary requires the demonstration of a direct linkage between the presence and action of ovarian IGFs. In the present report, we have used a neutralizing monoclonal antibody to IGF-I (6,7) in the porcine granulosa cell system to demonstrate a role for ovarian IGFs in the stimulation of progesterone production by FF, FSH, E_2 and GH, and in the stimulation of [3H]-thymidine incorporation by FF.

Methods

The hormones used for these studies included FSH (NIDDK oFSH-16) and GH (NIDDK oGH-14) from the National Hormone and Pituitary Program and estradiol from Sigma. Recombinant human IGF-I was from Amgen. A second IGF preparation was from Dr. R. Humbel, Zurich (lot 1932, contains both IGFs I and II in approximately equal amounts). The antibodies used were a monoclonal antibody to IGF-I (Sm 1.2B, Dr. J. Van Wyk, University of North Carolina, Chapel Hill) and a control monoclonal antibody, MOPC 21, from Sigma. The MOPC 21 preparation was dialyzed prior to use to remove the azide preservative. Epidermal growth factor (EGF, receptor grade) was from Collaborative Research.

Granulosa cells were isolated from small (1-3 mm) follicles of immature ovaries (7). The effects of FF on progesterone production were studied using experimental paradigms similar to those of Ledwitz-Rigby et al. (8). Granulosa cells were seeded (1.5x10E6 viable cells/well) in medium supplemented with porcine serum (30% v/v, Sigma) or FF (30% v/v) from large (6-10 mm) porcine follicles which had been treated with dextran-coated charcoal to remove steroids. Treatments with the monoclonal antibodies were begun with the 3-day medium change. Cultures were terminated on day 5. Medium from days 3 to 5 was analyzed for progesterone by RIA (7). In a second series of experiments, granulosa cells were seeded (2.25-3x10E6 viable cells/well) in a serum-free culture medium containing insulin (300 mU/ml) and platelet extract (2.5% v/v) (7). At the day 3 medium change, insulin was removed and treatments with hormones and Sm 1.2B were begun. At the day 5 medium change, platelet extract was removed and the hormone and antibody treatments continued. Cultures were terminated on day 7, and medium from days 5 to 7 was analyzed for progesterone. The incorporation of [3H]-thymidine into DNA was determined as previously described (5) with growth factors, FF and antibody treatments begun after a 30-h period of serum deprivation. All data were normalized by cell counts determined at the end of culture.

Results

The effects of Sm 1.2B on the production of progesterone by granulosa cells cultured with FF is shown in Figure 1. The monoclonal antibody had a significant inhibitory effect on progesterone production at a dilution of 1:5000. Further inhibition by lesser dilutions of the antibody was not significant. In a series of 7 experiments using a 1:500 dilution of Sm 1.2B, progesterone production was inhibited by 67.2% ± 6.3%. In agreement with the findings of Ledwitz-Rigby et al. (8), we observed rates of progesterone production by granulosa cells cultured with FF from large follicles to be markedly greater than those observed with serum (Fig. 1). The blocking antibody was not able to suppress progesterone production to levels observed in serum. The inhibitory effect of Sm 1.2B could be overcome by the addition of 500 ng/ml IGFs but not by 100 ng/ml (Fig. 2). In the absence of the monoclonal antibody, addition of 100 ng/ml IGFs did not further enhance progesterone production, suggesting that the levels of IGFs in FF are saturating. A biphasic dose-response relationship for IGFs is suggested by the observation that progesterone production is impaired by IGFs at 500 ng/ml. The inhibitory effect of Sm 1.2B was found to be specific for this antibody since a monoclonal antibody of the same subtype, IgGl kappa, with no known antigenic specificity, MOPC 21, did not inhibit progesterone production (Fig. 2).

Using the anti-IGF antibody, we have also demonstrated a role for IGFs produced by granulosa cells in culture. In these experiments, cultures were made dependent on endogenously produced growth factors. Granulosa cell cultures were initiated in medium supplemented with insulin and platelet extract. These supplements were withdrawn as cultures were treated with hormones with and without Sm 1.2B. We found that progesterone production stimulated by FSH, E_2, GH and combinations thereof was inhibited from 45 to 76% by Sm 1.2B (Table 1).

In addition to investigating the role of ovarian IGFs on the differentiated function of granulosa cells, we have probed the role of IGFs on granulosa cell growth using the blocking antibody in a [3H]-thymidine incorporation protocol. We have found that [3H]-thymidine incorporation is relatively insensitive to stimulation by single growth factors and that the highest levels of incorporation are observed with growth factor combinations and complex mixtures such as FF (7, and Table 2). Sm 1.2B produced a slight (12%) but significant inhibition of [3H]-thymidine incorporation stimulated by FF. We were unable to demonstrate

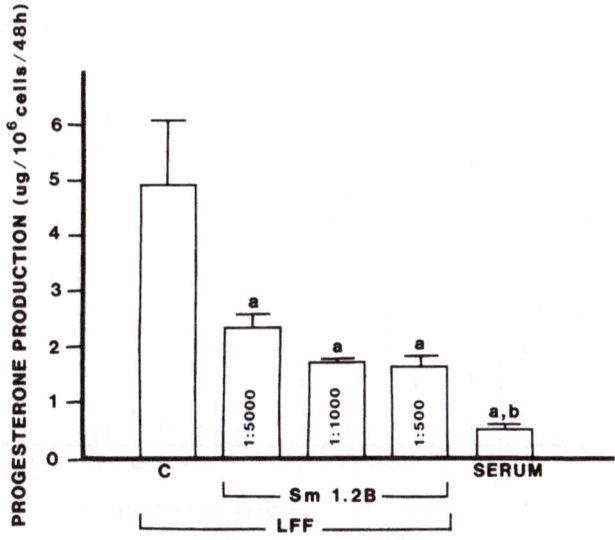

Fig. 1. Effects of a monoclonal antibody to IGF-I (Sm 1.2B) on progesterone production. Granulosa cells were cultured with pig serum or fluid from large porcine follicles (LFF) as described in Methods. Treatments with the indicated concentrations of antibody were begun at the day 3 medium change. Data are the means ± SE of quadruplicate cultures. a, P<.05 vs. control (C); b, P<.05 vs. other treatments.

Table 1. Effects of a monoclonal antibody to IGF-I (Sm 1.2B) on progesterone
production by porcine granulosa cells cultured in defined medium

Treatment		Progesterone Production (ng/10E6 cells/48 h)	
		No Antibody	Sm 1.2b(1:500)
Experiment A	Control	17 ± 1	16 ± 1
	FSH (200 ng/ml)	95 ± 13 a,c	36 ± 5 a,b,c
	E_2 (1 μg/ml)	79 ± 9 a,c	36 ± 1 a,b,c
	FSH + E_2	588 ± 61 a	276 ± 16 a,b,d
Experiment B	Control	38 ± 2	46 ± 13
	FSH + E_2	2264 ± 391 a,d	1271 ± 124 a,b
	GH (100 ng/ml)	222 ± 27 a,d	94 ± 7 a,b,d
	FSH + E_2 + GH	3492 ± 67 a	1659 ± 167 a,b

Granulosa cell cultures were initiated in supplemented medium, then cultured in defined
medium as described in Methods. Hormone and antibody treatments were begun with
the day 3 medium change. Data are the means ± SE of sextuplicate cultures. a, P<.05 vs.
control; b, P<.05 vs. no antibody; c, P<.05 vs. FSH + E_2 + GH.

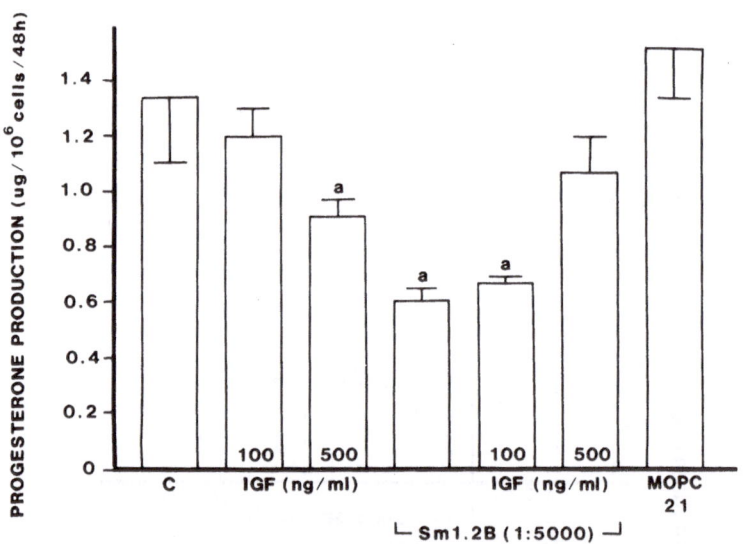

Fig. 2. Specificity of the inhibitory effect of Sm 1.2B on progesterone
production. Granulosa cells were cultured with fluid from large porcine
follicles (LFF) as described in Methods. Treatment with Sm 1.2B, MOPC 21
(9 μg protein/ml, equal to Sm 1.2B at 1:5000), and the indicated concentrations of IGF (Humbel 1932) were begun at the day 3 medium change. Data
are the means ± SE of sextuplicate cultures. a, P<.05 vs. control (C).

Table 2. Effect of a monoclonal antibody to IGF-I (Sm 1.2B) on [3H]-thymidine incorporation in porcine granulosa cell cultures

Treatment	[3H]-Thymidine Incorporated (cpm/10E6 cells)	
	No Antibody	SM 1.2B (1:500)
Control	226 ± 33	367 ± 16
Insulin (100 mU/ml)	387 ± 39	468 ± 71
IGF-I (10 ng/ml)	500 ± 32 a	596 ± 5 a
EGF (10 ng/ml)	1398 ± 90 a	1458 ± 119 a
LEF (3% v/v)	4667 ± 85 a	4119 ± 34 a,b

Granulosa cells were cultured as described in Methods with treatments begun after a 30-h period of serum deprivation. Follicular fluid from large porcine follicles (LFF) was not charcoal treated. Data are the means ± SE of quadruplicate cultures. a, $P<.05$ vs. control; b, $P<.05$ vs. no antibody.

the predicted inhibition of IGF-I stimulated [3H]-thymidine incorporation with Sm 1.2B, in part because the single growth factor was such a weak stimulator, and also, perhaps, because the antibody, as a nutrient source, had a tendency to stimulate [3H]-thymidine incorporation in the more spartan cultures.

Discussion

Although it has been recognized for nearly 10 years that FF from large follicles stimulates steroidogenesis, the identity of the stimulatory principle(s) has remained elusive (8). Since follicular fluid contains high levels of IGFs, we hypothesized that the stimulatory effect of FF might involve IGFs, at least in part. Our studies showing inhibition of FF-stimulated progesterone production by Sm 1.2B support this hypothesis. At present, our studies do not distinguish between the actions of FF IGFs and the actions of other FF factors which may enhance the action of IGFs or their production by granulosa cells. Because Sm 1.2B has approximately 50% cross-reactivity with IGF-II (10), it is not possible to distinguish between the actions of the 2 IGFs. For granulosa cells cultured in defined medium devoid of exogenous growth factors, FSH-, E_2-, and GH-stimulated progesterone production was markedly attenuated by Sm 1.2B, suggesting that the actions of these hormones is mediated, at least in part, by IGFs. That hormone-stimulated progesterone production could not be completely blocked by the anti-IGF antibody suggests that these hormones have actions independent of the IGFs and supports the concept of IGFs as amplifiers of the actions of other hormones (11). In contrast to the marked influence on differentiated function, the IGFs appeared to play a less important role in cell replication in these studies. Cell number was not influenced by Sm 1.2B (data not shown) and FF-stimulated [3H]-thymidine incorporation was inhibited only 12% by the antibody. Our studies provide the most conclusive evidence available supporting the concept of IGFs as autocrine/paracrine regulators in the ovary.

References

1. Adashi EY, Resnick CE, D'Ercole AJ, Svoboda ME, Van Wyk JJ. Insulin-like growth factors as intraovarian regulators. Endocr Rev 1985; 6:400-20.
2. Hsu CJ, Hammond JM. Gonadotropins and estradiol stimulate immunoreactive insulin-like growth factor-I production by porcine granulosa cells in vitro. Endocrinology 1987; 120:198-207.
3. Hsu CJ, Hammond JM. Concomitant effects of growth hormone on secretion of insulin-like growth factor I and progesterone by cultured porcine granulosa cells. Endocrinology 1987; 121:1343-8.
4. Mondschein JS, Hammond JM. Growth factors regulate immunoreactive insulin-like growth factor-I production by cultured porcine granulosa cells. Endocrinology 1988 (in press).
5. Mondschein JS, Canning SF, Hammond JM. Effects of transforming growth factor beta on the production of immunoreactive insulin-like growth factor-I and progesterone and on ^{3}H-thymidine incorporation in porcine granulosa cell cultures. Endocrinology 1988 (in press).
6. Burch WM, Weir S, Van Wyk JJ. Embryonic chick cartilage produces its own somatomedin-like peptide to stimulate cartilage growth in vitro. Endocrinology 1986; 119:1370-6.
7. Baranao JLS, Hammond JM. Multihormone regulation of steroidogenesis in cultured porcine granulosa cells: studies in serum-free medium. Endocrinology 1985; 116:2143-51.
8. Ledwitz-Rigby F, Petito SH, Tyner JK, Rigby BW. Follicular fluid effects on progesterone secretion are not due to follicle-stimulating hormone steroids. Biol Reprod 1985; 33:277-85.
9. Hammond JM, English HF. Regulation of deoxyribonucleic acid synthesis in cultured porcine granulosa cells by growth factors and hormones. Endocrinology 1987; 120:1039-46.
10. Han VKM, Hill DJ, Strain AJ, et al. Identification of somatomedin/insulin-like growth factor immunoreactive cells in the human fetus. Pediatr Res 1987; 22:245-9.
11. Veldhuis JD, Demers LM. A role for somatomedin C as a differentiating hormone and amplifier of hormone action on ovarian cells: studies with synthetically pure somatomedin C and swine granulosa cells. Biochem Biophys Res Commun 1985; 130:234-40.

16

Insulin-Like Growth Factor-I Regulates Δ5-3β-Hydroxysteroid Dehydrogenase Activity in Rat Granulosa Cells

James J. Bendell and Jennifer H. Dorrington

Banting and Best Department of Medical Research,
University of Toronto, Toronto, Ontario, Canada, M5G 1L6

Abstract. The objectives of this study were: (1) to examine the role of insulin-like growth factor-I (IGF-I) in the regulation of Δ5-3β-hydroxysteroid dehydrogenase (3β-HSD) in cultures of rat granulosa cells; and, (2) to determine if IGF-I was secreted by granulosa cells. Granulosa cells were isolated from 25-day-old diethylstilbestrol-primed rats and cultured under serum-free conditions. The 3β-HSD activity was measured by the conversion of [^{3}H]pregnenolone to [^{3}H]progesterone by granulosa cell sonicates under optimal conditions. Cells cultured in the presence of FSH for 48 h had elevated levels of 3β-HSD activity. Both insulin and IGF-I alone stimulated 3β-HSD activity and augmented the actions of FSH. The concentrations of insulin required to stimulate 3β-HSD were higher than physiological levels, whereas the concentrations of IGF-I were consistent with those found in follicular fluid. This suggested that IGF-I may play a physiological role in the regulation of 3β-HSD. Since growth factors usually act on cells in close proximity to their site of production, we looked for biological activity in conditioned medium generated by primary cultures of rat granulosa cells under serum-free conditions. The biological activity of the conditioned medium was similar to that described for IGF-I, in that it augmented the actions of FSH on aromatase activity and also acted alone in the absence of FSH to stimulate 3β-HSD activity. When granulosa cell-secreted proteins were separated by chromatography on a Sephadex G75 column, a peak of IGF-I immunoreactivity was found at 7,000 da corresponding to commercially available ^{125}I-IGF-I passed through the same column. In conclusion, the secretion of IGF-I by rat granulosa cells in culture and its actions on 3β-HSD suggest that the production and accumulation of IGF-I in follicular fluid may be important in the regulation of steroidogenesis during follicular development.

Introduction

The changes that take place in the ovary during each estrous cycle can be divided into the follicular and the luteal phase of growth and development. The LH surge is responsible for the initiation of luteinization of the cells of the follicle which then give rise to the corpus luteum. The acquisition of the ability to synthesize progesterone from cholesterol is necessary in order for a follicle to form a competent corpus luteum. Progesterone is formed from cholesterol by two enzyme systems; first, the cholesterol side-chain cleavage complex converts cholesterol to pregnenolone and secondly, $\Delta 5$-3β–hydroxysteroid dehydrogenase (3β-HSD) and $\Delta 5$-3-ketosteroid-isomerase convert pregnenolone to progesterone. Both of these enzyme systems are under hormonal regulation (1). FSH stimulates cholesterol side-chain cleavage activity in immature rat granulosa cells, and this is further enhanced by concomitant treatment with androgens, testosterone and dihydrotestosterone (2). FSH also stimulates 3β-HSD activity in immature rat granulosa cells but this activity does not appear to be modulated by androgens (1). In addition to FSH, other hormones such as gonadotropin releasing hormone (GnRH), epidermal growth factor (EGF) and insulin can influence progesterone synthesis (3-5). Of particular interest was the action of insulin since it was able to influence progesterone synthesis at a number of different sites, including cholesterol side-chain cleavage and the binding, internalization, and degradation of low density lipoprotein (6,7).

In this paper we have measured 3β-HSD activity under optimal conditions in cell sonicates of granulosa cells after treatment with insulin and IGF-I. This approach minimizes many of the possible sources of regulation by soluble cytoplasmic factors, thus allowing the amount of active enzyme to be estimated. Having established the modulatory effects of IGF-I and insulin on the 3β-HSD enzyme, we used a radioimmunoassay that was specific for IGF-I to identify the presence of IGF-I in the conditioned medium generated by rat granulosa cells cultured under serum-free conditions.

Materials and Methods

Ovine FSH (NIDDK oFSH-17; 2Ox NIH FSH S12 by the hCG augmentation bioassay of Steelman-Pohley) was provided by the National Hormone and Pituitary Program, NIDDK. Bovine insulin was purchased from Sigma Chemical Company (St. Louis, MO). ^{125}I-IGF-I, [7-^{3}H]pregnenolone and [^{14}C]progesterone were obtained from New England Nuclear, Boston, MA. Recombinant IGF-I was purchased from Kabigen, Stockholm, Sweden, while the specific antiserum to IGF-I (UB 286) was a gift of Drs. L. Underwood and J. Van Wyk, Division of Pediatric Endocrinology, University of North Carolina at Chapel Hill, and the National Hormone and Pituitary Program.

Immature Wistar Crl: (W1) BR rats were obtained from Charles River Canada (Montreal, Canada) and maintained with their mothers under conditions of controlled light and temperature. They were treated daily for 4 days with 1 mg diethylstilbestrol (DES) in 0.1 ml sesame oil by sc injection, killed at 25 days of age and the granulosa cells were prepared and plated as previously described (8). Addition of hormones was made 3 h after plating the cells at which time the cells were attaching to the culture surface. The medium was changed after 24 h and the cells were retreated with the appropriate hormones. For the generation of conditioned medium, granulosa cell suspensions were plated into 35-mm culture dishes in the presence of 10% calf serum for 24 h. The medium was discarded and the cells were washed with culture medium and maintained a further 24 h in the absence of serum. The medium was then replaced and conditioned medium was collected over three consecutive 48-h culture periods.

Preparation of Cell Sonicates and Enzyme Assay for Δ5-3β-Hydroxysteroid Dehydrogenase Activity

After 48 h, the medium was removed and the cell monolayers were washed twice with 1 ml phosphate-buffered saline at room temperature. The cells were disrupted by sonication and the activity of 3β-HSD was measured from the conversion of [^{3}H]pregnenolone to [^{3}H]progesterone under optimal conditions for the enzyme system (5).

Fractionation of Granulosa Cell-Conditioned Medium and RIA for IGF-I

Granulosa cell-conditioned medium (9 ml) was lyophilized and resuspended in 1.5 ml of 1.0 M acetic acid. Following a 1-h incubation at 37°C, the sample was centrifuged for 5 min at 10,000 g and the supernatant loaded onto a 75 cm x 1 cm Sephadex G-75 superfine column and eluted with 1 M acetic acid. The resulting 1.25 ml fractions were lyophilized and resuspended in 300 μl of RIA buffer with gentle agitation. Duplicate 50 μl aliquots of each fraction were assayed for IGF-I using the RIA assay procedure provided by Drs. Underwood and Van Wyk with the following modifications. Samples (also a standard curve of triplicate IGF-I samples from 0-1,000 pg/tube) were brought to a volume of 100 μl with RIA buffer in 12 x 75 mm silica tubes and preincubated in a volume of 450 μl for 24 h with IGF-I antiserum (1:8,000 in 500 μl RIA buffer). 50 μl of ^{125}I-IGF-I (approximately 10,000 cpm) in RIA buffer was added to each sample and, following a further 24-h incubation, the secondary antibody (anti-rabbit IgG, 1:8,000 in 500 μl RIA buffer) was added. At the completion of the final 24-h incubation, the volume of the incubates was brought to 3 ml with RIA buffer containing normal rabbit serum at a final dilution of 1:2,000. After a 30-min incubation, the samples were centrifuged for 1 h at 4,000 g, the supernatant removed and the precipitated radioactivity counted in a gamma counter. All incubations were conducted at 4°C.

Results and Discussion

Granulosa cells isolated from DES-primed immature rats and cultured for 48 h in serum-free medium had low levels of 3β-HSD activity as assessed by the conversion of [^{3}H]pregnenolone to [^{3}H]progesterone by cell sonicates incubated under optimal conditions for the enzyme complex. Cells cultured in the presence of FSH (5 ng/ml) for 48 h had an elevated level of 3β-HSD activity. Treatment with insulin (5 μg/ml) or with IGF-I (0.1 μg/ml) alone significantly stimulated 3β-HSD and these effects were augmented in the presence of a suboptimal concentration of FSH (5 ng/ml) (Fig. 1A).

To determine the range of concentrations of insulin that are effective in stimulating 3β-HSD, granulosa cells were cultured with levels of insulin ranging from 0.05 to 5 μg/ml. Insulin was minimally effective at 0.1 μg/ml and approached maximal response at 1 μg/ml (Fig. 1B). The dose-response curve for the effects of insulin on 3β-HSD was similar to that shown for the effects on fibronectin secretion (5). The high levels of insulin required to influence cytodifferentiation in granulosa cells suggest that insulin may be interacting at low affinity with IGF-I receptors and that IGF-I may be important from a physiological standpoint. Several lines of evidence support this hypothesis. Granulosa cells from a number of different species contain IGF-I receptors and IGF-I can promote the proliferation and cytodifferentiation of granulosa cells in vitro (9). Whereas the effective concentrations of insulin were supraphysiological, the levels of IGF-I required to stimulate both growth and differentiation of granulosa cells were within the physiological range (5). The dose-response curves (Fig. 1B) showed that although the concentration of insulin required to stimulate 3β-HSD activity were higher than those found physiologically in the follicle, the levels of IGF-I needed were comparable with those documented by Hammond in porcine follicular fluid (63 ng/ml in medium follicles [<3 mm] to 104 ng/ml in large follicles [>6 mm]) (10).

In contrast to the endocrine hormones, growth factors elicit their effects on cells that are in close proximity to their site of production. The concept of a short-range mode of action for IGF-I in the ovary led us to look for IGF-I-like bioactivity in the conditioned medium from rat granulosa cells cultured under serum-free conditions. The conditioned medium generated by rat granulosa cells augmented the actions of FSH on aromatase activity and was able to independently stimulate 3β-HSD activity, indicating the presence of IGF-I-like activity. To further characterize the IGF-I-like bioactivity, the peptides in the rat granulosa cell-conditioned medium were fractionated by elution through a Sephadex G-75 column. The fractions of secreted peptides were assayed for IGF-I using a radioimmunoassay. A peak of immunoreactive IGF-I was detected in fractions containing peptides with an apparent molecular weight of 7,000. This peak coincided with the location of ^{125}I-IGF-I fractionated under identical conditions (Fig. 2).

The data presented support our earlier observation that IGF-I is secreted by rat granulosa cells (5). It has been shown previously that IGF-I augments FSH-induced aromatase in rat granulosa cells, stimulates the proliferation of bovine, human and porcine granulosa cells and stimulates progesterone synthesis by rat and porcine granulosa cells (reviewed in 9). We have extended these observations further by showing that IGF-I alone stimulated 3β-HSD activity in rat granulosa cells.

This study reinforces our hypothesis that the dominant follicle acquires autonomy by generating mechanisms to amplify the signals received from LH and FSH (5). IGF-I is a growth factor synthesized by the follicle that can increase the number of granulosa cells and

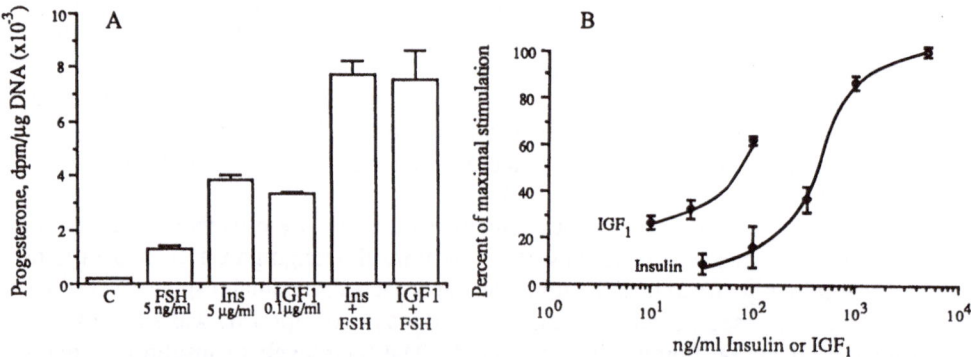

Fig. 1. Δ5-3β-HSD activity in rat granulosa cells cultured with 5 μg/ml insulin, 0.1 μg/ml IGF-I with or without 5 ng/ml FSH (A) and Δ5-3β-HSD activity in response to various concentrations of insulin or IGF-I expressed as the percent of the maximal stimulation obtained with insulin (5 μg/ml) (B). The error bars represent the standard error of triplicate samples and are representative of three independent experiments. (C, control.)

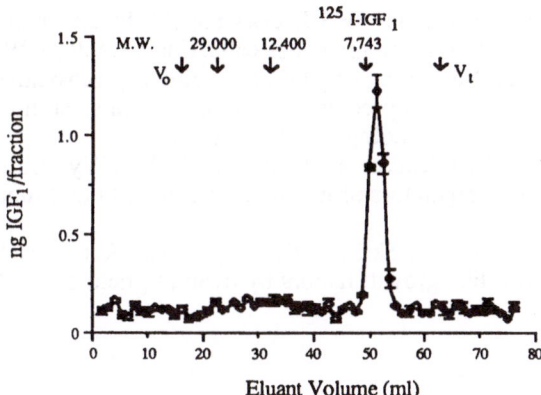

Fig. 2. Immunoreactive IGF-I present in concentrated rat granulosa cell-conditioned medium fractionated on a 75 x 1 cm Sephadex G-75 Superfine column eluted with 1 M acetic acid. IGF-I was detected using an IGF-I-specific RIA as described in Materials and Methods. The column was calibrated under identical running conditions using blue dextran (2,000 kda) at the void volume (Vo), carbonic anhydrase (29 kda), cytochrome c (12.4 kda), ^{125}I-IGF-I (7.7 kda) and N-3,5-DNPyr-glycine (242 da) for the total volume (Vt).

also stimulate differentiated functions, thereby amplifying the signals received from the gonadotropins. Through the follicular production of IGF-I and other peptides, the actions of the gonadotropins can be modulated at the level of the individual follicle. This mechanism of local control allows the coexistence of follicles at the various stages of development that are observed in the adult mammalian ovary.

Acknowledgments

The authors wish to thank H. McKeracher for excellent technical assistance.

References

1. Armstrong DT, Dorrington JH. Androgens augment FSH-induced progesterone secretion by cultured rat granulosa cells. Endocrinology 1976; 99:1411-4.
2. Dorrington JH, Armstrong DT. Effects of FSH on gonadal function. Recent Prog Horm Res 1979; 35:301-42.
3. Jones PBC, Hsueh AJW. Direct stimulation of progesterone metabolizing enzyme by gonadotropin-releasing hormone in cultured granulosa cells. J Biol Chem 1981; 256:1248-54.
4. Jones PBC, Welsh TH Jr, Hsueh AJW. Regulation of ovarian progestin production by EGF in cultured rat granulosa cells. J Biol Chem 1982; 257:11268-73.
5. Dorrington JH, Bendell JJ, Chuma A, Lobb DK. Actions of growth factors in the follicle. J Steroid Biochem 1987; 27:405-11.
6. Veldhuis J, Kolp LA, Toaff ME, Strauss JF III, Demmers LM. Mechanisms subserving the trophic actions of insulin on ovarian cells. In vitro studies using swine granulosa cells. J Clin Invest 1983; 72:1046-57.

7. Veldhuis J, Nestler JE, Strauss JF III, Gwynne JT. Insulin regulates low density lipoprotein metabolism by swine granulosa cells. Endocrinology 1986; 118:2242-53.
8. Dorrington JH, Moon YS, Armstrong DT. Estradiol-17β biosynthesis in cultured rat granulosa cells from hypophysectomized immature rats: stimulation by follicle-stimulating hormone. Endocrinology 1975; 97:1328-32.
9. Adashi EY, Resnick CE, D'Ercole AJ, Svoboda ME, Van Wyk JJ. Insulin-like growth factors as intraovarian regulators of granulosa cell growth and function. Endocr Rev 1985; 6:400-20.
10. Hammond JM, Baranao LS, Skaleris D, Knight AB, Romanus JA, Rechler MM. Production of insulin-like growth factors by ovarian granulosa cells. Endocrinology 1985; 117:2553-5.

17

Steroidogenic Effect of Insulin May Not Be Mediated Through Somatomedin-C/IGF-I Receptors

A. D. Gooneratne, P. A. Thacker, B. Laarveld, B. D. Murphy*
and K. Rajkumar*

Department of Animal and Poultry Science and *Department of
Obstetrics and Gynecology, University of Saskatchewan,
Saskatoon, Saskatchewan, Canada S7N OWO

Introduction

Insulin and Somatomedin-C/insulin-like growth factor-I (IGF-I) are capable of eliciting selective differentiative changes in ovarian granulosa cells of several species including growth promotion, enhanced steroidogenesis and induction of luteinizing hormone (LH) receptors (1-3). Insulin and IGF-I can also amplify the stimulatory effects of classical ovarian effector hormones and low-density lipoproteins (LDL) on progesterone (P4) biosynthesis in ovarian cells (3-5). IGF-I receptors have recently been shown to be present, and it is possible that the action of insulin may be mediated through the IGF-I receptors (2).

In the present study we compared the modulatory effects of insulin and IGF-I on the follicle-stimulating hormone (FSH)-induced responses in porcine granulosa cells under different culture conditions and further determined if the action of insulin is mediated through IGF-I receptors. Growth hormone (GH), which has been previously shown to stimulate ovarian IGF-I secretion (6), was included for comparative purposes.

Materials and Methods

Cell Cultures

Granulosa cells were collected by fine needle aspiration of medium follicles (3-5 mm) from nonpregnant sows at slaughter. The cells were recovered by centrifugation (200 x g), and approximately 2×10^6 viable cells were cultured in plastic multiwell plates, either in the presence or absence of 1% fetal bovine serum (FBS). The culture medium consisted of Eagle's minimum essential medium (MEM, Gibco) buffered with bicarbonate and HEPES (pH 7.4) containing penicillin (100 IU/ml), streptomycin (100 µg/ml) and Fungizone®

(1 μg/ml). To some culture wells, either 20 or 200 ng/ml porcine FSH was added on the day of plating. After 48 h (day 3), the medium was replaced with serum-free media with the same doses of FSH. To these cultures, either 100 ng/ml of insulin (Sigma), IGF-I (receptor grade, Imcera), porcine GH or no hormone was added. On day 5, the media was replaced with serum-free media with the same hormones included in the culture medium and LDL (100 μg) was provided as a substrate. Media was collected 24 h later for P4 estimation (7) and the cells were detached from the wells for protein estimation (8).

IGF-I Binding Studies

Granulosa cells (1×10^7) were incubated with saturating concentrations of $[^{125}I]IGF\text{-}I$ (1.1×10^5 cpm; 160 μCi/μg) in the presence or absence of increasing concentrations of either IGF-I or insulin (0.1 ng to 1.0 μg) in a final volume of 1 ml MEM containing 1% BSA. Following a 2-h incubation at 4°C, the cells were washed thrice in ice cold phosphate-buffered saline and the cell-associated radioactivity was counted. Scatchard plots were used to determine binding capacity and affinity (9).

Results

Granulosa cells exposed to 1% FBS during the initial 48 h of culture secreted 14.05 ± 0.88 ng P4/mg protein. The addition of insulin, but not IGF-I or GH, significantly enhanced P4 secretion to 49.73 ± 2.88 ng/mg protein (P<0.001). When LDL was provided as a substrate, P4 secretion increased threefold in all the cultures. In the presence of 20 or 200 ng FSH, P4 secretion was further increased 1.7- and twentyfold, respectively. The response to FSH was further increased in the presence of insulin, but not IGF-I, under these culture conditions (P<0.001, Fig. 1).

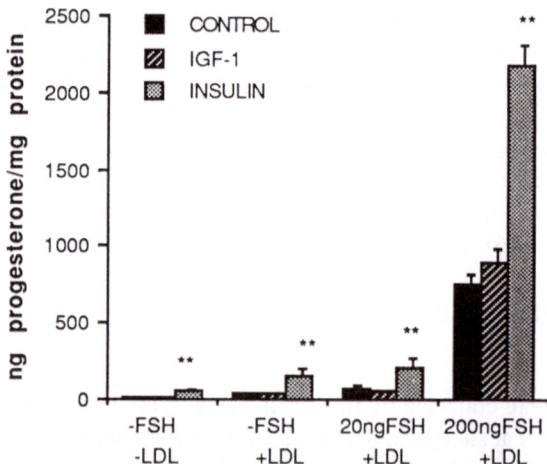

Fig. 1. Progesterone secretion by porcine granulosa cells plated with 1% FBS. Effect of treatment with insulin and IGF-I in the presence or absence of 20 or 200 ng FSH and 100 μg LDL. Significantly different from control, ** P<0.001.

Granulosa cells cultured in serum-free media from the time of plating secreted less P4 (0.78 ± 0.05 ng/mg protein) compared to cultures plated with 1% FBS during the initial 48 h (Figures 1 and 2). In the absence of FSH, insulin stimulated a significant increase ($P<0.001$) in P4 secretion compared to control cultures and those treated with IGF-I and GH (Fig. 2). However, in the presence of 20 or 200 ng FSH, P4 ($P<0.01$ and $P<0.001$, respectively; Fig. 2). GH treatment had no effect on FSH-induced responses (Fig. 2).

Receptor binding studies revealed the presence of specific IGF-I receptors with one class of binding sites in the granulosa cells. The Scatchard plot yielded a Kd estimate of 3.96 nM. The cross-reactivity of insulin and IGF-I with [^{125}I]IGF-I binding to granulosa cells is depicted in Figure 3, and the competition potency of the peptides was IGF-I > insulin. Insulin, at the dose of 100 ng/ml used in this study, had negligible cross-reactivity with IGF-I binding to granulosa cells.

Discussion

These results demonstrate that insulin has a direct effect on P4 secretion by porcine granulosa cells in vitro, which agrees with the findings of Veldhuis et al. (1). Although 100 ng insulin/ml was used in the present study, the stimulatory effects of insulin on antral granulosa cells have been observed in our laboratory with only 10 ng/ml (Rajkumar and Murphy, unpublished data). The concentration of insulin used in these in vitro studies cannot be extrapolated to that in follicular fluid which ranges between 0.45-0.63 ng insulin/ml (10), since insulin is added discontinuously to the cultures and is susceptible to degradation (11). Unlike insulin, the addition of IGF-I failed to stimulate P4 secretion in the absence of FSH. This is in agreement with the findings of Maruo et al. (3) using porcine granulosa cells and those of Adashi et al. (12) using rat granulosa cells. In contrast, Veldhuis et al. (2) showed that IGF-I can exert potent stimulatory effects on P4 secretion even in the absence of FSH.

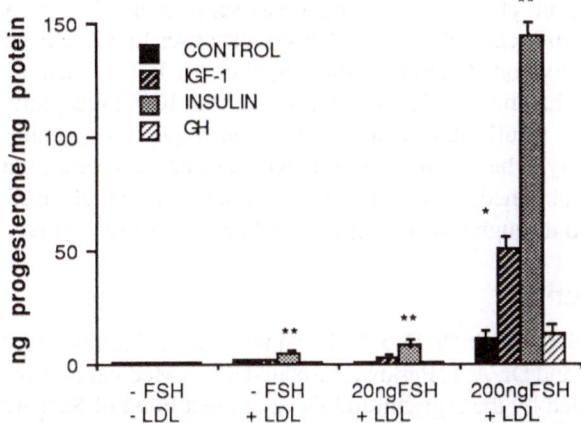

Fig. 2. Progesterone secretion by porcine granulosa cells plated without FBS. Effect of treatment with insulin, IGF-I and GH in the presence or absence of 20 or 200 ng FSH and 100 µg LDL. Significantly different from control, ** $P<0.001$, * $P<0.01$.

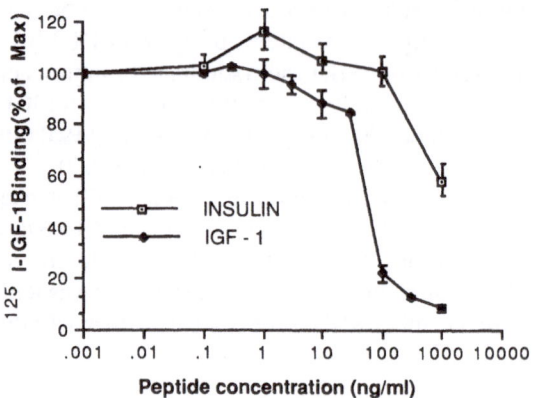

Fig. 3. Competition by insulin and IGF-I for [^{125}I]IGF-I binding to porcine granulosa cells. Granulosa cells were incubated at 4°C for 2 h with [^{125}I]IGF-I and increasing doses of insulin or IGF-I.

The role of FSH in granulosa cell differentiation is well established (13). The results from the present study indicate potentiating effects of insulin on FSH-stimulated P4 secretion under both culture conditions. Moreover, the potentiating effect was significantly greater in the cultures established in the absence of serum. Unlike insulin, IGF-I potentiated the FSH-induced P4 secretion only in granulosa cells cultured in the absence of serum from the time of plating. The reason for this is not clear.

The present study indicates that insulin is more potent than IGF-I in potentiating FSH responses in serum-free cultures, whereas previous studies (3) suggested that IGF-I was more potent. These differences could be attributed to the source of IGF-I and/or culture conditions. In the studies of Maruo et al. (3), the media was supplemented with hydrocortisone and platelet extract. The influence of these factors on responses to IGF-I is not known.

Granulosa cells exhibited saturable binding sites for IGF-I. Insulin, at the dose level studied (100 ng/ml), had negligible cross-reactivity with IGF-I receptors. The existence of specific receptors for insulin has been demonstrated in porcine granulosa cells (14). The results from this study, where a direct steroidogenic effect of insulin, but not of IGF-I, on granulosa cells was obtained, suggest that the stimulatory effect of insulin on P4 secretion may not be mediated through IGF-I receptors, but via its own receptors.

Acknowledgments

The authors wish to thank Dr. D. J. Bolt and the USDA National Hormone Program for providing the pFSH and Dr. A. F. Parlow, Harbour-UCLA Medical Centre, CA, for the pGH. This study was funded by the Agricultural Development Fund of Saskatchewan and Grant No. MA-9245 from MRC of Canada.

References

1. Veldhuis JD, Kolp LA, Juchter D, Veldhuis PP, Garmy JC. Mechanisms subserving insulins differentiating actions on progestin biosynthesis by ovarian cells: studies with cultured swine granulosa cells. Endocrinology 1985; 116:651-9.

2. Veldhuis JD, Furlanetto RW, Juchter D, Garmy JC, Veldhuis P. Trophic actions of human somatomedin C/insulin-like growth factor 1 on ovarian cells: in vitro studies with swine granulosa cells. Endocrinology 1985; 116:1235-42.

3. Maruo T, Hayashi M, Matsuo H, Ueda Y, Morikawa H, Mochizuki M. Comparison of facilitative roles of insulin and insulin-like growth factor-1 in the functional differentiation of granulosa cells; in vitro studies with the porcine model. Acta Endocrinol (Copenh) 1988; 117:230-40.

4. Veldhuis JD, Nestler JE, Straus JF, Gwynne JJ. Insulin regulates low-density lipoprotein metabolism by swine granulosa cells. Endocrinology 1986; 118:2242-53.

5. Veldhuis JD, Nestler JE, Strauss JF, Azimi P, Garmy J, Juchter D. The insulin-like growth factor, Somatomedin C, modulates low density lipoprotein metabolism by swine granulosa cells. Endocrinology 1987; 121:340-6.

6. Hsu C-J, Hammond JM. Concomitant effects of growth hormone on secretion of insulin like growth factor 1 and progesterone by cultured porcine granulosa cells. Endocrinology 1987; 121:1343-8.

7. Rajkumar K, Malinek J, Murphy BD. Effect of lipoproteins and luteotrophins on progesterone accumulation by luteal cells from the pregnant pig. Steroids 1986; 45:119-34.

8. Lowry OH, Rosebrough NJ, Farr AL, Randall RJ. Protein measurement with folin phenol reagent. J Biol Chem 1951; 193:265-73.

9. Scatchard G. The attraction of proteins for small molecules and ions. Ann NY Acad Sci 1949; 51:660-72.

10. Hammond JM, Baranao JLS, Skateris D, Knight AB, Romanus JS, Rechler MM. Production of insulin-like growth factors by ovarian granulosa cells. Endocrinology 1985; 117:2553-5.

11. Mather JP, Sato GH. Growth of mouse melanoma cells in hormone supplemented serum-free medium. Exp Cell Res 1979; 120:191-5.

12. Adashi EY, Resnick CE, Svoboda ME, Van Wyk J. A novel role for somatomedin-C in the cytodifferentiation of the ovarian granulosa cell. Endocrinology 1984; 115:1227-9.

13. Hsueh AJW, Adashi EY, Jones PBC, Welsh TH. Hormonal regulation of the differentiation of cultured ovarian granulosa cells. Endocr Rev 1984; 5:76-127.

14. Otani T, Maruo T, Mochizuki M. Effect of insulin on porcine granulosa cells: implication of a possible receptor mediated action. Acta Endocrinol (Copenh) 1985; 108:104-10.

18

Insulin-Like Growth Factor-I and Transforming Growth Factor-β Regulate the Differentiation of Purified Ovarian Theca-Interstitial Cells in Serum-Free Medium

Denis A. Magoffin and Gregory F. Erickson

Department of Reproductive Medicine, M-025
University of California, San Diego
La Jolla, California 92093

Introduction

The ovarian theca-interstitial cells (TIC) are the source of androgens which are essential for follicle estrogen synthesis (1). Regulation of TIC androgen synthesis is critical for normal follicle development and ovulation. Although luteinizing hormone (LH) is the principal regulator of TIC androgen production (1), recent evidence suggests that intraovarian factors may modulate LH action by autocrine and paracrine mechanisms. Two such factors are insulin-like growth factor-I (IGF-I) secreted by granulosa cells (2) and transforming growth factor-β (TGF-β) produced by TIC (3). Although it has been shown that IGF-I increases LH-stimulated TIC androgen synthesis (4,5), the effects of TGF-β on TIC are unknown. The purpose of these studies was to test the effect of TGF-β on LH and IGF-I stimulated TIC androgen synthesis.

Materials and Methods

Four days after hypophysectomy, 25-day-old Sprague-Dawley rats were killed by cervical dislocation and the ovaries dispersed into a cell suspension with collagenase/DNase solution (6). The TIC were purified by centrifugation through 1.055 g/ml Percoll (7) and then cultured (1×10^5 viable cells/well) up to 6 days in 96-well microtest plates (4) containing ovine LH (G3-330BR provided by Dr. H. Papkoff), human TGF-β (Collaborative Research) and/or IGF-I (AMGen). The medium, collected every 2 days, was assayed for androsterone (the principal androgen produced by this cell type), androstenedione, testosterone, progesterone and estradiol by specific radioimmunoassays (6). The dose-response curves were analyzed using the Allfit program (8).

Results and Discussion

Recently we developed the first model system in which highly purified and hormone responsive TIC can be cultured in serum-free medium (7). This important advance now permits us to study ovarian TIC without the complications of serum-derived or granulosa cell-secreted growth factors. In these experiments we utilized this model to study the effects of TGF-β and IGF-I on TIC androgen synthesis.

Figure 1 shows that TGF-β caused a dose-related inhibition of LH-stimulated androsterone synthesis. When TIC were treated with a saturating concentration of LH (50 ng/ml), androsterone synthesis was stimulated approximately 200-fold above basal levels. TGF-β alone (0.01-10 ng/ml) caused no change in basal androsterone production (Fig. 1). However, TGF-β caused a dose-related inhibition of LH-stimulated androsterone production which reached 65% at 10 ng/ml of TGF-β. The ED_{50} (0.1 ± 0.06 ng/ml) for TGF-β inhibition of LH-stimulated androsterone synthesis agreed with the ED_{50} observed for physiological effects of TGF-β in other tissues (9). This result suggests that the TGF-β inhibition is mediated by a TGF-β receptor on the TIC.

We next examined the time course of TGF-β action. As shown in Figure 2, TGF-β alone (10 ng/ml) had no effect on basal androsterone secretion. LH stimulated androsterone production 200-fold at 2 days, and 130-fold at 4 and 6 days. Treatment of the TIC with TGF-β

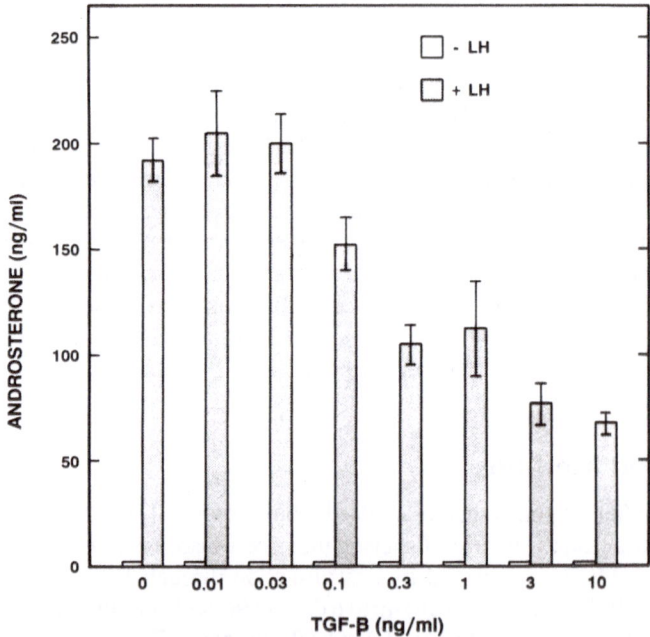

Fig. 1. Effect of TGF-β on TIC androgen synthesis. Purified TIC were cultured in the presence and absence of a saturating concentration of LH (50 ng/ml) with increasing concentrations of TGF-β (0-10 ng/ml) for 2 days. The data are the mean ± SEM of 3 experiments with 4 replicates each.

inhibited LH-stimulated androsterone production by 65% at each time period. Because TGF-β did not alter the DNA content and viability of the TIC cultures (data not shown), it seems clear that the inhibitory effect of TGF-β was not caused by decreases in the number of viable TIC. It should also be noted that TGF-β by itself does not appear to be a mitogen for TIC in serum-free medium.

To determine if the inhibitory effect of TGF-β might be caused by changes in steroid metabolism, we measured certain key steroid metabolites secreted by the TIC. As shown in Table 1, LH stimulated increases in progesterone and each of the androgens above basal levels. Although TGF-β did not affect basal steroid production, TGF-β inhibited androsterone (65%) and androstenedione (58%) production. In contrast, TGF-β increased LH-stimulated progesterone and testosterone production approximately 2.5-fold. These results indicate that TGF-β may selectively inhibit the $P450_{17\alpha}$ enzyme without decreasing

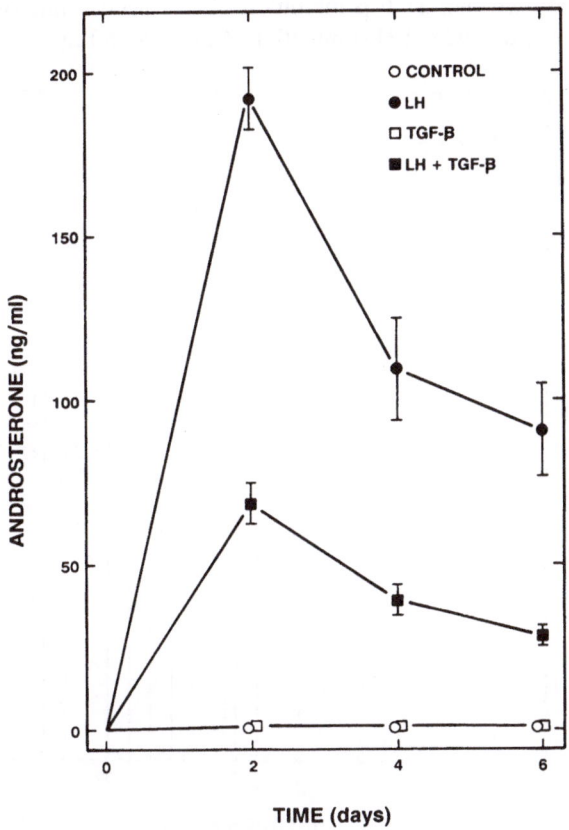

Fig. 2. Time course of TGF-β inhibition of androgen synthesis. Purified TIC were cultured for 6 days with and without LH (50 ng/ml) and/or TGF-β (10 ng/ml). The medium was collected and replaced every 2 days. The data are the mean ± SEM of 3 experiments with 4 replicates each.

Table 1. Effect of TGF-β TIC steroid metabolites

Steroid	Control	LH	TGF-β	LH + TGF-β
Progesterone	<0.1	5.4 ± 1.0	<0.1	13.6 ± 1.1
Androsterone	3.1 ± 0.6	280.6 ± 10.8	2.4 ± 0.2	161.1 ± 15.1
Androstenedione	<0.1	26.3 ± 3.3	<0.1	15.3 ± 1.8
Testosterone	<0.1	1.0 ± 0.1	<0.1	2.4 ± 0.2
Estradiol	<0.1	<0.1	<0.1	<0.1

$P450_{scc}$ activity. This observation could provide evidence for an autocrine/paracrine mechanism which may help to explain the shift from androgen to progesterone production as the TIC luteinize after the preovulatory surge of LH.

Next, we examined whether TGF-β inhibition of androgen synthesis was caused by changes in the sensitivity of TIC to LH stimulation. As shown in Figure 3, LH stimulated a

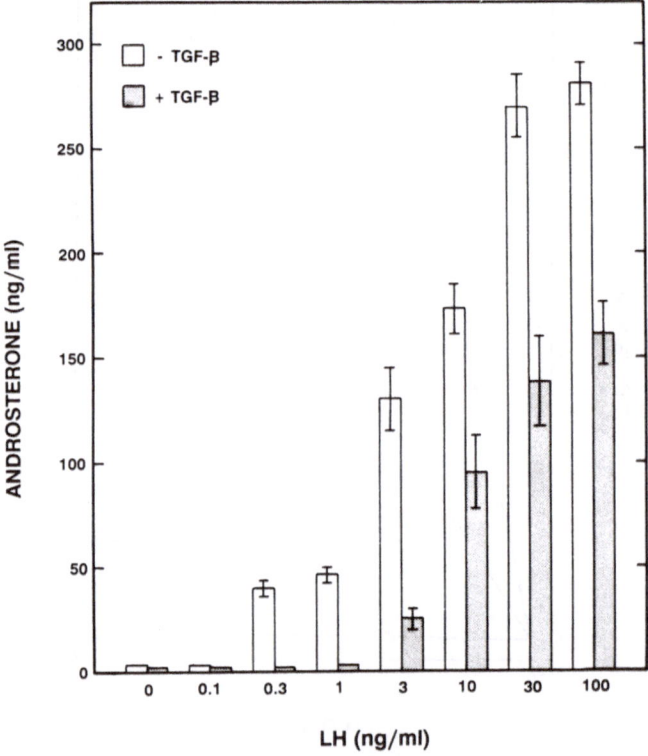

Fig. 3. Effect of TGF-β on the sensitivity of TIC to LH stimulation. Purified TIC were cultured for 2 days with increasing concentrations of LH (0-100 ng/ml) with and without a saturating concentration (3 ng/ml) of TGF-β. The data are mean ± SEM of 3 experiments with 4 replicates each.

dose-related increase in androsterone production (ED_{50} = 3.4 ± 0.04 ng/ml). When the TIC were treated with increasing concentrations of LH in the presence of TGF-β (3 ng/ml), the stimulatory effect of LH was inhibited at each dose tested. The ED_{50} for LH stimulation in the presence of TGF-β was 8.0 ± 0.5 ng/ml. These results suggest that a decrease in the efficiency of LH-stimulated intracellular signal transduction might play a role in the mechanism of TGF-β action.

New data demonstrate that IGF-I is a potent stimulator of TIC androgen synthesis (4,5). It was of interest, therefore, to determine if TGF-β can block IGF-I action in the TIC. As shown in Figure 4, treatment of the TIC with saturating concentrations of LH (50 ng/ml) and IGF-I (30 ng/ml) resulted in a threefold increase in androsterone production above that of LH alone. LH + IGF-I stimulation of androsterone was inhibited by TGF-β in a dose-related manner (ED_{50} = 0.2 ± 0.07 ng/ml), reaching 68% at 10 ng/ml. These results indicate that

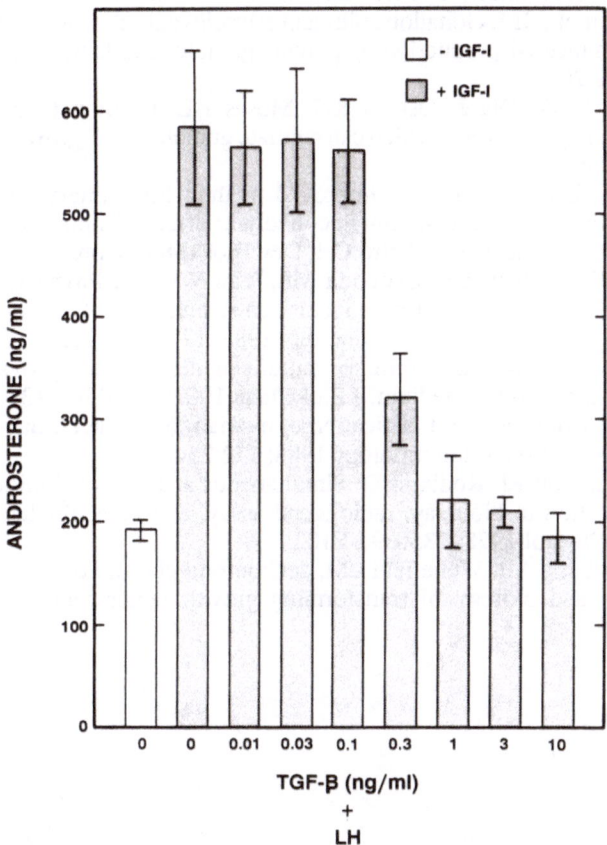

Fig. 4. Effect of TGF-β on LH plus IGF-I stimulated androgen biosynthesis. Purified TIC were cultured for 2 days with LH (50 ng/ml) and IGF-I (30 ng/ml) with increasing concentrations of TGF-β (0-10 ng/ml). The data are the mean ± SEM of 3 experiments with 4 replicates each.

IGF-I does not diminish TGF-β inhibition or alter the sensitivity of the TIC to TGF-β, suggesting that TGF-β and IGF-I act by separate mechanisms.

The results of our experiments demonstrate that (1) TGF-β does not affect basal steroidogenesis in TIC; (2) TGF-β causes a potent inhibition of LH-stimulated androgen synthesis and a stimulation of LH-stimulated progesterone production; (3) TGF-β appears to decrease the sensitivity of TIC to LH stimulation; and, (4) IGF-I does not block TGF-β inhibition of androgen synthesis. These observations are consistent with the hypothesis that TGF-β and IGF-I may be important autocrine/paracrine regulators of follicle development and atresia.

References

1. Erickson GF, Magoffin DA, Dyer CA, Hofeditz C. The ovarian androgen producing cells: a review of structure/function relationships. Endocr Rev 1985; 6:371-99.
2. Hsu C-J, Hammond JM. Gonadotropins and estradiol stimulate immunoreactive insulin-like growth factor-I production by porcine granulosa cells in vitro. Endocrinology 1987; 120:198-207.
3. Skinner MK, Keski-Oja J, Osteen KG, Moses HL. Ovarian thecal cells produce transforming growth factor-β which can regulate granulosa cell growth. Endocrinology 1987; 121:786-92.
4. Magoffin DA, Erickson GF. An improved method for primary culture of ovarian androgen-producing cells in serum-free medium: effect of lipoproteins, insulin, and insulin-like growth factor-I. In Vitro Cell Dev Biol 1988 (in press).
5. Hernandez ER, Resnick CE, Svoboda ME, Van Wyk JJ, Payne DW, Adashi EY. Somatomedin-C/insulin-like growth factor I as an enhancer of androgen biosynthesis by cultured rat ovarian cells. Endocrinology 1988; 122:1603-22.
6. Magoffin DA, Erickson GF. Primary culture of differentiating ovarian androgen-producing cells in defined medium. J Biol Chem 1982; 257:4507-13.
7. Magoffin DA, Erickson GF. Purification of ovarian theca-interstitial cells by density gradient centrifugation. Endocrinology 1988; 122:2345-7.
8. DeLean A, Munson PJ, Rodbard D. Simultaneous analysis of families of sigmoidal curves: application to bioassay, radioligand assay, and physiological dose-response curves. Am J Physiol 1978; 235:E97-E102.
9. Sporn MB, Roberts AB, Wakefield LM, deCrombrugghe B. Some recent advances in the chemistry and biology of transforming growth factor-beta. J Cell Biol 1987; 105:1039-45.

19

Bovine Thecal Cells Secrete Transforming Growth Factor α and β

Derek K. Lobb and Jennifer H. Dorrington

Banting and Best Department of Medical Research
University of Toronto, Toronto, Canada M5G 1L6

Abstract. The objective of the present study was to determine if the peptides secreted by bovine thecal cells influenced the growth and differentiation of bovine granulosa cells. Bovine thecal cells were cultured under serum-free conditions, the conditioned medium was concentrated and the peptides fractionated on a Bio-Gel P-60 column in 1.0 M acetic acid. Fractions were tested for their ability to stimulate [^{3}H]thymidine incorporation into bovine granulosa cell DNA. Growth-promoting activity was located in the 6,000-9,000 and the 16,000 molecular weight fractions. The peak fractions inhibited FSH-induced aromatase activity in rat granulosa cells, indicating the presence of TGFα-like peptides. A growth inhibitory activity was observed in fractions with a molecular weight of approximately 25,000. The inhibitory activity had the molecular weight of TGFβ, and TGFβ was found to inhibit [^{3}H]thymidine incorporation into bovine granulosa cell DNA. The presence of TGFβ-like activity was confirmed in two independent bioassays; stimulation of FSH-induced aromatase activity, and increased [^{3}H]thymidine incorporation into rat granulosa cell DNA in the presence of FSH. In summary, bovine thecal cells secrete TGFα- and TGFβ-like activities that have opposing actions on the growth of bovine granulosa cells. The relative amounts of these growth factors may determine the rate of growth of granulosa cells during follicular development.

Introduction

The adult mammalian ovary is a dynamic organ in which follicles undergo a cyclic pattern of regulated growth and development. Once a primordial follicle commences growth, it continues until it undergoes atresia or ovulates. During the development of a healthy follicle, the proliferation of the granulosa cells depends upon the size of the follicle. In the bovine ovary, the mitotic index of the granulosa cells in small follicles is low, increases in medium follicles and declines in large follicles (1). Even though follicle stimulating hormone (FSH), luteinizing hormone (LH) and gonadal steroids are required to promote normal follicular development to the stage of ovulation, none of these hormones are mitogens for granulosa cells in vitro. To explain the latter observations, it has been proposed that granulosa cell growth is regulated by nonsteroidal products secreted by thecal cells, and that thecal cell-granulosa cell interactions are essential for the development of the dominant follicles (2).

Growth factors, in particular epidermal growth factor (EGF), fibroblast growth factor (FGF), insulin-like growth factor-I (IGF-I), transforming growth factor α (TFGα) and transforming growth factor β (TGFβ) have been recognized as classes of potent peptides that may be involved in cell-cell interactions in the follicles since they have pronounced effects not only on the growth of granulosa cells but also on their cytodifferentiation (3,4). Production of growth factors by cells within the follicle is supported by the presence of IGF-I and EGF-like activities in porcine follicular fluid (5,6) and the synthesis of IGF-I by porcine granulosa cells (5) and an EGF-like factor by rat thecal/interstitial cells (7). We have shown that bovine thecal cells secrete a mitogen for bovine granulosa cells (8,9). In order to characterize the growth-promoting activity, the peptides secreted by bovine thecal cells were fractionated by column chromatography and tested for their ability to influence bovine granulosa cell DNA synthesis.

Materials and Methods

Healthy follicles, approximately 1 cm in diameter with a well vascularized theca, were isolated from bovine ovaries. Granulosa and thecal cells were isolated from the follicles and cultured as described previously (10). Thecal cells were plated in culture medium (9,10) containing 10% calf serum and grown to confluence, subcultured, replated at a 1:4 density and again grown to confluence. The serum was removed, and the cells were washed in serum-free medium and maintained in serum-free medium. Medium was collected every 48 h over a 6-day culture period, centrifuged and frozen until use.

Conditioned medium was concentrated approximately one hundredfold by ultrafiltration, lyophilized and resuspended in 1.0 M acetic acid. Thecal cell-secreted peptides were then applied to a Bio-Gel P-60 column and eluted with 1.0 M acetic acid. Lyophilized fractions were resuspended in 0.1 M HEPES-phosphate buffered saline.

Bioassays

The effects of the column fractions on [^{3}H]thymidine incorporation into bovine granulosa cell DNA were determined as described previously (9,10). EGF (Sigma Chemical Co., St. Louis, MO) and TGFβ (from porcine platelets; R and D Systems, Minneapolis, MN) were included as controls.

TGFβ bioactivity was examined in the fractions using a rat granulosa cell growth assay that is specified for TGFβ (11). All the cultures were treated with 10 ng FSH/ml.

The ability of the column fractions to influence FSH-induced aromatase in rat granulosa cells was assessed as described previously (12). After treatment of the cells with FSH (10 ng/ml), aliquots of the column fractions, EGF (10 ng/ml) and TGFβ (10 ng/ml) for 48 h, [1β-^{3}H]testosterone (0.2 µCi, 0.25 µM) was added for 3 h, and aromatase activity determined from the stereospecific release of tritium to give tritiated water.

Results and Discussion

The peptide fractions obtained from the elution of bovine thecal cell-conditioned medium through a Bio-Gel P-60 column were assayed for growth-promoting activity on bovine granulosa cells. Activity was localized in fractions that contained thecal cell-secreted peptides of molecular weight 6,000-9,000 and 16,000 (Fig. 1). EGF, FGF and IGF-I are all potent mitogens for the proliferation of bovine granulosa cells; and in order to characterize the thecal cell-derived growth factor, the effects on FSH-induced aromatase activity in rat granulosa cells were examined. The latter bioassay was selected to distinguish between IGF-I-like and EGF-like activities since IGF-I potentiated and EGF and TGFα inhibited aromatase activity. Fractions that contained growth-promoting activity inhibited FSH-induced aromatase activity (Fig. 2), indicating that the factors were EGF-like or TGFα-like. Since EGF and TGFα interact with the same receptor in equimolar amounts (13), the identity of the growth factors could not be determined from the above bioassays. To distinguish between EGF and TGFα, a radioimmunoassay using a monoclonal antibody that binds to TGFα and not to EGF was used. The fractions that had growth-promoting activity and inhibited FSH-induced aromatase activity contained TGFα-like immunoreactivity (14,15). Native TGFα is a polypeptide of approximately 6,000 molecular weight. A biologically active precursor of 17,000-19,000 molecular weight has also been identified (16).

Fractions containing peptides with an apparent molecular weight of 25,000 significantly suppress [^{3}H]thymidine incorporation into bovine granulosa cell DNA below that of untreated control cells. The reduction in the level of [^{3}H]thymidine incorporation was not due to a decrease in the viability of the cells or a decrease in the DNA content of the cells in each

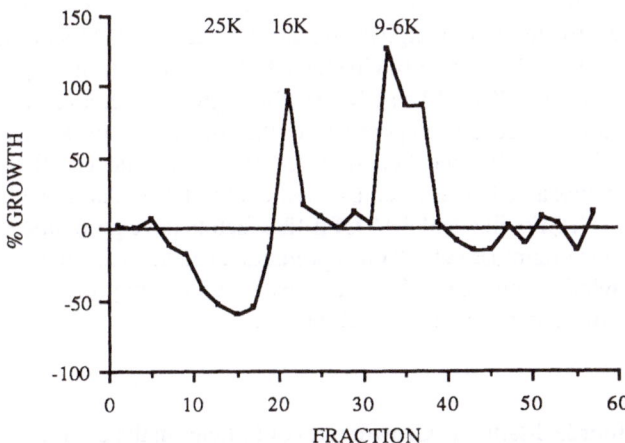

Fig. 1. Growth-promoting effects of bovine thecal cell-secreted proteins on bovine granulosa cells. Concentrated thecal cell-conditioned medium was size fractionated on a Bio-Gel P-60 column in 1.0 M acetic acid. Lyophilized fractions were then tested for the ability to stimulate granulosa cell growth. [^{3}H]Thymidine incorporation into bovine granulosa cell DNA was measured and represented as a percentage of untreated controls.

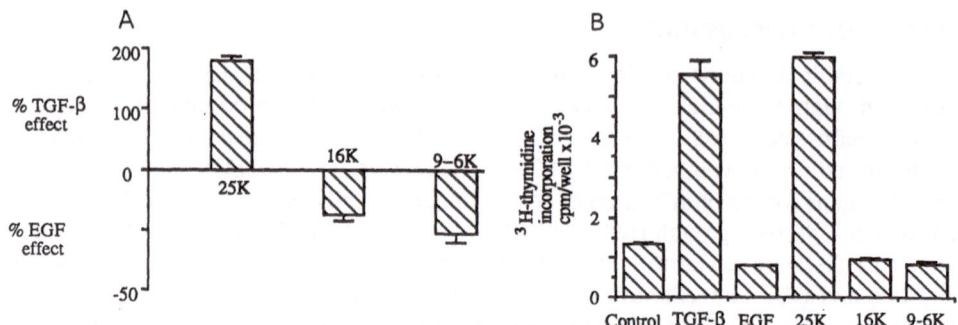

Fig. 2. Effects of fractions of bovine thecal cell-secreted peptides on (A) FSH-induced aromatase activity in rat granulosa cells; and, (B) [³H]thymidine incorporation into rat granulosa cell DNA in the presence of FSH (10 ng/ml). Aromatase activity was expressed as the percentage of the effect of 10 ng/ml TGFβ or 10 ng/ml EGF.

culture well. In the same experiments, TGFβ, which has a molecular weight of 25,000, inhibited [³H]thymidine incorporation into bovine granulosa cell DNA, suggesting that the bovine thecal cells were secreting TGFβ. This notion was supported by the ability of the fractions containing peptides in the 25,000 molecular weight range to augment FSH-induced aromatase activity, a previously demonstrated property of TGFβ (4) (Fig. 2A). The presence of TGFβ in these fractions was confirmed using a rat granulosa cell growth assay that was specific for TGFβ (11). In this assay, rat granulosa cells cultured in the presence of FSH responded to TGFβ with increased incorporation of [³H]thymidine into DNA. Fractions containing bovine thecal cell-secreted peptides in the 25,000 molecular weight range also stimulated [³H]thymidine incorporation to rat granulosa cell DNA (Fig. 2B). Skinner et al. (17) have also shown by immunoprecipitation that TGFβ is secreted by bovine thecal cells.

In this study, we have shown that bovine thecal cells isolated from large antral follicles secrete both TGFα-like and TGFβ-like activities. Since growth factors can be considered to be "inducer molecules" that act on cell populations that are in close proximity to their source of production, the effects of the thecal cell-derived TGFα-like and TGFβ-like activities on the neighboring granulosa cells was of considerable importance. As shown in the bioassay used in this study, the TGFα-like and the TGFβ-like factors have pronounced effects on the proliferation of bovine granulosa cells, TGFα promoting cell growth whereas TGFβ inhibits cell growth. The relative amounts of these growth factors may determine the rates of granulosa cell growth during follicular development.

References

1. Lussier J, Dufour JJ, Matton P. Growth rates of follicles in the bovine ovary [Abstract]. J Anim Sci 1983; 57(suppl 1):353.
2. Dorrington JH, McKeracher H, Garzo G, Skinner MK. Granulosa cell-theca cell interactions during follicular development. In: Labrie F, Proulx L, eds. Endocrinology. Amsterdam: Elsevier Science Publishers B.V., 1984:807-10.
3. Gospodarowicz D, Ill CR, Birdwell CR. Effects of fibroblast and epidermal growth factors on ovarian cell proliferation in vitro. I. Characterization of the response of granulosa cells to FGF and EGF. Endocrinology 1977; 100:1108-20.

4. Adashi EY, Resnick CE. Antagonistic interactions of transforming growth factors in the regulation of granulosa cell differentiation. Endocrinology 1986; 1879-81.

5. Hammond JM, Baranao JLS, Skaleris D, Knight AB, Romanus JA, Rechler MM. Production of insulin-like growth factors by ovarian granulosa cells. Endocrinology 1985; 117:2553-5.

6. Hsu C-J, Holmes SD, Hammond JM. Ovarian epidermal growth factor-like activity. Concentrations in porcine follicular fluid during follicular enlargement. Biochem Biophys Res Commun 1987; 147:242-7.

7. Skinner MK, Lobb D, Dorrington JH. Ovarian thecal/interstitial cells produce an epidermal growth factor-like substance. Endocrinology 1987; 121:1892-9.

8. Lobb DK, Bendell JJ, Dorrington JH. Bovine thecal cells secrete a growth factor which stimulates granulosa cell proliferation [Abstract]. Biol Reprod 1986; 34(1):78.

9. Bendell JJ, Lobb DK, Chuma A, Gysler M, Dorrington JH. Bovine thecal cells secrete factor(s) that promote granulosa cell proliferation. Biol Reprod 1988; 38:790-7.

10. Lobb DK, Skinner MK, Dorrington JH. Rat thecal/interstitial cells produce a mitogenic activity that promotes the growth of granulosa cells. Mol Cell Endocrinol 1986; 55:209-17.

11. Dorrington JH, Chuma AV, Bendell JJ. Transforming growth factor β and follicle-stimulating hormone promote rat granulosa cell proliferation. Endocrinology 1988 (in press).

12. Gore-Langton RE, Dorrington JH. FSH induction of aromatase in cultured rat granulosa cells measured by a radiometric assay. Mol Cell Endocrinol 1981; 22:135-51.

13. Massague J. Epidermal growth factor-like transforming growth factor. II. Interaction with epidermal growth factor receptors in human placenta membranes and A431 cells. J Biol Chem 1983; 258:13614-20.

14. Kobrin MS, Samsoondar J, Kudlow JE. α-Transforming growth factor secreted by untransformed bovine anterior pituitary cells in culture. II. Identification using a sequence-specific monoclonal antibody. J Biol Chem 1986; 261:14414-9.

15. Lobb DK, Kobrin MS, Kudlow JE, Dorrington JH (in preparation).

16. Ignotz RA, Kelly B, Davis RJ, Massague J. Biologically active precursor for transforming growth factor type α, released by retrovirally transformed cells. Proc Natl Acad Sci USA 1986; 83:6302-11.

17. Skinner MK, Keski-Oja J, Osteen KG, Moses HL. Ovarian thecal cells produce transforming growth factor-β which can regulate granulosa cell growth. Endocrinology 1987; 121:786-92.

20

Variations in the Level of Transforming Growth Factor-Alpha (TGFα) mRNA During the Human Menstrual Cycle

R. S. Williams, G. S. Schultz, T. E. Geoghegan, M. C. Steffan, and M. A. Yussman

University of Louisville School of Medicine, Louisville, KY 40292

Introduction

Transforming growth factor alpha (TGFα) is a peptide growth factor which is highly homologous to epidermal growth factor (EGF) and shares the epidermal growth factor receptor (EGF-R) to affect its action. These growth factors may play a role in the normal physiology of the human reproductive system.

TGFα was thought originally to be an embryonic growth factor which was replaced in the adult by EGF. When induced in the adult, TGFα was thought to function as an oncogene to induce tumorigenesis. However, TGFα was recently identified in normal human keratinocytes (1) and ovarian theca and interstitial cells of the adult rat (2).

We have previously reported the levels of mRNA for EGF and EGF-R in human female reproductive tissues during the menstrual cycle and postmenopausally (3). Because TGFα shares the EGF-R, it is also important to evaluate the role of TGFα in these tissues. The current study was undertaken to determine the presence of mRNA for TGFα in the human female reproductive tract and variations of mRNA levels for TGFα during the menstrual cycle and postmenopausally.

Methods

One or more tissues, including cervix, endometrium, myometrium, fallopian tube, and ovary, were collected at the time of hysterectomy from 44 women. Tissues were immediately dissected and frozen in liquid nitrogen. They were stored at -70°C until the assays were performed.

Tissues were divided into four groups: (1) early follicular, days 1-7; (2) late follicular, days 8-14; (3) luteal, days 15-27; and, (4) postmenopausal phases. Classification was based on the patient's menstrual history and confirmed by pathologic examination of the endometrium.

Samples from 2 to 3 patients were pooled and RNA extracted by the guanidinium thiocyanate method. Dot blots were made with total RNA and hybridized with a cDNA probe for TGFα under stringent conditions. Specificity of hybridization was confirmed by Northern blot analysis.

TGFα Probe

The TGFα probe was kindly supplied by Oncogen Corporation, Seattle, WA. This rat cDNA probe encodes for the 50 amino acid mature rat TGFα coding sequence, as well as an 85 amino acid polypeptide, NH2-flanking region, a 71 polypeptide COOH-flanking region, and a 3′ untranslated sequence.

Results

Northern blot analysis showed the presence of the expected 4.3 kb transcript for TGFα as well as bands of 6.8, 3.7, and 1.85 kb.

Each dot blot contained all of the menstrual phases for that tissue, and equal amounts of total RNA were used for each menstrual phase. Relative levels of mRNA may not be comparable between blots of different tissues. The results are displayed in the accompanying graph (Fig. 1).

Discussion

We have demonstrated the presence of mRNA for TGFα in normal human cervix, uterus, fallopian tube, and ovary throughout the menstrual cycle and postmenopausally. This finding supports the possible role of TGFα in reproductive tissues. In general, mRNA levels were lowest in the luteal phase and higher in the follicular phases and postmenopausally. This suggests that the transcription rate or the stability of TGFα mRNA may be partially controlled

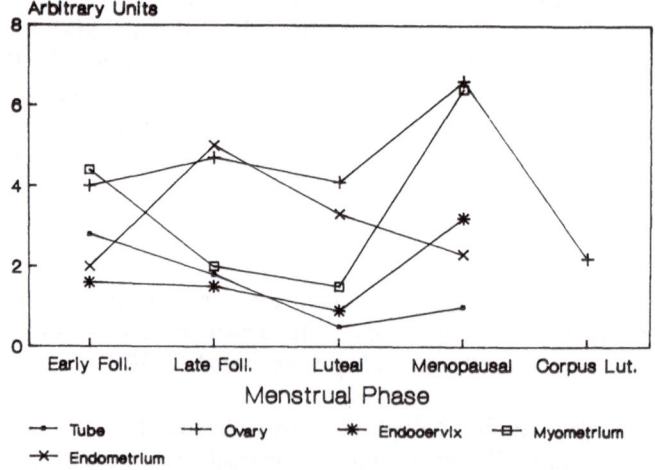

Fig. 1. TGFα mRNA levels during the menstrual cycle and postmenopausally as determined by quantitative densitometric analysis of dot blots.

by steroid hormones and gonadotropins in human reproductive tissues. It is doubtful that the TGFα mRNA is being processed postmenopausally into mature proteins since these tissues are atropic after the menopause. However, it is possible that the presence of estrogen is required for the processing of these mRNAs into mature growth factors. The failure to process prepro-EGF in the mouse kidney has been described previously (4).

The physiologic role of EGF and TGFα in female reproductive tissues is suggested by several lines of evidence. First, paracrine factors appear to mediate the mitogenic action of estrogen in many tissues. Although estrogen is a well-known mitogen in vivo in the female reproductive tract, in vitro cultures of uterine or vaginal epithelial cells do not show proliferative responses to estrogen stimulation unless stromal cells are also included in the culture (5). Similarly, mammary epithelial cells and prostatic epithelial cells require adjacent stromal cells for a mitogenic response when stimulated by estrogen and testosterone, respectively. (5) These studies suggest that the mitogenic response of sex steroids in these issues depends partly on the local production of paracrine factors.

There is now strong evidence that EGF and TGFα are the mitogenic factors produced by stromal cells. EGF and TGFα are known mitogens for many epithelial cells and have been shown to be mitogens in vitro for granulosa cells (6). Furthermore, it was recently shown that estrogen-induced mitogenesis in uterine cell cultures could be blocked by antibodies to EGF (7).

Specific high-affinity binding sites for EGF and TGFα have been identified in many reproductive tissues (8), and we have previously demonstrated mRNA for EGF and EGF-R in human myometrium, endometrium, endocervix, fallopian tube, and ovary. These studies further support a physiologic role for these growth factors in human reproduction.

Consistent with our findings, levels of TGFα have been previously shown to be partially controlled by steroid hormones and gonadotropins in the rat ovary (2) and mammary tumor cells (9).

By demonstrating the mRNA for TGFα in normal human female reproductive tissues, we have shown that these tissues are capable of producing these peptides, a fact that supports the concept that TGFα functions as an autocrine/paracrine regulator in female reproduction.

References

1. Coffey RJ Jr, Derynck R, Wilcox JN, et al. Production and auto-induction of transforming growth factor-α in human keratinocytes. Nature 1987; 328:817-20.
2. Kudlow JE, Kobrin MS, Purchio AF, et al. Ovarian transforming growth factor-α gene expression: immunohistochemical localization to the theca-interstitial cells. Endocrinology 1987: 121:1577-9.
3. Williams RS, Schultz GS, Geoghegan TE, Steffan M, Yussman MA. Variations in the transcription of epidermal growth factor (EGF) and EGF-receptor during the human menstrual cycle [Abstract]. Society for Gynecologic Investigation Scientific Program and Abstracts, 35th Annual Meeting Baltimore, March 17-19, 1988; 248.
4. Rall LB, Scott J, Bell GI, et al. Mouse prepro-epidermal growth factor synthesis by the kidney and other tissues. Nature 1985; 313:228-31.
5. Bigsby RM, Cunha GR. Estrogen stimulation of deoxyribonucleic acid synthesis in uterine epithelia cells which lack estrogen receptors. Endocrinology 1986; 119:390-6.

6. Gospodarowicz D, Ill GR, Birdwell CR. Effects of fibroblast and epidermal growth factors on ovarian cell proliferation in vitro. I. Characterization of the response of granulosa cells to FGF and EGF. Endocrinology 1977; 100:108-20.

7. McLachlan JA, DiAugustine RP, Newbold RR. Estrogen induced uterine cell proliferation in organ culture is inhibited by antibodies to epidermal growth factor [Abstract]. 67th Endocrine Society Meeting, 1985; 169.

8. Hofmann GE, Rao CV, Barrows G, Schultz GS, Sanfilippo JS. Binding sites for epidermal growth factor in human uterine tissues and leiomyomas. J Clin Endocrinol Metab 1984: 58:880-4.

9. Liu SC, Sanfilippo B, Perroteau I, Erynck R, Salomon DS, Kidwell WR. Expression of transforming growth factor α (TGFα) in differentiated rat mammary tumors: estrogen induction of TGFα production. Mol Endocrinol 1987; 1:683-92.

21

Transforming Growth Factor-β Inhibits the LH-Induced Maturation of Rat Oocytes

Alex Tsafriri and Aaron J. W. Hsueh

Department of Reproductive Medicine
University of California, San Diego
La Jolla, CA 92093

Introduction

Recent studies demonstrated the expression of the transforming factor-β (TGFβ) gene in the rat ovary (1). In addition, the production of TGFβ by theca and granulosa cells was detected by radioreceptor- and radioimmunoassays (2).

TGFβ inhibits EGF-stimulated granulosa cell growth (2). In addition to its effects on granulosa cell growth, TGFβ modifies ovarian cell differentiation in vitro. TGFβ enhances FSH-stimulated estradiol and progesterone production by granulosa cells (3-6), modifies FSH induction of LH receptors in a biphasic manner (7), and inhibits androgen production by ovarian theca-interstitial cells (8).

In view of these effects of TGFβ and other members of the TGFβ family on ovarian cells in vitro (reviewed by 9), we have examined their effects on the preovulatory rat follicles in vitro (in preparation). While these studies were in progress, a paper was published giving evidence for acceleration of the meiotic maturation of rat oocytes in culture by TGFβ (10). Here our studies on the actions of TGFβ on the resumption of meiosis of rat oocytes in vitro will be summarized. Two model systems were employed in this study: potential inhibitory activity of TGFβ was tested using cumulus-enclosed oocytes or preovulatory graafian follicles cultured in the presence of LH (1 μg/ml) and the suggested stimulatory activity of TGFβ was examined in similar graafian follicles cultured without LH.

Experimental

Both cumulus-enclosed oocytes and preovulatory follicles were obtained from 27- to 28-day-old rats pretreated 48 h earlier with PMSG (10-15 IU). The oocytes and follicles were isolated and cultured as previously described (11) in Falcon organ culture dishes. The data were analyzed by the chi square test; $P<0.05$ was considered significant.

The Effect of TGFβ on Spontaneous Maturation of Cumulus-Enclosed Oocytes

Spontaneous maturation of rat oocytes cultured for 2 h was lower (P<0.001) as compared to those cultured for 4 h. TGFβ (0.1-30 ng/ml) did not significantly affect the spontaneous maturation of oocytes cultured for 2 or 4 h (Table 1).

The Effect of TGFβ on the Maturation of Follicle-Enclosed Oocytes

TGFβ (1-50 ng/ml) did not stimulate the maturation of follicle-enclosed oocytes during a 24-h culture period (Table 2; P>0.5). By contrast, addition of TGFβ (10-50 ng/ml) in the presence of LH resulted in partial inhibition (P<0.035) of the gonadotropin-triggered resumption of meiosis (Table 2). In addition to its inhibitory action of meiosis, TGFβ increased dose-dependently the percentage of degenerating oocytes (P>0.035).

Concluding Remarks

In contrast to the action of TGFβ on differentiation of granulosa cells (2-9), the mature preovulatory follicles seem relatively refractory to its action. Addition of TGFβ to cultures of preovulatory follicles did not alter significantly basal or LH-stimulated steroid production in vitro (data not shown). Furthermore, we were unable to find any stimulatory action of TGFβ on the maturation of rat oocytes in vitro. The growth factor could neither accelerate the spontaneous maturation of cumulus-enclosed rat oocytes or induce maturation in follicle-enclosed rat oocytes cultured without LH. This is in contrast to the recently published results of Feng et al. (10). In their study, TGFβ (25 pg-2.5 ng/ml) accelerated the spontaneous maturation of both cumulus-enclosed as well as follicle-enclosed rat oocytes. It was shown that 20-85% of follicle-enclosed oocytes matured during the 2- to 8-h culture period

Table 1. Effect of TGFβ on the spontaneous maturation of
rat oocytes in culture

Treatment (ng/ml)	Culture Duration (h)	No. Oocytes Examined	Mature Oocytes (%)
Control	2	197	56.8[a]
TGFβ (10)	2	171	59.1[a]
(30)	2	197	62.4[a]
Control	4	180	81.1[b]
TFGβ (0.1)	4	103	84.5[b]
(10)	4	147	72.8[b]
(30)	4	152	77.6[b]

[a,b]Data with different superscripts differ significantly (P<0.001).

Table 2. Effect of TGFβ on the LH-induced maturation of
follicle-enclosed oocytes

Treatment (ng/ml)	No. Oocytes Examined	Immature Oocytes (%)	Mature Oocytes (%)	Degenerated Oocytes (%)
Control	61	95.1[a]	1.6[a]	3.3[a]
TGFβ (1-3)	36	100.0[a]		
(10)	40	95.5[a]	2.5[a]	5.0[a]
(30-50)	83	89.1[a]	4.8[a]	6.0[a]
LH (1 µg/ml)	62	11.3[b]	87.1[b]	1.6[b]
+TGFβ (1-3)	89	19.1[b]	75.2[b]	5.6[b]
+ (10)	81	29.6[c]	61.7[c]	8.6[c]
+ (30-50)	92	29.3[c]	51.1[c]	19.6[c]

[a,b,c]Data with different superscripts differ significantly (P<0.035).

and TGFβ accelerated the resumption of meiosis even further. It should be noted, however, that in the vast majority of the published studies (reviewed by 12-14), resumption of oocyte meiosis in follicle-enclosed oocytes is dependent upon hormonal stimulation. Follicles which were not stimulated in vivo or in vitro retain oocytes arrested at the meiotic prophase, i.e., at the germinal vesicle stage.

By contrast, resumption of meiosis triggered by LH in follicle-enclosed oocytes was partially inhibited by the addition of TGFβ. The arrest at the germinal vesicle stage was accompanied by an increased incidence of oocyte degeneration. It is not clear whether this inhibitory action of TGFβ on LH stimulation is due to its modulation of LH-induced responses of the preovulatory follicle or indirectly through unspecific adverse effects on the explanted follicles.

In conclusion, while TGFβ does not induce or accelerate the resumption of oocyte maturation, it exerts a significant inhibition of LH-stimulated meiosis in follicle-enclosed rat oocytes. Whether this is a pharmacological effect of TGFβ or related to its paracrine role in follicular development and atresia remain to be determined.

References

1. Hernandez ER, Twardzik DR, Purchio A, Adashi EY. Gonadotropin-dependent ovarian transforming growth factor-β gene expression. Biol Reprod 1987; 36:58A.
2. Skinner MK, Keski-Oja J, Osteen KG, Moses HL. Ovarian thecal cells produce transforming growth factor-β which can regulate granulosa cell growth. Endocrinology 1987; 121:786-92.
3. Ying S-Y, Becker A, Ling N, Ueno N, Guillemin R. Inhibin and β type transforming growth factor have opposite modulating effects on FSH induced aromatase activity of cultured rat granulosa cells. Biochem Biophys Res Commun 1986; 136:969-75.

4. Adashi EY, Resnick CE. Antagonistic interactions of transforming growth factors in the regulation of granulosa cell differentiation. Endocrinology 1986; 119:1879-81.
5. Hutchinson LA, Findlay JK, de Vos FL, Robertson DM. Effects of bovine inhibin, transforming growth factor-β and bovine activin-A on granulosa cell differentiation. Biochem Biophy Res Commun 1987; 146:1405-12.
6. Dodson WC, Schomberg DW. The effect of transforming growth factor-β on follicle stimulating hormone induced differentiation of cultured rat granulosa cells. Endocrinology 1987; 120:512-6.
7. Knecht M, Feng P, Catt KJ. Bifunctional role of transforming growth factor-β during granulosa cell development. Endocrinology 1987; 120:1243-9.
8. Hernandez ER, Adashi EY. Transforming growth factor β (TGFβ) inhibits ovarian androgen productions: a novel autocrine loop. Endocrinology 1988; 122:300A.
9. Fauser BCJM, Galway B, Hsueh AJW. Differentiation of ovarian and testicular cells: intragonadal regulation by growth factors. 5th European Workshop on Molecular and Cellular Endocrinology of the Testis. New York: Raven Press (in press).
10. Feng P, Catt KJ, Knecht M. Transforming growth factor-β stimulates meiotic maturation of the rat oocyte. Endocrinology 1988; 122:181-6.
11. Tsafriri A, Lindner HR, Zor U, Lamprecht SA. In vitro induction of meiotic division in follicle-enclosed rat oocytes with LH, cyclic AMP and prostaglandin E2. J Reprod Fertil 1972; 31:39-50.
12. Tsafriri A. Oocyte maturation in mammals. In: Jones RE, ed. The vertebrate ovary. New York: Plenum Press, 1987:409-33.
13. Tsafriri A, Reich R, Abisogun AO. The ovarian egg and ovulation. In: Lamming GE, ed. Marshall's physiology of reproduction; vol II. London: Churchill Livingston (in press).
14. Schuetz AW. Local control mechanisms during oogenesis and folliculogenesis. In: Browder LW, ed. Developmental biology. A comprehensive synthesis, vol I. Oogenesis. New York: Plenum Press, 1985:3-83.

22

Light and Electron Microscope Immunocytochemical Localization of Epidermal Growth Factor Receptors in Bovine Corpora Lutea of Pregnancy

N. Chegini, Z. M. Lei, and C. V. Rao

Department of Obstetrics/Gynecology, University of Louisville
School of Medicine, Louisville, KY 40292

Summary

Both luteal and nonluteal cells, i.e., macrophages, fibroblasts, vascular smooth muscle and endothelium, contain EGF receptors. Small luteal and nonluteal cells, however, contain more receptors than large luteal cells. The nuclei of both luteal and nonluteal cells also seem to contain EGF receptors. However, the pattern of nuclear receptor distribution differed with the receptor antibodies specific to the carbohydrate moiety and the binding sites on the extracellular domain of EGF receptor molecules. At the electron microscope level using the receptor antibody specific to the carbohydrate moiety, EGF receptors were found not only in plasma membranes, but also in rough endoplasmic reticulum, lysosomal vesicles, mitochondria and nuclei. The nuclear receptors are associated with nuclear membranes, condensed chromatin and the border between the condensed and dispersed chromatin. In conclusion, our results suggest that EGF may have steroidogenic and nonsteroidogenic roles in bovine corpora lutea and that transduction of EGF signals may also involve nuclear receptors.

Introduction

As in other tissues (1), EGF has mitogenic and nonmitogenic roles in gonadal cells (2,3). EGF can act on theca interna (4) and granulosa (2) cells. When granulosa cells differentiate into luteal cells, EGF receptors double in number with a loss of mitogenic influence (5). Although the functional relevance remains to be investigated, the presence of EGF receptors in corpora lutea of various species has been demonstrated (5-9).

The majority of the cells found in corpora lutea are nonluteal cells (10). There are small and large luteal cells which differ in some of the morphological and functional characteristics

(10). It is not known whether nonluteal as well as small and large luteal cells contain EGF receptors. Also not known is whether intracellular organelles of these cells also contain EGF receptors as there is growing evidence that transduction of EGF signals may also involve the intracellular receptors (11-18). The present studies were undertaken to obtain this information.

Materials and Methods

A monoclonal antibody to human EGF receptors (clone 29.1) was purchased from Sigma Chemical Company. This antibody is specific to the carbohydrate moiety of the extracellular domain of the receptor molecules. It does not inhibit ^{125}I-EGF binding to the receptors but selectively immunoprecipitates them (19). A monoclonal antibody to human EGF receptors (528 IgG) specific to binding sites on the extracellular domain of receptors was kindly provided by Dr. Hideo Masui from the Memorial Sloan-Kettering Cancer Center in New York City.

Three bovine corpora lutea of early pregnancy collected from a local slaughterhouse were processed immediately. For light microscopy, the tissues were fixed in Bouin's solution overnight at 22°C and processed according to Koay et al. (20). Hydrogen peroxide (H_2O_2)-treated 5 micron thick sections were washed for 30 min with phosphate buffered physiological saline (PBS), pH 7.3 and sequentially exposed to:

1. 1:50 dilution of normal horse serum in PBS for 30 min to saturate all the nonspecific binding sites for IgG.
2. 1:100 dilution of EGF receptor antibodies in PBS containing 0.5% BSA for 2 h.
3. 1:250 dilution of biotinylated horse anti-mouse IgG in PBS for 1 h.
4. 1:100 dilution of avidin-biotinylated horseradish peroxidase complex in PBS for 1 h.
5. Incubation with 0.1% 3,3'-diaminobenzidine (w/v) and 0.02% H_2O_2 (v/v) in PBS for 5 min for chromogenic reaction.

After each step, the sections were rinsed 3 times for 5 min each with PBS. All the steps were carried out in a humidified chamber at 22°C.

For electron microscopy, the tissue pieces (1 mm across) were fixed for 30 min at 4°C with 0.1% EM grade glutaraldehyde and 2% paraformaldehyde buffered with PBS. The tissue pieces were washed, dehydrated and embedded in either Spurr's resin (21) or Lowicryl K4M (22). Thin sections were cut and placed on 200 mesh-coated nickel grids. The grids were etched with 10% H_2O_2 for 10 min. Then the grids were sequentially exposed to drops of:

1. 1:100 dilution of normal goat serum in PBS for 10 min at 22°C.
2. 1:100 dilution of EGF receptor antibody in PBS containing 0.5% BSA overnight in a humidified chamber.
3. 1:100 dilution of normal goat serum for 10 min at 22°C.
4. 1:20 dilution of goat anti-mouse IgG gold (15 nm) in PBS.

The grids were fixed with 0.1% glutaraldehyde in PBS for 30 min and stained with uranyl acetate for 30 min. After each step, the grids were washed 3 times with PBS. Controls for light and electron microscopy included the use of receptor antibodies preabsorbed for 24 h at 4°C with placental microvilli followed by centrifugation at 100,000 x g for 1 h and omission of receptor antibodies during the immunostaining procedure.

Results

Figures 1A and 1B show immunostaining in both luteal (>15 μm) and nonluteal (<15 μm) cells following exposure to two different receptor antibodies. These figures also show that small luteal cells (15-18 μm) and nonluteal cells immunostained more than large luteal cells (19-45 μm). The nuclei of both luteal and nonluteal cells were also immunostained. However, the pattern of nuclear immunostaining was different with these two receptor antibodies. Using the receptor antibody specific to the carbohydrate moiety, immunostaining in nuclei was found to be greater than that in cytoplasmic organelles and plasma membranes (Fig. 1A). Using the receptor antibody specific to binding sites, the immunostaining in cytoplasmic organelles and plasma membranes was found to be greater than that in nuclei (Fig. 1B).

Figures 1C and 1D show that immunostaining considerably decreased from all the cells when preabsorbed receptor antibodies were used. Similar results were obtained when the receptor antibodies were omitted during the immunostaining procedure (data not shown).

The subcellular distribution of EGF receptors was investigated using the receptor antibody specific to the carbohydrate moiety of the receptor molecule. Figure 2 shows that immunogold particles are present in plasma membranes (A), nuclei (A & F), lysosomal vesicles (C & E), mitochondria (A & C) and rough ER (D). The nuclear gold particles are associated with nuclear membranes, condensed chromatin and the border between condensed and dispersed chromatin (F). Dispersed chromatin contain very few gold particles (F).

The studies on subcellular distribution of EGF receptors using the receptor antibody specific to binding sites are in progress.

Preabsorption of the receptor antibody (Fig. 3) or omission of unabsorbed receptor antibody (data not shown) during the immunostaining procedure resulted in dramatic reduction of gold particles from all the cellular organelles.

Discussion

The resolution of light microscope immunocytochemistry is adequate for revealing that nuclei of both luteal and nonluteal cells also contain receptors. However, the pattern of nuclear distribution is different with the two receptor antibodies. This difference in nuclear receptor distribution raises two possibilities. First, receptor antibody specific to the carbohydrate moiety cross-reacted with the other nuclear glycoproteins. Second, nuclei is the major site of a form of receptor which lacks EGF binding sites. There is no indication from the previous studies, however, that this receptor antibody cross-reacts with any other cellular glycoproteins (19,23).

In agreement with some previous studies (12-14), the present studies demonstrate the presence of EGF receptors not only in plasma membranes but also rough ER, lysosomal vesicles, mitochondria and nuclei. The nuclear sites are associated with nuclear membranes, condensed chromatin and the border between condensed and dispersed chromatin where transcriptionally active genes are known to be present (24). The present findings, along with those from previous studies (11-18), strongly suggest that the transduction of EGF signals involves nuclear receptors.

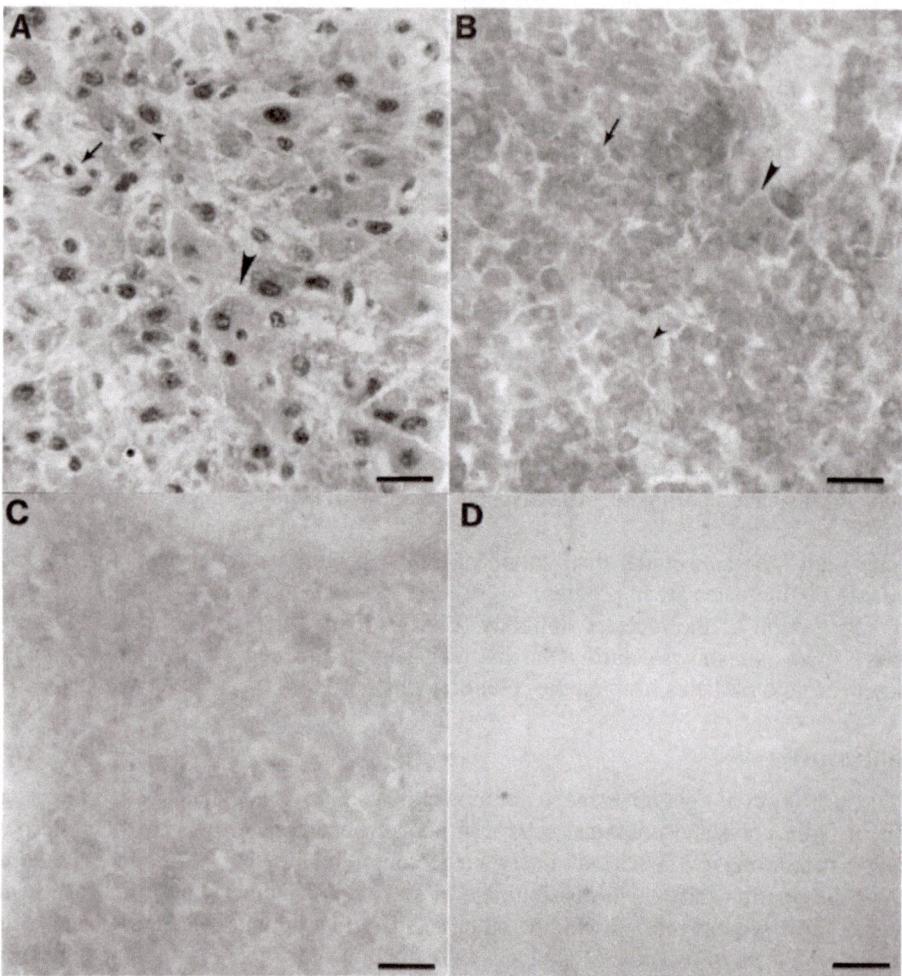

Fig. 1. Light microscope immunocytochemical localization of EGF receptors in bovine corpora lutea using the unabsorbed (A & B) and preabsorbed (C & D) receptor antibodies specific to the carbohydrate moiety (A & C) and binding sites (B & D) on the extracellular domain of the receptors. Large and small luteal cells are pointed out by large and small arrow heads, respectively. Arrows point out nonluteal cells. Bars, A = 20 μm; B & C = 40 μm; and, D = 80 μm.

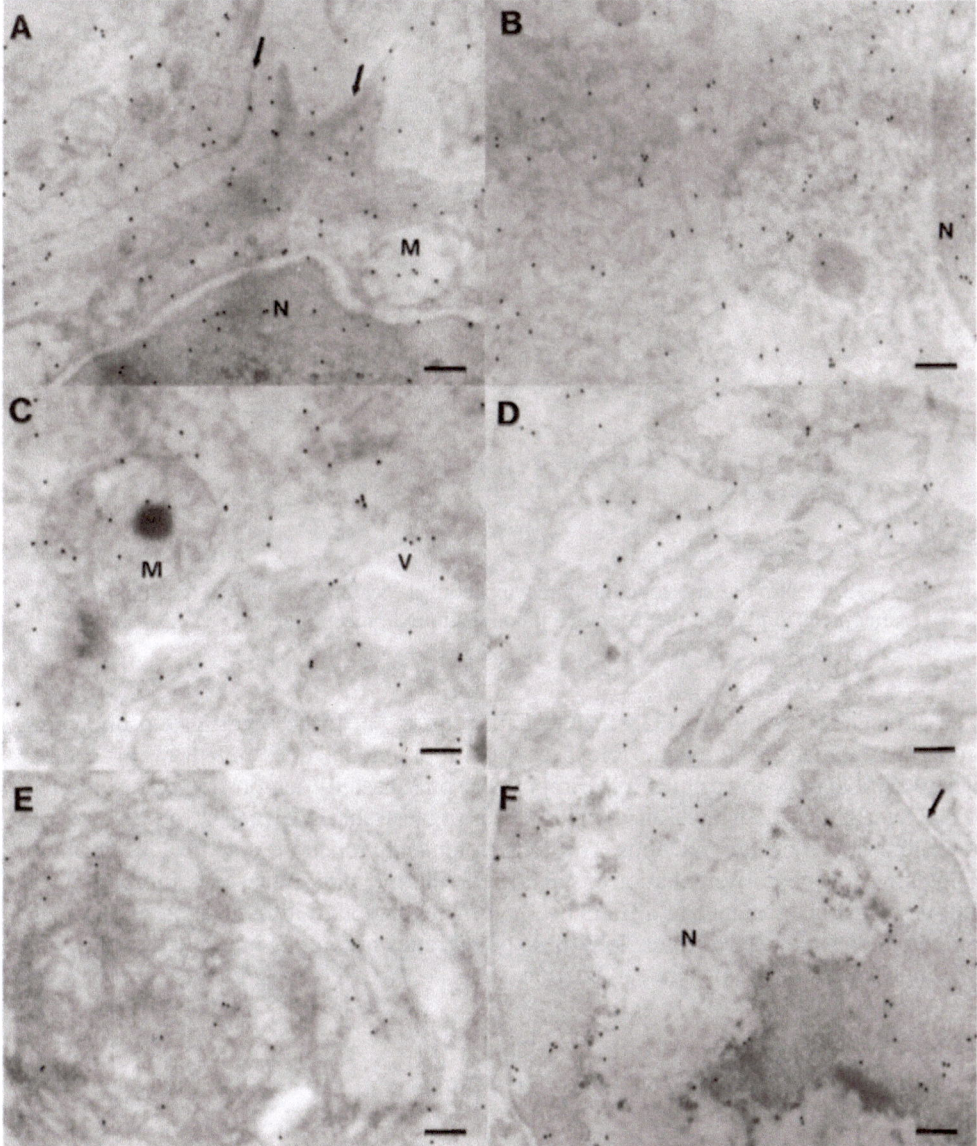

Fig. 2. Electron microscope immunocytochemical localization of EGF receptors in bovine corpora lutea using the receptor antibody specific to the carbohydrate moiety. Arrows in A indicate the plasma membranes of two adjacent luteal cells and nuclear membrane in F. N = nucleus, V = presumed lysosomal vesicles, M = mitochondria. Bar = 0.25 μm.

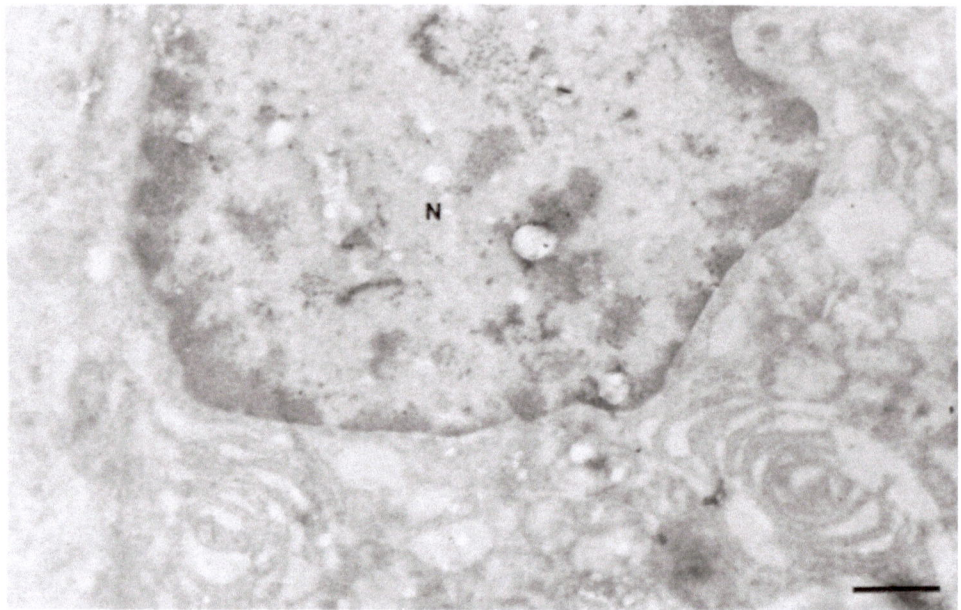

Fig. 3. Electron microscope immunocytochemical localization of EGF receptors after preabsorption of the receptor antibody with EGF receptors. N = nucleus. Bar = 0.25 μm.

Although the role(s) of EGF in luteal function is yet to be investigated, one could probably eliminate a mitogenic role because corpus luteum does not grow by cellular hyperplasia but rather by cellular hypertrophy. The present study demonstrating the presence of EGF receptors in both luteal and nonluteal cells suggests that EGF may have steroidogenic as well nonsteroidogenic functions. The nonsteroidogenic functions could be, for example, cellular hypertrophy, differentiation of small luteal cells into large luteal cells, morphological and functional maintenance of different cell types, regulation of intraluteal blood flow, etc. Further studies are needed to explore these possibilities as well as interrelationships with other hormones that regulate luteal function.

Acknowledgment

This work is supported by NIH grant HD 14697.

References

1. Carpenter G, Cohen S. Epidermal growth factor. Annu Rev Biochem 1979; 48:193-216.
2. Gospodarowicz D, Bialecki H. Fibroblast and epidermal growth factors are mitogenic agents for cultured granulosa cells of rodent, porcine and human origin. Endocrinology 1979; 104:757-64.
3. Hsueh AJW, Welsh TH, Jones PBC. Inhibition of ovarian and testicular steroidogenesis by epidermal growth factor. Endocrinology 1981; 108:2002-4.

4. Erickson GF, Case E. Epidermal growth factor antagonizes ovarian theca-interstitial cytodifferentiation. Mol Cell Endocrinol 1983; 31:71-6.
5. Vlodavsky I, Brown KD, Gospodarowicz D. A comparison of the binding of epidermal growth factor to cultured granulosa and luteal cells. J Biol Chem 1978; 253:3744-50.
6. Mock EJ, Niswender GD. Differences in the rates of internalization of ^{125}I-labeled chorionic gonadotropin, luteinizing hormone and epidermal growth factor by ovine luteal cells. Endocrinology 1983; 113:259-64.
7. Homm RJ, Osuampke CO, Rao CV, Sanfilippo JS. Epidermal growth factor binding to human ovaries. Fertil Steril 1984; 41:75.
8. Chabot J-G, StArnaud R, Walker P, Pelletier G. Distribution of epidermal growth factor receptors in the rat ovary. Mol Cell Endocrinol 1986; 44:99-108.
9. Ayyagari RR, Khan-Dawood FS. Human corpus luteum: presence of epidermal growth factor receptors and binding characteristics. Am J Obstet Gynecol 1987; 156:942-6.
10. Chegini N, Ramani N, Rao CV. Morphological and biochemical characterization of small and large bovine luteal cells during pregnancy. Mol Cell Endocrinol 1984; 37:89-102.
11. Savion N, Vlodavsky I, Gospodarowicz D. Nuclear accumulation of epidermal growth factor in cultured bovine corneal endothelial and granulosa cells. J Biol Chem 1981; 256:1149-54.
12. Lev-Ran A, Hwang D, Josefsberg Z, et al. Binding of epidermal growth factor and insulin to human liver microsomes and Golgi fractions. Biochem Biophys Res Commun 1984; 119:1181-5.
13. Ramani N, Chegini N, Rao CV, Woost PG, Schultz GS. The presence of epidermal growth factor binding sites in the intracellular organelles of term human placenta. J Cell Sci 1986; 84:19-40.
14. Rakowicz-Szulczynska EM, Rodeck U, Herlyn M, Koprowski H. Chromatin binding of epidermal growth factor and platelet derived growth factor in cells bearing the appropriate receptors. Proc Natl Acad Sci USA 1986; 83:3728-32.
15. Lai WH, Guyada HJ, Bergeron JJM. Binding and internalization of epidermal growth factor in human term placental cells in culture. Endocrinology 1986; 118:413-23.
16. Schindler M, Jiang L-N. Epidermal growth factor and insulin stimulate nuclear pore-mediated macromolecular transport in isolated rat liver nuclei. J Cell Biol 1987; 104:849-53.
17. Raper SE, Burwen SJ, Barker ME, Jones AL. Translocation of epidermal growth factor to the hepatocyte nucleus during rat liver regeneration. Gastroenterology 1987; 92:1243-50.
18. Green MR, Mycock C, Smith CG, Couchman JR. Biochemical and ultrastructural processing of [^{125}I]epidermal growth factor in rat epidermis and hair follicles: accumulation of nuclear label. J Invest Dermatol 1987; 88:259-65.
19. Yarden Y, Harari I, Schlessinger J. Purification of an active EGF receptor kinase with monoclonal antireceptor antibodies. J Biol Chem 1985; 260:315-9.
20. Koay ES, Bagnell CA, Bryant-Greenwood GD, Lord SB, Cruz AC, Larkin LH. Immunocytochemical localization of relaxin in human decidua and placenta. J Clin Endocrinol Metab 1985; 60:859-63.
21. Chegini N, Rao CV. Quantitative electron microscope autoradiographic studies on ^{125}I-epidermal growth factor internalization in term human placenta. J Cell Sci 1986; 84:41-52.
22. Bendayan M. Ultrastructural localization of nucleic acids by the use of enzyme-gold complexes. J Histochem Cytochem 1981; 29:531-41.

23. Carpentier J-L, Rees AR, Gregoriou M, Kris R, Schlessinger J, Orci L. Subcellular distribution of the external and internal domains of the EGF receptor in A-431 cells. Exp Cell Res 1986; 166:312-26.
24. Fakan S, Puvion E. The ultrastructural visualization of nucleolar and extranucleolar RNA synthesis and distribution. Int Rev Cytol 1980; 65:255-99.

23

Maturation of the Oocyte-Cumulus Cell Complex in Mice: Specificity of Epidermal Growth Factor Activity

Stephen M. Downs

Biology Department, Biological and Biomedical Research Institute
Marquette University, Milwaukee, WI 53233

Introduction

Fully grown mammalian oocytes within the ovary remain arrested in prophase 1 of meiosis until the preovulatory gonadotropin surge, at which time the resumption of meiotic maturation is stimulated in a specific group of graafian follicles. This event is heralded by dissolution of the nucleus, a process termed germinal vesicle breakdown (GVB). The mechanism by which oocytes are induced to mature in vivo is poorly understood. Because GVB occurs spontaneously when meiotically competent oocytes are removed from the ovary and placed in culture, it appears that the ovary provides inhibitory input that maintains meiotic arrest. Indeed, various follicular fluid components have been shown to suppress the spontaneous maturation of oocytes (1,2).

Within the follicle, the oocyte is metabolically coupled to the surrounding follicle cells by gap junctions, facilitating direct transfer of instructional signals from somatic to germ cells (3-5). Following the preovulatory gonadotropin surge, gap junctional communication is terminated between the oocyte and cumulus cells (6,7) and between the cumulus cells and membrana granulosa (8). Such uncoupling has been proposed as a mechanism for resumption of meiosis in vivo. According to this hypothesis, the loss of gap junctional communication separates the oocyte from follicle cell inhibitory signals, thereby permitting GVB (9,10).

Evidence for a Positive Stimulus for GVB

We have recently presented evidence in support of an alternative mechanism for oocyte maturation in vivo, that of positive stimulation (11). When cumulus cell-enclosed oocytes (CEO) from 21-23-day-old, pregnant mare serum gonadotropin-primed mice were maintained in meiotic arrest in vitro with hypoxanthine (HX) guanosine (Guo), the cyclic AMP analog, dbcAMP, or the cAMP phosphodiesterase inhibitor, 3-isobutyl-1-methylxanthine (IBMX), addition of follicle-stimulating hormone (FSH) or epidermal growth factor (EGF) stimulated GVB (Table 1). Moreover, the frequency of GVB in the FSH- or EGF-treated groups was significantly higher than that in oocytes cultured in the absence of cumulus cells (denuded oocytes). Neither hormone had any effect on denuded oocytes. Consequently, the induction of maturation in cumulus cell-enclosed oocytes in response to FSH or EGF cannot be due simply to termination of coupling or gap junction-mediated inhibitory somatic cell input. Rather, the data argue in favor of a positive stimulus, generated in the cumulus cells in response to hormone treatment, that promotes GVB. Similar results were obtained when meiotically incompetent oocytes with 1-3 layers of granulosa cells were isolated from 10-day-old mice and grown in vitro for 12 days in the presence of HX. FSH induced maturation in a manner consistent with the generation of a positive stimulus (12).

Specificity of the EGF Response

The efficacy of EGF in promoting oocyte maturation raised the question of specificity, e.g., were other growth factors as effective? To test this question, ten different growth factors were compared for their ability to induce GVB in CEO from primed mice when meiotic arrest was maintained 21-22 h in vitro with HX. Each growth factor was tested in a separate experiment, with four different doses of growth factor. The range of GVB in the HX control groups (no growth factor present) was 44-65%. As shown in Table 2, GVB occurred in 100% of EGF-treated oocytes. While most of the remaining growth factors demonstrated a positive

Table 1. Induction of mouse oocyte maturation by FSH and EGF

Treatment*	CEO			Denuded		
	n	GVB	(%)	n	GVB	(%)
HX	717	251	(35)	402	246	(61)
HX + FSH	591	526	(89)	308	183	(59)
HX + EGF	617	523	(85)	336	190	(57)
Guo	307	100	(36)	424	187	(44)
Guo + FSH	327	241	(74)	312	101	(32)
Guo + EGF	338	300	(89)	317	98	(31)
dbcAMP	303	69	(23)	357	170	(48)
dbcAMP + FSH	273	258	(95)			
dbcAMP + EGF	279	256	(92)			
IBMX	272	5	(2)	298	94	(32)
IBMX + FSH	271	200	(74)			
IBMX + EGF	246	188	(76)			

*CEO and denuded oocytes from PMSG-primed, immature mice were cultured 21-22 h in medium (MEM supplemented with 3 mg/ml BSA) containing 4 mM HX, 2 mM Guo, 300 μM dbcAMP or 100 μM IBMX, plus or minus oFSH (0.1 μg/ml) or EGF (1 ng/ml). Data from Downs et al. (11).

effect on oocyte maturation, the frequency of GVB produced by the optimal dose of growth factor was, in every instance, still significantly below that of the EGF group. Thus, the meiotic response to growth factor appears to be most specific for EGF. A recent study has demonstrated a stimulatory action of TGF-β on rat oocyte maturation (13). In this light, it is interesting that TGF-β was the least effective growth factor tested on mouse oocyte maturation. However, it must be emphasized that the effect of a particular growth factor may be influenced by the presence or absence of other growth factors.

The optimal dose obtained for each growth factor in the previous experiment was tested on cumulus cell expansion in medium containing 5% fetal bovine serum. The degree of expansion was assessed according to a subjective scale from "0" (no expansion) to "+4" (complete expansion). After 17-18 h in culture, EGF stimulated expansion to "+4" in 100% of the oocyte-cumulus cell complexes. Fewer than 12% of the FSH-treated complexes had expanded to a similar extent by this time (68% at "+3"). Ninety-nine percent of controls were at "0." None of the other growth factors stimulated expansion; in all cases, ≥94% of the complexes were at "0." The effect of EGF was striking in that the appearance of the complexes was identical to that of freshly ovulated ova. While FSH-treated complexes were expanded, they rarely achieved the degree of expansion and "stickiness" observed in cumuli of EGF-treated or ovulated ova. In addition, when compared to the effect of FSH, EGF accelerated the kinetics of cumulus expansion (data not presented).

Table 2. Effect of growth factors on hypoxanthine-maintained meiotic arrest

Treatment*	% GVB in Control (HX alone)	Optimal Dose (ng/ml)	% GVB	% Increase
EGF	49	0.1	100	51
FGF	51	10.0	76	25
NGF	48	1.0	68	20
TGF-β	62	1.0	69	7
Insulin	52	1.0	74	22
IGF-1	44	100.0	66	22
IGF-2	48	100.0	75	27
Bombesin	53	100.0	69	16
PDGF	65	1.0	73	8
Orthovanadate	52	0.1 μM	76	24

*Cumulus cell-enclosed oocytes from PMSG-primed, immature mice were cultured 21-22 h in medium (supplemented with 3 mg/ml BSA) containing 4 mM HX. Four different doses of each growth factor were tested and the maturation data for the optimal dose are reported in the table. The % GVB is given as the mean of at least three separate experiments. Fifty oocytes were assayed per group per experiment. FGF, fibroblast growth factor; NGF, nerve growth factor; TGF-β, transforming growth factor-β; IGF-1,2, insulin-like growth factors-1,2; PDGF, platelet-derived growth factor.

Mechanism of Action

It is possible that the action of FSH and EGF are mediated by cAMP. Both hormones stimulated cAMP synthesis in oocyte-cumulus cell complexes, but the effect of FSH was 3.4-fold greater than that of EGF (11). This might explain the observation that the action of FSH on oocyte maturation is initially inhibitory and later stimulatory (11,14), while that of EGF is always stimulatory (11). However, if cAMP were the principal mediator of EGF action, one would expect at least a transient inhibition of spontaneous oocyte maturation in response to EGF treatment. In addition, cAMP has been shown to stimulate cumulus expansion (15,16), but the greater potency of EGF in eliciting this response suggests a different mechanism must be responsible for the action of this growth factor on cumulus expansion. Also, preliminary data show that the sulfated glycosaminoglycan, heparin, prevents both FSH- and EGF-stimulated cumulus expansion but has no suppressive effect on meiotic maturation induced by these hormones. The above data are consistent with the idea that the actions of FSH and EGF are mediated by separate second messengers that converge more distally on common mechanisms for meiotic maturation and cumulus expansion. For example, hormone stimulation may provoke the synthesis of specific proteins involved in meiotic maturation because protein synthesis inhibitors prevent both FSH- and EGF-induced oocyte maturation (17). While cAMP is the likely mediator of FSH action, EGF and other growth factors may elicit their response through phospholipid turnover, with a subsequent increase in intracellular calcium and activation of protein kinase C (18). Consistent with this idea are the findings that protein kinase C activators stimulate GVB in follicle-enclosed rat oocytes (19) and elevation of calcium levels induces GVB in oocytes of several rodent species (20-22). The possibility that FSH action may be mediated, at least in part, in a similar manner cannot be discounted.

References

1. Tsafriri A, Dekel N, Bar-Ami S. J Reprod Fertil 1982; 64:541-51.
2. Eppig JJ, Downs SM. In: Haseltine FP, First NL, eds. Meiotic inhibition: molecular control mechanisms. New York: Alan R. Liss, Inc., 1988 (in press).
3. Amsterdam A, Josephs R, Lieberman ME, Lindner HR. J Cell Sci 1976; 21:93-105.
4. Anderson E, Albertini DF. J Cell Biol 1976; 71:680-6.
5. Gilula NB, Epstein ML, Beers WH. J Cell Biol 1978; 78:58-75.
6. Moor RM, Osborn JC, Cran DG, Walters DE. J Embryol Exp Morphol 1981; 61:347-65.
7. Eppig JJ. Dev Biol 1981; 89:268-72.
8. Larsen WJ, West SE, Brunner GD. Dev Biol 1986; 113:517-21.
9. Dekel N, Beers WH. Proc Natl Acad Sci USA 1978; 75:4369-73.
10. Dekel N, Beers WH. Dev Biol 1980; 75:247-54.
11. Downs SM, Daniel SAJ, Eppig JJ. J Exp Zool 1988; 245:86-96.
12. Eppig JJ, Downs SM. Dev Biol 1986; 119:313-21.
13. Feng P, Catt KJ, Knecht M. Endocrinology 1988; 122:181-6.
14. Downs SM, Eppig JJ. Gamete Res 1985; 11:83-97.
15. Eppig JJ. J Exp Zool 1979; 208:111-20.
16. Dekel N, Phillips DM. Biol Reprod 1980; 22:289-96.
17. Downs SM. Biol Reprod 1988; 38(suppl 1):67 (Abstract 57).

18. Nishizuka Y, Takai Y, Kishimoto A, Kikkawa U, Kaibuchi K. Recent Prog Horm Res 1984; 40:301-45.
19. Aberdam E, Dekel N. Biochem Biophys Res Commun 1985; 132:570-4.
20. Tsafriri A, Bar-Ami S. J Exp Zool 1978; 205:293-9.
21. Powers RD, Paleos GA. J Reprod Fertil 1982; 66:1-8.
22. Racowsky C. J Exp Zool 1986; 239:263-75.

24

Multifactorial Regulation of Granulosa Cell (GC) Proliferation: Interactions Among Polypeptide Growth Factors

Jeffrey V. May

Department of Obstetrics and Gynecology, The University of Kansas School of Medicine-Wichita, and The Women's Research Institute
2903 E. Central, Wichita, KS 67214

Introduction

Proliferation of the mural granulosa cells is a requisite component of the folliculogenic process. Our understanding of the regulation of this process at the level of the cell is limited. Although FSH and estradiol stimulate granulosa cell proliferation in vivo, they have a limited effect in vitro which suggests that they may act indirectly by stimulating the production of local, intraovarian mitogens, i.e., growth factors. Indeed, the ovary may be a site for the production of insulin-like growth factor-I (IGF-I, 1,2), epidermal growth factor (EGF, 3,4), and transforming growth factor-beta (TGFβ, 5). Studies by Gospodarowicz and colleagues suggested that EGF and fibroblast growth factor (FGF) were mitogens for many but not all granulosa cells (6-8). The actions of these growth factors could be enhanced markedly by serum which suggested that other factors, perhaps other growth factors, could synergize with EGF and FGF to promote granulosa cell proliferation. Accordingly, studies were initiated in this laboratory to investigate interactions among growth factors with respect to the regulation of granulosa cell proliferation.

Methods

It became necessary to develop a model system which supported cell attachment during active cell proliferation but which was growth factor restricted. This was accomplished using platelet-poor plasma-derived serum (PPPDS). Platelets are a major source of serum growth factors including EGF, PDGF, and TGFβ (9-11). During the preparation of PPPDS, the platelets are removed prior to the formation of the clot, thus reducing the endogenous growth factor content. EGF, present at 1-2 ng/ml in serum, is <0.1 ng/ml in PPPDS (12).

Porcine granulosa cells (pGC, 50,000/cm2 well, 4 wells/group) were cultured in 0.5 ml of medium (Ham's F12:DMEM, 1:1) supplemented with 5% fetal calf serum (FCS) for 2 days (37°C, 95%/5% air/CO_2) to facilitate cell attachment. This was replaced by medium + 0.1% PPPDS +/- growth factors (as given) +/- human low density lipoprotein (LDL, 10 μg/ml). Cells were maintained in their respective media for 6 days with a medium change on day 3. Thus, the cells were allowed to attach and proliferate for 2 and 6 days, respectively. Following culture, the cells were trypsinized and the cell content determined using a Coulter Counter.

Results

Previous studies in this laboratory have shown that in the 0.1% PPPDS model system, EGF alone has little proliferative activity toward pGC, but when combined with IGF-I/Sm-C can stimulate pGC proliferation (13). These studies were expanded to include platelet-derived growth factor (PDGF). Furthermore, it was determined that medium containing 0.1% PPPDS is rate-limiting with respect to cholesterol for the maintenance of pGC proliferation (14). Accordingly, the effects of LDL upon growth factor-stimulated pGC proliferation were investigated. The results given in Figure 1 are derived from 9 separate experiments, and the results are presented as the percent of media controls (0.1% PPPDS). Neither EGF, IGF-I, nor PDGF alone stimulated pGC proliferation relative to controls. Although PDGF + IGF-I had no effect upon pGC proliferation, the levels of proliferation obtained using EGF + IGF-I and EGF + PDGF were identical to those obtained having 10% fetal calf serum in the medium throughout the culture period. When EGF, IGF-I, and PDGF are combined at 10, 10, and 5 ng/ml, respectively, the extent of pGC proliferation was significantly greater than that obtained with 10% FCS (P<0.05) and was 55% of that obtained with 10% FCS + EGF (10 ng/ml). Thus, the regulation of pGC proliferation is multifactorial involving several facilitative growth factors acting synergistically.

LDL alone had no effect upon pGC proliferation nor did it facilitate proliferation mediated by any single growth factor (Fig. 1). LDL did markedly enhance the proliferative actions of EGF, IGF-I, and PDGF when used in dual growth factor combinations. The combinations of EGF + IGF-I + LDL and EGF + PDGF + LDL were particularly effective. When optimum doses of EGF, IGF-I, PDGF and LDL were combined, the proliferation rate equalled 90% of that obtained with FCS + EGF. Thus, pGC population growth is governed both by the availability of facilitative growth factors such as EGF, IGF-I, and PDGF, and the availability of cholesterol, presumably to facilitate plasma membrane biosynthesis.

Although most growth factors promote cell proliferation, this is not uniformly the case. TGFβ has been shown to inhibit proliferation of numerous cell types, especially those of epithelial origin (15). Indeed, TGFβ may have a dual role with respect to granulosa cell function. TGFβ has been shown to enhance processes associated with granulosa cell differentiation such as FSH-stimulated estrogen production and LH/hCG receptor induction (16,17). Alternatively, TGFβ has been shown to inhibit granulosa cell proliferation (5). To determine if TGFβ attenuated pGC proliferation mediated by the facilitative growth factors in the 0.1% PPPDS system described above, cultures were established using combinations of EGF, IGF-I, PDGF, and LDL and increasing doses of TGFβ. The results are presented in Figure 2 where the data are presented as cell counts per culture. As indicated in Figure 1, pGC proliferation could be increased by the addition of specific growth factor combinations. TGFβ dose-dependent attenuated pGC proliferation by all growth factor combinations with

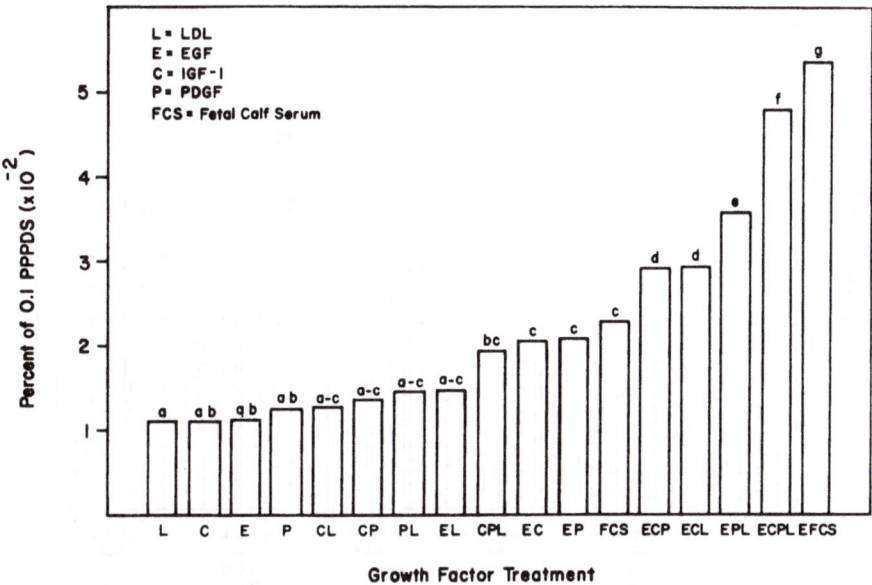

Fig. 1. The regulation of pGC proliferation. PGC were cultured as described in Methods with combinations of growth factors, LDL, and serum as indicated and the cell counts expressed as a percent of media controls (0.1% PPPDS). The concentrations of supplements were: hEGF (E), 10 ng/ml; hIGF-I (C), 10 ng/ml; hPDGF (P), 5 ng/ml; hLDL (L) 10 µg/ml; fetal calf serum (FCS), 10%. Data bars having no common letters are significantly different at P<0.05 (one-way ANOVA and Duncan's new multiple range tests).

an optimum inhibitory dose of 2.5-5 ng/ml. At low doses of TGFβ (0.1-1 ng/ml), however, the level of proliferation could be increased as the complement of growth-promoting factors was increased (i.e., EGF + IGF-I + PDGF + LDL > EGF + IGF-I + LDL > EGF + IGF-I + PDGF, etc.).

Discussion

The results presented above suggest that the regulation of granulosa cell proliferation is complex and is not mediated by any single factor but rather by the interaction of several factors including facilitative growth factors such as EGF, PDGF, and IGF-I, and inhibitory factors such as TGFβ. With respect to EGF, IGF-I and TGFβ, regulation may involve intraovarian expression at the level of the gene since each growth factor appears to be produced in the ovary (1-5). EGF appears to play a dominant proliferative role based upon the need for this growth factor for optimum granulosa cell proliferation and its negative impact upon granulosa cell differentiation (18). The actions of TGFβ are directly opposite to those of EGF. TGFβ inhibits growth factor-mediated granulosa cell proliferation but enhances granulosa cell differentiation (16,17). IGF-I is unique in that it can enhance both EGF-stimulated proliferation and enhance FSH-mediated granulosa cell differentiation (19). PDGF enhances markedly the proliferative actions of EGF. Its role with respect to granulosa

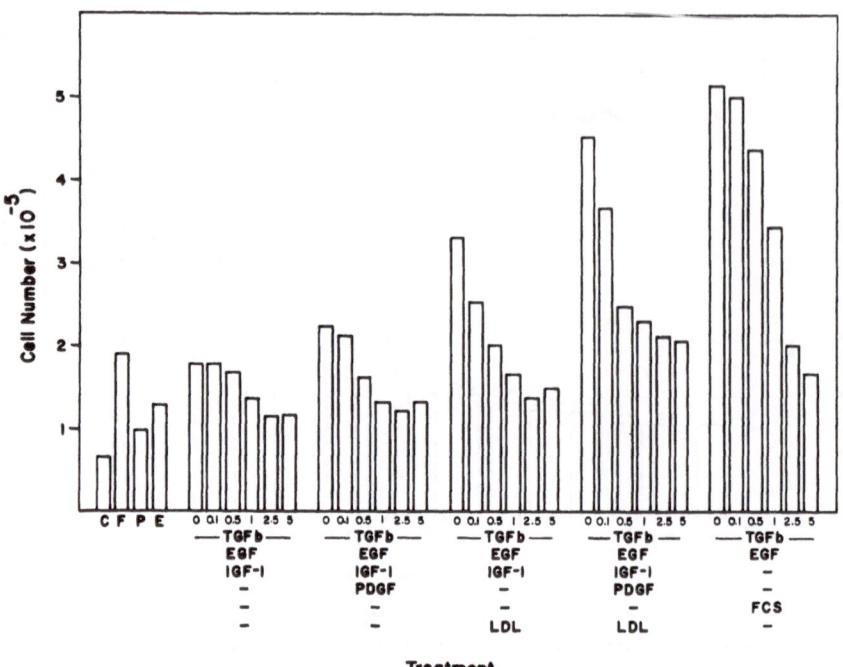

Fig. 2. Inhibitory action of TGFβ upon growth factor-stimulated pGC proliferation.
Cells were cultured as described in Methods with growth factor combinations given
in the presence of TGFβ at 0-5 ng/ml. C = day 2 cell counts; F = 10% FCS control;
P = 0.1% PPPDS control; E = EGF, 10 ng/ml; IGF-I, 10 ng/ml; PDGF, 5 ng/ml;
LDL, 10 μg/ml; FCS, 10%.

cell differentiation is largely unknown. Although originally thought to enhance granulosa
cell differentiation, it is believed that this action was due to TGFβ contamination of the PDGF
preparations. PDGF expression in the ovary has yet to be demonstrated. However, since the
follicular fluid is a transudate of plasma, it may be available to granulosa cells from systemic
sources. The necessity of exogenous cholesterol for gonadotropin-stimulated granulosa cell
steroidogenesis is well documented. Granulosa cells make little if any cholesterol de novo.
The availability of lipoprotein-derived cholesterol also appears to be important for sustained
granulosa cell proliferation.

The roles of growth factors upon granulosa cell proliferation and differentiation are
summarized in Table 1. It is clear that the regulation of granulosa cell proliferation is
multifactorial. The extent of proliferation in the follicle would appear to be dependent upon
both the complement and levels of growth regulatory factors present available from intraovarian and/or systemic sources.

Table 1. The roles of growth factors in granulosa cell
differentiation and proliferation

	Effect upon granulosa cell:	
Growth Factor	Differentiation	Proliferation
EGF	Attenuates	Stimulates
IGF-I	Facilitates	Facilitates
PDGF	?	Facilitates
TGFβ	Facilitates	Attenuates
LDL	Facilitates	Facilitates

References

1. Hernandez ER, Hoyt E, Van Wyk JJ, Adashi EY. The Somatomedin-C/insulin-like growth factor-I (Sm-C/IGF-I) gene is expressed in the rat ovary [Abstract]. Endocrinology 1987; 120(1):821A.
2. Hsu CJ, Hammond JM. Gonadotropins and estradiol stimulate immunoreactive insulin-like growth factor-I production by porcine granulosa cells in vitro. Endocrinology 1987; 120:198-207.
3. Rall LB, Scott J, Bell GI, et al. Mouse prepro-epidermal growth factor synthesis by the kidney and other tissues. Nature 1985; 313:228-31.
4. Skinner MK, Lobb D, Dorrington JH. Ovarian thecal/interstitial cells produce an epidermal growth factor-like substance. Endocrinology 1987; 121:1892-9.
5. Skinner MK, Keski-Oja J, Osteen KG, Moses HL. Ovarian thecal cells produce transforming growth factor-beta which can regulate granulosa cell growth. Endocrinology 1987; 121:786-92.
6. Gospodarowicz D, Bialecki H. Fibroblast and epidermal growth factors are mitogenic agents for cultured granulosa cells of rodent, porcine, and human origin. Endocrinology 1979; 104:757-64.
7. Gospodarowicz D, Ill CR, Birdwell CR. Effects of fibroblast and epidermal growth factors on ovarian cell proliferation in vitro. I. Characterization of the response of granulosa cells to FGF and EGF. Endocrinology 1977; 100:1108-20.
8. Savion N, Lui G-M, Laherty R, Gospodarowicz D. Factors controlling proliferation and progesterone production by bovine granulosa cells in serum-free medium. Endocrinology 1981; 109:409-20.
9. Antoniades HN, Scher CD, Stiles CD. Purification of human platelet-derived growth factor. Proc Natl Acad Sci USA 1979; 76:1809-13.
10. Assoian RK, Komoriya A, Meyers CA, Miller DM, Sporn MB. Transforming growth factor-B in human platelets: identification of a major storage site, purification, and characterization. J Biol Chem 1983; 7155-60.
11. Oka Y, Orth DN. Human plasma epidermal growth factor/B-urogasterone is associated with blood platelets. J Clin Invest 1983; 72:249.
12. Biomedical Technologies Inc., Stoughton, MA, 02072, personal communication.
13. May JV, Frost JP, Schomberg DW. Differential effects of epidermal growth factor (EGF), somatomedin C/insulin-like growth factor I (Sm-C), and transforming growth

factor-beta (TGFβ) upon porcine granulosa cell DNA synthesis cell proliferation. Endocrinology 1988 (in press).

14. May JV, Frost JP. Rate-limiting effect of low-density lipoprotein (LDL) upon growth factor-stimulated proliferation of porcine granulosa cells (pGC) [Abstract]. Biol Reprod 1988; 38(1):177A.

15. Sporn MB, Roberts AB, Wakefield LM, Assoian RK. Transforming growth factor-B: biological function and chemical structure. Science 1986; 233:532-4.

16. Adashi EY, Resnick CE. Antagonistic interactions of transforming growth factors in the regulation of granulosa cell differentiation. Endocrinology 1986; 119:1879-81.

17. Dodson WC, Schomberg DW. The effect of transforming growth factor-beta on follicle-stimulating hormone-induced differentiation of cultured rat granulosa cells. Endocrinology 1987; 120:512-6.

18. Mondschein JS, Schomberg DW. Growth factors modulate gonadotropin receptor induction in granulosa cell cultures. Science 1981; 211:1179-81.

19. Adashi EY, Resnick CE, D'Ercole AJ, Svoboda ME, Van Wyk JJ. Insulin-like growth factors as intraovarian regulators of granulosa cell growth and function. Endocr Rev 1985; 6:400-20.

25

Gonadotropins Enhance the Cytoplasmic Maturation of Mouse Oocytes Under the Influence of Growth Factors

Masao Jinno, Bruce A. Sandow, Rihachi Iizuka,* and Gary D. Hodgen

The Jones Institute for Reproductive Medicine, Department of Obstetrics and Gynecology, Eastern Virginia Medical School, Medical College of Hampton Roads, 855 W. Brambleton Avenue, Suite B, Norfolk, Virginia 23510. *Keio University School of Medicine, Department of Obstetrics and Gynecology, Tokyo, Japan

Introduction

Although germinal vesicle (GV) stage oocytes collected before the gonadotropin surge can resume meiosis relatively easily and reach metaphase II in vitro, the potential for fertilization and embryonic development of these in vitro matured oocytes is usually poor. To understand the role of the gonadotropin surge in controlling the physiological maturation of oocytes, we attempted to mature GV stage mouse oocytes, which had not been exposed to a gonadotropin surge, in medium supplemented by gonadotropins, and then assessed the physiological maturity of the oocytes by examining their potential for fertilization and embryonic development in vitro.

Materials and Methods

Cumulus cell-enclosed GV stage oocytes were collected from 21- to 24-day-old B6SJL F_1 hybrid mice primed with 5 IU of pregnant mare serum gonadotropin (PMSG) 48-52 h earlier. In the first experiment, the oocytes were matured in vitro for 15-17 h in modified minimum essential medium (1) containing 10% fetal bovine serum (or serum replacement with growth factors: CPSR-1, Sigma) without (no hormone group) or with the following gonadotropins: 2.5 µg/ml follicle-stimulating hormone (FSH), 10 µg/ml luteinizing hormone (LH), 2.5 µg/ml FSH + 10 µg/ml LH, or 0.25 µg/ml FSH + 10 µg/ml LH. In the second experiment, a sequential combination of FSH and LH was tested. After 15 min, 2 h, or 3.5 h from the beginning of the maturation culture, 10 µg/ml LH was added into the maturation medium containing 2.5 µg/ml FSH. No LH was added in the control group. Ovine FSH

(NIADDK-oFSH-17, 20 U/mg) and ovine LH (NIADDK-oLH-25, 2.3 U/mg, FSH contamination <0.5%) were kindly provided by NIDDK and NHPP.

Some females were injected with 5 IU of human chorionic gonadotropin (hCG) 48-52 h after PMSG, and the ovulated oocytes were collected from the oviducts 15-17 h after hCG (in vivo matured group).

The in vitro matured and in vivo matured oocytes were fertilized in vitro by epididymal sperm from B6SJL F_1 males in Whitten's medium (WM) (2), then embryo culture was carried out in WM. The rates of development to the 2-cell stage and the blastocyst stage were determined at 26-28 h and 5 days post-insemination, respectively. All the cultures were performed under a humidified atmosphere of 5% CO_2, 5% O_2 and 90% N_2 at 37°C. The data were analyzed by the Chi-square test. A P value less than 0.05 was considered significant.

Results

Effects of FSH alone, LH alone or the simultaneous combination of FSH and LH on oocyte maturation in vitro are summarized in Table 1. FSH or LH supplementation of the oocyte maturation medium significantly improved the rate of development to the 2-cell stage. There was no significant difference between FSH and LH. However, the combination of FSH and LH at the same dose eliminated the beneficial effect of FSH or LH alone on 2-cell development.

There was no significant difference in the rate of development from 2-cell embryos to blastocysts among the in vitro matured groups, either with or without gonadotropin supplementation.

FSH or LH supplementation increased the rate of blastocyst development from inseminated oocytes twofold compared with that in the no hormone group. There was no significant difference between the FSH and LH groups. In the FSH + LH group there was a tendency for a decrease in the beneficial effect of FSH or LH alone on blastocyst development from inseminated oocytes, although the difference was not statistically significant (P=0.22, P=0.053, respectively).

Table 1. Effects of FSH alone, LH alone or simultaneous combination of FSH and LH on oocyte maturation in vitro

	No. Inseminated Oocytes	% 2-cell Embryos from Oocytes	% Blastocysts from 2-cell Embryos	% Blastocysts from Oocytes
No hormone	119	24%	54%	13%
FSH	110	45%*	55%	25%*
LH	114	46%*	62%	29%*
FSH + LH	96	29%**	57%	17%
Low FSH + LH	74	42%	61%	26%
In vivo matured	181	47%	86%	40%

The data are the sum of 3 replicate experiments, except the FSH + LH and low FSH + LH groups (2 replicates). *P < 0.05 vs. no hormone. **P < 0.05 vs. FSH or LH.

Effects of the sequential combination of FSH and LH on oocyte maturation in vitro are summarized in Table 2. Delayed addition of LH following FSH priming enhanced 2-cell embryo development as well as blastocyst development from 2-cell embryos, with maximal enhancement after 3.5- and 2-h delays, respectively. Consequently, the "FSH → FSH + LH after 2-h" regimen significantly improved the rate of blastocyst development from inseminated oocytes more than twofold compared with that in FSH alone. This rate was near that in the in vivo matured oocytes.

Discussion

This study has shown the following: (a) Supplementation with FSH or LH alone of the oocyte maturation medium increases the rate of blastocyst development from inseminated oocytes twofold compared with no hormone supplementation; (b) There is no significant difference in blastocyst development between FSH and LH supplementation; (c) The beneficial effect of FSH or LH appears to be abolished when both are present simultaneously; and, (d) When LH is given 2 h after FSH priming, blastocyst development is further increased twofold compared with FSH alone.

FSH has previously been reported to have a positive effect on fertilization and preimplantation development of oocytes matured in vitro (3). To our knowledge, no such positive effects of LH have been reported. The positive effect of LH on fertilization and/or embryonic development, reported in this study, does not appear to be due to FSH contamination in the LH preparation because <0.5% of FSH contamination cannot account for the results observed with the simultaneous and sequential combination of FSH and LH.

Salustri et al. showed that FSH initially increases the cAMP level in GV stage oocytes and prolongs the meiotic arrest, followed by a drop in the cAMP level, then by GV breakdown (4). Also, the cAMP degradation rate in oocytes appeared to be increased dramatically as the cAMP level in the oocytes was elevated (4). Therefore, it was proposed that an initial increase in oocyte cAMP by FSH induces an increase in cAMP degradation, and the resulting drop in cAMP induces oocyte maturation (4). Schultz et al. reported that following hCG admin-

Table 2. Effects of sequential combination of FSH and LH
on oocyte maturation in vitro

	No. Inseminated Oocytes	% 2-cell Embryos from Oocytes	% Blastocysts from 2-cell Embryos	% Blastocysts from Oocytes
FSH alone	46	39%	50%	20%
FSH → FSH + LH				
15 min	41	51%	71%	37%
2 h	48	58%	75%	44%*
3.5 h	47	64%*	57%	36%
In vivo matured	91	64%	91%	58%

The data are the sum of 2 replicate experiments. *P < 0.05 vs. FSH alone.

istration, a decrease in oocyte cAMP precedes GV breakdown in vivo, and speculated that LH might inactivate a maturation inhibitor involved in regulating the oocyte cAMP level (5).

It is unknown why the simultaneous combination of FSH and LH eliminated the beneficial effect seen with FSH or LH alone in this study. It is possible that when FSH and LH were simultaneously combined, LH inhibited the initial elevation of oocyte cAMP by FSH, resulting in a failure to increase the rate of cAMP degradation, followed by an inadequate decline of cAMP for maturation induction.

When LH was given 2 h after FSH priming in this study, LH may have synchronously accelerated the drop in oocyte cAMP level induced by FSH. Because the oocyte cAMP level appears to reach a peak 1 h after FSH addition and to return to the initial level in 3 h (4), addition of LH 15 min or 3.5 h after FSH priming, as in this study, may be either too early or too late to allow LH to synchronously accelerate the cAMP drop induced by FSH.

Acknowledgments

The authors would like to thank Ms. Dara Leary for her assistance in the preparation of this manuscript. This work was supported, in part, by grants from Serono Laboratories, Inc.

References

1. Schroeder AC, Eppig JJ. The developmental capacity of mouse oocytes that matured spontaneously in vitro is normal. Dev Biol 1984; 102:493-7.
2. Whitten WK. Nutrient requirements for the culture of preimplantation embryos in vitro. Adv Biosci 1971; 6:129-41.
3. Downs SM, Schroeder AC, Eppig JJ. Developmental capacity of mouse oocytes following maintenance of meiotic arrest in vitro. Gamete Res 1986; 15:305-16.
4. Salustri A, Petrungaro S, De Felici M, Conti M, Siracusa G. Effect of follicle-stimulating hormone on cyclic adenosine monophosphate level and on meiotic maturation in mouse cumulus cell-enclosed oocytes cultured in vitro. Biol Reprod 1985; 33:797-802.
5. Schultz RM, Montgomery RR, Belanoff JR. Regulation of mouse oocyte meiotic maturation: implication of a decrease in oocyte cAMP and protein dephosphorylation in commitment to resume meiosis. Dev Biol 1983; 97:264-73.

26

Initial Characterization of a Luteal Growth Factor for Ovarian Mesothelial Cells

Santo V. Nicosia and Beatriz O. Saunders

Department of Pathology, University of South Florida
College of Medicine, Tampa, FL 33612

The ovarian surface epithelium is a modified mesothelial tissue which undergoes species-dependent morphogenetic events throughout life (1,2). The mechanisms regulating such events are poorly understood in spite of the relevance of this tissue in reproduction and cancer (3,4). We have postulated that ovarian mesothelial cells may be influenced by underlying growth signals based on the observation of highly polarized DNA synthesis and morphogenesis in the postovulatory rabbit ovary (5). In the present study, we report on the isolation, biological activity and initial characterization of a recently discovered intraluteal growth factor for rabbit ovarian mesothelial cells (6).

Materials and Methods

Animals

New Zealand White rabbits (age 4-5 months) were the source of ovarian mesothelia (OM) cells and corpora lutea (CL). Animals were individually caged for 3 weeks prior to use and sacrificed by barbiturate overdose.

Preparation of Corpora Lutea Tissue Extract (CLE)

CL were obtained 5 days after induction of ovulation with 50 IU of hCG (Sigma, St. Louis, MO). After dissection from surrounding tissues, CL were resuspended in 1 ml of ice-cold medium 199 (GIBCO, Grand Island, NY) and mechanically homogenized in a tissue grinder. The entire homogenate was centrifuged at 40,000 rpm for 1 h at 4°C. After discarding fat and unhomogenized tissue residues, the supernatant (CLE) was sterilized through a 0.22 μm filter and stored at -20°C until use for determination of protein content (7), evaluation of biological activity and initial characterization.

Growth Assay

OM cells were obtained from estrous rabbits (n=2/assay) by a previously described enzymatic and unit gravity sedimentation procedure (8). Cells were seeded at an original density of 2×10^5 into T_{25} flasks (n=10/group) and maintained for 7.5 days in antibiotic-rich medium 199 containing the following concentrations of fetal bovine serum (GIBCO): day 0-2.5 = 15%; day 2.5-5 = 2%; day 5-7.5 = 0.5%. CLE (60 µg/ml) was added at each change of medium (days 2.5 and 5) with control cultures receiving equivalent amounts of rabbit serum proteins. Cell growth was evaluated by assessing the percent change in cell number, the number of cell population doublings (CPD) and the cell population doubling time in hours (CPDT) (9). Growth values were expressed as mean ± SEM and statistically evaluated by analysis of variance.

Initial Characterization of CLE

In order to evaluate its dose-dependent growth effects, CLE was added to OM cell cultures (n=12/group) at the following concentrations: 1, 10, 30, 60 and 100 µg/ml. To assess its specificity, the growth effects of CLE were compared with those of crude tissue extracts (60 µg/ml) obtained from 5 days post-hCG ovaries (OE) after removal of corpora lutea, from extraovarian pelvic mesothelia (ME) and from kidneys (KE). Temporal changes in growth activity were evaluated by adding to OM cell cultures (n=10/group) 60 µg/ml of CLE obtained from 0, 1, 5, 12, 18 and 21 days after hCG. Finally, additional OM cell cultures (n=6/group) were utilized to assess the sensitivity of CLE (60 µg/ml) to the following treatments: (a) 1% activated charcoal for 45 min at 4°C; (b) pronase (Sigma), 225 U/ml for 2 h at 37°C; (c) heat, 56°C for 45 min or 100°C for 10 min; (d) freeze-thawing; (e) lyophilization; (f) storage at 4°C for >24 h or at -20°C for >4 weeks; (g) dialysis and ultrafiltration (Amicon, Lexington, MA) utilizing membranes with a respective retentivity of 10,000 and 30,000 daltons.

Results

An average of 40 corpora lutea was obtained from each CLE preparation procedure equivalent to a total protein content varying from a minimum of 2.8 mg at day 0 to a maximum of 20 mg or to an individual CL protein content varying from 73.30 ± 7.99 day 0 (mature follicles) to 513.56 ± 57.74 at day 12 post-hCG (Fig. 1). Protein recovery averaged 90%.

OM cells grown in control medium formed dyshesive monolayers, exhibited a low nucleo-cytoplasmic ratio (Fig. 2A) and underwent only a 1.5-fold increase in number with respective CPD and CPDT values of 0.59 ± 0.08 and 117.29 ± 6.43 h (Fig. 3). In contrast, OM cells exposed to 5-day-old CLE formed cohesive monolayers with high nucleo-cytoplasmic ratios (Fig. 2B) and grew over threefold with respective CPD and CPDT values of 1.71 ± 0.07 and 53.43 ± 2.93 h (Fig.3). The growth effects of CLE were dose dependent with the active factor titrating at 30 µg/ml and being most potent at 60 µg/ml (Fig. 4). CLE was unique among all tested tissue extracts in significantly stimulating the growth of OM cells (Fig. 5).

The activity of CLE was temporally related with significant growth effects only at days 5, 12 and 18 (Fig. 6). The active factor in CLE withstood charcoal extraction, freeze-thawing and lyophilization, was stable for several weeks at -20°C, unstable at 4°C for over 24 h and after heating and was sensitive to proteolysis. The factor was not dialyzable and larger than 30,000 daltons as estimated by ultrafiltration (Table 1).

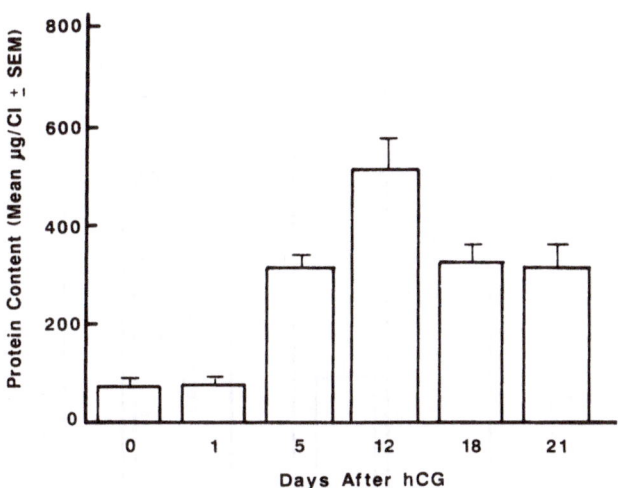

Fig. 1. Protein content of corpora lutea (CL) at various post-hCG intervals.

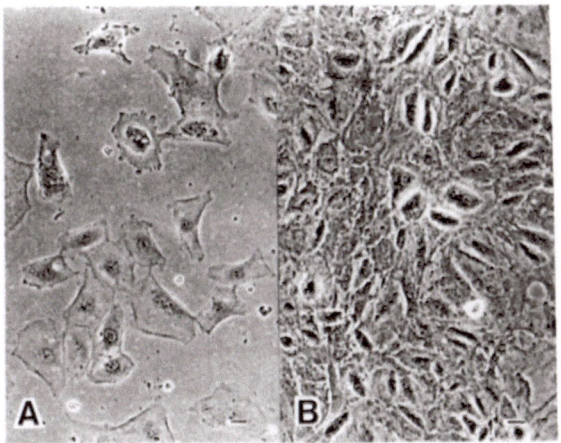

Fig. 2. Morphology of OM cells cultured for 7 days without (A) and with CLE (B). — 10 μm.

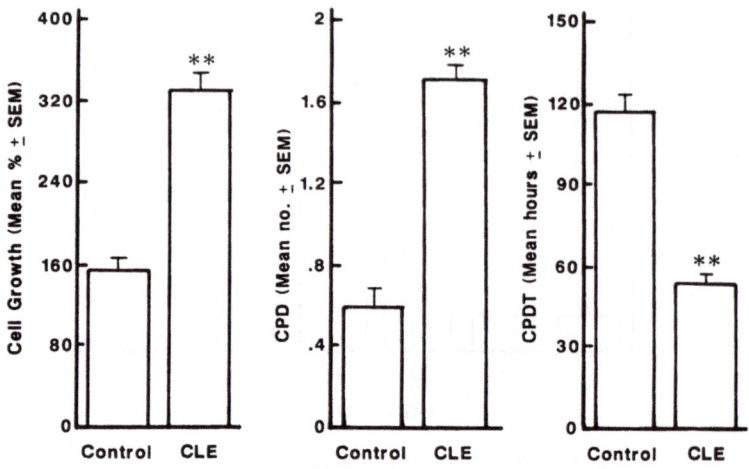

Fig. 3. Growth parameters of control and CLE-enriched OM cells. **P<0.001.

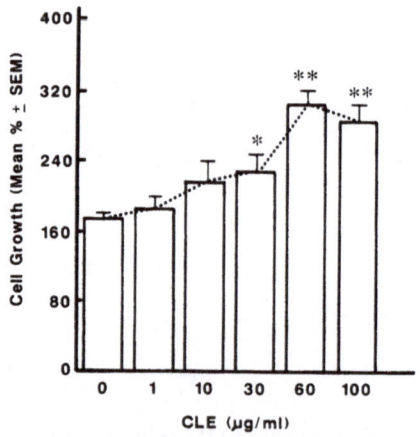

Fig. 4. Dose response effect CLE on
OM cell growth. *P<0.05; **P<0.001.

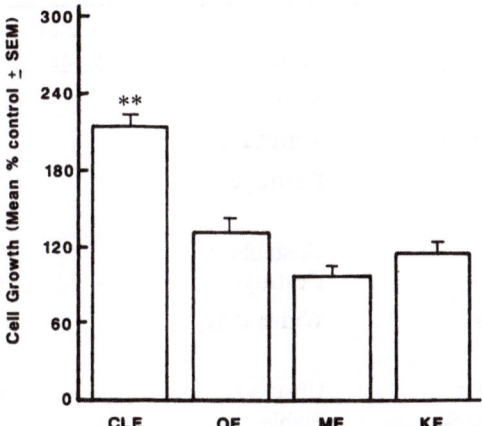

Fig. 5. Growth response of OM cells to ovarian
and extraovarian tissue extracts. **P<0.001.

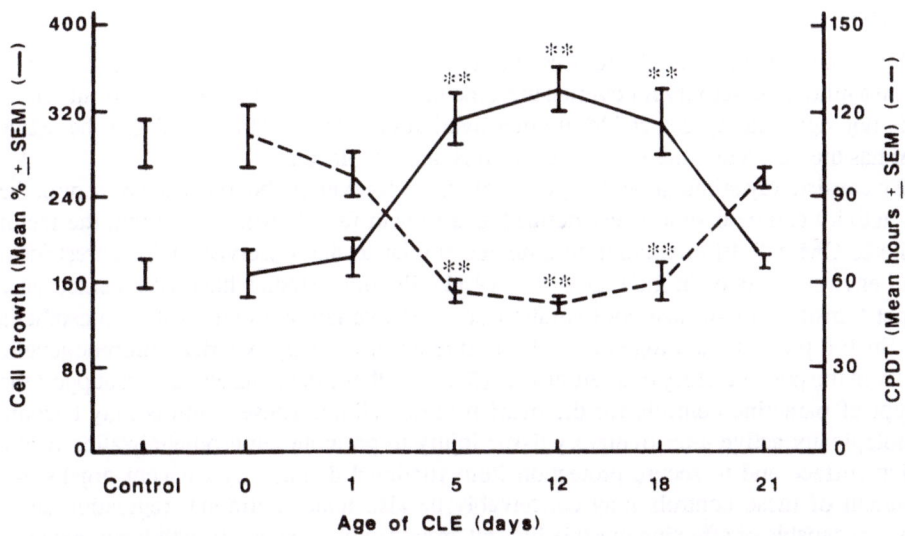

Fig. 6. Growth response of OM cells to CLE of different developmental ages.
**P<0.001.

Table 1. Some characteristics of the ovarian mesothelial
growth factor in 5-day-old CLE

Treatment	Factor	Cell Proliferation as % of Untreated CLE
None	Stable	100
Activated Charcoal	Withstands	103
Pronase	Destroyed	58
Heat		
56°C	Unstable	73
100°C	Destroyed	63
Freeze-thawing	Withstands	113
Shelf-life		
4°C >24 h	Unstable	64
-20°C 4 weeks	Stable	100
Lyophilization	Withstands	94
Dialysis	Retained	85
Amicon PM30	Retained	106

Discussion

The results obtained in this study can be summarized as follows: (1) rabbit corpora lutea contain a mitogenic activity for ovarian mesothelial cells; (2) this activity is temporally finite and is not significantly detectable in other ovarian or extraovarian tissues; (3) the active factor has the characteristics of a proteinaceous macromolecule.

By consistently stimulating the growth of OM cells even in the presence of serum, the CLE activity can be operationally defined as a growth factor (10). In addition, the factor facilitates OM cell differentiation to a degree similar to that observed under unrestricted serum environments or in the native state (9,11). Previous studies have commented on a distinct transition in surface configuration between ovarian and extraovarian mesothelia (11). Such a phenomenon together with the finding of a highly polarized morphogenetic activity in the postovulatory ovarian surface (5) and with the data presented here support the concept of paracrine controls for the ovarian mesothelium. These controls may become physiologically active after ovulatory tissue injury to promote remesothelialization of the ovarian surface and to secure protection from frictional damage by adjacent organs (4). Activation of these controls may conceivably be also under hormonal regulation since hormones capable of affecting mesothelial cell growth may also alter growth factor receptor levels (12,13).

Several growth factors have been recently described in ovarian tissues including angiogenic or fibroblast growth factors (14), transforming growth factors (15) and insulin-like growth factors (16). Based on the initial characterization data reported here and on recent evidence indicating lack of heparin affinity (Saunders and Nicosia, unpublished work), the

CLE activity appears to be different from such factors. The presence of platelet-derived and other growth factors in immediately postovulatory ovaries is also plausible in view of the local influx of cellular and noncellular blood elements. In the present study, the CLE activity was, however, temporally correlated only with mature and not with hemorrhagic corpora lutea where such influx is most prominent (2). Identification of the exact nature and intraluteal localization of this activity should provide a currently unavailable tool to gain insight into the pathobiology of the ovarian mesothelium.

Acknowledgments

Thanks are due to Mr. R. Narconis and Mrs. M. Alojipan. This work was supported by VA Merit Grant.

References

1. Motta PM, Van Blerkom J, Makabe S. Changes in the surface morphology of ovarian germinal epithelium during the reproductive cycle and in some pathological conditions. J Submicrosc Cytol 1980; 12:407-15.
2. Nicosia SV. Morphological changes of the human ovary throughout life. In: Serra GB, ed. The ovary. New York: Raven Press, 1983:57-81.
3. Bjersing L, Cajander S. Ovulation and the mechanism of follicle rupture. III. Transmission electron microscopy of rabbit germinal epithelium prior to induced ovulation. Cell Tissue Res 1974; 149:313-27.
4. Nicosia SV, Nicosia RF. Neoplasms of the ovarian mesothelium. In: Azar HA, ed. Pathology of human neoplasms. New York: Raven Press, 1988:435-86.
5. Osterholzer HO, Johnson JH, Nicosia SV. An autoradiographic study of the rabbit ovarian surface epithelium before and after ovulation. Biol Reprod 1985; 33:729-38.
6. Nicosia SV, Saunders BO. Corpus luteum extract stimulates the growth of ovarian surface epithelial cells. Lab Invest 1986; 54:47a.
7. Bradford MN. A rapid and sensitive method for the quantitation of microgram quantities of proteins utilizing a principle of protein-dye binding. Ann Biochem 1976; 72:238-54.
8. Nicosia SV, Johnson JH, Streibel EJ. Isolation and ultrastructure of rabbit ovarian mesothelium (surface epithelium). Int J Gynecol Pathol 1984; 3:338-60.
9. Nicosia SV, Johnson JH, Streibel EJ. Growth characteristics of rabbit ovarian mesothelial (surface epithelial) cells. Int J Gynecol Pathol 1985; 4:58-74.
10. Goustin AS, Leof EB, Shipley GD, Moses HL. Growth factors and cancer. Cancer Res 1986; 46:1015-29.
11. Nicosia SV, Johnson JH. Surface morphology of ovarian mesothelium (surface epithelium) and of other pelvic and extrapelvic mesothelial sites in the rabbit. Int J Gynecol Pathol 1984; 3:249-60.
12. Mukku VR, Stancel GM. Regulation of epidermal growth factor receptor by estrogen. J Biol Chem 1985; 260:9820-4.
13. Osterholzer HO, Streibel EJ, Nicosia SV. Growth effects of protein hormones on cultured rabbit ovarian surface epithelial cells. Biol Reprod 1985; 33:247-58.
14. Gospodarowicz D, Cheng J, Lui GM, Baird A, Esch F, Bohlen P. Corpus luteum angiogenic factor is related to fibroblast growth factor. Endocrinology 1985; 117:2283-391.
15. Lobb DK, Kobrin MC, Kudlow JE, Dorrington JH. Transforming growth factor-alpha production by bovine thecal cells. Biol Reprod 1988; 38(1):191a.

16. Mondschein JS, Hammond JM, Canning SF. Profiles of immunoreactive insulin-like growth factors I and II in porcine follicular fluid and granulosa cell conditioned medium. Biol Reprod 1988; 38(1):191a.

27

Gap Junctions in Transformed Rat Granulosa Cells

T. A. Fitz,[1] M. M. Marr,[1] T. L. Walden,[2] W. A. Schmidt,[3] and C. A. Winkel[3]

[1]Department of Obstetrics and Gynecology
Uniformed Services University of the Health Sciences
Bethesda, MD 20814; [2]AFRRI, Bethesda, MD 20814
[3]University of Texas Health Sciences Center, Houston, TX 77030

Introduction

Granulosa cells perform a variety of functions essential for ovarian cyclicity, ovulation, fertilization and maintenance of pregnancy. Because of their diverse functions and crucial roles in reproduction, granulosa cells are among the most intensively studied endocrine cells (1). However, the properties of granulosa cells in vitro are not necessarily indicative of their properties in vivo because of their marked propensity toward luteinization. Granulosa cells in culture undergo rapid luteinization following treatments with gonadotropins or other agents which stimulate the intracellular formation of cyclic adenosine monophosphate (cAMP) (2), following incubation in media containing serum (3) or even in the absence of known differentiation factors (4,5). The luteinized granulosa cell acquires properties that are quite different from the nonluteinized precursor, losing mitotic and aromatase activities and producing greatly increased amounts of progesterone. Therefore, the properties of luteinized granulosa cells are in many ways more relevant to functions of corpora lutea than to follicles.

We previously evaluated the utility of SV40-transformed rat granulosa (DC3) cells as a model for studies of granulosa cell functions. We determined that DC3 cells were steroid active, producing estradiol, estrone and progesterone, and steroidogenesis was stimulable by provision of the steroidogenic substrate 25-hydroxycholesterol (25-OHC) or treatment with agents that stimulated activation of adenylate cyclase, including isoproterenol, vasoactive intestinal peptide, cholera toxin (CT), and forskolin (FSK). Specific binding sites were detected for follicle-stimulating hormone and luteinizing hormone, but treatments with gonadotropins did not alter the rate of steroidogenesis (manuscript submitted).

Gap junctions are believed to be a ubiquitous feature in multicelled organisms (6) of importance for control of cell proliferation, tissue metabolism and synchrony (6-8). Gap junctions are prominent features among the granulosa cells in ovarian follicles, where they are believed to facilitate transport of ions and small molecules throughout the avascular environment of the follicle as well as to coordinate granulosa cell functions and interactions with the oocyte (7,9,10). Gap junctions also form readily in cultured granulosa cells (9). While some cancers are characterized by impaired or lost capacity for cell-cell communication (11), gap junctions were evident in electron photomicrographs of DC3 cells (12).

Evidence acquired by electrical measurements and increased abundance of junctions after freeze-fracture is suggestive that elevated intracellular levels of cAMP cause the formation of new channels for intercellular communication (13). Since the morphology of DC3 cells is markedly altered by treatment with FSK or CT, by media supplementation with 25-OHC, or by gamma-irradiation, we monitored intercellular communication during basal culture conditions as well as following treatments which altered cell morphology and secretory properties.

Materials and Methods

DC3 cells were maintained at 37°C under 95% air:5% CO_2 in culture flasks containing Iscoves Modified Dulbeccos Medium (IMDM)-20% fetal calf serum (FBS), and seeded onto 35 mm culture dishes before experiments. Before analyses of fluorescence transfer, cells were incubated in IMDM-5% FBS containing secretagogues for 24-96 h. One group of fluorescence transfer experiments was conducted using DC3 cells which were adapted to and grown in a serum-free, defined medium. Nontransformed granulosa cells were harvested from prepubertal rats. Donors were primed with 40 IU of pregnant mare serum gonadotropin, then ovaries were removed 40 h later. Ovaries were macerated with a sterile 24-gauge needle and expressed cells were incubated in IMDM-5% FBS for 48 h before use in experiments.

Intercellular communication was monitored in DC3 cells by observing transfer of carboxyfluorescein (CF) between abutting cells. Plated cells were incubated for 20 min at 4 C with 10 μg/ml 5(6)-carboxyfluorescein diacetate, which is rapidly internalized and hydrolyzed into CF. CF is fluorescent and impermeant through cell membranes. Following fluorescence loading, dishes were extensively washed to remove noninternalized CF. Cells were inspected microscopically, and fields were selected which contained both isolated and abutting cells. Three to five pairs of abutting cells were selected from each field for monitoring of fluorescence transfer. In addition, one isolated cell in each field was designated as a positive control and one isolated cell as a negative control. The positive control was not photobleached, while the negative control and one cell of each selected abutting pair were bleached using a directed laser microbeam. Subsequent redistribution of intracellular fluorescence was monitored and evaluated.

Quantitative fluorescence and photobleaching were accomplished using the Meridian ACAS 470 Workstation. The Workstation is an integrated unit containing a 5 W argon laser, dual photomultiplier capacity and microscope, which is driven and coordinated by a computer. Parameters of laser intensity for photobleaching and fluorescence quantification were adjusted daily to produce ca. 90% bleaching of selected cells and minimal bleaching of abutting cells. Typically, cells were irradiated using a 488 nm directed laser microbeam at bleaching intensity of 9 mW and scanning intensity of 1 mW. Fluorescence emission was quantified using a 510 nm dichroic filter.

Some DC3 cells were irradiated with 4 or 20 Gy at 37°C in a bilateral ^{60}Co gamma-irradiation field at a dose rate of 1 Gy/min. Following irradiation, media were replaced and cells were returned to the incubator. Irradiated cells were maintained in culture for 4 or 96 h before use in fluorescence experiments. To determine the effects of irradiation upon rate of mitosis, cells were removed from culture dishes using 0.02% EDTA and counted using a hemocytometer.

To enhance intracellular cAMP, dishes containing plated DC3 cells were incubated with 10 μM FSK or 10 ng/ml CT. In preliminary experiments these concentrations of secretagogue caused multifold elevations in intracellular and extracellular cAMP. Dishes were also incubated with dibutyryl cAMP (dbcAMP) to mimic the effects of elevated cAMP. Dishes of cells were incubated with one of two concentrations of 25-OHC; 100 ng/ml which caused slight elevation of steroidogenesis and 10 μg/ml which caused near maximal stimulation of steroidogenesis and pronounced morphological changes.

Results and Discussion

Fluorescence transfer has been widely used as evidence of cell-cell communication, providing demonstrations of intercellular communication equivalent to that obtained using electrical coupling (14). Intercellular transfer of CF using the Meridian ACAS Workstation was used previously to demonstrate intercellular communication in human teratocarcinoma cells (8).

The abundance of intercellular communication between abutting cells is depicted in Table 1. All cells tested from gonadotropin-primed rats exhibited fluorescence transfer. The incidence of fluorescence transfer between abutting DC3 cells was 35-40% following treatment with 100 μM dbcAMP, 10 μM FSK, 10 ng/ml CT, 10 μg/ml 25-OHC, or 4 h after either 5 or 20 Gy of irradiation. The incidence of fluorescence transfer was decreased by treatment with 100 ng/ml 25-OHC (P<.03 by Chi^2 analysis). It is unknown why intercellular communication appeared to be disrupted by a low concentration of 25-OHC which has minimal effects upon steroidogenesis but not by higher concentrations which maximally stimulate steroidogenesis. The incidence of intercellular communication appeared to be diminished 96 h after either irradiation regimen; however, due possibly to low numbers of cells evaluated after irradiation, this effect was not significant (P=0.1).

The pattern of fluorescence transfer between DC3 cells during basal culture conditions is depicted in Figure 1. Two of five abutting, photobleached cells recovered fluorescence. Intracellular fluorescence was essentially constant in an isolated unbleached cell (triangle) and in an isolated bleached cell (circle). The rate of fluorescence transfer and confidence levels are depicted beside each plot.

In our experiments, intercellular communication appeared to be a ubiquitous feature of normal rat cells but only among 35-40% of abutting DC3 cell pairs. Since the doubling time of DC3 cells is ca. 18 h, at any one time in our experiments a large proportion of DC3 cells would be undergoing or preparing for cell division. It is possible that intercellular communication is disrupted during one or more stages of cell division. Conversely, normal rat granulosa cells have ceased mitosis after 48 h of incubation in medium containing serum.

Treatments were selected which have pronounced effects upon morphology of DC3 cells, in the expectation that these would alter intercellular communication. During basal

Table 1. Incidence of fluorescence transfer among abutting cells

Cells/Treatment	Pairs Communicating Cells	
	Total No. Pairs	(%)
Nontransformed rat		
granulosa cells	19/19	100
DC3 cells		
Basal control	49/130	38
Defined medium	6/15	40
100 μM dbcAMP	8/25	32
10 μM FSK	12/33	36
10 ng/ml CT	14/44	32
10 μg/ml 25-OHC	13/37	35
100 ng/ml 25-OHC	3/25	12
4 h post 5 Gy	4/9	44
96 h post 5 Gy[1]	1/9	11
4 h post 20 Gy	7/18	39
96 h post 20 Gy[2]	3/16	19

[1]Growth rate inhibited by 40%. [2]Growth rate inhibited by 72%

incubations, DC3 cells have a polygonal shape and confluent cultures have a cobblestone appearance. Following incubations with CT or FSK, DC3 cells acquire a marked spindle shape with long processes. Following incubations with 25-OHC, DC3 cells become rounded, tend to become detached from the substrate and associate into clusters of cells. Treatment

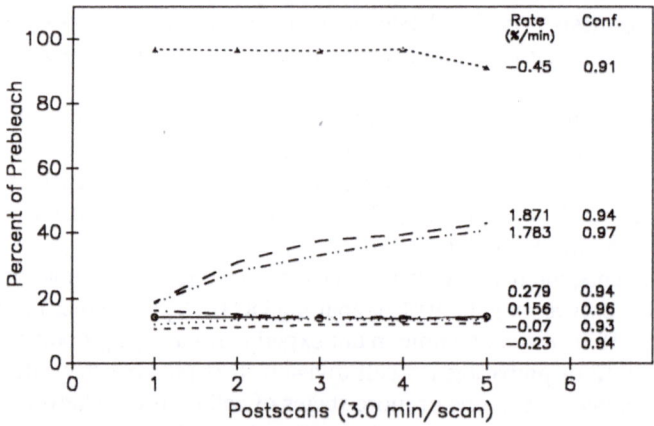

Fig. 1. Fluorescence recovery after photobleaching in untreated DC3 cells. ▲ - - - ▲ unbleached isolated cell; o—o bleached isolated cell; others are bleached cells abutting unbleached cells.

with a low, but not a high, concentration of 25-OHC decreased the incidence of fluorescence transfer, while treatments which elevated cAMP levels had no apparent effect on cell-cell communication.

Irradiation of DC3 cells resulted in inhibition of mitosis and appearance of giant cells. Ninety-six h after irradiation with 20 Gy, the growth rate was decreased by 72% and most cells were enlarged. The appearance of giant cells following irradiation is a well-known phenomenon that may be related to impaired mitosis (15). Although the incidence of fluorescence transfer was decreased following irradiation, intercellular communication was not abolished and some abutting cell pairs exhibited remarkably rapid transfer of fluorescence.

Acknowledgments

We are grateful to Ms. Ivonne Caicedo for expert technical support and Dr. R. Burghardt (Texas A&M University) for electron microscopy. Supported by USUHS Protocols GM8522 and CO8519.

References

1. Hsueh AJW, Adashi EY, Jones PBC, Welsh TH Jr. Hormonal regulation of the differentiation of cultured ovarian granulosa cells. Endocr Rev 1984; 5:76-127.
2. Channing CP, Ledwitz-Rigby F. Methods for assessing hormone-mediated differentiation of ovarian cells in culture and in short term incubations. Methods Enzymol 1975; 39:182-230.
3. Bernard J. Effects of follicular fluid and oestradiol on the luteinization of rat granulosa cells in vitro. J Reprod Fertil 1975; 43:453-60.
4. Channing CP. Effects of stage of the menstrual cycle gonadotropins on luteinization of Rhesus monkey granulosa cells in culture. Endocrinology 1970; 87:49-60.
5. Channing CP. Effect of stage of the estrous cycle and gonadotrophin upon luteinization of porcine granulosa cells in culture. Endocrinology 1970; 87:156-64.
6. Finbow ME, Yancey SB. The roles of intercellular junctions. In: Knox, P, ed. Biochemistry of cellular regulation. IV. The cell surface. Boca Raton: CRC Press, 1981:215-49.
7. Larsen WJ. Biological implications of gap junction structure, distribution and composition: a review. Tissue Cell 1983; 15:645-71.
8. Wade MH, Trosko JE, Schindler M. A fluorescence photobleaching assay of gap junction-mediated communication between human cells. Science 1986; 232:525-8.
9. Beers WH, Olsiewski PJ. Junctional communication and oocyte maturation. In: Bennet MVL, Spray DC, eds. Gap junctions. New York: Cold Spring Harbor Laboratory, 1985:307-14.
10. Gilula NB, Epstein ML, Beers WH. Cell-to-cell communication and ovulation. J Cell Biol 1978; 78:58-75.
11. Sutherland RM. Cell and environment interactions in tumor microregions: the multicell spheroid model. Science 1988; 240:177-84.
12. Burghardt R. Personal communication.
13. De Robertis EDP, De Robertis EMF. Cellular interactions. In: Cell and molecular biology. New York: Lea and Febiger, 1987:130-53.

14. Petersen OH. Importance of electrical cell-cell communication in secretory epithelia. In: Bennet MVL, Spray DC, eds. Gap junctions. New York: Cold Spring Harbor Laboratory, 1985:315-24.
15. Okada S. Radiation effects on cell progress through the life cycle. In: Altman KI, Gerber GB, Okada S, eds. Radiation biochemistry. I. Cells. New York: Academic Press, 1970:190-246.

28

PMSG Induction of C-Fos and C-Myc Proteins Within Granulosa Cells of Immature Rat Ovaries

John J. Peluso and Anna Pappalardo

Department of Obstetrics and Gynecology, University of Connecticut Health Center, Farmington, CT 06032

Introduction

In order for gonadotropins to stimulate granulosa cells, they must first bind to their respective receptors which are located on the surface membrane (1). This binding initiates a cascade of yet undefined events which ultimately leads to a signal being sent to the nucleus which, in turn, induces mitosis and steroidogenesis. These two physiological processes could be the result of differential activation of "mitogenic" and "steroidogenic" gene systems.

Recent work with various cell lines and tissues have suggested that mitogens induce the expression of the proto-oncogenes, c-fos and c-myc, as part of the molecular mechanism by which they induce mitosis (2). The c-fos protein is thought to act as a transducer conveying either a mitogenic or a differentiating signal from the cell membrane to the nucleus (3), while the c-myc protein stimulates DNA polymerase activity and the incorporation of nucleotides into DNA and thereby promoting mitosis (4). The present study was undertaken to determine whether Pregnant Mare's Serum Gonadotropin (PMSG): (1) increases the synthesis of c-fos and c-myc proteins within granulosa cells; and, (2) to correlate these changes with granulosa cell mitosis and serum estradiol-17β and progesterone levels.

Materials and Methods

Animals

Immature female rats were injected with 25 IU of PMSG. At 0, 30, 60, and 120 min after treatment, 5 rats from each group were autopsied and trunk blood collected. The ovaries were removed and placed in chilled phosphate-buffered saline (PBS, pH 7.4). The large antral follicles were pricked with a 25-gauge needle and compressed to release the granulosa cells into the PBS. The granulosa cells were collected from both ovaries, pooled, then centrifuged at 600 g for 10 min at 4°C. The cell pellet was resuspended in 1 ml of PBS and a 0.1 ml aliquot taken. From this 0.1 ml sample, the number of cells/ml was determined using a hematocytometer and the percentage of mitotically active cells estimated by staining the cells with hydroethidine and examining the cells under fluorescent optics.

The remainder of the cells were transferred to individual microfuge tubes and centrifuged in a microfuge for 15 sec at 7,000-12,000 g. The supernate from each tube was aspirated and the resulting cell pellet used to assess the presence of c-fos or c-myc proteins.

Detection of C-Fos and C-Myc Proteins

Granulosa cells were fixed in cold 2% para-formaldehyde in PBS for 5 min. The cells were then centrifuged at 600 g for 10 min and resuspended in 0.1 ml of distilled water. Ten μl of fixed cells were spotted onto microscope slides and the samples air dried, incubated with 0.3% hydrogen peroxide solution for 30 min and then incubated with an affinity-purified antibody to either the c-fos or c-myc protein. The antibodies to these proto-oncogene proteins were purchased from Cambridge Research Biochemicals (Valley Stream, NY). The proto-oncogene proteins were localized using the peroxidase-antiperoxidase procedure with reagents supplied in the vectastain ABC kit (Vector Labs, Burlingame, CA). The specific protein was revealed within the cells by the presence of a blue-purple stain. One hundred cells from each sample were examined and the percentage of stained cells for each protein determined. The relative intensity of the staining reaction within each cell was determined with a video densitometer. The number of cells showing nonspecific staining was estimated by replacing the antibody to the specific protein with normal sheep serum.

Percentage of Mitotically Active Cells

In order to estimate mitotic activity, granulosa cells were stained with hydroethidine. For this procedure, 0.5 ml of hydroethidine (14 μg/ml of PBS) was added to 0.1 ml of cells and staining allowed to continue for 15 min at room temperature. The cell suspensions were then centrifuged at 600 g for 10 min to remove the stain and resuspended in 0.1 ml of PBS. A drop of the suspended cells was placed on a slide and covered with a coverslip. The cells were then observed with a fluorescent microscope with an excitation filter of 535 nm and a barrier filter of 585 nm. At these settings, the chromatin stains red and condensed chromosomes can be easily identified (5). One hundred cells of each granulosa cell suspension were scored and those cells with condensed chromosomes were classified as mitotically active cells.

Serum Steroids

Serum prepared from the blood samples taken at autopsy was assayed for progesterone and estradiol-17β by radioimmunoassay. All samples were assayed in duplicate.

Statistical Evaluations

All treatments were replicated between 5 and 6 times. The data were expressed as a mean ± one standard error and analyzed using a one-way analysis of variance. All relevant comparisons were made using the Student-Neuman-Keuls multiple range test. Differences between groups was considered significant if $P<0.05$.

Results

In all groups tested, some granulosa cells stained for c-fos protein (Fig. 1) but the percentage of cells varied with time after PMSG. At 0 min, 5 ± 2 % of the cells stained for c-fos protein with a relative intensity of 6 ± 0.2 units/cell. By 30 min, the percentage of stained cells increased eightfold ($P<0.05$) while the staining intensity/cell decreased ($P<0.05$). Both the percentage of c-fos stained cells and the staining intensity/cell returned to basal levels by 60 min after PMSG. The staining pattern for c-myc was similar to c-fos with the exception that the percentage of cells stained for c-myc was maintained at an elevated level for 1 h before returning to 0 h values (Table 1).

In addition to changing the staining patterns for these proto-oncogene proteins, PMSG increased serum progesterone levels from 75 ± 15 pg/ml at 0 min to 120 pg/ml at 120 min ($P<0.05$). Serum estradiol-17β was not altered and remained between 10 and 20 pg/ml. The percentage of mitotically active granulosa cells was also increased from 25 ± 0.8 % at 0 min to 42 ± 2 % by 120 min ($P<0.05$).

Discussion

The present data demonstrate that both the c-fos and c-myc proto-oncogene products are normally present in a few granulosa cells and PMSG increases the percentage of granulosa cells that express these gene products. The percentage of cells staining for c-fos protein is only increased at 30 min after PMSG then rapidly declines, while the percentage of cells that stain for c-myc protein is elevated for up to 60 min before returning to baseline. Follicle-stimulating hormone induces a similar pattern of c-fos expression in cultured Sertoli

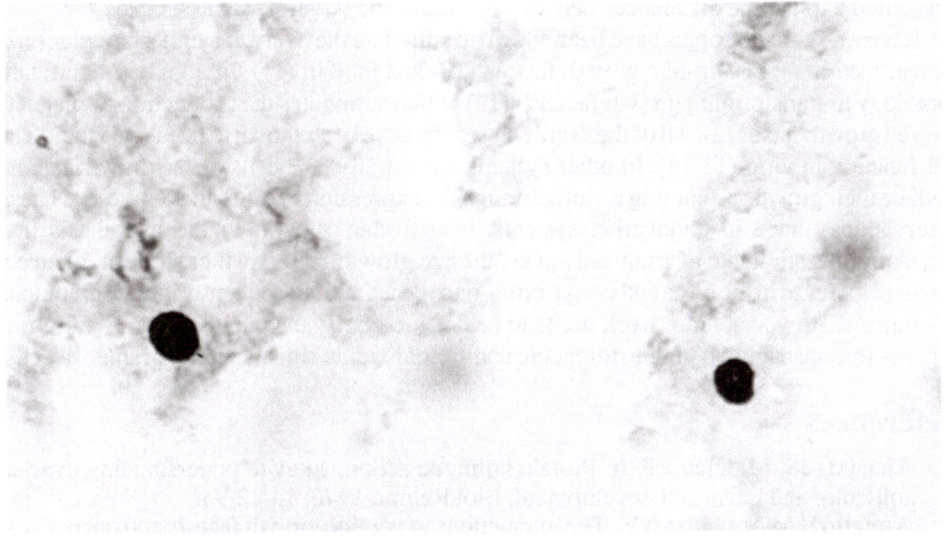

Fig. 1. Immunocytochemical localization of c-fos protein within granulosa cells. Note the stained cells in the top-half and the nonstained cells in the lower center section of the figure.

Table 1. Effect of PMSG on the percentage of granulosa cells and
staining intensity for c-fos and c-myc protein

Protein		Time After PMSG (min)			
		0	30	60	90
C-fos	% stained	5 ± 2	39 ± 6*	13 ± 5	10 ± 2
	Intensity/cell	6 ± .3	4 ± .1*	6 ± .3	5 ± .2
C-myc	% stained	1 ± 1	40 ± 3*	17 ± 6*	8 ± 3
	Intensity/cell	6 ± .2	5 ± .2*	6 ± .2	6 ± .2

* Indicates value is different from 0 min ($P<0.05$).

cells (6). Further, the transient presence of these proteins precedes changes in both mitotic activity and steroid secretion, suggesting that part of molecular mechanism by which PMSG mediates its effects is through the expression of these two proto-oncogenes. This observation contradicts a recent report that failed to show a correlation between the expression of mRNA's for c-fos and c-myc and the increased follicular development associated with unilateral ovariectomy (7). Although tissue was collected during the time of the presumed surge release of follicle-stimulating hormone associated with unilateral ovariectomy (8), gene expression was assessed within the entire ovary and not just the granulosa cells. Since the granulosa cell comprise a relatively small proportion of ovary, it is possible that the transient expression of c-fos and c-myc within granulosa cells that was observed in our study may not have been able to be detected by assessing gene expression within the entire ovary. This could explain the differences between our study and Alvarez and associates.

Recently, gonadotropins have been shown to stimulate the ovary to synthesize epidermal growth factor (9), insulin-like growth factors (10) and inhibin (11). Inhibin has significant homology to transforming growth factor β (12) which stimulates the production of platelet-derived growth factor (2). All of these growth factors have been shown to influence granulosa cell function in vitro (13-15). In other systems, principally 3T3 cells, these growth factors mediate their growth-promoting actions through the expression of c-fos and c-myc (2). These observations, made in nonovarian systems, lend further support to the hypothesis that gonadotropins stimulate ovarian cells to synthesize growth factors which, in turn, induce a transient increase in the c-fos and c-myc proto-oncogenes and subsequently induce granulosa cell mitosis. However, more work needs to be done to clarify the putative role of proto-on-cogenes in transducing both the mitogenic and steroidogenic signals within granulosa cells.

References

1. Richards JS, Midgley AR Jr. Protein hormone action: a key to understanding ovarian follicular and luteal cell development. Biol Reprod 1976; 14:82-94.
2. Armelin HA, Armelin MCS. The interactions of peptide growth factors and oncogenes. In: Guroff G, ed. Oncogenes, genes and growth factors. New York: John Wiley & Sons, 1987; 331-72.
3. Sambucetti LC, Curran T. The fos protein complex is associated with DNA in isolated nuclei and binds to DNA cellulose. Science 1986; 234:1417-9.

4. Studzinski GP, Brelvi ZS, Feldman SC, Watt RA. Participation of c-myc protein in DNA synthesis of human cells. Science 1986; 234:467-70.

5. Bucana C, Saiki I, Nayar R. Uptake and accumulation of the vital dye hydroethidine in neoplastic cells. J Histochem Cytochem 1986; 34:1109-15.

6. Hall SH, Joseph DR, French FS, Conti M. Follicle-stimulating hormone induces transient expression of the proto-oncogene c-fos in primary Sertoli cell cultures. Mol Endocrinol 1988; 2:55-61.

7. Alvarez RD, Smith LJ, Miller DM, Grizzle WE. Proto-oncogene expression in compensatory ovarian hypertrophy [Abstract]. Biol Reprod 1988; 38(suppl 1):149.

8. Butcher RL. Changes in gonadotropins and steroids associated with unilateral ovariectomy of the rat. Endocrinology 1977; 101:830-40.

9. Skinner MK, Lobb D, Dorrington JH. Ovarian thecal/interstitial cells produce an epidermal growth factor-like substance. Endocrinology 1987; 121:1892-9.

10. Hsu CJ, Hammond JM. Gonadotropins and estradiol stimulate immunoreactive insulin-like growth factor-I production by porcine granulosa cells in vitro. Endocrinology 1987; 120:198-207.

11. Zhang ZW, Carson RS, Herington AC, Lee VW, Berger HG. Follicle-stimulating hormone and somatomedin-C stimulate inhibin production by rat granulosa cells in vitro. Endocrinology 1987; 120:1633-8.

12. Mason AJ, Hayflick JS, Ling N, et al. Complimentary DNA sequences of ovarian follicular fluid inhibin show precursor structure and homology with transforming growth factor-β. Nature 1985; 318:659-63.

13. May JV, Buck PA, Schomberg DW. Epidermal growth factor enhances [125 I] iodo-follicle-stimulating hormone binding by cultured porcine granulosa cells. Endocrinology 1987; 120:2413-20.

14. Knecht M, Feng P, Catt K. Bifunctional role of transforming growth factor-β during granulosa cell development. Endocrinology 1987; 120:1243-9.

15. Hammond JM, Englaish HF. Regulation of deoxyribonucleic acid synthesis in cultured porcine granulosa cells by growth factors and hormones. Endocrinology 1987; 120:1039-46.

29

E-Cadherin May Be Involved in Mediating FSH-Stimulated Responses in Rat Granulosa Cells

Riaz Farookhi and Orest W. Blaschuk

Departments of Physiology and of Urology
and the Center for the Study of Reproduction
McGill University, Montreal, Quebec, Canada H3G 1Y6

The complex morphogenesis of tissues and their subsequent participation in successful homeostatic regulation in an organism requires both intercellular and extracellular interactions of the cells. The influence of hormones and growth factors on these interactions has been studied extensively and has been fairly well characterized. Less well appreciated and understood is the nature and influence of direct cell to cell contact on the development, differentiation, and responsiveness of tissue cells.

There are few tissues in the adult mammal that undergo extensive morphological development and differentiation under physiological conditions. A notable exception is the female gonad, the ovary. In this organ, follicular growth, and differentiation of the membrana granulosa of the follicle is a repeating process which continues throughout the reproductive life span of the animal. Most of the growth and development of the ovarian follicle is regulated by hormones. These are not sufficient, however, to explain the exquisite topographical or position-specific differentiation of the granulosa cells that occurs within the membrana granulosa of the follicle (1-3).

In many respects, the events leading to the maturation of the ovarian follicle resemble the processes that occur during embryogenesis. Both follicular maturation and embryogenesis are characterized by such events as cell division, cell movement, and cell restructuring (4,5). As a result of these events, the total cell number of both the embryo and of the follicle are increased in comparison to their original numbers; the relationships of the cells to one another within both the embryo and the follicle are altered, and diverse populations of cells are created within both the embryo and the follicle.

Recent studies have shown that cell adhesion molecules (CAMs) play an important role during embryogenesis (5). These molecules seem to be directly involved in modulating both the movement of embryonic cells and the ultimate segregation of these cells into distinct, cohesive populations (5-7). For example, the epithelial, calcium-dependent CAM known as

E-cadherin has been shown to mediate the compaction of mouse blastomeres (5,8). Antibodies directed against E-cadherin prevent the compaction event from occurring, thus preventing the blastomeres from forming a functional blastocyst. Although all of the blastomeres display E-cadherin on their surfaces, the distribution of this CAM becomes more restricted as development proceeds. All epithelial cells continue to display E-cadherin in the adult animal, but neural and muscle cells cease to exhibit this CAM and instead replace it with a related CAM known as N-cadherin (5,9-11). In general, the expression of E-cadherin and N-cadherin appears to be mutually exclusive. The switch in expression from one cadherin to the other correlates with the differentiation and segregation of either neural or mesodermal cells from ectodermal cells (5-7,9).

In view of the similarities between embryogenesis and follicular development, the hypothesis emerges that CAMs may contribute significantly to the process by which the primordial follicle develops into the mature follicle. These molecules could, conceivably, modulate the establishment of diverse granulosa cell populations within the stratified epithelium of the mature follicle from the single-cell layer of granulosa cells found within the primordial follicle. On another level, CAMs must certainly be involved in maintaining the structural integrity of the follicle, as the epithelium would not remain intact unless the granulosa cells were capable of adhering to one another, as well as adhering to the basal lamina and to the oocyte. Indeed, electron microscopic studies have shown that adherans junctions and gap junctions are present between adjacent granulosa cells, and that gap junctions are present between these cells and the oocyte (4,12,13). E-cadherin has been shown to be capable of mediating the formation of adherans junctions by epithelial cells in several different tissues (14), but the presence of this CAM in the mammalian follicle has not been demonstrated.

Studies from our laboratory (15) have shown that granulosa cell aggregation is important for the expression of at least one specific differentiation event, the FSH-stimulated induction of LH receptors on granulosa cells. Disaggregated granulosa cells fail to induce receptors in response to FSH. The inclusion of estradiol (or an aromatizable substrate) with FSH, however, restores this property (15). Estradiol promotes granulosa cell aggregation (15).

In view of the observations described above, we have initiated a series of studies designed to elucidate the role of CAMs in the process of follicular maturation. Our objectives for the studies reported here were twofold. One was to demonstrate that rat granulosa cells express E-Cad on their cell surface; the other was to determine whether or not our procedure for preparing disaggregated granulosa cells removes E-Cad from these cells. Our results demonstrate that granulosa cells from preantral rat follicles express E-Cad on their surface and that our procedure for preparing disaggregated cells removes this CAM. These results suggest that the responsiveness of granulosa cells to hormonal stimuli may be modulated by CAMs.

Materials and Methods

Preparation of Aggregated and Disaggregated Granulosa Cells

The procedures for the preparation of aggregated and disaggregated granulosa cells have been described previously (15). Granulosa cells were obtained from ovaries of diethylstilbestrol (DES)-primed immature rats (15). Nonviable cells were removed by a mild trypsin treatment (16). LH receptor induction in cultures of granulosa cells (aggregated or disaggregated) was examined as described previously (15).

Purification of Granulosa Cell Plasma Membranes

Granulosa cells (either aggregated or disaggregated) were used as the starting material. Approximately 150-200 million cells (equivalent to 40 rat ovaries) of each preparation were utilized. The freshly isolated cell preparations were suspended in 2 ml of ice-cold PBS containing 1 mg/ml of sulfosuccinimidobiotin (Pierce Chemical Co., Rockford, IL). This compound selectively labels membrane proteins (17). The cell suspension was incubated on ice for 2 min, and then centrifuged at 4°C for 10 min at 1,000 rpm. The cell pellet was then suspended in 5 ml ice-cold PBS containing 10 mM glycine in order to quench the biotinylation reaction. An aliquot of 100 µl was withdrawn from this cell suspension and centrifuged at 4°C for 1 min at 11,000 x g. The pellet was suspended in 75 µl distilled water and frozen at -20°C until needed. This preparation was designated as the total cell fraction. The rest of the cell suspension was subjected to a second centrifugation, and then the cell pellet was suspended in 8 ml 0.1 M citrate, pH 2.6 containing 6 M guanidine HCl. The cell suspension was homogenized by hand (2 strokes), and the resulting homogenate was transferred into two polyallomer ultracentrifuge tubes. The homogenate in each tube was overlaid with approximately 0.5 ml of 0.1 M citrate, pH 2.6, and centrifuged at 100,000 x g in an SW56 rotor for 60 min at 4°C. After this centrifugation period, the material visible at the interface and in the citrate buffer was collected (total volume 1 ml), and diluted to 8 ml with a fresh solution of 0.1 M citrate, pH 2.6 containing 8 M guanidine HCl. This suspension was centrifuged as before, except that the duration of centrifugation was increased to 12 h. Upon completion of the centrifugation, the material was collected and dialyzed against one liter of 10 mM ethanolamine containing 3 mM $CaCl_2$ for 24 h at 4°C. Finally, the dialysate was centrifuged at 11,000 x g for 5 min at 4°C. The pellet was suspended in 150 µl distilled water and frozen at -20°C until needed. This material was designated as the plasma membrane fraction.

Electrophoretic Procedures

The total cell and plasma membrane fractions were analyzed by SDS-PAGE under reducing conditions according to the procedures described by Laemmli (17). The stacking gels contained 5% acrylamide and the separating gels were composed of 7.5% acrylamide. The gels were stained for protein with the Bio-Rad silver staining kit. Proteins resolved by SDS-PAGE were electrophoretically transferred to nitrocellulose by the procedure of Towbin et al. (18) when immunoblots were to be employed.

Western Blot Procedures

Biotinylated proteins transferred onto nitrocellulose were detected as follows. The nitrocellulose blots were incubated for 30 min in 25 mM tris HCl, pH 8 containing 150 mM NaCl (TBS) and 20% fetal calf serum (FCS). This solution was then removed, and egg white avidin conjugated to alkaline phosphatase (Cedarlane Labs, Ontario) diluted 1:500 in the same buffer was added to the blots. The blots were incubated an additional 60 min, after which they were subjected to three washes with TBS containing 0.05% Tween 20 (TBS-Tween). The duration of each wash was 10 min. Control blots were incubated with D (+)

biotin (1 mg/ml) in conjunction with the alkaline phosphatase conjugate. Alkaline phosphatase activity was detected utilizing the substrates 5-bromo-4-chloro-3 indolylphosphate (BCIP) and nitro blue tetrazolium (NBT) (Promega Biotec, Madison, WI) according to the manufacturer's instructions.

Nitrocellulose blots were also probed with a rabbit polyclonal antiserum directed against E-cadherin (kindly provided by M. Takeichi, Kyoto University, Japan). The blots were first incubated in TBS containing 20% FCS (TBS-FCS) as described above. They were then probed with the antiserum diluted 1:300 in TBS-FCS for 24 h. The blots were subsequently washed three times with TBS-Tween, and then probed with goat anti-rabbit immunoglobulins conjugated to alkaline phosphatase (Promega) diluted 1:5000 in TBS-FCS for 30 min. Finally, the blots were again washed with TBS-Tween, and the alkaline phosphatase activity was detected utilizing the substrates BCIP and NBT.

Results

Representative examples of the preparations of aggregated and disaggregated granulosa cells are illustrated in Figures 1A and 1B, respectively. The ability to induce LH receptors on these cells, after 72 h of culture in defined media containing either FSH alone or FSH and

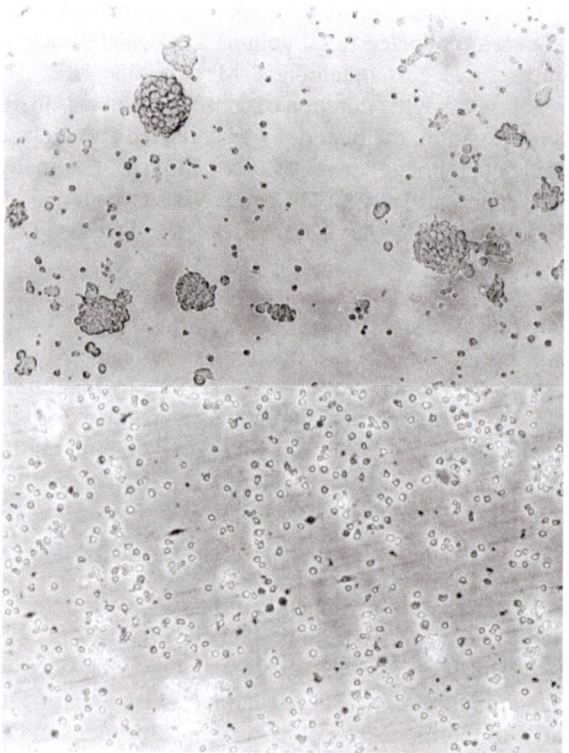

Fig. 1. Granulosa cells obtained after either (A) trypsin treatment or (B) incubation with EGTA followed by trypsin treatment.

estradiol, is depicted in Figure 2. LH receptors are induced by FSH in aggregated cells whether or not estradiol is present. In contrast, the induction of LH receptors in disaggregated cells required both FSH and estradiol. Note that even with estradiol present, disaggregated granulosa cells do not express as much LH receptor as their aggregated counterparts.

Silver-staining of the proteins separated by SDS-PAGE of the total cell fraction and of the plasma membrane fraction of granulosa cells are shown in Figure 3. The inability to detect staining of the membrane fraction is due to the lower protein concentration in the membranes. Development of the stain for a longer period (Fig. 4, lane E), however, reveals that all of stained bands seen in the PAGE of the membrane fraction are present in the total cell fraction.

The integrity of the plasma membrane proteins is revealed by probing the blots of the SDS-PAGE separated membrane proteins with avidin-alkaline phosphatase (Fig. 4, lanes A-D). There is a one-to-one correspondence of the bands in the blot for the plasma membrane fraction (lane A) with that of the total cell extract (lane B). Lanes C and D of Figure 4 indicate that exogenous biotin blocks the binding of the avidin reporter probe to the biotinylated membrane proteins.

The immunoblot depicted in lane B of Figure 5 shows that E-Cad is detectable in the SDS-PAGE of the plasma membrane fraction of aggregated granulosa cells. E-Cad was not detectable in the corresponding fraction from disaggregated granulosa cells (lane A).

Discussion

The overall objective of our studies is to determine the role of CAMs in follicular maturation. Our goal was to investigate the influence of CAMs on the processes mediated by granulosa cells. Granulosa cells expressed from ovaries treated with EGTA can be totally dispersed by treatment with trypsin (Fig. 1B). In contrast, granulosa cells expressed from ovaries not exposed to EGTA, but treated with trypsin, remained adherent to one another (Fig. 1A). These results demonstrate that granulosa cell adhesion is mediated by calcium-dependent CAMs.

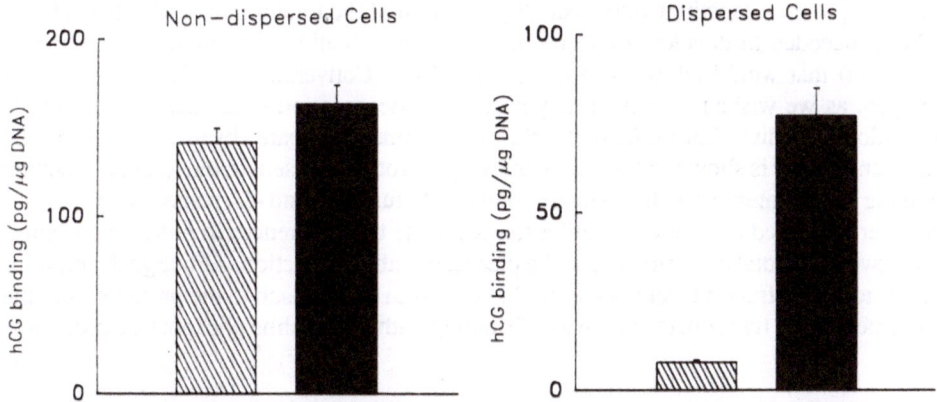

Fig. 2. LH receptor induction in nondispersed or dispersed granulosa cells cultured for 72 h with either FSH alone (hatched bars) or FSH and estradiol (solid bars). Receptor content was assessed by the measurement of specific ^{125}I-hCG binding.

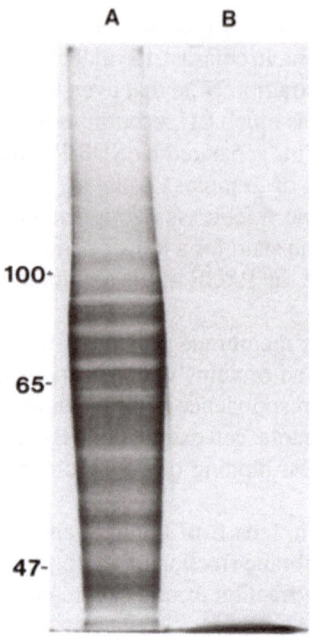

Fig. 3. Silver stain of SDS-PAGE resolved proteins
from: (A) total granulosa cell fraction; (B) plasma
membrane fraction.

The major calcium-dependent CAM present in all epithelial cells is E-cadherin (11).
This CAM is extremely sensitive to proteolysis in the absence of calcium (20,21). We could
not detect the presence of E-cadherin in total extracts of either dispersed or nondispersed
granulosa cells by immunoblotting techniques. This is not an unexpected observation, as
membrane proteins constitute only a small proportion of the total proteins within a cell.

We proceeded to develop a plasma membrane purification procedure (manuscript in
preparation) that would allow us to detect this CAM. Conventional techniques were not
employed, as we wished to prevent any proteolytic degradation of E-cadherin during the
purification procedure. The purity of the plasma membranes prepared by this procedure from
nondispersed cells is shown in Figures 3 and 4. The proteins present in the total cell fraction
and in the plasma membrane fraction are shown in Figures 3A and 4E, respectively. The gel
was underdeveloped in Figure 3 in order to accentuate the differences in protein concentrations between the total cell fraction and the plasma membrane fraction. Although the proteins
from the total cell fraction were twentyfold in excess in comparison to the proteins from the
plasma membrane fraction, the intensity of staining with the alkaline phosphatase probe was

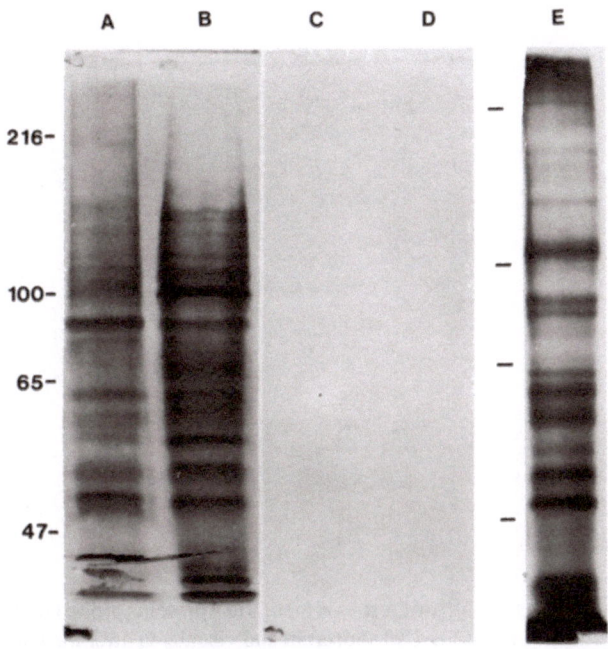

Fig. 4. Avidin-alkaline phosphatase reacted blots of SDS-PAGE resolved: (A) biotin-labeled membrane proteins; (B) biotin-labeled total cell proteins; (C) and (D) same as A and B with exogenous biotin; and (E) silver-stained membrane proteins.

identical. This result indicates that a significant purification of the granulosa cell plasma membranes was achieved. Figure 3B is identical to Figure 4E, with the exception that the silver-staining reaction was allowed to proceed for a longer duration for Figure 4E. The major protein constituents of the plasma membrane fraction are shown in Figure 4E. Note that these protein constituents have also been specifically labeled with sulfosuc-cinimidobiotin, as they are all stained with the alkaline phosphatase probe (compare Figures 4A and 4E).

Plasma membranes were also prepared from dispersed cells. Western blots containing the plasma membrane protein components of both dispersed and nondispersed granulosa cells were then probed with a rabbit antiserum directed against E-cadherin (Fig. 5). Nondis-persed granulosa cell plasma membranes were found to possess this CAM (Fig. 5B), whereas E-Cad was not detectable in the plasma membrane fraction prepared from dispersed granulosa cells (Fig. 5A).

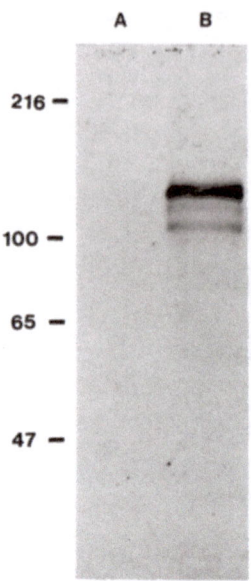

Fig. 5. Western blots of resolved membrane proteins probed with
rabbit anti-mouse E-Cad antiserum and visualized after incubation with alkaline phosphatase-linked goat anti-rabbit antisera.
(A) EGTA and trypsin-treated cells; (B) trypsin-treated cells.

In summary, our results indicate that granulosa cell aggregation is mediated by a CAM
which displays all of the properties of E-cadherin. Furthermore, the removal of this CAM
by EGTA-trypsin treatment renders the granulosa cells incapable of LH receptor induction
by FSH. Since LH receptor induction can be restored by including estradiol in the culture
medium, and since this is preceded by granulosa cell aggregation, we predict that E-cadherin
expression may be regulated by estradiol.

References

1. Amsterdam A, Koch Y, Lieberman ME, Lindner HL. Distribution of binding sites for
   human chorionic gonadotropin in the preovulatory follicle of the rat. J Cell Biol 1975;
   67:894-902.
2. Kasson BG, Meidan R, Davoran JB, Hseuh AJ. Identification of subpopulations of rat
   granulosa cells: sedimentation properties and hormonal responsiveness. Endocrinology
   1985; 117:1027-34.
3. Weisz J, Zoller LC. Quantitative cytochemistry in the study of regional specialization
   in the membrana granulosa of the ovulable type of follicle. In: Pattison JR, Bitensky L,
   Chayen J, eds. Quantitative cytochemistry and its applications. New York: Academic
   Press, 1979:269-83.
4. Caveney S. The role of gap junctions in development. Annu Rev Physiol 1985;
   47:319-35.
5. McClay DR, Ettensohn CA. Cell adhesion in morphogenesis. Annu Rev Cell Biol 1987;
   3:319-445.

6. Thiery JP, Duband JL, Tucker GC. Cell migration in the vertebrate embryo. Annu Rev Cell Biol 1985; 101:91-114.

7. Edelman GM. Cell adhesion molecules in the regulation of animal form and tissue pattern. Annu Rev Cell Biol 1986; 2:81-116.

8. Yoshida-Noro C, Suzuki N, Takeichi M. Molecular nature of the calcium-dependent cell-cell adhesion system in mouse teratocarcinoma and embryonic cells studied with a monoclonal antibody. Dev Biol 1984; 101:19-27.

9. Duband JL, Dufour S, Hatta K, Takeichi M, Edelman E, Thiery JP. Adhesion molecules during somitogenesis in the avian embryo. J Cell Biol 1987; 104:1361-74.

10. Hatta K, Takagi S, Fujusawa H, Takeichi M. Spatial and temporal expression pattern of N-cadherin cell adhesion molecules correlated with morphogenetic processes of chicken embryos. Dev Biol 1987; 120:215-27.

11. Hatta K, Nose A, Nagafuchi A, Takeichi M. Cloning and expression of cDNA encoding a neural calcium-dependent cell adhesion molecule: identity in the cadherin gene family. J Cell Biol 1988; 106:873-81.

12. Czernobilsky B, Moll R, Levy R, Franke WW. Co-expression of cytokeratin and vimentin filaments in mesothelial, granulosa, and rete ovarii cells of the human ovary. Eur J Cell Biol 1985; 37:175-90.

13. Czernobilsky B, Moll R, Leppien G, Schweikhart G, Franke WW. Desmosomal plaque-associated vimentin filaments in human ovarian granulosa cell tumors of various histologic patterns. Am J Pathol 1987; 126:476-86.

14. Volk T, Cohen O, Geiger B. Formation of heterotypic adherens-type junctions between L-CAM-containing liver cells and A-CAM-containing lens cells. Cell 1987; 50:987-94.

15. Farookhi R, Desjardins J. Luteinizing hormone receptor induction in dispersed granulosa cells requires estrogen. Mol Cell Endocrinol 1986; 47:13-24.

16. Farookhi R. Granulosa cell fusion allows heterologous receptor stimulation of adenylate cyclase and progesterone accumulation. Endocrinology 1982; 110:1061-3.

17. Roffman E, Meromsky L, Ben-Hur H, Bayer EA, Wilchek M. Selective labeling of functional groups on membrane proteins or glycoproteins using reactive biotin derivatives and ^{125}I-strepavidin. Biochem Biophys Res Commun 1986; 136:80-5.

18. Laemmli UK. Cleavage of structural proteins during the assembly of the head of bacteriophage T4. Nature 1970; 227:680-5.

19. Towbin H, Staehelin T, Gordon G. Electrophoretic transfer of proteins from polyacrylamide gels to nitrocellulose sheets and some application. Proc Natl Acad Sci USA 1979; 76:4350-4.

20. Hyafil F, Babinet C, Jacob F. Cell-cell interactions in early embryogenesis: molecular approach to the role of calcium. Cell 1981; 26:447-54.

21. Ogou S-I, Okada TS, Takeichi M. Cleavage stage mouse embryos share a common cell adhesion system with teratocarcinoma cells. Dev Biol 1982; 92:521-8.

30

In Vitro Secretion of Angiogenic Activity by Ovine Follicles

T. Taraska, L. P. Reynolds, and D. A. Redmer

Department of Animal and Range Sciences
North Dakota State University, Fargo, ND 58105

Introduction

Earlier investigators noted the tremendous vascularity of ovarian follicles (1-3). This rich blood supply is reflected by the large rate of blood flow to ovarian follicles compared with other tissues (4). During the estrous cycle, growth of vascular beds and increased blood flow accompanies tissue growth of developing follicles (1,2,4), whereas degeneration of follicular blood vessels occurs during atresia (1,5). These observations suggest that angiogenesis is an important component of follicular function.

Dominant follicles appear to have increased uptake of plasma gonadotropin and a more vascular theca compared with other antral follicles (6-8). Atretic follicles from ewes regenerate when placed in vitro, suggesting that access to gonadotropins may be limited in vivo (9). Thus, vascularity of developing follicles may be an important determinant of selective gonadotropin uptake.

Angiogenic activity has been detected in extracts of porcine nonluteal ovaries (10) and ovaries from PMSG-treated rats (11) and mice (12) as well as in media from culture of whole rabbit follicles (13). The purpose of this investigation was to determine the relationships between follicular development and angiogenic activity in ewes.

Materials and Methods

In Experiment 1, ewes had ovaries removed on day 8 or 9 postestrus (Controls, n=3) or received 0.9% saline (2 injections IM, 3 h apart) on day 8 or 9 and ovaries were removed 22 (n=2) or 44 (n=3) h after the first injection. Additional ewes received prostaglandin $F_2\alpha$ (PGF, UpJohn; 2 injections IM, 5 mg each, 3 h apart) on day 8 or 9 postestrus and ovaries were removed 22 (n=9) or 44 (n=9) h later. A blood sample was obtained from each ewe immediately before ovariectomy.

Each ovary was placed into a 100-mm Petri dish containing serum-free medium (DMEM:HAM's F-10, 1:1; 4). For each follicle ≥4 mm, follicular fluid was aspirated with a Hamilton syringe (25-gauge needle) and volume (µl) of follicular fluid recorded. Follicular fluid was centrifuged (8700 x g, 5 min) and supernatant stored at -70°C. The pellet of granulosa cells was resuspended in 100 µl medium and returned to the dish containing the ovary. Theca was peeled from each follicle, the ovary and follicular cavity were rinsed with medium and the ovary was then transferred to another Petri dish for dissection of the next follicle. Granulosa cells were removed from each theca by teasing with forceps and trituration with a siliconized Pasteur pipette. Medium containing granulosa cells was centrifuged (400 x g, 10 min), and granulosa cells were resuspended in 500 µl medium, placed into a well of a 24-well plate and incubated (5% CO_2, 95% air, 37°C) for 24 h. Theca was blotted on sterile gauze, weighed on a torsion balance, placed into a screw-top tube containing 500 µl medium and incubated (5% CO_2, 95% air, 37°C) in a shaking water bath (30 cycles/min) for 6 h. After incubation, conditioned media were centrifuged (400 x g, 10 min) and supernatants stored at -70°C. Angiogenic activity of conditioned media was evaluated by determining ability to stimulate proliferation of endothelial cells (15).

In Experiment 2, ewes (n=12) received a subcutaneous progestin implant (Synchro-Mate B, Ceva) on day 7-11 of the estrous cycle. Implants were removed 11-14 days later. Beginning 2 days before implant removal, ewes were injected IM twice daily with FSH (FSH-P, Schering) for 3 days (decreasing daily doses of 10, 8 and 6 mg, respectively). Ewes were slaughtered 12 h after the last FSH injection. A blood sample was obtained from each ewe immediately before slaughter. Ovaries were collected and processed as in Experiment 1, and follicular fluid, granulosa cells and theca were pooled within each ewe. Granulosa cells (2.5 x 10^5 viable cells) and theca (10 mg) were incubated (5% CO_2, 95% air, 37°C) in 500 µl medium in 24-well plates for 24 h with no hormone, luteinizing hormone (100 ng/ml, NIADDK-oLH-25), follicle stimulating hormone (100 ng/ml, oFSH AFP-1343A), or LH + FSH. Conditioned media were assayed for effects on proliferation of endothelial cells as in Experiment 1. Ovaries from 3 ewes that were primed with progestin and treated with FSH as above were evaluated histologically and follicles were classified as nonatretic or atretic according to Hay et al. (5).

Estradiol-17β (E) was measured in 50 µl or less of follicular fluid diluted 1:100 with PBS (0.01 M sodium phosphate, 0.14 M NaCl, pH 7.4). Known amounts (2-500 pg) of E added to 100 µl diluted follicular fluid from which steroids had previously been removed (C-18 reverse-phase column, J. T. Baker) were assayed and regression of pg E measured (y) vs. Pg E added (x) was y = 5.9 + 0.9x, r = 0.99. The within-assay coefficient of variation (cv) was 11.7%. Progesterone (P) was measured in follicular fluid diluted 1:25 with PBS. Progesterone (50-5000 pg) added to 100 µl C-18 extracted follicular fluid was assayed, and regression of pg P measured (y) vs. pg P added (x) was y = 166.9 + 0.7x, r = 0.99. Within- and between-assay cv were 7.0 and 7.6%. Progesterone was measured in 100 µl of plasma after extraction with 20 volumes benzene: hexane (1:2). Known amounts of P (50-500 pg) added to 100 µl plasma from an ovariectomized ewe were assayed, and regression of pg P measured (y) vs. pg P added (x) was y = -38.3 + 1.5x, r = 0.98. The within- and between-assay cv were 2.2 and 16.7%. Luteinizing hormone (LH) was measured in 100 µl unextracted plasma. A curve established by assaying plasma (from an ewe in early lactation) to which LH (NIADDK-oLH-25, 10-78 pg/100 µl) had been added had a regression equation of y = -1.0 + 1.0x, r = 0.99 (y = pg luteinizing hormone measured, x = pg luteinizing hormone added). The within-assay cv was 15.9%.

Relationships between E:F ratio in follicular fluid and proliferation-stimulating (angiogenic) activity of conditioned media were evaluated by using linear regression procedures (16). Individual (Experiment 1) and pooled (Experiment 2) follicles were classified estrogen active or estrogen inactive based upon E:P in follicular fluid (17). Difference among treatment groups in frequency of estrogen active follicles were evaluated by using Chi-square (18). Effects of treatment, classification of follicles and cell type were evaluated by using general linear models procedures and differences between specific means were evaluated with orthogonal contrasts (16).

Results

In Experiment 1, P concentrations in plasma were greater (P<0.01) for midluteal (Control and saline-treated) than for follicular (PGF-treated) ewes (Table 1). Concentrations of LH were greater (P<0.01) in plasma of ewes at 44 h after PGF than in plasma of other ewes (Table 1). In Experiment 2, plasma concentrations of LH and P were 4.3 ± 1.9 and 0.8 ± 0.1 ng/ml, respectively.

In Experiment 1, 58% of 66 follicles were classified estrogen active (follicular fluid E:P $\geq$ 1). However, the percentage of follicles classified estrogen active was less (P<0.02) in midluteal (control and saline-treated) ewes (16%) than in follicular phase (PGF-treated) ewes (84%). Compared with unconditioned media (58 ± 4 x 10^3 cells/well), theca-conditioned media stimulated (P<0.01) proliferation of endothelial cells ($152 \pm 5\%$). Although no treatment effects were observed, at 44 h after PGF angiogenic activity of theca from estrogen inactive follicles ($118 \pm 4\%$) was less (P<0.01) than that of theca from estrogen active follicles ($163 \pm 10\%$). When compared across all treatments and both classes of follicles, granulosa cell-conditioned media had no effect on proliferation of endothelial cells ($101 \pm 2\%$). However, at 44 h after PGF, granulosa cell-conditioned media from estrogen active follicles stimulated (P<0.01) proliferation of endothelial cells ($113 \pm 4\%$) compared with unconditioned media.

In Experiment 2, 8 of 10 pools of follicular fluid that were assayed were classified estrogen active. In addition, for 3 ewes in which 82 follicles were evaluated histologically, 86% were classified nonatretic and 14% atretic. In vitro treatment with gonadotropins had no effect on angiogenic activity of theca- or granulosa cell-conditioned media. However, compared with unconditioned media (58 ± 2 x 10^3 cells/well), granulosa cell-conditioned

Table 1. Hormone concentrations (ng/ml) in plasma of ewes in Experiment 1 *

Hormone	Treatment				
	Control	Saline 22 h	Saline 44 h	PGF 22 h	PGF 44 h
Progesterone	5.4 ± 0.7	3.6 ± 1.1	7.6 ± 1.9	0.7 ± 0.3	1.1 ± 0.4
Luteinizing hormone	0.5 ± 0.2	0.3 ± 0.1	0.5 ± 0.2	0.9 ± 0.2	12.9 ± 8.2

*Mean ± SEM

media stimulated (P<0.01) proliferation of endothelial cells (133 ± 10%). Theca-conditioned media also stimulated (P<0.01) proliferation of endothelial cells (161 ± 8%). Proliferation-stimulating activity of granulosa cells was less (P<0.02) than that of theca, and these activities were not significantly correlated with E:P ratio in follicular fluid.

Discussion

Angiogenesis (formation of new blood vessels) includes at least three processes: digestion of basement membrane of the preexisting vessel, migration of endothelial cells from the preexisting vessel, and proliferation of endothelial cells (19). In the present study, ability of ovine follicles to secrete activity that stimulates proliferation of endothelial cells was evaluated. In Experiment 1, angiogenic activity was secreted only by theca and not granulosa cells from a mixed population (i.e., estrogen active and estrogen inactive) of follicles. However, as antral follicular development progressed (i.e., 44 h after PGF), granulosa cells of estrogen active follicles began to secrete angiogenic activity. In Experiment 2, in which follicles were primarily preovulatory, nonatretic and estrogen active, both theca and granulosa cells secreted angiogenic activity. Therefore, we suggest that theca, the site of the dense capillary network of growing follicles (1,2,20), may be capable of secreting angiogenic activity throughout antral follicular growth, whereas granulosa cells, which are avascular until after ovulation (21), may not begin to secrete angiogenic activity until just before ovulation. In support of these conclusions, angiogenic activity has been detected in extracts of porcine theca (10) and in media conditioned by theca of primate dominant follicles (22) but not in extracts of granulosa cells from porcine nonluteal ovaries (10). Angiogenic activity was detected, however, in media from culture of granulosa cells from PMSG-treated rats (23). In addition, media from cultures of granulosa cells of primate dominant follicles released angiogenic activity only when cultured with FSH and LH (22). In the present investigation, angiogenic activity was detected in granulosa cell-conditioned media when concentrations of endogenous LH were elevated (Experiment 1, 44 h after PGF) and also when ewes were stimulated with exogenous FSH (Experiment 2). In addition, preovulatory, "dominant" follicles may be capable of recruiting a greater vascular supply and also appear to have increased uptake of plasma gonadotropins compared with other antral follicle (6-8). Secretion of angiogenic activity by granulosa cells of preovulatory follicles may, therefore, enhance recruitment of a vascular supply and contribute to maintaining these follicles in a nonatretic, preovulatory state.

Acknowledgments

The authors thank Dr. A. F. Parlow, Pituitary Hormones and Antisera Center, for highly purified oFSH; and National Hormone and Pituitary Program, NIADDK and University of Maryland School of Medicine for oLH. The authors acknowledge Dr. M. H. Smith for providing access to necropsy and histological facilities; Dr. W. D. Slanger for assistance with statistical analyses; Mr. J. D. Kirsch and Mr. K. C. Kraft for technical assistance; and, J. Berg for typing the manuscript. Published as Journal Article No. 1654 of the North Dakota Agricultural Experiment Station; Project 1780. Supported, in part, by Competitive Research Grant 87-CRCR-1-2573 from the U.S. Department of Agriculture.

References

1. Clark JG. The origin, development and degeneration of blood-vessels of the human ovary. John Hopkins Hosp Rep 1900; 9:593-676.
2. Bassett DL. The changes in the vascular pattern of the ovary of the albino rat during the estrous cycle. Am J Anat 1943; 73:251-91.
3. Burr JH Jr, Davies JI. The vascular system of the rabbit ovary and its relationship to ovulation. Anat Rec 1951; 111:273-92.
4. Bruce NW, Moor RM. Capillary blood flow to ovarian follicles, stroma and corpora lutea of anesthesized sheep. J Reprod Fertil 1976; 46:299-304.
5. Hay MF, Cran DG, Moor RM. Structural changes occurring during atresia in sheep ovarian follicles. Cell Tissue Res 1976; 169:515-29.
6. DiZerega GS, Hodgen GD. Fluorescence localization of luteinizing hormone/human chorionic gonadotropin uptake in the primate ovary. II. Changing distribution during selection of the dominant follicle. J Clin Endocrinol Metab 1980; 51:903-7.
7. McNatty KP, Dobson C, Gibb M, Kieboom L, Thurley DC. Accumulation of luteinizing hormone, oestradiol and androstenedione by sheep ovarian follicles in vivo. J Endocrinol 1981; 91:99-109.
8. Zeleznik AJ, Schuler HM, Reichert LE Jr. Gonadotropin-binding sites in the rhesus monkey ovary: role of the vasculature in the selective distribution of human chorionic gonadotropin to the preovulatory follicle. Endocrinology 1981; 109:356-62.
9. Hay MF, Moor RM, Cran DG, Dott HM. Regeneration of atretic sheep ovarian follicles in vitro. J Reprod Fertil 1979; 55:195-207.
10. Makris A, Ryan KJ, Yasumizu T, Hill CL, Zetter BR. The nonluteal porcine ovary as a source of angiogenic activity. Endocrinology 1984; 115:1672-7.
11. Koos RD, LeMaire WJ. Evidence for an angiogenic factor from rat follicles. In: Greenwald GS, Terranova PF, eds. Factors regulating ovarian function. New York: Raven Press, 1983:191-5.
12. Sato E, Ishibashi T, Koide SS. Inducement of blood vessel formation by ovarian extracts from mice injected with gonadotropins. Experientia 1982; 38:1248-9.
13. Rone JD, Goodman AL. Detection of angiotropic activity from intact rabbit follicles cultured in serum-free media [Abstract]. Biol Reprod 1985; 32(suppl 1):184.
14. Redmer DA, Grazul AT, Kirsch JD, Reynolds LP. Angiogenic activity of bovine corpora lutea at several stages of luteal development. J Reprod Fertil 1988; 82:627-34.
15. Reynolds LP, Millaway DS, Kirsch JD, Infeld JE, Redmer DA. Angiogenic activity of placental tissues of cows. J Reprod Fertil 1987; 81:233-40.
16. SAS User's Guide: Statistics. 5th ed. Cary, NC: SAS Institute Inc., 1985.
17. Moor RM, Hay MF, Dott HM, Cran DG. Macroscopic identification and steroidogenic function of atretic follicles in sheep. J Endocrinol 1978; 77:309-18.
18. Steel RGD, Torrie JH. Principles and procedures of statistics: a biometrical approach. New York: McGraw-Hill, 1980.
19. Shepro D, D'Amore PA. Physiology and biochemistry of the vascular wall endothelium. In: Renken EM, Michel CC, eds. Handbook of physiology. Bethesda: Am Physiol Soc, 1984:103-64.
20. Kitai H, Yoshimura Y, Wright KH, Santulli R, Wallach EE. Microvasculature of preovulatory follicles: comparison of in situ and in vitro perfused rabbit ovaries following stimulation of ovulation. Am J Obstet Gynecol 1985; 152:889-95.
21. Reynolds SRM. Blood and lymph vascular systems of the ovary. In: Greep RO, Astwood EB, eds. Handbook of physiology. Bethesda: Am Physiol Soc, 1973:261-316.

22. Redmer DA, Rone JD, Goodman AL. Detection of angiotropic activity from primate dominant follicle [Abstract]. 67th Annu Mtg Endocrine Soc 1985:151.
23. Koos RD. Stimulation of endothelial cell proliferation by rat granulosa cell-conditioned medium. Endocrinology 1986; 119:481-9.

31

Localization of Tumor Necrosis Factor (TNF) in the Rat and Bovine Ovary Using Immunocytochemistry and Cell Blot: Evidence for Granulosal Production

K. F. Roby and P. F. Terranova

Department of Physiology, University of Kansas Medical Center
Kansas City, Kansas 66103

A protein fraction recently isolated from the bovine ovary has in vitro activity similar to tumor necrosis factor-α (TNF) and was thus hypothesized to be a tumor necrosis-like factor (TNLF) (1). In another related study, rabbit corpora lutea (CL) incubated in vitro in the presence of lipopolysaccharide (LPS) secrete a substance with bioactivity similar to TNF (2). In addition, macrophages which produce TNF (3) are present within the ovary. To investigate the cellular sources of TNF in the ovary, TNF was localized in bovine and rat ovaries using polyclonal antibodies to human recombinant TNFα with a Biotin-StreptAvidin immunostaining technique. Granulosal cells were examined by cell blot technique to ascertain the presence and/or secretion of TNF using a similar Biotin-StreptAvidin immuno-staining technique. This study reveals the presence of immunoreactive TNF (I-TNF) in the bovine and rat ovary localized primarily to three regions: the CL, the antral layer of granulosal cells in small antral and large preovulatory follicles, and throughout the granulosal layer of atretic follicles. Cell blot analyses indicate the presence and secretion of TNF by bovine and rat granulosa cells in vitro.

Methods

Bovine ovaries were obtained from beef cattle and placed on ice. For im-munocytochemistry, selected pieces of ovary were embedded in OCT tissue embedding compound (Baxter Health Care Corp., North Kansas City, MO) and snap frozen on dry ice. While the remaining ovaries were at 4°C, granulosal cells were aspirated from small (<5 mm) and large (>5 mm) antral follicles and subjected to cell blot analysis (methods described below). Holtzman rats (Madison, WI) were maintained in 22-24°C rooms on a 14 h:10 h light:dark schedule (lights on at 0500 h) and given food and water ad libitum. Estrous cycles were monitored by the appearance of cornified cells in the vaginal smear on day 1 (estrus).

Animals were used after at least 3 consecutive 4- to 5-day estrous cycles. Ovaries were removed at 0900 h on proestrus, trimmed of adhering tissues, and either embedded in OCT and snap frozen for subsequent immunocytochemistry or placed in Medium 199 (Gibco, Grand Island, NE) containing 0.1% bovine serum albumin (M199-BSA), whereby granulosal cells were harvested from preovulatory follicles for cell blot analysis.

Immunocytochemistry

Bovine and rat ovaries sectioned in a cryostat (-20°C) at 6 microns were placed on precleaned, subbed glass microscope slides and then warmed at room temperature. The sections were fixed in ice-cold acetone for 5 min and then air dried at room temperature. I-TNF was localized in the bovine and rat ovary using a Biotin-StreptAvidin immunostaining kit (BioGenex Laboratories, Dublin, CA) and a rabbit polyclonal antibody to human recombinant tumor necrosis factor-α (PAb-HuTNF) supplied by Genentech Inc., South San Francisco, CA. Sections were incubated with PAb-HuTNF, 1:100 dilution (1 part Ab: 100 parts PBS), PAb-HuTNF plus excess human recombinant TNF (supplied by Genentech), or preimmune rabbit serum as a control. Incubations were performed at room temperature in a humidified chamber and 1-2 drops of the incubating solutions were placed directly on the tissue sections. The chromogenic sites formed a red to brownish-red stain on the tissue. 5 x 10^5 neutralizing units/ml of Pab-HuTNF was preincubated with 5 x 10^7 or 5 x 10^8 units/ml of TNF; this represented 100x and 1000x TNF, respectively, and was used as a control.

Cell Blot

Granulosal cells were harvested by puncturing follicles with a needle and expressing the granulosal cells with gentle pressure into M199-BSA. According to a method described by Kendall and Hymer (4), granulosal cells were washed and applied in 100 µl media to the gridded side of a 1 x 1 cm piece of Immobilon, polyvinyldiene difluoride (PVDF) transfer membrane (Millipore, Bedford, MA). The membrane was placed on a coverslip in a humidified Petri dish and incubated at 37°C, in 5% CO_2 and air for 5 h. Then, media were removed and the membrane was subjected to immunostaining (4) using the Biotin-Strept-Avidin technique with PAb-HuTNF described for frozen sections (see above). Following immunostaining, membranes were rinsed with distilled water and air dried.

Results

Immunocytochemistry

Bovine Ovaries. I-TNF was observed in the CL and antral and atretic follicles. I-TNF in the CL was contained primarily in the thecal cords radiating into the center of the CL from the periphery (Fig. 1A). A few lightly-staining TNF positive cells (Fig. 1A, arrow) were also distributed throughout the CL in relatively low numbers compared to thecal cords. The granulosal cells of antral follicles contained I-TNF which was observed predominantly within the layers of granulosal cells lining the antral cavity and appeared to be in the follicular fluid surrounding the granulosal cells. I-TNF was observed in atretic follicles throughout the granulosal layer and also appeared to be in the fluid surrounding the granulosal cells (Fig. 1G). Sections incubated with preimmune rabbit serum showed no immunoreaction in any region of the ovary (Fig. 1B and H). PAb-HuTNF neutralized with 100x excess TNF resulted in a reduction in the intensity of immunostaining. In the presence of 1000x excess TNF, no immunostaining was apparent.

Rat Ovaries. I-TNF was localized in CL, throughout the granulosal layer in atretic follicles, and only in the more antral layers of granulosal cells in small and large preovulatory follicles. I-TNF was not apparent in preantral follicles. I-TNF in the CL was localized to the more diffuse cells in the central core. Qualitatively, the most intense I-TNF occurred in the granulosal layer of atretic follicles and in the granulosal cells lining the antral cavity (Fig. 1C), whereby I-TNF appeared to be in follicular fluid surrounding the granulosal cells (Fig. 1C). Sections of rat ovaries incubated with preimmune rabbit serum contained no immunostaining (Fig. 1D) and in the presence of 1000x excess TNF, immunostaining in response to the PAb-HuTNF was not apparent.

Cell Blot Analysis

Bovine Granulosa. Bovine granulosal cells subjected to cell blot contained and released I-TNF. TNF positive cells exhibited a range in staining intensity from a pink to brownish-red; intense staining was observed in granulosal cells. Release of I-TNF from the granulosa cells was observed as a "halo" of immunostaining (Fig. 1E) surrounding and extending from the

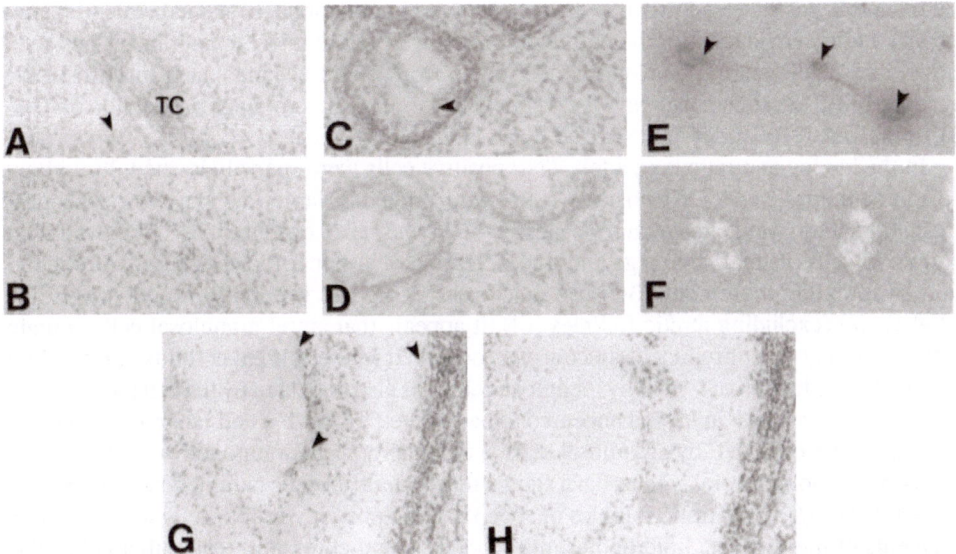

Fig. 1. Localization of I-TNF in the bovine and rat ovary and cell blot analysis of bovine granulosa cells (A) I-TNF in the thecal cord (TC) of the bovine CL; also a few scattered TNF positive cells can be seen (arrow). (C) A small antral follicle from the rat I-TNF can be seen in the antral layer of granulosa cells and in the follicular fluid surrounding the granulosa (arrow). (E) Cell blot analysis of bovine granulosa cells. Secreted TNF can be seen as an intense stain extending from the centrally located granulosa cell (arrows). (G) I-TNF in an atretic bovine follicle surrounds pyknotic granulosa cells and also appears to be present in the follicular fluid (arrows). Immunocytochemistry of adjacent sections performed in the presence of preimmune rabbit serum resulted in no immunostaining (B,D,F,H).

cells. Positive cells were observed singly and in groups. Groups of granulosal cells generally contained a more brilliantly intense staining although all cells within a group were not TNF positive.

Granulosal cells from small antral follicles contained fewer TNF positive cells than did the large antral follicles although strict quantitative measurements were not performed. Granulosal cells incubated with preimmune rabbit serum contained no immunoreaction. The negative TNF-containing cells appeared as white spots on the PVDF membrane (Fig. 1F).

Rat Granulosa. Cell blots with rat granulosal cells revealed similar results as seen with bovine granulosal cells. Intense immunostaining and the appearance of red cytoplasmic grains were present in both single cells and groups of cells. Groups of cells exhibited more intense immunostaining than singlets. Release of I-TNF from the granulosal cells was also observed as a "halo" surrounding the granulosal cells.

Discussion

I-TNF was localized in the luteal and follicular compartments of bovine and rat ovaries. I-TNF was observed in cells of the thecal cords penetrating deep into the CL, and in cells scattered throughout the bovine and rat CL. It is possible that these cells were macrophages because alternating sections of bovine and rat CL stained immunocytochemically for TNF, and macrophages revealed that I-TNF was observed in macrophagic stained cells (data not shown). Indirect evidence for the production of TNF by rabbit luteal macrophages has been shown in a recent study (2). Conditioned media from rabbit CL incubated in vitro in the presence of LPS, a substance previously shown to stimulate macrophage production of TNF (5), contained TNF activity as assessed by an in vitro cell lytic assay (2).

In the bovine and rat ovary, a few TNF positive cells were sparsely located throughout the interstitium. These TNF positive cells were relatively large and polyhedral shaped, suggesting they were also macrophages. I-TNF was also observed in bovine and rat granulosal cells of small and large antral follicles and of atretic follicles and in the follicular fluid surrounding these cells. Because macrophages are not generally present within the antral cavity (excluding atretic follicles [6]), it appears that antral granulosal cells contain I-TNF and may even produce it since it was observed in the follicular fluids surrounding these cells. Production of I-TNF by granulosa cells was also indicated by the cell blot analysis where I-TNF was present in, and appeared to be secreted by, bovine and rat granulosal cells.

Production of I-TNF by granulosal cells, a nonmacrophage/nonmonocyte cell type, is a novel observation. Several studies have shown that granulosal cells exhibit macrophage-like characteristics (6-10). Atretic follicles of sheep contain phagocytic-like cells which contain fragments of membranes, lipid bodies, mitochondria, and chromatin from other cells. The origin of these phagocytic-, macrophage-like cells is unknown; however, their ultrastructural appearance strongly suggests a granulosal cell origin (7). Regeneration of atretic sheep follicles cultured in vitro is associated with a decrease in the numbers of pyknotic nuclei and atretic bodies due, in part, to phagocytosis of these cellular remnants by granulosal cells (8). Macrophages have also been observed in the follicular fluid of atretic rat follicles (11). In many nonmammalian vertebrates, granulosal cells transform into phagocytic cells during follicular atresia and engulf degenerative components of the dying follicles (10). Therefore, it is possible that macrophage-like granulosal cells could produce I-TNF. The TNF positive cells observed in the central core of the CL might originate from either blood born monocyte/macrophages, and/or from antral granulosal cells that were TNF positive.

Preantral follicles of bovine and rat ovaries did not exhibit I-TNF; however, antral follicles from both species exhibited I-TNF. The observation that TNF appears during antrum formation in the antral granulosa cells might indicate a hormonal control of TNF production. Since FSH induces antrum formation in estrogen-primed immature rats, it is possible that these hormones might also regulate the production of TNF by antral granulosal cells. The granulosa cells surrounding the antrum have the morphology of protein-producing cells, e.g., an abundance of rough endoplasmic reticulum (12), and would thus presumably have the capability to produce TNF. The appearance of TNF during antrum formation might also indicate that TNF participates in the formation of the antrum. The mechanism by which this occurs is unknown, but may be related to TNF's cytolytic/cytostatic actions (3,13).

TNF may participate in follicular atresia and luteal regression. Atresia is associated with degeneration of the membrana granulosa, dissolution of the basement membrane and the disruption of the vasculature (for review, see Greenwald and Terranova [14]), all of which might be mediated, at least in part, by TNF. TNF is cytolytic, causing degeneration of several cell types in vitro and in vivo (4,13). TNF also inhibits endothelial cell proliferation (13), enhances procoagulant activity (15) and increases the adhesiveness of leukocytes to the endothelium (16). These processes could mediate the degeneration of the membrana granulosa, retard and/or inhibit growth of the vasculature and block small vessels with cellular debris, thus disrupting the blood supply to the growing follicle. TNF also stimulates collagenase production (17) and, therefore, another possible role for TNF in atresia is breakdown of the basement membrane. As in atresia, an inhibitor of endothelial proliferation such as TNF might function in limiting and/or disrupting the vasculature in the CL during regression. Changes observed in endothelial cells during luteal regression include nuclear pyknosis and cellular disintegration (18) similar to the actions of TNF on endothelial cells (13). Also, TNF stimulates phospholipase A_2 (19), the enzyme that cleaves the prostaglandin substrate, arachidonic acid, from triglycerides. Therefore, TNF might stimulate $PGF_{2\alpha}$ production and participate in demise of the CL.

I-TNF was localized in bovine and rat ovaries to three primary regions: the CL (thecal cords of the cow and the central core of the rat), throughout the granulosal layer of atretic follicles, and only in the most antral granulosal cells in small and large healthy antral follicles. Single TNF positive macrophage-like cells were also located throughout the interstitium and in some areas of the CL. Preantral follicles did not contain I-TNF. Cell blot analysis of bovine and rat granulosal cells substantiated the presence of I-TNF in granulosa cells and their ability to release the I-TNF.

References

1. Roby KF, Terranova PF. Inhibition of endothelial cell growth by a tumor necrosis-like fraction from the bovine ovary. Biol Reprod (submitted).
2. Bagavandos P, Kunkel SL, Wiggins RC, Keyes PL. Tumor necrosis factor a (TNF a) production and localization of macrophages and T lymphocytes in the rabbit corpus luteum. Endocrinology 1988; 122:1185-7.
3. Old LJ. Tumor necrosis factor (TNF). Science 1985; 230:630-2.

4. Kendall ME, Hymer WC. Cell blotting: a new approach to quantify hormone secretion from individual rat pituitary cells. Endocrinology 1987; 121:2260-2.

5. Mannel DN, Moore RN, Mergenhagen SE. Macrophages as a source of tumoricidal activity (tumor-necrotizing factor). Infect Immun 1980; 30:523-30.

6. Byskov AG. Atresia. In: Midgley AR, Sadler WA, eds. Ovarian follicular development and function. New York: Raven Press, 1979.

7. Hay MF, Cran DG, Moor RM. Structural changes occurring during atresia in sheep ovarian follicles. Cell Tissue Res 1976; 169:515-29.

8. Hay MF, Moor RM, Cran DG, Dott HM. Regeneration of atretic sheep ovarian follicles in vitro. J Reprod Fertil 1979; 55:195-207.

9. Peluso JJ, England-Charlesworth C, Bolender DL, Steger RW. Ultrastructural alterations with the initiation of follicular atresia. Cell Tissue Res 1980; 211:105-15.

10. Saidapur SK. Follicular atresia in the ovaries of nonmammalian vertebrates. Int Rev Cytol 1978; 54:225-44.

11. Braw RH, Tsafriri A. Effect of PMSG on follicular atresia in the immature rat ovary. J Reprod Fertil 1980; 59:267-72.

12. Christensen AK, Gillim SW. The correlation of fine structure and function in steroid-secreting cells, with emphasis on those of the gonads. In: McKerns KW, ed. The gonads. New York: Appleton-Century-Crofts, 1969.

13. Sato N, Goto T, Haranaka K, et al. Actions of tumor necrosis factor on cultured vascular endothelial cells: morphologic modulation, growth inhibition and cytotoxicity. J Natl Cancer Inst 1986; 76:1113-21.

14. Greenwald GS, Terranova PF. Follicular selection and its control. In: Knobil E, Neil JD, eds. The physiology of reproduction. New York: Raven Press, 1988.

15. Nawroth PP, Stern DM. Modulation of endothelial cell hemostatic properties by tumor necrosis factor. J Exp Med 1986; 163:740-5.

16. Gamble JR, Harlan JM, Klebanoff SJ, Vadas MA. Stimulation of adherence of neutrophills to umbilical vein endothelium by human recombinant tumor necrosis factor. Proc Natl Acad Sci USA 1985; 82:8667-71.

17. Dayer JM, Beutler B, Cerami A. Cachectin/tumor necrosis factor stimulates collagenase and prostaglandin E_2 production by human synovial cells and dermal fibroblasts. J Exp Med 1985; 162:2163-8.

18. Lobel BL, Levy E. Enzymatic correlates of development, secretory function and regression of follicles and corpora lutea in the bovine ovary. Acta Endocrinol (Copenh) 1968; 59(suppl 132):7-63.

19. Hepburn A, Boeynaems J, Fiers W, Dumont JE. Modulation of tumor necrosis factor cytotoxicity in L929 cells by bacterial toxins, hydrocortisone and inhibitors of arachidonic acid metabolism. Biochem Biophys Res Commun 1987; 149:815-22.

32

Direct Action of Gonadotropin Releasing-Hormone and Visualization of Its Receptors on Porcine Ovaries

Florence Ledwitz-Rigby and Pamela Dement-Liebenow

Department of Biological Sciences, Northern Illinois University
DeKalb, Illinois 60115

Gonadotropin releasing hormone (GnRH) has direct actions on the rat ovary (1). Specific GnRH receptors have been demonstrated on rat (2) and human (3) ovaries. While hypothalamic GnRH is not believed to reach the ovary in sufficient concentration to influence its function, evidence exists for a locally made rat ovarian GnRH-like molecule (4). A GnRH-like molecule may play a role in the local control of follicular response to gonadotropins. Specific receptors for GnRH have not been detected by radioreceptor assays in porcine, equine or bovine ovaries (5). The experiments presented in this paper were aimed at examining whether GnRH or a GnRH-like molecule might play a role in regulation of follicular development in the porcine ovary.

Materials and Methods

Porcine ovaries were obtained from a local slaughterhouse within 20 min of death. Granulosa cells were collected from small (1-2 mm), medium (3-5 mm), or large (6-12 mm) antral follicles and cultured as described by Ledwitz-Rigby (6). A GnRH agonist (GnRHa) ([des Gly^{10} dlys^6 Na Met-Leu^7 Pro-NHET]-GnRH) was used in the cell culture experiments. Progesterone content of the culture media was determined by radioimmunoassay (7).

GnRH receptors were visualized on frozen sections of freshly collected porcine ovaries. Ten- to 15-micron sections were incubated at room temperature with 10^{-6} or 10^{-5} M biotinylated d-lys^6-GnRH (Bio-GnRHa) for 3-5 min. Sections were rinsed in phosphate buffer with 0.1% BSA at 4°C followed by a 20-min exposure to 25 µg/ml of streptaviden-phycoprobe (Biomeda) at 37°C. Control sections were exposed to phycoprobe and either buffer alone, or to bio-GnRHa and fifty- or one hundredfold excess unlabeled D-lys^6-GnRH. The fluorescence of the sections was analyzed at magnifications of 100x and 250x using a Leitz I1-2 filter cube on a Leitz laborlux fluoresence microscope. Phycoprobe fluoresced golden orange. Autofluorescence appeared yellow to green.

Results

GnRHa Inhibition of Progesterone Secretion by Porcine Granulosa Cells

10^{-11} to 5×10^{-8}M GnRHa reduced LH (500 ng N1H LH S19/ml) stimulated progesterone secretion by porcine granulosa cells during 3-day incubations. Basal progesterone secretion was suppressed only at concentrations of 10^{-9}M GnRHa or higher. Results were similar for granulosa cells from all size antral follicles (8).

Time Course for GnRHa Inhibition of LH Stimulation of Progesterone Secretion

Incubation of granulosa cells with GnRHa for 1 day or less did not reduce LH-stimulated progesterone secretion during the first day of incubation. Culture media collected from the first 48 h of exposure to both LH and GnRHa contained significantly less progesterone than that of media from 2-day incubations with LH alone, in about half of our experiments. Three-day incubations with both LH and GnRHa consistently reduced the progesterone content of the media compared to media collected after 3 days with LH alone. Cells exposed to GnRHa for 2 days were inhibited in their response to LH on the third day even in the absence of GnRHa (9). A more recent experiment has shown that even a one-half hour exposure of freshly collected granulosa cells to 10^{-8} or 5×10^{-8}M GnRHa, followed by a 2-day incubation in 10% serum in medium 199 alone, reduced LH-stimulated progesterone secretion on day 3 to the same extent as a 2-day incubation with GnRHa (Ledwitz-Rigby unpublished observation). Two- or 3-day preincubations of freshly collected granulosa cells in 10% serum in medium 199 prior to exposing the cells to GnRHa had no effect on the time course for GnRHa action. Thus, it appears that receptors that bind GnRHa and mediate its action are present in porcine granulosa cells in vivo. The reduced response to LH provoked by a brief exposure of these cells to GnRHa, however, requires an extended time (24-48 h) to develop.

Visualization of GnRH Receptors on Porcine Ovaries

To date, we have examined 19 ovaries including 6 early luteal phase ovaries. The other ovaries were pubertal ovaries with their largest follicles ranging from 2 mm to 10 mm. Specific binding of GnRHa was identified by a golden-orange fluorescence of the phycoerythrin which appeared only on the sections incubated with 10^{-6} to 10^{-5}M bio-GnRHA. Control sections incubated with buffer alone or with bioGnRHa in the presence of 50- to one hundredfold excess unlabeled GnRHa did not exhibit the orange fluorescence but did exhibit a nonspecific yellow fluorescence.

The specific orange fluorescence was observed primarily on small atretic-appearing follicles (Figures 1 and 2). To date, we have not found evidence of GnRH receptors on corpora lutea or on larger healthy follicles.

Discussion

The results of our studies on GnRHa actions on progesterone secretion suggest that receptors which bind GnRHa and mediate GnRHa effects on granulosa cells are present in freshly collected antral granulosa cells. Moreover, the ability of GnRHa to suppress proges-

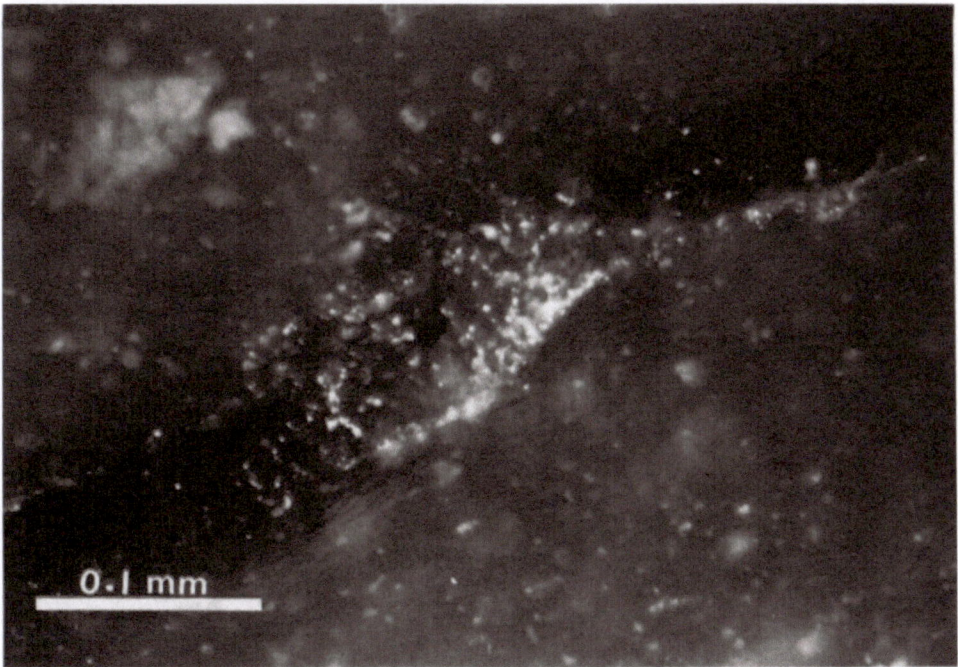

Fig. 1. GnRH receptors on a frozen section of a pig ovary treated with 10^{-6}M bioGnRHa and phycoprobe. The cluster of spots in the center were golden orange and represent the streptavidon phycoprobe bound to the biotinylated GnRHa bound to an atretic follicle. 250x.

terone secretion appears to require substantial changes in the granulosa cells, as an effect cannot be observed until 2 days after exposure to GnRHa. GnRHa may induce the loss of LH receptors (or reduce the rate at which they are maintained in culture). The steroidogenic machinery may also be altered, as basal progesterone secretion was reduced. In addition, GnRHa has been shown to decrease the adenyl cyclase response of rat ovaries to gonadotropins (1).

The presence of a GnRH-like molecule within specific follicles could explain the failure of these follicles to respond to LH with appropriate changes leading to maturation, ovulation and luteinization. One difference between "dominant follicles" and follicles destined for atresia might be the local rate of production or delivery of GnRH or a GnRH-like molecule to these follicles. Alternatively, those follicles with the largest number of GnRH receptors might be the most susceptible to atretogenic actions of a GnRH-like molecule. In our in vitro incubations, even concentrations as high as 5×10^{-8}M GnRHa did not totally suppress LH-stimulated progesterone secretion. As we do not distinguish between maturing, atretic or preatretic follicles in our collection of granulosa cells, it is possible that only cells collected from atretic or preatretic follicles possess sufficient GnRH receptors to be influenced by the GnRHa added to the cultures.

Our studies on the visualization of GnRH receptors in ovarian slices have allowed us to distinguish between healthy and atretic follicles. The majority of GnRHa receptors have been

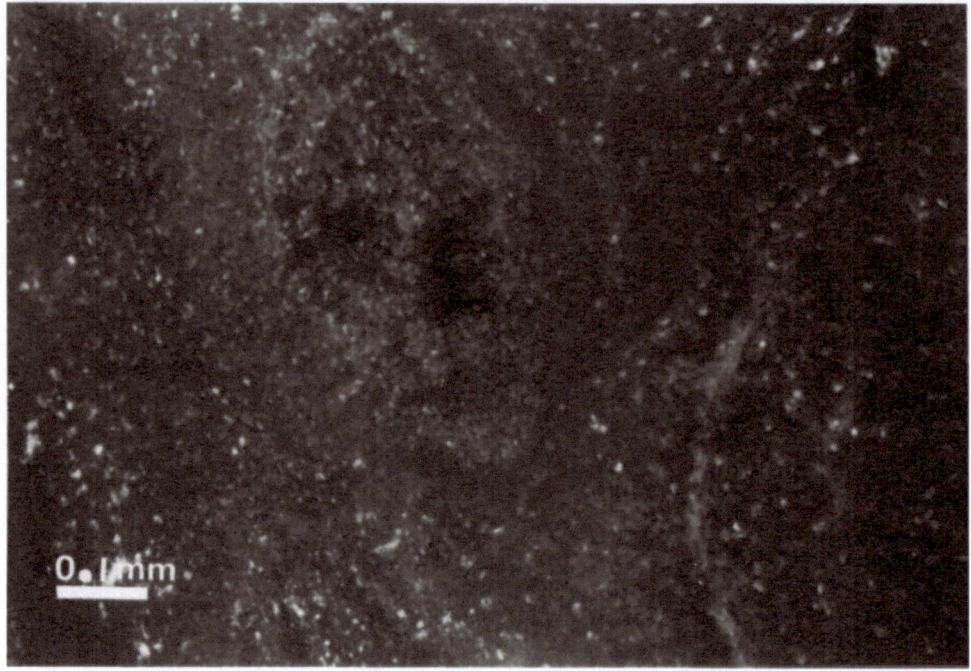

Fig. 2. Control frozen section of the same pig ovary as in Figure 1 incubated with unlabeled 5 x 10^{-5}M GnRHa, 10^{-6}M bioGnRHa and phycoprobe. All scattered spots were yellow autofluorescence. No specific binding of the phycoprobe was observed. 100x.

observed on atretic follicles. This has led us to hypothesize that the development of receptors for a GnRH-like molecule might predispose a follicle toward atresia. The factors controlling the production of GnRH receptors within a follicle are not known, but are under investigation in our laboratory.

The visualization of GnRH receptors in the porcine ovary indicates that only a small proportion of porcine ovarian tissue contains GnRH receptors. This may explain why radioreceptor assays of whole porcine ovaries (5) or preparations of granulosa cells from specific sized antral follicles (10) fail to detect statistically significant amounts of specifically bound radioactive GnRH.

Acknowledgments

This research was supported, in part, by BRSG 507 R20 7116 awarded by the Biomedical Research Support Grant Program, Division of Research Resources, National Institutes of Health, grants from the N.I.U. Graduate School, NSF grant RCD 8758085 and Sigma Xi Grants-In-Aid.

The technical assistance of Darryl Beckett in preparing the tissue sections and Mark Grzeszkowiak in preparation of the prints is gratefully acknowledged. Valuable advice on microscopy was received from Dr. R. Toth.

References

1. Knecht M, Amsterdam A, Catt KJ. Inhibition of granulosa cell differentiation by gonadotropin-releasing hormone. Endocrinology 1982; 110:865-72.
2. Clayton RN, Harwood JP, Catt KT. GnRH analogue binds to luteal cells and inhibits progesterone production. Nature, Land 1979; 282:90-2.
3. Bramley TA, Menzies GS, Baird DT. Specific binding of GnRH and an agonist to human corpus luteum homogenates: characterization, properties and luteal phase levels. J Clin Endocrinol Metab 1985; 61:834-41.
4. Aten RF, Williams AT, Behrman HR. Ovarian GnRH-like protein(s): demonstration and characterization. Endocrinology 1986; 118:961-7.
5. Brown JL, Reeves JJ. Absence of specific LHRH receptors in ovine, bovine, and porcine ovaries. Biol Reprod 1983; 29:1179-82.
6. Ledwitz-Rigby F. Local regulation of granulosa cell maturation. J Steroid Biochem 1987; 27:385-91.
7. Ledwitz-Rigby F. Reversal of follicular fluid inhibition of granulosa cell progesterone secretion by manipulation of intracellular cyclic AMP. Biol Reprod 1980; 23:324-30.
8. Ledwitz-Rigby F, Petito SH, Gross TM, et al. A comparison of the actions of GnRH agonist, antagonist and follicular fluids on granulosa cell progesterone secretion. Excerpta Med Int Cong Ser 1984; 652:903.
9. Ledwitz-Rigby F. GnRH analogs alter LH but not FSH stimulation of progesterone secretion by porcine granulosa cells in vitro. Biol Reprod 1986; 34(suppl 1):221.
10. Ledwitz-Rigby F, Thau RB (unpublished observations).

33

Role of Calcium in the Action of LHRH on Ovarian Progesterone Production

Peter C. K. Leung and Jian Wang

Department of Obstetrics and Gynecology
University of British Columbia, Vancouver, B.C., Canada V6H 3V5

Abstract. In fura-2AM-loaded rat granulosa cells, $[Ca^{++}]i$ rapidly increased after addition of LHRH ($10^{-6}M$). The effect of LHRH on $[Ca^{++}]i$ changes could be completely blocked by an LHRH antagonist. In a 5-h incubation, combined treatment of granulosa cells with LHRH and EDTA caused a 45% decrease in P production induced by LHRH. Concomitant treatment with EDTA plus TPA caused a 30% reduction in P accumulation when compared with TPA treatment alone. In a 24-h incubation, concomitant treatment with FSH plus LHRH markedly decreased P accumulation induced by FSH. Addition of EDTA to the cells partially reversed the inhibitory effect of LHRH upon FSH-induced P formation, by ca. 25%. Likewise, the inhibitory effect of TPA on P production could be partially reversed by the concomitant presence of 1 mM EDTA. Further, the reversal effect of EDTA could be completely abolished by the simultaneous addition of 1 mM Ca^{++}, and P production went down to the same levels as those induced by TPA alone. These data further support the hypothesis that the action of LHRH on ovarian steroidogenesis is mediated, at least in part, by a Ca^{++}-dependent protein kinase C.

Introduction

In previous studies, LHRH has been shown to stimulate polyphosphoinositide turnover in ovarian granulosa cells (1,2). Inositol 1,4,5-triphosphate (IP_3), a product of phosphatidylinositol 4,5 biphosphate (PIP_2) hydrolysis, has been proposed as a mediator for intracellular Ca^{++} mobilization (3). 1,2-Diacylglycerol, another product of polyphosphoinositide hydrolysis, activates protein kinase C (4). On the other hand, phosphoinositide turnover is believed to be involved in Ca^{++} gating as well (5). The aim of this study was to investigate the role of calcium in the action of LHRH on ovarian hormone production.

Materials and Methods

Immature Sprague-Dawley female rats purchased from Charles River Canada, Inc. (Montreal, Canada) were injected sc with 12 IU pregnant mare's serum gonadotropin. After

48 h, the rats were killed by cervical dislocation on the morning of day 25 of age. Granulosa cells were harvested as previously described (1). Aliquots of the granulosa cells (2×10^5/ml) were added to 24-well culture pates (Falcon, Oxnard, CA) and incubated at 37°C under an atmosphere of 5% CO_2 in air.

Progesterone (P) Production

Granulosa cells were treated with various hormones and drugs. LHRH and FSH were dissolved in saline. 12-O-Tetradecanoylphorbol-13-acetate (TPA) was dissolved in dimethylsulfoxide (DMSO). All treatments were diluted to their respective working concentrations with MEM medium before use and added in 5-10 µl aliquots to a total incubation volume of 1 ml. Control incubations received the same volume of DMSO. The final concentration of ethanol or DMSO in the incubations did not exceed 0.5%. At the end of a 5-h or 24-h incubation period, the culture medium was collected and stored at -20°C until assay. Cell viability, as determined by trypan blue exclusion, was not affected by the various treatments. The P concentration in the culture medium was determined by RIA. The intraassay coefficient of variation was 5.0% and the coefficient of interassay variation was 5.9%.

Intracellular Calcium Measurement

For intracellular calcium measurement, granulosa cells were cultured on cover glass with 5% FBS. After 2-3 days culture, cells were loaded with fura-2AM (5 µM fura-2/ml, Molecular Probes Inc.) for 60 min. When the excess of fura-2AM was washed away, the cover glass was mounted on a specially designed cell chamber which allows the free exchange of the culture medium. The fluorescent images from single cells were recorded by fluorescent microscope (6) with the assistance of Dr. K. Baimbridge. TPA, LHRH and calcium chloride were purchased from Sigma.

Results

LHRH-Induced $[Ca^{++}]i$ Alterations

Figure 1 shows the representative example of a single granulosa cell loaded with fura-2AM. When the cell was stimulated with 10^{-6}M LHRH, $[Ca^{++}]i$ increased from a basal level of 235 nM to 664 nM. By 2 min following LHRH addition, $[Ca^{++}]i$ fell towards basal level. A dose of 10^{-5}M of LHRH antagonist totally blocked the subsequent effect of LHRH on $[Ca^{++}]i$ increase.

Effect of EDTA on LHRH Stimulation of P Production

Addition of LHRH to rat granulosa cells stimulated P production during a 5-h incubation. To investigate the role of Ca^{++} in the action of LHRH, a calcium chelator, EDT (1 mM) was used. Combined treatment of granulosa cells with LHRH and EDTA caused a 45% reduction in P production (P<0.01) when compared with that induced by LHRH. Incubation of granulosa cells with TPA resulted in a significant increase in P formation, but concomitant treatment of the cells with EDTA plus TPA caused a 30% reduction (P<0.05) in P accumulation when compared with TPA treatment alone. Addition of 1 mM EDTA alone to granulosa cells had no effect on basal P production (Fig. 2).

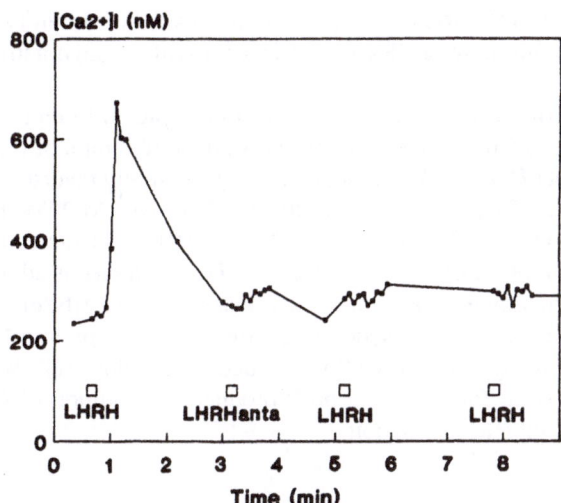

Fig. 1. Effect of LHRH or LHRH antagonist (LHRHanta) on intracellular calcium ion concentrations, $[Ca^{++}]i$, in rat granulosa cells loaded with fura-2AM.

Inhibitory Action of LHRH or TPA on P Production: Partial Reversal by EDTA

During a 24-h culture period, treatment of granulosa cells with FSH caused a significant increase in P production (Fig. 3). Concomitant treatment of the cells with FSH plus LHRH markedly decreased P accumulation when compared with that induced by FSH. Interestingly,

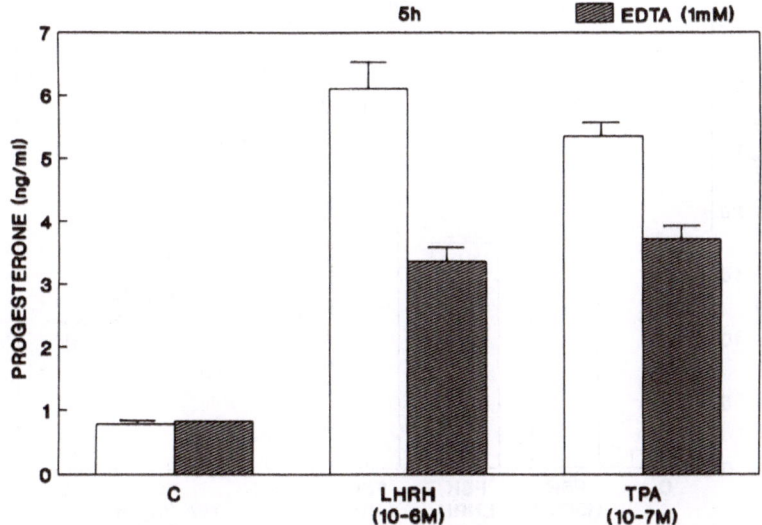

Fig. 2. Effect of EDTA on stimulation of progesterone production by LHRH or TPA in rat granulosa cells during a 5-h incubation.

the addition of 1 mM EDTA to the cells partially reversed the inhibitory effect of LHRH on FSH-induced P formation, by ca. 25% (P<0.01). EDTA alone did not influence FSH-stimulated P production.

Likewise, incubation of granulosa cells with FSH plus different doses of TPA, from 10^{-11}M to 10^{-9}M, for 24 h resulted in a dose-dependent inhibition of P production (Fig. 3). The inhibitory effect of TPA on P production could be partially reversed by the concomitant presence of 1 mM EDTA, 19% over that inhibited by 10^{-11}M TPA (P<0.05), 37% over 10^{-10}M TPA (P<0.01), and 23% over 10^{-9}M TPA (P<0.01). It is interesting that the reversal effect of EDTA could be completely abolished by the simultaneous addition of 1 mM Ca^{++} and P production went down to the same level as that inhibited by the different doses of TPA. In order to examine the possible synergistic effect between protein kinase C and Ca^{++} pathways, extra amount of Ca^{++} (1 mM) was added to granulosa cells without the presence of EDTA. There was no further effect on P production. Addition of Ca^{++} alone did not influence FSH-induced P accumulation.

Discussion

In this study, we presented direct evidence that LHRH caused a rapid increase of $[Ca^{++}]i$. The effect on LHRH on $[Ca^{++}]i$ changes was completely blocked by a specific LHRH receptor antagonist, which indicates an LHRH receptor-mediated mechanism. Since LHRH induces the rapid breakdown of membrane inositol lipids (1,2), the subsequent alterations in $[Ca^{++}]i$ likely participates in the action of LHRH on ovarian hormone production.

In the 5-h incubations, the effect of LHRH alone on P production is stimulatory. In order to investigate the role of extracellular Ca^{++} in the action of LHRH, a calcium chelator, EDTA,

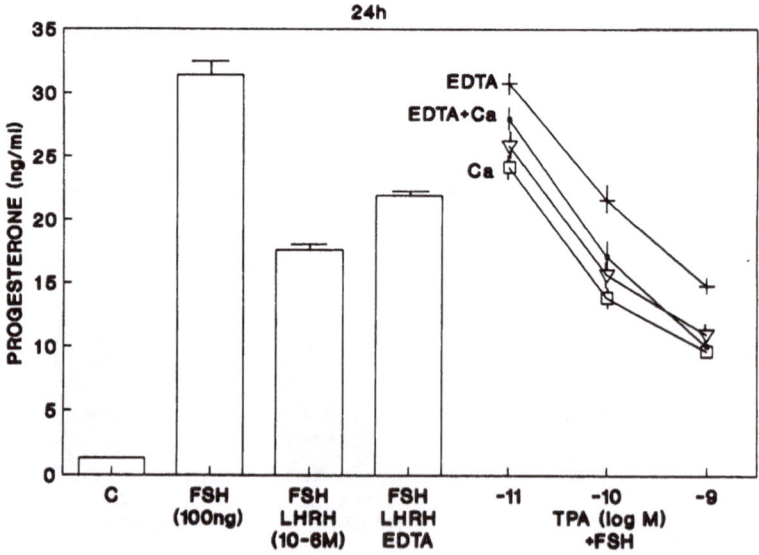

Fig. 3. Effect of EDTA (with or without calcium chloride) on LHRH/TPA inhibition of FSH-induced progesterone production during a 24-h incubation.

is used. The addition of EDTA (1 mM) in the culture medium can diminish LHRH-induced increase in P production. This result is similar to that reported by Eckstein et al. (7). In addition, we observe that TPA-stimulated P production can also be decreased by EDTA. Interestingly during a 24-h incubation, the well-established inhibitory effect of LHRH on FSH-induced P production can also be reversed by the presence of EDTA, at least partially. Likewise, the dose-dependent inhibitory effect of TPA on P production can be partially reversed by EDTA. When 1 mM Ca^{++} is added back to granulosa cells which have been treated with 1 mM EDTA, the reversal by EDTA of TPA-inhibited P production is completely abolished. Together, these data support the hypothesis that LHRH action on ovarian steroidogenesis is mediated, at least in part, by protein kinase C, and that the activation of protein kinase C is Ca^{++} dependent.

Acknowledgments

A potent LHRH antagonist, Ac-D-Nal(2)[1], 4 Cl-D-Phe[2], D-Trp[3], D-Arg[6], D-Ala[10]-LHRH, was obtained as a gift from Dr. M. V. Nekola of Tulane University. Bovine FSH (NIH-oFSH-16) and pregnant mare's serum gonadotropin were obtained from the NIDDK and the National Hormone and Pituitary Program (University of Maryland School of Medicine).

References

1. Ma F, Leung PCK. Luteinizing hormone-releasing hormone enhances polyphosphoinositide breakdown in rat granulosa cells. Biochem Biphys Res Commun 1985; 130:1201-8.
2. Davis JS, West LA, Farese RV. Gonadotropin-releasing hormone (GnRH) rapidly stimulates the formation of inositol phosphates and diacylglycerol in rat granulosa cells: further evidence for the involvement of Ca^{2+} and protein kinase C in the action of GnRH. Endocrinology 1986; 118:2561-71.
3. Burgess GM, Godfrey PP, McKinney JS, Berridge MJ, Irvine RF, Putney JW Jr. The second messenger linking receptor activations to internal Ca^{2+} release in liver. Nature 1984; 309:63-6.
4. Nishizuka Y, Takei Y, Kishimoto A, Kikkawa U, Kaibuichi K. Phospholipid turnover in hormone actions. Recent Prog Horm Res 1984; 40:301-41.
5. Berridge MJ. Inositol trisphosphate and diacylglycerol as second messengers. Biochem J 1984; 820:345-60.
6. Grynkiewicz G, Poenie M, Tsien RY. A new generation of Ca^{2+} indicators with greatly improved fluorescence properties. J Biol Chem 1985; 260:3440-50.
7. Eckstein N, Eshel A, Eli Y, Ayalon D, Naor Z. Calcium-dependent actions of gonadotropin-releasing hormone agonist and luteinizing hormone upon cyclic AMP and progesterone production in rat ovarian granulosa cells. Mol Cell Endocrinol 1986; 47:91-8.

34

Modulation of Rat Inhibin mRNAs in Preovulatory and Atretic Follicles

Teresa K. Woodruff, JoBeth D'Agostino, Neena B. Schwartz and Kelly E. Mayo

Department of Biochemistry, Molecular Biology and Cell Biology, and Department of Neurobiology and Physiology Northwestern University, Evanston, Illinois 60208

Summary

Inhibin α and β_A mRNA levels can be correlated with the maturational status of the antral follicle. Two distinct classes of follicles in which the levels of inhibin α and β_A mRNAs decrease have been identified by in situ hybridization. They are preovulatory follicles found on the evening of proestrus, and atretic follicles found at all times during the rat estrous cycle. Inhibin α and β_A mRNA levels decline in mature follicles following the preovulatory gonadotropin surges on the evening of proestrus. Administration of a GnRH antagonist to block the primary gonadotropin surges results in elevation of both inhibin α and β_A subunit mRNAs through the following morning (estrus). Replacement of exogenous LH or FSH causes a decline in inhibin α and β_A subunit mRNA levels 4 h following treatment. We conclude that the primary gonadotropin surges are important for appropriate regulation of inhibin gene expression. In addition to the late proestrus decrease in inhibin mRNA levels, we have observed that inhibin mRNA levels decrease in atretic follicles. Follicles of the type 1a class entering the earliest stages of atresia express α mRNA at low levels and β_A at levels not significantly greater than background. Follicles in later stages of atresia do not express detectable levels of either inhibin subunit mRNA.

Ovarian hormones function as feedback modulators to ensure precise communication between the ovary, pituitary, and hypothalamus. Inhibin is one such gonadal hormone. Inhibin is a dimeric glycoprotein, composed of an α subunit and one of two highly related β subunits (β_A or β_B), that acts to suppress the secretion of the pituitary hormone FSH (1,2). We have examined the expression of inhibin in the rat ovary, using in situ hybridization to measure the levels of α and β_A subunit mRNAs under a variety of physiological conditions.

We previously demonstrated that expression of the inhibin subunit mRNAs is precisely modulated throughout the rat estrous cycle (3,4). The levels of inhibin subunit mRNAs increase progressively from estrus to proestrus, culminating in mature, healthy, graafian follicles on the afternoon of proestrus, and decline between 1800 and 1900 h of the same day. The dramatic decline of the inhibin mRNAs on the evening of proestrus is coincident with stimulation of the follicles by the primary gonadotropin surges. We, therefore, investigated the role of LH and FSH in the negative regulation of the inhibin α and β mRNAs.

A second class of follicles was identified in which the inhibin subunit mRNA levels decreased, the atretic follicles. We have characterized expression of the inhibin subunit mRNAs in these follicles, and find evidence for differential expression of inhibin α and β subunit mRNAs.

Materials and Methods

Adult female Sprague-Dawley rats (proestrus) were divided into 4 experimental groups: Group I = untreated control; Group II = GnRH antagonist/vehicle [100 μg WY45760 [AcB92-D-Nal^1-4-F-D-Phe^2-D-Arg^6-LHRH] 1200 h proestrus subcutaneous injection (sc)/saline 1530 h proestrus tail vein injection (tv)]; Group III = antagonist/LH [100 μg WY45760 1200 h proestrus (sc)/16 μg oLH 1530 h proestrus (tv)]; Group IV = antagonist/FSH [100 μg WY45760 1200 h Pro (sc)/oFSH 1530 h Pro (tv)]. Animals were decapitated at times listed in Table 1. Ovaries were removed and 20-μm frozen sections were processed for in situ hybridization utilizing ^{32}P-labeled antisense α and β_A inhibin riboprobes as described (3-5). Sections were hybridized for 18 h at 42°C, washed, processed for autoradiogphy, and stained with hematoxylin and eosin for histological analysis. Serum LH (S16) and FSH (RP1) amounts were determined by RIA.

Results

Intact animals displayed typical serum LH and FSH values during the evening of proestrus (LH-1830 h, 24 ng/ml; 2400 h, 2 ng/ml; FSH-1830 h, 370 ng/ml; 2400 h, 371 ng/ml) (6). Hybridization to the inhibin probes remained elevated until 1830 h and was dramatically reduced in stimulated follicles following 1930 h (Table 1 and Figure 1, A-B). Data for the β_A subunit is not shown in the figure but is similar to that presented for the α subunit. When the GnRH antagonist has administered at 1200 h proestrus, the release of FSH and LH from the anterior pituitary was blocked, as indicated by RIA. In these animals, the inhibin mRNA levels remained elevated throughout the evening and following morning (Table 1 and Figure 1, C-D). Replacement with ovulatory doses of LH or FSH in animals receiving the GnRH antagonist resulted in stimulation of mature graafian follicles and a decrease in inhibin mRNA levels 4 h following injection (Table 1).

Table 1. Summary of detection of inhibin α and β_A mRNAs in preovulatory follicles of the rat ovary

Experimental Group	Time of Autopsy (proestrus)				
	1830 h	1930 h	2030 h	2400 h	0700 h
Intact	+	−	−	−	−
Antag/Veh	+	+	+	+	+
Antag/LH	+	+	−	−	−
Antag/FSH	+	+	−	−	−

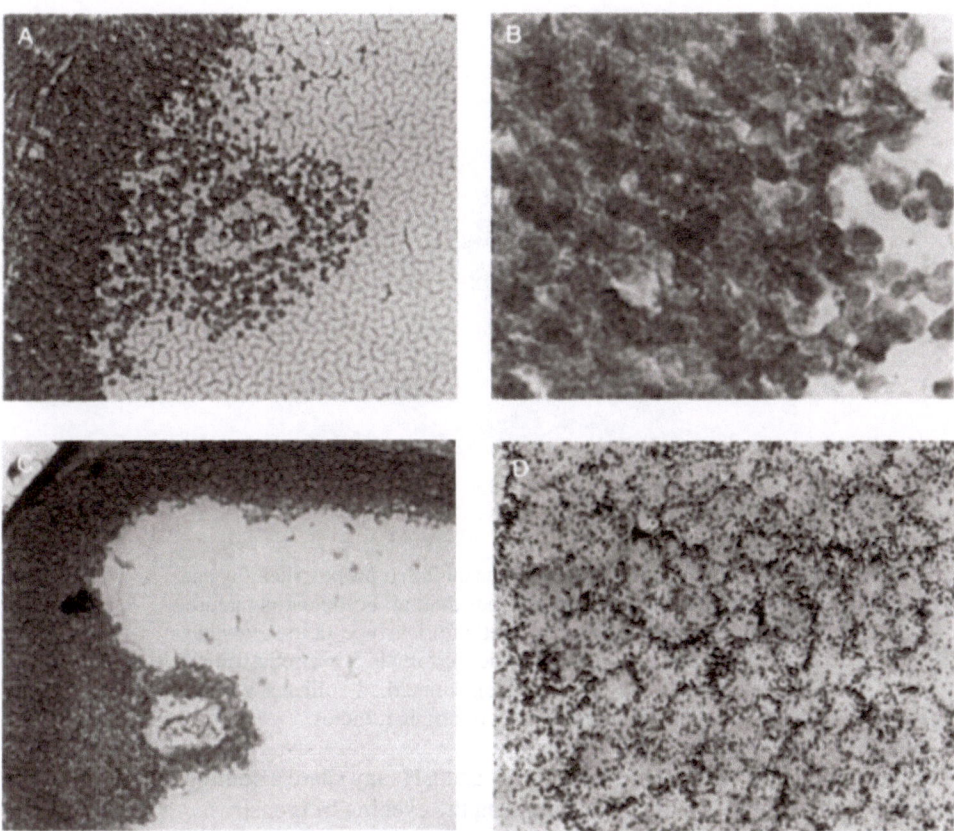

Fig. 1. In situ hybridization to detect α inhibin mRNA in preovulatory follicles. *Panel A*, intact at 2400 h proestrus, 100x magnification. *Panel B*, intact at 2400 h proestrus, 500x magnification. *Panel C*, antagonist-treated at 2400 h proestrus, 100x magnification. *Panel D*, antagonist-treated at 2400 h proestrus, 500x magnification.

A second class of follicles in which we have observed changes in inhibin subunit mRNAs is atretic follicles. As Figure 2 indicates, there is a striking decrease in inhibin mRNA in all types of atretic follicles vs. a healthy, mature graafian follicle. Moreover, these follicles display a subtle divergence in expression of the α and β_A subunit mRNAs. Follicles of the type 1a class (7) express α mRNA at low but detectable levels, and β_A mRNA at levels not significantly greater than background (data not shown). Follicles in later stages of atresia express neither of the inhibin subunit mRNAs above background.

Discussion

Inhibin subunit mRNAs decline on the evening of proestrus in normal preovulatory follicles. We have established the involvement of LH and FSH in this decline by employing a GnRH antagonist. When LH and FSH stimulation of graafian follicles is prevented, inhibin mRNA levels remain elevated through the morning of estrus. Replacement of these animals with exogenous LH or FSH causes a decline in inhibin subunit mRNA levels coincident with

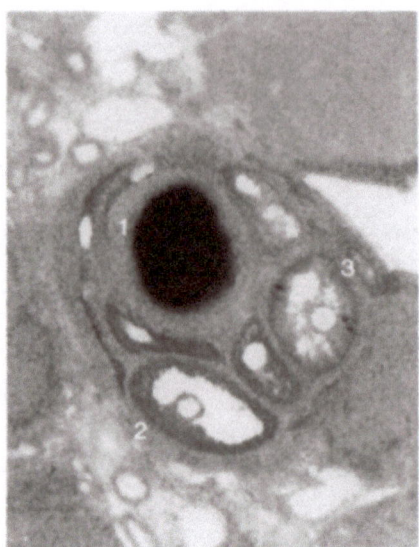

Fig. 2. In situ hybridization of the inhibin α probe to healthy and atretic follicles from a proestrous animal. Follicle 1 = mature, healthy follicle; follicle 2 = atretic follicle type 1a (note distinct beads around periphery of follicle); follicle 3 = atretic follicle type 1b (note lacy appearance). Unmarked follicles without oocytes are also various classes of atretic follicles.

follicular stimulation. This suggests that FSH and LH may share a common mechanism for directing the decline of inhibin mRNAs during the evening of proestrus.

Inhibin subunit mRNA levels were also found to decrease dramatically in follicles undergoing atresia. While mRNA levels are significantly reduced compared to healthy follicles, follicles in early stages of atresia retain α subunit mRNA while the β_A subunit mRNA is either turned off transcriptionally, has an enhanced turnover rate, or is simply below the detection threshold of our experiments. The reason for this divergent modulation is not known, but it represents an interesting pattern of inhibin mRNA expression in follicles of the nonovulatable pool.

The modulation of inhibin subunit mRNA expression may be related to altered sensitivity of the granulosa cell to the actions of FSH and LH at different times in the development of the follicle. Richards (8) and Hunzicker-Dunn (9) have demonstrated distinct differences in developing follicles with respect to responsiveness and activation of adenylate cyclases by FSH and LH. Further experiments directed at correlating the mechanisms of gonadotropin action on granulosa cells of the intact follicle with inhibin mRNA levels in follicles of different developmental stages must be undertaken to fully understand the interplay of inhibin, FSH, and LH in maintaining mammalian reproduction.

Acknowledgments

William Talley and Brigitte Mann contributed greatly to the animal work and the radioimmunoassays, respectively. Dr. Harold Papkoff kindly contributed oLH and oFSH for the replacement experiments. This work was supported by NIH grant HD-07504 (NBS), the NSF Presidential Young Investigators Program grant DCB-8552977 and the Chicago Community Trust Searle Scholars Program grant 87-G-113 (KEM), and NICHHD Program Project HD-219121.

References

1. Rivier J, Spiess J, McClintock R, Vaughan J, Vale W. Purification and partial characterization of inhibin from porcine follicular fluid. Biochem Biophys Res Commun 1985; 133:120-7.
2. Ling N, Ying S-Y, Ueno N, Esch F, Denoroy L, Guillemin R. Isolation and partial characterization of a Mr 32,000 protein with inhibin activity from porcine ovarian fluid. Proc Natl Acad Sci USA 1985; 82:7217-21.
3. Woodruff T, D'Agostino J, Schwartz N, Mayo K. Dynamic changes in inhibin messenger RNAs in rat ovarian follicles during the reproductive cycle. Science 1988; 239:1296-9.
4. D'Agostino J, Woodruff T, Mayo K, Schwartz N. Unilateral ovariectomy increases inhibin mRNA levels in newly recruited follicles. Submitted for publication.
5. Woodruff T, Meunier H, Jones P, Hsueh A, Mayo K. Rat inhibin: molecular cloning of α and β subunit complementary deoxyribonucleic acids and expression in the ovary. Mol Endocrinol 1987; 1:561-8.
6. Nequin L, Alvarez J, Schwartz N. Measurement of serum steroid and gonadotropin levels and uterine variables throughout 4 day and 5 day estrous cycles in the rat. Biol Reprod 1979; 20:658-70.
7. Osman P. Rate and course of atresia during follicular development in the adult cyclic rat. J Reprod Fertil 1985; 73:261-70.
8. Richards J, Hedin L. Molecular aspects of hormone action in ovarian follicular development, ovulation, and luteinization. Annu Rev Physiol 1988; 50:441-63.
9. Hunzicker-Dunn M, LaBarbera A. Unique properties of the follicle-stimulating hormone and cholera toxin-sensitive adenylyl cyclase of immature granulosa cells. Endocrinology 1986; 118:302-11.

35

Vasoactive Intestinal Peptide (VIP) Has an LH-Like Action on In Vitro Follicular Steroidogenesis But Not on Ovulation in the Cyclic Hamster

Y. Nakamura, B. K. Gangrade, and P. F. Terranova

Department of Physiology, University of Kansas Medical Center
Kansas City, Kansas 66103

Introduction

In vitro Vasoactive Intestinal Peptide (VIP) (but not Substance P) increases ovarian progesterone (P), androstenedione (A) and estradiol (E_2) production in the prepubertal rat (1); the source of P and A was interstitium and/or theca. VIP also stimulates in vitro granulosa cell production of P and E_2 (2). The VIP-induced E_2 secretion was mediated by an increase in granulosa cell aromatase activity (2). These steroidogenic actions of VIP are similar to FSH and LH. The in vitro effects of VIP on steroidogenesis of various types of follicles, i.e., preantral, preovulatory and atretic, are unknown. Thus, our aims were to determine whether VIP altered steroidogenesis in thecae and/or granulosa cells of follicles in various stages of development.

Materials and Methods

Preantral and Preovulatory Follicles

Cyclic hamsters were decapitated under ether anesthesia on day 4 at 0900 h (preovulatory group) and on day 1 at 0900 h (preantral group); 14L:10D (lights on 0500 h). The ovaries were removed, and follicles were dissected and cleaned of adhering tissues in cold (4°C) Krebs Ringer Bicarbonate buffer containing 1 mg/ml Glucose (KRBG). Each follicle in 1 m KRBG was preincubated at 37°C for 1 h in 95% O_2-5% CO_2. After preincubation, media were changed to fresh KRBG containing VIP (10^{-9}-10^{-6}M) or Substance P (10^{-7}-10^{-4}M) and incubated under the same conditions continuously for 5 h. Each group contained 6-7 follicles. At 1 h, 2 h and 3 h of incubation, 20 μl of incubation media were removed and saved at -20°C for E_2 RIA. At the 5th h of incubation, the entire medium was saved at -20°C for steroid RIA.

Thecae and Granulosa Cells

Preovulatory follicles were dissected and ruptured with fine forceps, and granulosa cells were removed by gentle pressure. The ruptured follicles were partially bisected in another dish containing fresh KRBG and theca cleaned as previously described. Two thecae in 1 ml KRBG were preincubated as mentioned above for preovulatory follicles. After preincubation, media were changed and VIP (10^{-7}, 10^{-6}M) was added. Granulosa cells were centrifuged at 40xG for 3 min at 4°C and supernatant fluid was decanted. Fresh media were added to the cells and incubations were performed as described above. 10^5 viable granulosa cells were incubated for 5 h in 1 ml KRBG containing VIP (10^{-7}, 10^{-6}M). Media were saved for steroid assay.

Experimentally Induced Atretic Follicles

To delay ovulation for 2 days, cyclic hamsters were injected sc at 1300 h on proestrus with 6.5 mg phenobarbital and again at 1200 h of the next day with 13 mg phenobarbital (4). On the morning following the last injection, the ovaries were removed, checked for blockage of ovulation and absence of corpora lutea. Large delayed preovulatory follicles were incubated with 10^{-6}M VIP and media were saved for steroid assay.

VIP Autoradiography

VIP autoradiography was performed as described earlier (5). Ovaries were rapidly frozen in OCT medium (Baxter Health Care Corp., North Kansas City, MO). Sections (12 μm) were cut in a cryostat, preincubated for 15 min at room temperature in 20 mM Tris-HCl buffer (pH 7.4), containing 2 mM MgCl 1% BSA and 0.25% bacitracin. This was followed by incubation in ^{125}I-VIP (approximately 10,000 cpm) with or without 1 μM unlabelled VIP. Sections were washed in ice-cold Tris buffer, air dried, fixed in formaldehyde vapors at 60°C for 2 h and then coated with Kodak NTB-2 autoradiographic emulsion. The slides were developed using Dektol developer.

Injection of VIP

Hamsters were injected sc at 1300 h on proestrus with 6.5 mg phenobarbital. One group was injected with 1 μg VIP into the jugular vein, the other was injected intercardiac with 5 μg VIP and the control groups were injected with the same volume of saline. The next morning, the oviducts were irrigated with saline in order to determine the number of ova shed.

Steroid Assay

P, A and E_2 in media were determined by an unextracted radioimmunoassay (6).

Statistics

Data from hormone assays were analyzed by ANOVA and Duncan's Multiple Range test. Differences were considered significant if $P \leq 0.05$.

Results

Effects of Substance P and VIP on In Vitro Steroidogenesis of Preantral and Preovulatory Follicles

Substance P (10^{-9}-10^{-6}M) did not alter P, A and E_2 production in vitro (data not shown) by preovulatory follicles. VIP, however, exhibited potent stimulatory effects on steroidogenesis of preovulatory follicles in a dose-dependent manner (Fig. 1). The time course of E_2 production revealed a significant increase after 2-h incubation at 10^{-7} and 10^{-6}M VIP; thereafter, E_2 production continued to increase throughout the 5-h incubation. Also in preovulatory follicles, VIP at 10^{-7} and 10^{-6}M increased production of A (270 pg/follicle/5 h) and 992 pg/follicle, respectively; control <45 pg/follicle). Most interestingly, VIP at 10^{-6}M (but not at 10^{-7}M) stimulated production of P by preovulatory follicles (2185 pg/follicle; control <40 pg/follicle) (Fig. 2). In preantral follicles, in vitro VIP at 10^{-6}M (but not 10^{-7}M) increased production of P (2736 pg/follicle; control 61 pg/follicle) but not A and E_2.

Effects of VIP on Steroidogenesis of Thecae and Granulosa Cells of Preovulatory Follicles

Thecae of preovulatory follicles produced P and A in response to 10^{-6}M VIP but not to 10^{-7}M (Table 1). In contrast, granulosa cells produced P (11 and 17 ng/10^5 viable cells/5 h; control <55 pg/10^5 cells) with both doses of VIP (10^{-7} and 10^{-6}M, respectively).

In Vitro Effects of VIP on Steroidogenesis of Experimentally Induced Atretic Preovulatory Follicles

Hamsters given phenobarbital to delay ovulation for 2 days induced atresia of preovulatory follicles. In vitro VIP at 10^{-6}M induced a large increase in P production (15 ng/follicle/5 h; control 180 pg/follicle) but only small amounts of A (113 pg/follicle; control <80 pg/follicle) and E_2 (110 pg/follicle; control <40 pg/follicle).

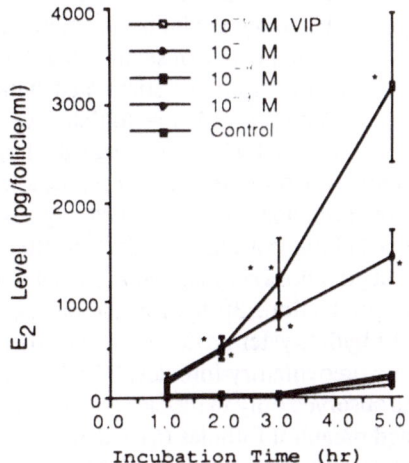

Fig. 1. In vitro effects of VIP on E_2 production by preovulatory follicles of the cyclic hamster (*P<0.01; **P<0.025; vs. control).

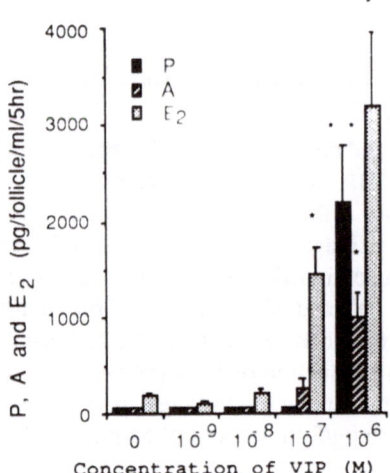

Fig. 2. In vitro effects of VIP on P, A and E_2
production by preovulatory follicles of the
cyclic hamster (*P<0.01; **P<0.025; vs. 0).

VIP Autoradiography

^{125}I-VIP binding was observed in the ovarian interstitium and thecae of preantral and
antral preovulatory follicles. Granulosa layers of large antral follicles but not small preantral
follicles exhibited moderate degree of VIP binding. Corpora lutea in estrous ovaries also
exhibited a significant degree of ^{125}I-VIP binding sites.

Discussion

These results demonstrated that VIP (but not Substance P) induced in vitro synthesis of
P, A and E_2 by preovulatory follicles in the cyclic hamsters in a dose- and time-dependent
manner. The VIP-induced steroidogenic response in vitro was similar to the in vitro
steroidogenic response of preovulatory follicles stimulated with ovine LH in the cyclic
hamster (4). The source of P and A by preovulatory follicles was presumably thecae since
thecae of preovulatory follicles incubated with VIP revealed a large increase in production
of P and A and ^{125}I-VIP binding was observed on thecae; these results are similar to those
using ovine LH (3). In addition, granulosa cells produced large amounts of P but not A and
E_2 in response to VIP in vitro and this correlated with ^{125}I-VIP binding to granulosa cells.
A recent study with cultured rat granulosa cells also showed that VIP stimulated P production
by increasing pregnenolone production, 3β-hydroxysteroid dehydrogenase activity and
decreasing metabolism of 20α-hydroxysteroid dehydrogenase (2). In preantral follicles and
experimentally induced atretic preovulatory follicles, VIP also induced production of P by
thecae; ^{125}I-VIP binding was observed only in thecae (not granulosa). These results are also
similar to those LH-stimulated preantral follicles (6) and atretic preovulatory follicles (4).

A recent study has shown that immunoreactive VIP fibers did not originate in the ovary,
but were of extrinsic origin, the abdominal vagus; the nerve fibers were located around blood

Table 1. Effects of VIP on thecal steroidogenesis

	Control (n=5)	10^{-7}M VIP (n=6) (pg/ml/2 thecae/5 h)	10^{-6}M VIP (n=6)
Progesterone	<55	<55	1346 ± 864
Androstenedione	113 ± 29	115 ± 15	1677 ± 317
Estradiol	31 ± 3	3 ± 8	55 ± 10

vessels, in the interstitial tissue and thecal layers of developing follicles (1). In rats, abdominal vagotomy disrupts the estrous cycle (7) and decreased the number of ova shed (8). The ovarian responsiveness to PMSG is also reduced in cyclic hamsters after abdominal vagotomy (Nakamura Y and Terranova PF, unpublished). Thus, it appears that VIP may play an important role during follicle development, steroidogenesis and ovulation.

The ovulation-inducing capacity of VIP was investigated in vivo using phenobarbital-blocked proestrus hamsters. Neither 1 µg nor 5 µg VIP injected IV or intracardiac caused ovulation. There may be an explanation as to why VIP did not induce ovulation. First is the short half-life of VIP, averaging 1-2 min in circulation (9). Presumably, the amount of VIP reaching the ovary is not sufficient to cause ovulation since the VIP concentration in blood would have been <1 µg/ml; this would be in a low range (10^{-7}-10^{-6}M) for stimulating steroidogenesis. Secondly, VIP is a neurotransmitter and reaches the ovary through nerve fibers. In this experiment, however, VIP entered the ovary through the ovarian circulation. Thus, the deposition of VIP at the follicle would be different and the cellular stimulation may be less. Lastly, in granulosa cells of the hen, Plasminogen Activator (PA) activity was inhibited by VIP (10), but VIP stimulated PA activity in cultured rat granulosa cells and cumulus-oocyte complexes (11). It is not known whether VIP stimulates or inhibits PA activity in the cyclic hamster.

In summary, these results revealed that VIP stimulated in vitro steroidogenesis of preantral, preovulatory and experimentally induced atretic follicles in cyclic hamsters. The steroidogenic action of VIP was similar to LH. Thecae of preovulatory follicles were a primary target of VIP in stimulating A production. However, in vivo injection of VIP did not induce ovulation in proestrus phenobarbital-blocked cyclic hamsters.

References

1. Ahmed CE, Dees WL, Ojeda SR. The immature rat ovary is innervated by vasoactive intestinal peptide (VIP)-containing fibers and responds to VIP with steroid secretion. Endocrinology 1986; 118(4):1682-9.
2. Davoren JB, Hsueh AJW. Vasoactive intestinal peptide: a novel stimulator of steroidogenesis by cultured rat granulosa cells. Biol Reprod 1985; 33:37-52.
3. Terranova PF, Martin NC, Chien S. Theca is the source of progesterone in experimentally induced atretic follicles of the hamster. Biol Reprod 1982; 26:721-7.
4. Terranova PF. Steroidogenesis in experimentally induced atretic follicles of the hamster: a shift from estradiol to progesterone synthesis. Endocrinology 1981; 108(5):1885-90.

5. Poulin O, Suzuki Y, Lederis K, Rorstad OP. Autoradiographic localization of binding sites for vasoactive intestinal peptide (VIP) in bovine cerebral arteries. Brain Res 1986; 381:382.

6. Terranova PF, Garza F. Relationship between the preovulatory luteinizing hormone (LH) surge and androstenedione synthesis of preantral follicles in the cyclic hamster: detection by in vitro responses to LH. Biol Reprod 1983; 29:630-6.

7. Burden HW, Lawrence IE Jr, Louis TM, Hadson CA. Effects of abdominal vagotomy on the estrous cycle of the rat and the induction of pseudopregnancy. Neuroendocrinology 1981; 33:218-22.

8. Cruz ME, Chavez R, Dominguez R. Ovulation, follicular growth and ovarian reactivity to exogenous gonadotropins in adult rats with unilateral or bilateral section of the vagi nerves. Rev Invest Clin 1986; 38:167-71.

9. Straus E, Keltz TN, Yalow RS. Enzymatic degradation of VIP. In: Said SI, ed. Vasoactive intestinal peptide. New York: Raven Press, 1982:333-9.

10. Johnson AL, Tilly JL. Effects of vasoactive intestinal peptide on steroid secretion and plasminogen activator activity in granulosa cells of the hen. Biol Reprod 1988; 38:296-303.

11. Liu YX, Kasson BG, Dahl KD, Hsueh AJW. Vasoactive intestinal peptide stimulates plasminogen activator activity by cultured rat granulosa cells and cumulus-oocyte complexes. Peptides (Fayetteville) 1987; 8:29-33.

36

Mechanisms by Which Vasoactive Intestinal Peptide Regulate Baboon Granulosa Cell Steroidogenesis

Susan L. Silavin

Department of Obstetrics and Gynecology, University of Oklahoma
Health Sciences Center, P.O. Box 26901, Oklahoma City, OK 73190

Introduction

Vasoactive intestinal peptide (VIP) has been shown to enhance steroid production in vivo in rabbits (1) and humans (2) and in vitro in prepubertal rat ovaries (3), isolated rat granulosa cells (4), as well as cultured baboon granulosa cells (5). In addition, Gozes and Tsafriri (6) have found VIP-encoding mRNA in rat ovaries, suggesting a local ovarian synthesis of VIP.

The effects of VIP appear to be mediated via a cAMP-dependent pathway. Increased intracellular and extracellular cAMP in response to VIP have been measured in various endocrine systems, including mouse adrenal tumor cells (7), rat granulosa (4) and testicular cells (8), and human thyroid tissue (9).

Insulin also enhances ovarian steroidogenesis in numerous species. In granulosa cells from DES-primed rats, insulin had no effect on basal steroid production but enhanced gonadotropin-stimulated steroidogenesis (10). In contrast, insulin was shown to enhance basal as well as tropic hormone-stimulated steroid production in cultured porcine granulosa cells (11,12). It was, therefore, of interest to determine if insulin affected steroidogenesis in baboon granulosa cells and if VIP acting via a cAMP-dependent pathway modulated these responses.

Materials and Methods

Adult, cycling female baboons (*Papio anubis* and *P. cynocephalus*) received clomiphene citrate (Serophene®, Serono Laboratories, Norwell, MA) 50 mg on cycle days 2-5 (day 1 is the first day of menses). This drug was administered orally in a small banana section that was readily consumed. On cycle days 6-9, animals received 75, 150, 300 and 375 IU hMG (Pergonal®, Serono Laboratories, Norwell, MA), respectively. Additionally, 37.5 and 75 IU hFSH (Metrodin®, Serono Laboratories, Norwell, MA) was administered on days 6 and 7, respectively. On cycle day 10, animals received 5000 IU hCG (Profasi®, Serono Laboratories, Norwell, MA), and laparotomy for follicular aspiration was performed 24 h later. Blood was drawn daily through day 11 and then 3 days per week until the next menses for quantification of serum estradiol and progesterone concentrations.

Granulosa cells were aspirated into 12 ml of sterile Dulbecco's phosphate-buffered saline (PBS; GIBCO, Grand Island, NY) and cells from no more than 8 follicles were placed into each tube of PBS. Cells were washed once in sterile Dulbecco's Modified Eagle's Medium (DMEM; GIBCO, Grand Island, NY) and resuspended in DMEM containing hMG (30 mIU/ml), estradiol (1 µg/ml) and 20% (vol: vol) male baboon serum. Approximately 250,000-500,000 cells/ml were plated into 16-mm diameter culture wells (Nunclon, Nunc/Intermed, Roskilde, Denmark) and cultured at 37°C in an atmosphere of humidified 95% air: 5% CO_2. After 48 h, cells were washed once with serum-free DMEM followed by the addition DMEM containing 10^{-7}M androstenedione. Twenty-four to 48 h later, medium was replaced with serum-free, hormone-free DMEM and various treatments.

Proteins were measured by the method of Bradford (13). Progesterone and estradiol were determined by specific, solid-phase ^{125}I-RIA as previously described (14). CAMP was determined by a specific RIA (Amersham, Arlington Heights, IL).

Results

As shown previously (5), hCG (500 mIU/ml) or 8-bromo-cAMP (1.5 mM) stimulated progesterone production 1.5- to twofold in cultured baboon granulosa cells. Also VIP (10^{-6}M) was shown to enhance baseline progesterone and estradiol production (Table 1). Due to the variability in baseline steroid production among individual experiments, all results are expressed as percent increase over respective control. Subsequent values were obtained 24 h after initiation of treatment.

Treatment of granulosa cells with 10^{-6}M VIP resulted in a 39.6 ± 7.0% (n=9) increase over control in extracellular cAMP. In addition, VIP enhanced hCG-stimulated cAMP by 35.0 ± 5.7% (n=4). These results correlated well with the VIP enhancement of hCG-stimulated progesterone production (Table 2). The stimulation of cAMP by VIP was 40 ± 16% of that seen by hCG.

Insulin (1 µg/ml) enhanced baseline estradiol production by 36.2 ± 9.2% (n=5) over control and the addition of VIP resulted in a further increase in estradiol of 40.8 ± 10.9% (n=5) over that seen in the presence of insulin alone. Insulin also increased baseline

Table 1. Effect of VIP (10^{-6}M) on baseline steroid production
by cultured baboon granulosa cells *

Time after addition of VIP	Increased Steroid Production (%)	
	Progesterone (n=4)	Estradiol (n=6)
24 h	45 ± 9	37 ± 10
48 h	43 ± 8	65 ± 5

*Data are expressed as % increase in steroid production above control in response to VIP (mean ± SEM).

Table 2. Effect of VIP (10^{-6}M) on hormone-stimulated progesterone
production by cultured baboon granulosa cells *

Treatment	% Increase in progesterone production above that seen by agent alone
VIP + hCG (500 mIU/ml)	34.6 ± 4.9 (n=5)
VIP + 25-hydroxycholesterol (25 µg)	49.3 ± 8.9 (n=3)
VIP + 8-bromo-cAMP (1.5 mM)	26.3 ± 2.0 (n=4)
VIP + insulin (1 µg/ml)	2.2 ± 6.8 (n=6)

*Data are expressed as percent increase in progesterone production above that seen in
the presence of the tropic agent alone (mean ± SEM).

progesterone production by baboon granulosa cells by 37.5 ± 6.7% (n=6) and VIP augmented
the effect of insulin (Table 2).

The hydroxysterol, 25-hydroxycholesterol, a sterol shown to be more soluble than
cholesterol and representative of cholesterol side-chain cleavage enzyme activity (15), was
added to baboon granulosa cells following a 24-h incubation in the presence or absence of
VIP.

Preincubation with VIP consistently enhanced the conversion of 25-hydroxycholesterol
(25 µg) to progesterone (Table 2).

The addition of VIP to the incubation medium resulted in a small but consistent increase
in 8-bromo-cAMP-stimulated progesterone production (Table 2).

Discussion

VIP, originally isolated from porcine duodenum (16), was thought to be a gut hormone
involved in smooth muscle relaxation and vasodilation. However, VIPergic nerve fibers have
been found in female genital tracts of laboratory animals and humans (17-19), and VIP has
been shown to enhance steroid production by endocrine tissues including rat (4) and primate
(baboon; 5) granulosa cells.

The widespread effects of VIP appear to be mediated by a cAMP-dependent pathway.
VIP was shown to increase cAMP production by rat granulosa cells (4) and testicular cells
(8) to a lesser degree than that seen in response to tropic stimuli. In baboon granulosa cells,
VIP also stimulated extracellular cAMP production, but to a lesser extent than that seen by
hCG stimulation.

The enhancement of 25-hydroxycholesterol-stimulated progesterone production by VIP
indicates that this agent induces cholesterol side-chain cleavage enzyme (CSCC) activity in
baboon granulosa cells. These results are in agreement with data showing that in rat granulosa
cells, VIP treatment enhanced synthesis of all three components of CSCC (20) and increased
the mRNA for cytochrome P450$_{SCC}$ (21). The increased CSCC seen with VIP treatment in
rat granulosa cells was 60% less than that seen in the presence of cAMP alone (20). Yet the
synthesis of the cytochrome P450$_{SCC}$ and adrenodoxin components of CSCC in the presence
of VIP plus cAMP was nearly additive (20). Similarly, in baboon granulosa cells, VIP
enhanced cAMP-stimulated progesterone production. Taken together, these data indicate

that VIP enhances steroidogenesis by increasing the amount of available CSCC and that this occurs, in part, via a cAMP-dependent mechanism, but that another mechanism of action of VIP is likely in both rat and primate granulosa cells.

Similar to results in porcine granulosa cells (11,12), insulin stimulated basal estrogen and progesterone production by baboon granulosa cells. The augmentation of insulin-enhanced progesterone production by VIP suggests that in the primate ovary, interactions among local and systemic modulators of ovarian steroidogenesis occur. These interactions may represent an important mechanism for the preparation of granulosa cells for increased steroid production during early luteal development.

References

1. Fredericks CM, Lundquist LE, Mathur RS, Ashton SH, Landgrebe SC. Effects of vasoactive intestinal polypeptide upon ovarian steroid, ovum transport, and fertility in the rabbit. Biol Reprod 1983; 28:1052-60.
2. Otteson B, Pedersen B, Nielsen J, Dalgaard D, Fahrenkrug J. Effect of vasoactive intestine polypeptide (VIP) on steroidogenesis in women. Regul Pept 1986; 16:299-304.
3. Ahmed CE, Dees WL, Ojeda SR. The immature rat ovary is innervated by vasoactive intestinal peptide (VIP)-containing fibers and responds to VIP with steroid secretion. Endocrinology 1986; 118:1680-9.
4. Davoren BJ, Hsueh AJW. Vasoactive intestinal peptide: a novel stimulator of steroidogenesis by cultured rat granulosa cells. Biol Reprod 1985; 33:37-52.
5. Silavin SL. Role of vasoactive intestinal peptide (VIP) in steroidogenesis by cultured baboon granulosa cells. Biol Reprod 1987; 36(suppl 1):49.
6. Gozes I, Tsafriri A. Detection of vasoactive intestinal peptide-encoding messenger ribonucleic acid in the rat ovaries. Endocrinology 1986; 2606-10.
7. Kowal J, Horst I, Pensky J, Alfonzo M. A comparison of the effects of ACTH, vasoactive intestinal peptide and cholera toxin on adrenal cAMP and steroid synthesis. Ann NY Acad Sci 1977; 297:314-28.
8. Kasson BG, Lim P, Hsueh AJW. Vasoactive intestinal peptide stimulates androgen biosynthesis by cultured neonatal testicular cells. Mol Cell Endocrinol 1986; 48:21-9.
9. Toccafondi RS, Brandi ML, Melander A. Vasoactive intestinal peptide stimulation of human thyroid cell function. J Clin Endocrinol Metab 1984; 58:157-60.
10. Davoren JG, Hsueh AJW. Insulin enhances FSH-stimulated steroidogenesis by cultured rat granulosa cells. Mol Cell Endocrinol 1984; 35:97-105.
11. May JV, Schomberg DW. Granulosa cell differentiation in vitro: effect of insulin on growth and functional integrity. Biol Reprod 1981; 25:421-31.
12. Veldhuis JD, Kolp LA, Toaff ME, Strauss JF III, Demers LM. Mechanisms subserving the tropic actions of insulin on ovarian cells: in vitro studies using swine granulosa cells. J Clin Invest 1983; 72:1046-57.
13. Bradford MM. A rapid and sensitive method for the quantitation of microgram quantities of protein utilizing the principle of protein-dye binding. Anal Biochem 1976; 72:248-54.
14. Kubasik NP, Halluer GD, Bradows RG. Evaluation of a direct solid-phase radioimmunoassay for progesterone, useful for monitoring luteal function. Clin Chem 1984; 30:284-6.

15. Silavin SL, Strauss JF III. Progesterone production by hamster granulosa and luteal cells during short-term incubation. Effects of lipoproteins, compactin and 25-hydroxycholesterol. Biol Reprod 1983; 29:1163-71.
16. Said SI, Mutt V. Polypeptide with broad biological activity: isolation from small intestine. Science 1970; 169:1217-8.
17. Larsson LI, Fahrenkrug J, Schaffalitzky de Muckadell OB. Vasoactive intestinal peptide occurs in nerves of the female genitourinary tract. Science 1977; 197:1374-5.
18. Alm P, Alumets J, Hakanson R, et al. Origin and distribution of VIP (vasoactive intestinal peptide)-nerves in the genito-urinary tract. Cell Tissue Res 1980; 205:337-47.
19. Alm P, Alumets J, Hakanson R, Owman C, Sjoberg N-O, Sundler F. Vasoactive intestinal polypeptide nerves in the human female genital tract. Am J Obstet Gynecol 1980; 136:349-51.
20. Trzeciak WH, Ahmed CE, Simpson ER, Ojeda SR. Vasoactive intestinal peptide induces the synthesis of the cholesterol side-chain cleavage complex in cultured rat ovarian granulosa cells. Proc Natl Acad Sci USA 1986; 83:7490-4.
21. Trezeciak WH, Waterman MR, Simpson ER, Ojeda SR. Vasoactive intestinal peptide regulates cholesterol side-chain cleavage cytochrome P-450 (P450$_{SCC}$) gene expression in granulosa cells from immature rat ovaries. Molec Endocrinol 1987; 1:500-4.

37

Heparin-Binding Proteins in Purified Plasma Membranes of Bovine Granulosa Cells

Martin A. Winer and Roy L. Ax

Department of Dairy Science and the Endocrinology-Reproductive
Physiology Program, University of Wisconsin, Madison, WI 53706

Introduction

During follicular development, granulosa cells produce glycosaminoglycans (GAGs) as constituents which are secreted into follicular fluid (1). GAGs stimulate appearance of gonadotropin receptors on granulosa cells cultured in vitro (2). Conversely, follicular GAGs inhibit gonadotropin binding to cell surface receptors (2,3). They inhibit progesterone secretion (4,5) and may inhibit steroidogenesis indirectly by altering the binding and degradation of lipoproteins (4).

The commercially available GAGs heparin has biochemical characteristics similar to heparan sulfate and chondroitin sulfate-B, the two predominant follicular GAGs. Bovine granulosa cells are capable of binding [^{3}H]heparin in a fashion typical for receptor-ligand interactions. Binding is saturable, reversible, and dependent on factors such as pH and ionic strength of the medium (6). Other factors which influence GAG binding to granulosa cells include the maturation state of the follicle from which the cells are obtained (6-8), and the presence of GAGs already associated with the cell surface (9).

In order for follicular fluid GAGs to modulate granulosa cell function directly, they must interact with the cell surface. The purpose of these studies was to identify specific heparin-binding proteins associated with isolated plasma membranes from granulosa cells, and to determine if such proteins changed during follicular development.

Materials and Methods

Granulosa Cell Plasma Membrane Isolation

Bovine ovaries were obtained within 30 min of slaughter and follicular contents were aspirated from small (<5 mm dia), medium (5-10 mm dia), or large (10-20 mm dia) follicles. Granulosa cells were pelleted, resuspended in isolation buffer (40 mM Tris, 150 mM NaCl, 2 mM ethylene diamine tetra-acetic acid, 10 mM benzamidine, 2 μM phenyl methyl sulfonyl fluoride, 2 μM pepstatin A, 0.01% sodium azide, pH 7.35), and separated from red blood cells by centrifugation through a Percoll cushion (isolation buffer:Percoll, 2:1) at 1750 x g for 15 min. The diffuse band of material on top of the cushion was aspirated and washed by centrifugation at 1750 x g for 15 min. Washed granulosa cells were diluted to 5 ml with isolation buffer and subjected to nitrogen cavitation in a Parr Cell Disruption Bomb for 5 min at 600 psi (10). The suspension of cavitated cells was centrifuged at 1000 x g, 10 min. The supernatant fluid was decanted and the pellet washed twice with isolation buffer by centrifugation at 1000 x g, 10 min. The pooled supernatant fractions were adjusted to a final volume of 12.5 ml with isolation buffer and mixed with 6.8 ml Percoll and 0.7 ml 1.5 M NaCl. The suspension was centrifuged for 30 min at 60,000 x g_{ave}. The top band resolved by the self-generating Percoll gradient was aspirated and washed from the Percoll by centrifugation at 150,000 x g_{ave} for 1 h. The resulting pellets of purified plasma membrane were resuspended in distilled water and lyophilized.

Identification of Heparin-Binding Proteins

Samples were solubilized in electrophoresis sample buffer in the presence or absence of 5% 2-mercaptoethanol. Ten to 40 mg of membrane protein were subjected to one-dimensional sodium dodecyl sulfate polyacrylamide gel electrophoresis (11). Proteins were visualized by silver staining (12) or transferred electrophoretically to nitrocellulose paper (13). The nitrocellulose sheets were incubated 2 h with 2 µg/ml [125I]heparin (0.224 mCi/mg) (14,15) in labeling buffer (40 mM Tris, 0.05% Tween-20, pH 6.5) (15,16). The sheets were washed with labeling buffer, dried, and subjected to autoradiographic analysis. Specificity of binding was assessed by subsequent reincubation with 1 mg/ml unlabeled heparin. Proteins adsorbed to nitrocellulose were visualized by staining with Coomassie Brilliant Blue (13).

Results

Silver staining of the nonreduced samples indicated that plasma membranes purified from granulosa cells obtained from small bovine follicles contained a protein doublet of 59-60 kDa which was present in reduced amounts in gel profiles of membranes obtained from large follicles (Fig. 1). As follicles matured, there was an increase in the intensity of staining of a doublet of 50-53 kDa. Membranes from granulosa cells obtained from medium follicles exhibited gel patterns intermediate between those purified from small and large follicles. There was also a dramatic increase in the intensity of staining of the low molecular weight (13-18 kDa) proteins with follicular maturation. Autoradiography of nonreduced samples indicated 3 bands with molecular weights of 14, 15, 16 kDa labeled most intensely with [125I]heparin in membranes from medium and large follicles, corresponding to the apparent increase in the amounts of these proteins visualized by silver staining (Fig. 1). These proteins labeled with [125I]heparin despite the fact that insufficient quantities were present on nitrocellulose blots to visualize by Coomassie staining. Binding was specific for these proteins, as several higher molecular weight proteins identifiable on the silver stained gels remained unlabeled. Furthermore, radiolabeled heparin was completely displaced by incubation with a 500-fold excess of unlabeled heparin. There were no significant differences in the pattern of those low molecular weight heparin-binding proteins produced by cells at different stages of development. However, granulosa cell membranes from small follicles appeared to bind heparin much less intensely than membrane proteins from medium or large follicles. Disulfide reduction had no effect on the apparent molecular weights or heparin-binding abilities of the three major proteins (Fig. 2).

Discussion

These studies identify three low molecular weight proteins present in plasma membranes purified from granulosa cells at various stages of maturation. While the pattern of heparin-binding proteins did not change with increasing follicular size, the intensity of labeling did. It is unclear from the one-dimensional gels if this is due to increased amounts of existing proteins or new proteins of similar molecular weight. However, previous studies have indicated that granulosa cells from small follicles bind more heparin than granulosa cells from large follicles (6-8). Pretreatment of granulosa cells with heparatinase to remove heparan sulfate already associated with the membranes permitted increased binding of heparin to granulosa cells from bovine large follicles, but had no effect on the binding of heparin to granulosa cells from small follicles (9). This suggests that the lower binding observed in untreated cells from large follicles is due to occupation of the binding sites with heparan sulfate. Since any GAGs associated with binding proteins would be dissociated during electrophoretic separation, the more intense labeling of membrane proteins from granulosa cells from large follicles observed in the present study suggests that there are, in fact, more binding sites per unit total membrane protein in granulosa cells from large follicles

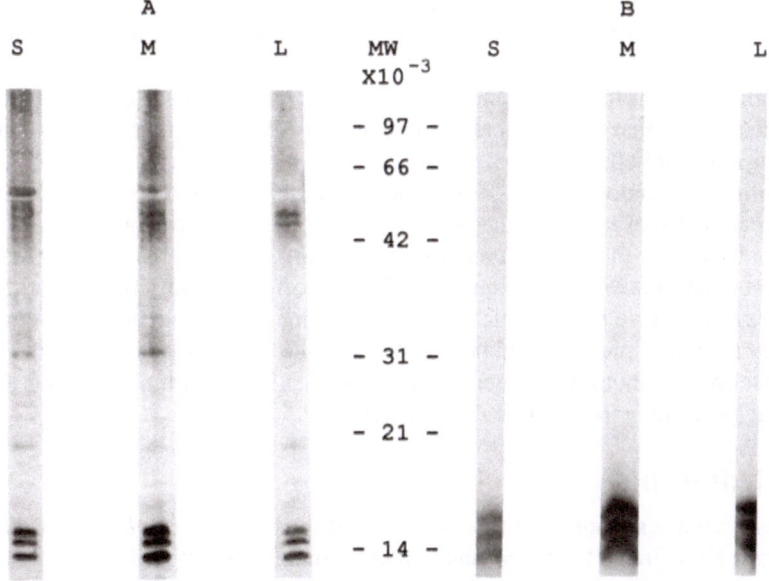

Fig. 1. Proteins present in plasma membranes purified from granulosa cells obtained from small (S), medium (M), or large (L) bovine follicles, separated under nonreducing conditions. *Panel A:* Silver stained sodium dodecyl sulfate polyacrylamide gel. *Panel B:* Autoradiogram of nitrocellulose blot probed with [125I]heparin.

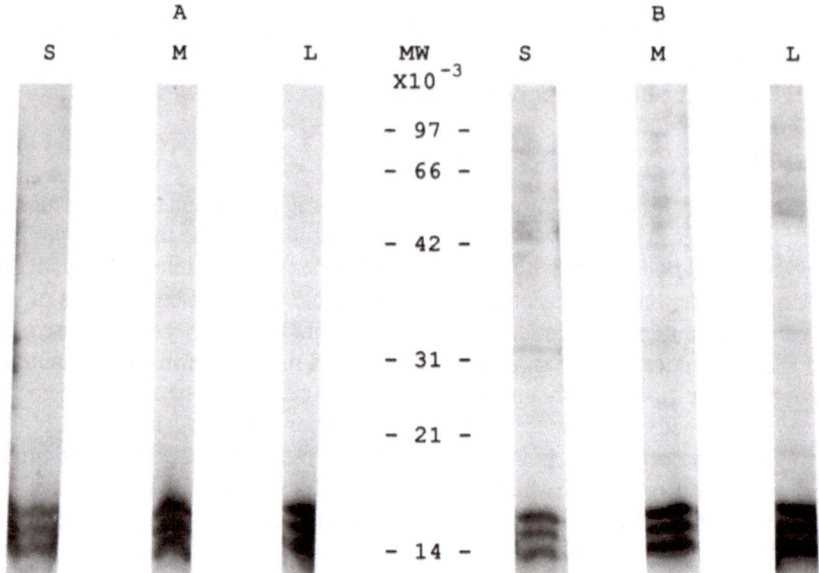

Fig. 2. Autoradiogram of [^{125}I]heparin-labeled proteins present in plasma membranes purified from granulosa cells obtained from small (S), medium (M), or large (L) bovine follicles, separated under nonreducing *(Panel A)* and reducing *(Panel B)* conditions.

than from small. In Chinese hamster ovary cells, mitotic activity is inversely related to the amount of surface-associated heparan sulfate (17), and in bovine granulosa cells the highest rate of mitotic activity is found in granulosa cells from small follicles (18). The current study supports the concept that nonproliferating granulosa cells from larger follicles have more total binding sites for heparin.

The ability of granulosa cell plasma membrane proteins to bind heparin after treatment with 2-mercaptoethanol indicates that binding is not dependent on the presence of intact disulfide bonds, nor are the binding proteins disulfide-linked fragments of a larger molecule. The apparent molecular weights are similar to those reported for a variety of heparin-binding polypeptides which have been implicated in stimulating cell growth and differentiation in other tissues (19). It is presently unknown what role the interactions between the heparin-binding proteins in granulosa cell membranes identified in the current study and follicular fluid proteoglycans play in follicular development.

Acknowledgments

This research was supported by the University of Wisconsin College of Agricultural and Life Sciences, NIH Grant HD-13964 and USDA Grant 85-CRCR-1-1864.

References

1. Ax RL, Bellin ME, Grimek HJ. Properties and synthesis of glycosaminoglycans by the ovary. In: Toft DO, Ryan RJ, eds. Proceedings of the 5th Ovarian Workshop, Champaign, IL, 1985:451-80.

2. Nimrod A, Lindner HR. Heparin facilitates the induction of LH receptors by FSH in granulosa cells cultured in serum-enriched medium. FEBS Lett 1980; 119:155-7.

3. Amsterdam A, Riesel R, Mintz Y, Shemesh M, Salomon Y. Inhibition of gonadotropin sensitive adenylate cyclase by ovarian follicular fluid. Biochem Biophys Res Commun 1979; 87:505-12.

4. Bellin ME, Veldhuis JD, Ax RL. Follicular fluid glycosaminoglycans inhibit degradation of low density lipoproteins and progesterone production by porcine granulosa cells. Biol Reprod 1987; 37:1179-84.

5. Ledwitz-Rigby F, Gross TM, Schjeide OA, Rigby BW. The glycosaminoglycan chondroitin-4-sulfate alters progesterone secretion by porcine granulosa cells. Biol Reprod 1987; 36:320-7.

6. Bushmeyer SM, Bellin ME, Ax RL. Specific binding of [^{3}H]heparin to bovine granulosa cell membranes. Mol Cell Endocrinol 1985; 42:135-44.

7. Ax RL, Bushmeyer SM, Boehm SK, Bellin ME. Binding of the glycosaminoglycan [^{3}H]heparin to bovine granulosa cells varies with size and estrogen content of ovarian follicles. Endocr Res 1984; 10:63-72.

8. Bellin ME, Wentworth BC, Ax RL. Comparisons of the ability of follicular fluid glycosaminoglycans and chemically desulfated heparin to compete for heparin binding sites on granulosa cells. Biol Reprod 1987; 37:293-300.

9. Ax RL, Stodd CM, Boehm SK, Bellin ME. Removal of glycosaminoglycans from bovine granulosa cells contributes to increased binding of hydrogen-3 heparin. J Dairy Sci 1986; 69:531-4.

10. Hunter MJ, Commerford SL. Pressure homogenization of mammalian tissues. Biochim Biophys Acta 1961; 47:580-6.

11. Laemmli UK. Cleavage of structural proteins during the assembly of the head of bacteriophage T4. Nature 1970; 277:680-5.

12. Wray W, Boulikas T, Wray VP, Hancock R. Silver staining of proteins in polyacrylamide gels. Anal Biochem 1981; 118:197-203.

13. Burnette WN. "Western blotting:" electrophoretic transfer of proteins from sodium dodecyl sulfate-polyacrylamide gels to unmodified nitrocellulose and radiographic detection with antibody and radioiodinated protein A. Anal Biochem 1981; 112:195-203.

14. Bolton AE, Hunter WM. The labelling of proteins to high specific radioactivities by conjugation to a ^{125}I-containing acylating agent. Biochem J 1973; 133:529-39.

15. Cardin AD, Witt KR, Jackson RL. Visualization of heparin-binding proteins by ligand blotting with ^{125}I-heparin. Anal Biochem 1984; 137:368-73.

16. Smith JW, Knauer DJ. Ligand blotting with ^{125}I-fluoresceinamine-heparin. Anal Biochem 1987; 160:105-14.

17. Kraemer PM, Tobey RA. Cell-cycle dependent desquamation of heparan sulfate from the cell surface. J Cell Biol 1972; 55:713-7.

18. Priedkalns J, Weber AF, Zemjanis R. Qualitative and quantitative morphological studies of the cells of the membrana granulosa, theca interna and corpus luteum of the bovine ovary. Z Mikrosk Anat Forsch 1968; 85:501-20.

19. Lobb RR, Harper JW, Fett JW. Purification of heparin-binding growth factors. Anal Biochem 1986; 154:1-14.

38

Variations in the Interaction Between Follicular Glycosaminoglycans and Fibronectin Relative to the LH Surge in Cattle

R. J. Vanderboom,[1] T. H. Wise,[2] R. R. Maurer,[2]
and R. L. Ax[1]

University of Wisconsin,[1] Madison, WI 53706, and USDA
Agricultural Research Services,* Roman L. Hruska U.S.
Meat Animal Research Center,[2] Clay Center, NE 68933

Introduction

Follicle stimulating hormone exerts divergent effects on production of fibronectin (Fn) and proteoglycans by granulosa cells (GC) (1,2). Fn is a glycoprotein constituent of the extracellular matrix and its production decreases when GC are exposed to FSH (3). In contrast, addition of FSH to GC enhances production of high molecular weight proteoglycans. Proteoglycans consist of a core protein with covalently attached glycosaminoglycan (GAG) side-chains (4). GAGs can inhibit gonadotropin binding and steroidogenesis, but the exact loci where those inhibitions occur are not known.

Follicular GAGs interact with Fn (5), and those interactions are characterized by the type of GAG and the size of the follicle from which the GAG is isolated. Research conducted in our laboratory indicated that dermatan sulfate (DS) from pooled samples of follicular fluid exhibited the greatest affinity for Fn, with 55% of a 100 µg sample bound to Fn. DS from large follicles or heparan sulfate from large or small follicles exhibited between 14% and 21% binding to Fn. Although follicular fluid pooled from sized follicles obtained at a slaughterhouse served to define significantly different interactions between small or large follicle GAG types and Fn, the pooling of antral fluid preempts definition of physiological effects such as atresia or hormonal influences at different times of the estrous cycle.

The objective of this study was to ascertain whether any variation existed in the ability of GAGs isolated from individual follicles collected at various times relative to the LH surge to interact with the extracellular matrix component Fn.

---

*Mention of a trade name, priority product or specific equipment does not constitute a guarantee or warrantee by the USDA and does not imply its approval to the exclusion of other products that may also be suitable.

Materials and Methods

Follicle Collection

Follicles from crossbred heifers (n=23) at the USMARC, Clay Center, NE, were individually collected. Those heifers represented a subset from 103 animals that were synchronized with prostaglandin $F_{2\alpha}$ (PGF$_{2\alpha}$; Lutalyse, Upjohn Co.) and superovulated with FSH (FSH-P; Burns Biotech) by methods of Wise et al. (6). Heifers were ovariec-tomized every 12 h (12-108 h post-PGF$_{2\alpha}$) and the follicles were aspirated individually. The diameter of each follicle >4 mm was measured, and the follicular fluid was aspirated. Luteinizing hormone (LH) concentrations in peripheral serum, as well as estradiol, progesterone and prolactin concentrations in the follicular fluid, were quantified by radioim-munoassay.

Follicular GAG Isolation

Composite follicular fluid GAGs were isolated and purified by the method of Bellin and Ax (7) with minor modifications from 32 follicles collected from 23 heifers. Aliquots of 750 μl from each follicle were individually incubated with 1 mg/ml protease (Type XIV; from *Streptomyces griseus*, Sigma, St. Louis, MO) at 37°C for 18 h under toluene. Trichloroacetic acid was added to each sample (final concentration of 5% TCA) and allowed to equilibrate for 20 min at room temperature. The supernatant was then decanted into 3 ml of ethanol containing 5% potassium acetate at -20°C. Samples were refrigerated at -20°C for 24 h to allow GAG precipitation. Samples were then centrifuged at 200 x g for 15 min at 4°C. Alcohol was decanted and GAG pellets were suspended in 0.5 ml distilled water/ml follicular fluid equivalent, frozen and lyophilized. The resultant powder was then dissolved in 750 μl 0.5 mM Tris buffer and was added to 3 ml chloroform/methanol (3:1, v:v) or lipid extraction. Samples were inverted repeatedly for thorough mixing, then centrifuged at 100 x g for 15 min at 4°C. The clear aqueous layer was aspirated into a fresh tube, frozen and then lyophilized. Sample powders were stored in a desiccator until total GAGs were individually quantified.

Each sample of GAG powder was dissolved in 220 μl GAG buffer (5 mM KH$_2$PO$_4$, 5 mM K$_2$HPO$_4$, 100 mM Na$_2$SO$_4$, pH 6.67), and 200 μl aliquots were applied to a gel filtration high performance liquid chromatography column (Protein Pak I-125, Waters Associates, Bedford, MA). Absorbance was monitored at 205 nm on a Perkin-Elmer LC-75 spectrophotometer. Results were expressed as areas integrated under elution peaks. Total GAG per 200 μl injection was determined by comparison to integrated areas of elution peaks obtained from a standard of commercial chondroitin sulfate isomers (CS, Sigma Chemical, St. Louis, MO). GAG samples were individually collected, frozen, lyophilized, and stored in a desiccator until application to the Fn-affinity chromatography column.

Fibronectin Affinity Chromatography

Fn was conjugated to CnBr-Sepharose (0.25 g dry weight) using the method recom-mended by Pharmacia (52-1153-00-08, Uppsala, Sweden). Of the 4 mg of Fn added, 30% was covalently linked to the Sepharose. GAG powder samples were dissolved in 50 mM Tris buffer (50 mM Tris, 1 mM MgCL$_2$, 1 mM CaCl$_2$, 0.01% NaN$_3$, pH 7.35). An aliquot of each sample containing 100 μg GAG was applied to the Fn affinity column and allowed to equilibrate for 1 h. GAG which did not bind to Fn was eluted with 10 ml Tris buffer. GAG which did bind to Fn was purged from the column with a stepwise gradient of 1 M NaCl in 5 ml of Tris buffer. Both the bound and unbound fractions were separately frozen and lyophilized, then dissolved in GAG buffer. The samples were applied to a gel filtration HPLC column (Protein Pak I-125, Waters Associates, Bedford, MA) in 200 μl injections and quantified as previously noted. Results were expressed as percent of GAG applied which bound to Fn.

Results

Figure 1A depicts the variation in the ability of GAGs isolated from follicles aspirated at different intervals from the LH surge to interact with Fn. Analysis of variance of these data suggests a trend (P=0.09) in the manner that GAGs present in follicular fluid at different times from the LH surge interact with Fn. Multiple comparison using Fisher's protected least significant difference test indicated significant differences among the means of those GAGs which bound to Fn from various time intervals from the LH surge. Follicles harvested from heifers at 30 h prior to the LH surge contained GAGs which bound significantly less to Fn (P<0.05) than follicles harvested 6, 12, or 54 h post-LH surge. GAGs from follicles harvested 18 h post-LH surge bound significantly less to Fn (P<0.05) than did GAGs from follicles aspirated at 6 h pre- and 6, 12, 30 and 54 h post-LH surge.

Figure 1B depicts the average concentration of GAGs in follicles collected at each time interval from the LH surge. The concentration of GAGs present in follicles at different times from the LH surge was not related to the amount of GAGs isolated from those follicles that bound to Fn (r = -.13, P>0.47).

The hormone profiles for estradiol, progesterone and prolactin were consistent with changes in hormone profiles from normally developing follicles prior to and after the LH surge (Fig. 2). There were no significant correlations (P>0.05) between temporal hormone concentrations and the Fn-binding ability of follicular GAGs isolated at various times relative to the LH surge.

Conclusions

The collection of individual follicles timed from the $PGF_{2\alpha}$ luteolysis afforded an excellent opportunity to inspect the ability of GAGs isolated from follicles at identified stages within the estrous cycle to interact with Fn. The data from this experiment expands upon information from a previous report that the manner in which follicular GAGs interacted with Fn was related to the size of follicles from which the GAGs were isolated (5). In this case, however, the utilization of individual follicles revealed that GAG binding ability was dependent upon follicular maturity. By eliminating the effect of pooling follicular fluid samples, GAG:Fn affinities due to follicular maturity or GC differentiation were more precisely estimated.

Previous studies have shown variation in the chemical composition of GAGs from follicles of differing size (8,9). DS is characteristically composed of repeating units of disaccharides containing N-acetyl galactosamine as the primary hexosamine sugar. DS from large follicles is known to have a galactosamine:glucosamine ratio 4 times greater than DS from small follicles (2). Whether that physicochemical variation contributes to the enhanced

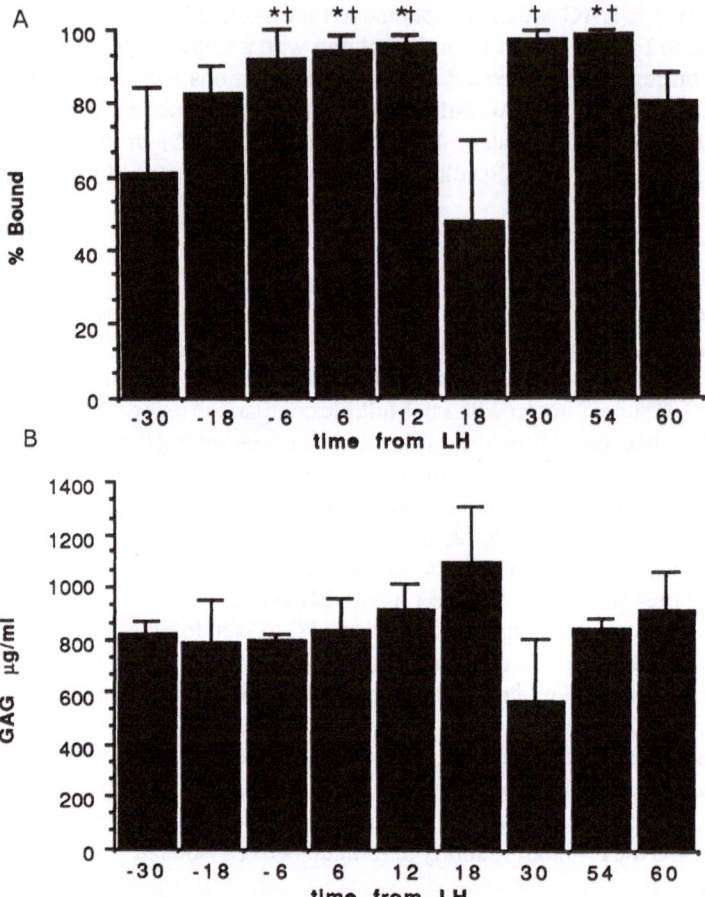

Fig. 1. (A) The percentage of glycosaminoglycans (GAGs) which bound
to fibronectin (Fn) varied depending on when the follicles from which the
GAGs were isolated were collected in relation to the LH surge. ANOVA
indicated a trend (P=0.09) in the manner that GAGs bound to Fn. Asterisks
(*) indicate samples in which the GAGs exhibited significantly different
binding ability to Fn than from the proportion of GAGs which bound to
Fn at 30 h prior to the LH surge. Crosses (†) indicate samples in which
the GAGs exhibited significantly different binding ability to Fn than from
the proportion of GAGs which bound to Fn at 18 h post-LH surge. (B)
Concentrations of GAGs isolated from follicles collected at various times
relative to the LH surge were not related to the ability of those GAGs to
bind to Fn (r = -.13, P>0.47).

ability of DS from large follicles to displace [^{3}H]-heparin from granulosa cell membranes
is not known. Other studies have noted higher concentration of GAGs in atretic follicles, but
no significant correlation was observed in this study between the concentration of the
follicles and the ability of the GAGs from those follicles to bind to Fn.

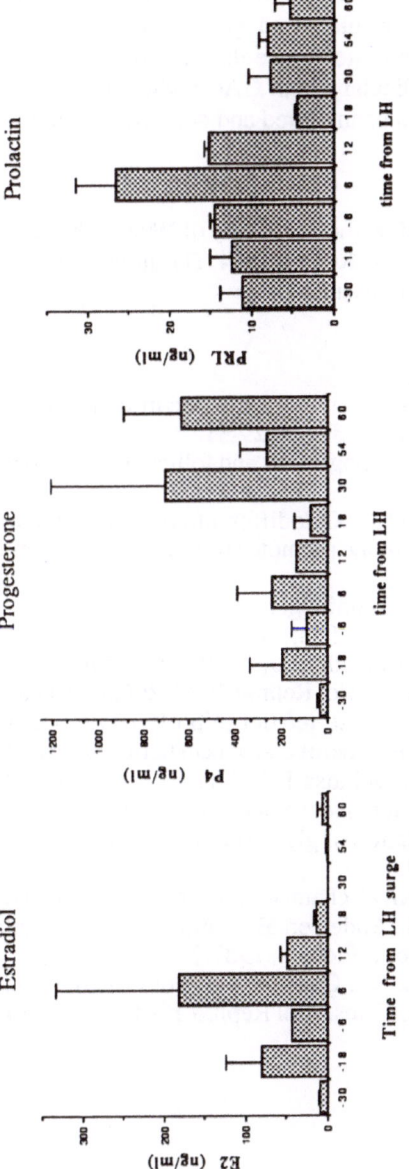

Fig. 2. Concentrations of estradiol, progesterone and prolactin from individual follicles at various times from the LH surge. The variation in the temporal hormone profile from follicles was consistent with expected changes relative to the LH surge, but did not correlate with the ability of follicular GAGs to bind to Fn (P>0.05).

The results of this experiment suggest the need for further chemical characterization of the GAGs from the follicles at respective times throughout follicular development. It is of particular interest to note the enhanced Fn-binding ability of GAGs from follicles 18 h post-LH surge. Perhaps this phenomenon is due to redirected synthesis action on proteoglycan/GAG production by luteinized granulosa cells. Or, perhaps it reflects the breakdown of follicular basement membrane during a time of vascular development that allows an infiltration of nonfollicular origin GAGs which have reduced ability to interact with Fn. These questions remain unanswered and deserve further attention.

Acknowledgments

This research was supported by the University of Wisconsin College of Agriculture and Life Sciences and USDA Grant 85-CRCR-1-1864. The authors are grateful to Ramona Dana and Claire Huebert for technical assistance.

References

1. Skinner MK, Dorrington JH. Control of fibronectin synthesis by rat granulosa cells in culture. Endocrinology 1984; 115(5):2029-31.
2. Ax RL, Bellin ME. Glycosaminoglycans and follicular development. J Anim Sci 1988; 66:(suppl 2):32-49.
3. Dorrington JH, Skinner MK. Cytodifferentiation of granulosa cells induced by gonadotropin-releasing hormone promotes fibronectin secretion. Endocrinology 1986; 118(5):2065-71.
4. Lindahl U, Hook M. Glycosaminoglycans and their binding to biological macro-molecules. Annu Rev Biochem 1978; 47:385-417.
5. Vanderboom RJ, Bellin ME, Miller DJ, Ax RL. Follicular fluid glycosaminoglycans bind to fibronectin [Abstract]. Biol Reprod 1987; 36(suppl 1):88.
6. Wise T, Suss U, Mauer RR. The relationship of oocyte quality and follicular fluid prolactin and progesterone in superovulated beef heifers with and without Norgestomet implants. In: Mahesh VB, Dhindsa DS, Anderson E, Kalra SP, eds. Regulation of ovarian and testicular function. New York: Plenum, 1987:697-701.
7. Bellin ME, Ax RL. Purification of glycosaminoglycans from bovine follicular fluid. J Dairy Sci 1987; 70:1913-9.
8. Bellin ME, Ax RL. Chemical characteristics of follicular glycosaminoglycans. In: Mahesh VB, Dhindsa DS, Anderson E, Kalra SP, eds. Regulation of ovarian and testicular function. New York: Plenum, 1987:731-5.
9. Grimek HJ, Bellin ME, Ax RL. Characteristics of proteoglycans isolated from small and large bovine ovarian follicles. Biol Reprod 1984; 30:397-409.

39

Differences in the Ovulatory Ability Between the Right and Left Ovary Are Related to Ovarian Innervation

Roberto Dominguez, Maria Esther Cruz, and Rebeca Chavez

Laboratorio de Biologia de la Reproduccion, E.N.E.P.Zaragoza U.N.A.M. a.p.9-020, c.p. 15000, Mexico D.F., Mexico

Peripheral innervation plays a role in the regulation of the function of the ovary. Both ovulation and endocrine functions can be modified by the alteration of ovarian innervation. Blockade or stimulation of ovarian nerves produce changes in ovarian function depending on the neural pathway and the experimental model used (1-3). Follicular development is modulated by catecholaminergic innervation, and the effects of its stimulation or blockade depends on the stage of follicular differentiation (4,5). Bilateral section of the vagus nerve induced an increase in the number of ova shed by the ovulating animal (2), while the same experiment performed in prepubertal animals induced a delay in puberty and in estrogen synthesis without changes in serum gonadotropin levels (6).

There are several indications that the neuroendocrine mechanisms related to gonadal regulation display lateralization, both in normal and hemispayed rats, and at central and peripheral levels (7-9,19,11). In the present study, we present evidence indicating that differences in the ovulatory ability of the right and left ovary partially depends on ovarian catecholaminergic and vagal innervation.

Material and Methods

Adult virgin rats of the C II Z-V strain from our stock were maintained in conditions of controlled lighting (lights on from 05.00 to 19.00 h), with free access to food and tap water. Estrous cycles were monitored by daily vaginal smears, and only those animals with 4-day cycles were used. All animals were autopsied on the morning of the expected day of estrus after 3 consecutive 4-day estrous cycles.

Ether anesthetized animals were laparotomized on each day of the estrous cycle and divided in the following groups: with unilateral or bilateral vagotomy, performed as previously described (2); with unilateral or bilateral superior ovarian nerve section following the method of Weiss et al. (12) or sutured and used as sham operated group.

In another group of rats, an ovulatory test was performed by the administration of 45 IU of ovine follicle stimulating hormone (FSH) (Prolan A, Bayer, Mexico) on diestrus, followed 56 h later by 30 IU of luteinizing hormone-human chorionic gonadotropin (LH-hCG) (Prolan E, Bayer, Mexico), and autopsy 20 h later. In some animals, an acute catecholaminergic blockade was performed by the administration of reserpine (125 µg/kg or 1 mg/kg) 3 h before FSH or LH-hCC administration. Groups of rats with bilateral section of the vagus nerves received reserpine (1 mg/kg) before they were injected with FSH or LH-hCG. In another group of rats, a peripheral noradrenergic denervation was performed injecting guanethidine, 20 mg/kg every second day, for 30 days followed by autopsy on the first day of estrus after ending the treatment.

The animals were decapitated, oviducts dissected and ova counted. The ovaries were dissected and weighed with a precision balance. Data were analyzed by multivariate analysis of variance (MANOVA) followed by Duncan's test or Student's t test or chi square test. A probability value less than 0.05 was considered significant.

Results

Unilateral section of the vagus nerve or superior ovarian nerve modified the estrous cycle; the effects of vagal section were more serious than those induced by superior ovarian nerve section (27/79 were cyclic vs. 46/76, $P<0.05$). Ovulation rate (number of ovulating/number of treated rats) diminished in those animals with either section of the left vagus nerve or right superior ovarian nerve section (Table 1). No differences in the weight of the ovaries were observed in the animals with vagal or superior ovarian nerve unilateral section.

The number of ova shed by the right and left ovaries of the animals with different nerve sections is presented in Table 2. In the control group, the left ovary released more ova than the right one. In the sham operated animals, the total number of ova shed was similar to the control group (9.0 ± 0.3 vs. 10.2 ± 0.3, NS); however, the left ovary released significantly less ova than in the untouched control group. Unilateral section of the vagus nerve also decreased the number of ova shed by the left ovary, while bilateral section reversed the effects of stress on the left ovary's ovulation ability. Left superior ovarian nerve section induced a significant diminution in the number of ova shed (6.3 ± 0.6 vs. 9.0 ± 0.3, $P<0.05$), while right

Table 1. Effects of unilateral section of the vagus nerve (VN) or superior ovarian nerve (SON), performed on each day of the estrous cycle, on estrous cyclicity (number of cyclic/number of treated rats) and ovulation rate (number of ovulating/number of treated rats)

	Estrous Cyclicity		Ovulation Rate	
Sham operation	43/54		50/54	
	SON	VN	SON	VN
Right nerve section	22/36*	13/32*	28/36*	25/32
Left nerve section	24/40*	14/47*†	36/40	32/47*†

*P<0.05 vs. sham operation group (chi square test).
†P<0.05 vs. superior ovarian nerve section (chi square test).

Table 2. Means ± SEM of the number of ova shed by the right or left ovaries of control animals, sham operated, with left, right or bilateral vagus nerve section (LVN, RVN, BVN) or left, right or bilateral superior ovarian nerve section (LSON, RSON, BSON) autopsied on the day of vaginal estrus after 3 consecutive 4-day cycles

	Right ovary	Left ovary
CONTROL	4.4 ± 0.2	5.8 ± 0.5*
SHAM	4.9 ± 0.3	4.1 ± 0.3†
LVN	4.9 ± 0.5	4.6 ± 0.4†
RVN	4.5 ± 0.5	4.6 ± 0.6
BVN	5.2 ± 0.3	6.4 ± 0.3‡
LSON	3.6 ± 0.4‡	2.7 ± 0.4†‡
RSON	2.6 ± 0.5†‡	4.8 ± 0.5
BSON	3.0 ± 0.4‡	4.0 ± 0.5†

*$P<0.05$ vs. right ovary (Student's t test).
†$P<0.05$ vs. control (Duncan's test after MANOVA).
‡$P<0.05$ vs. sham (Duncan's test after MANOVA).

superior ovarian nerve section did not induce changes compared with the sham operated group ($7.5 ± 0.7$ vs. $9.0 ± 0.3$, NS). While right superior ovarian nerve section affected only the ipsilateral ovary, left superior ovarian nerve section affected ovulation in both ovaries.

In those animals injected with reserpine (125 mg/kg) before they were subjected to an ovulatory test, the number of ova shed by the left ovary was higher than by the right one ($6.4 ± 0.7$ vs. $4.0 ± 0.8$, $P<0.01$). No difference was observed when a higher dose of reserpine was injected before FSH (right ovary released $10.8 ± 1.5$ ova and left ovary $10.7 ± 1.6$) or LH-hCG ($6.3 ± 1.0$ and $6.8 ± 0.8$). Bilateral section of the vagus nerves before reserpine administration (1 mg/kg) modified that picture: when reserpine was injected before FSH, the blockade of ovulation was similar in the right and left ovary ($2.3 ± 1.0$ ova and $2.8 ± 1.0$); when reserpine was injected before LH-hCG, ovulation by the right ovary was higher than by the left one ($6.0 ± 1.4$ vs. $3.7 ± 0.7$). Chronic peripheral pharmacological noradrenergic denervation induced by guanethidine, diminished spontaneous ovulation ($6.3 ± 0.5$ vs. $10.2 ± 0.4$, $P<0.05$). However, when compared with untouched control animals, the left ovary presented a significant drop in the number of ova shed ($2.9 ± 0.7$ vs. $5.8 ± 0.5$ $P<0.05$), while the right ovary did not ($3.4 ± 0.7$ vs. $4.1 ± 0.3$).

Discussion

Present results add further support to the hypothesis that there exists peripheral lateralization in the neuroendocrine mechanisms modulating ovarian function (2,3). Both cyclicity and ovulation rate depend on the integrity of vagal and superior ovarian nerve innervation. The information carried by the vagus nerves seems to be more necessary to maintain normal cyclicity than that carried by the superior ovarian nerve. According to various studies, bilateral section of the vagus nerves altered the estrous cycle length while bilateral superior ovarian nerve section did not (1,2,14). The present results show that to maintain estrous cyclicity, the presence of both vagus nerves is necessary since the integrity of one of them is not enough to compensate for the loss of information provoked by section of one of them. Differences in the estrogen secretion may explain the differences between the effects of section of the superior ovarian nerve and vagus nerve; the superior ovarian nerve is related to the regulation of progesterone secretion (12), while section of the vagus nerve alters estrogen production (6).

The ovulation rate seems to depend on the integrity of the left vagus nerve and right superior ovarian nerve. On the other hand, the number of ova shed by an ovulating animal was not affected by unilateral section of the vagus nerve; however, the superior ovarian nerve section affected this parameter. In the present study, the number of ova shed by the right ovary was altered by bilateral or unilateral (ipsi- and contralateral) section of the superior ovarian nerve, while the left ovary was affected only by the ipsilateral ovarian nerve section. These differences point to the existence of lateralization in the neuroendocrine mechanisms regulating ovulation. Ovulation ability reflects follicular growth and differentiation, and unpublished results from our laboratory show that the distribution of the follicular population in the right ovary is different from the left one.

Results presented herein indicate that catecholaminergic denervation (pharmacological and surgical) affects ovulatory ability of the ovaries in a different way. In those animals with pharmacological blockade of the catecholaminergic and serotoninergic systems by reserpine, induced ovulation of the left ovary was affected. The same picture was observed when spontaneous ovulation occurred in guanethidine-treated animals. In every case, the number of ova shed by ovulating animals was lower in the the left than in the right ovary.

We have previously proposed that ovarian innervation plays a double role in the regulation of ovarian function. Afferent ovarian innervation modulates the reactivity of the ovarian compartments (follicular, luteal and interstitial) to gonadotropins, and efferent ovarian innervation carries information to the hypothalamus on the performance of those compartments (13). Taken together, the present results suggest that the vagus nerve is one of the ovarian efferent pathways since its section affected estrous cyclicity, and the effects on the number of ova shed by ovulating animal did not present lateralization. On the other hand, the superior ovarian nerve, and other fibers through which information is transduced by catecholamines (noradrenaline?) would be one of the afferent pathways since their alteration by surgical or pharmacological procedures affected the number of ova shed, principally ipsilateral to the lesion or the left one. In the hemispayed animal, the left ovary has less ability to ovulate than the right one (3).

According to Wylie et al. (14) and Selstan et al. (15), ovarian sympathetic innervation does not affect ovulation; however, our results suggest a stimulatory role. These differences could be related to the fact that in other studies an extra-stimulatory stimuli was used (coitus [14] and gonadotropins [15]), while our results were obtained in spontaneously ovulating animals. This possibility is supported by the fact that bilateral section of the vagus nerve increased the number of ova shed in spontaneously ovulating animals and it was diminished when ovulation was induced with gonadotropins (2).

Acknowledgments

Supported by CONACYT, grant PCSACNA 50972 and PUIC. Reserpine and guanethidine were a generous gift by Ciba-Geigy, Mexico.

References

1. Burden WH. Ovarian innervation. In: Jones RE, ed. The vertebrate ovary: comparative biology. New York: Plenum Press, 1978:615-38.

2. Cruz ME, Chavez R, Dominguez R. Ovulation, follicular growth and ovarian reactivity to exogenous gonadotropins in adult rats with unilateral or bilateral section of the vagi nerves. Rev Invest Clin 1986; 38:167-71.

3. Chavez R, Cruz ME, Dominguez R. Differences in the ovulation rate of the right or left ovary in unilaterally ovariectomized rats: effect of ipsi- and contralateral vagus nerve on the remaining ovary. J Endocrinol 1987; 113:397-401.

4. Ben-Jonathan N, Braw RH, Reich LR, Bahr JM, Tsafriri A. Norepinephrine in graafian follicles is depleted by follicle stimulating hormone. Endocrinology 1982; 110:457-61.

5. Ayala ME, Flores A, Morales L, Dominguez R. Diferencias en la respuesta ovulatoria a la administracion de FSH-LH a lo largo del ciclo estral de la rata adulta. Bol Estud Med Biol Mex 1987; 35:Abstract 56.

6. Ojeda SR, White SS, Aguado IL, Advis JP, Andersen JM. Abdominal vagotomy delays the onset of puberty and inhibits ovarian function in the female rat. Neuroendocrinology 1987; 36:261-7.

7. Gerandai I, Rotsytein W, Marchetti B, Scapagnini V. LH-RH content changes in the mediobasal hypothalamus after unilateral ovariectomy. In: Pollery A, MacLeod R, eds. Neuroendocrinology: biological and clinical aspects. New York: Academic Press, Proceeding of Serono Symposia 1979; 19:97-102.

8. Nance DM, Moger WH. Ipsilateral hypothalamic deafferentation blocks the increase in serum FSH following hemicastration. Brain Res Bull 1982; 8:299-302.

9. Nance DM, White JP, Moger WH. Neural regulation of the ovary: evidence for hypothalamic assymetry in endocrine control. Brain Res Bull 1983; 10:353-5.

10. Bakalkin GY, Tsibezov VV, Sjutkin EA, Veselova SP, Novilov ID, Drivosheev OG. Lateralization of LH-RH in the rat hypothalamus. Brain Res 1984; 296:361-4.

11. Fukuda M, Yamanouchi K, Nakano Y, Fukuya H, Arai Y. Hypothalamic laterality in regulating gonadotropic function: unilateral hypothalamic lesion and ovarian compensatory hypertrophy. Neurosci Lett 1984; 51:365-70.

12. Weiss GK, Dail GW, Ratner A. Evidence for direct neural control of ovarian steroidogenesis in rats. J Reprod Fertil 1982; 65:507-11.

13. Dominguez R, Riboni L. Failure of ovulation in autografted ovary of hemispayed rat. Neuroendocrinology 1971; 7:164-70.

14. Wylie SN, Roche PJ, Gibson WR. Ovulation after sympathetic denervation of the rat ovary produced by freezing its nerve supply. J Reprod Fertil 1985; 213:369-72.

15. Selstan G, Norjavaara E, Tegenfelt T, Lundberg S, Sandstrom C, Persson S. Partial denervation of the ovaries by transection of the suspensory ligament does not inhibit ovulation in rats treated with pregnant mare serum gonadotropin. Anat Rec 1985; 213:392-5.

40

Differential Responses in the Component Cells of Graafian Follicles Perifused with Large and Small Doses of LH

D. Olson, C. J. Hubbard, and B. A. Oxberry

Department of Biological Sciences, Northern Illinois University,
DeKalb, IL 60115, and Department of Anatomy, Temple University
School of Medicine, Philadelphia, PA 19140

Oocytes in developing graafian follicles remain arrested at the prophase stage of meiosis I until the follicles are exposed to the preovulatory LH surge. The LH surge triggers the resumption of meiosis and the oocytes progress to the metaphase stage of meiosis II through the process of oocyte maturation.

Numerous studies have suggested that cAMP plays an important role in the regulation of oocyte maturation. However, the manner in which the LH surge induces maturation in follicle-enclosed oocytes has not been determined. In graafian follicles exposed to LH in vitro, concentrations of cAMP have been shown to increase in a dose-response manner (1,2). However, cAMP levels generated in the different tissue components of these follicles in response to high and low doses of LH have not been completely determined. Both the theca and the mural granulosa cells of hamster graafian follicles possess abundant receptors for LH (3). However, the distribution of LH receptors that are actually occupied when intact follicles are exposed to high and low doses of LH is not clear.

Concentration-dependent differential binding of LH to the component cells of graafian follicles may generate corresponding changes in cAMP levels in these cell types, which could trigger oocyte maturation. The objectives of this study were to: (a) determine the relative number of receptors in each of the tissue components of graafian follicles that bind LH when these follicles are exposed to a high and low dose of LH; (b) determine the subsequent cAMP changes that occur in each of the tissue components of these follicles; (c) correlate these findings with the initiation of oocyte maturation.

Materials and Methods

Mature female hamsters (30 days old) were injected with 30 IU of pregnant mare serum gonadotropin on day 1 (estrus) and killed during the morning of day 4 (proestrus). Intact graafian follicles (about 30 per animal) were dissected and incubated with various additives in defined medium (2).

Isolated follicles were incubated in a perifusion system consisting of two microprocessor controlled (Endotronics) pumps which feed a mixing chamber. A multichannel roller pump conveys incubation medium to tissue chambers in a 37°C water bath which drain into a waste container or fraction collector. The system is capable of generating mathematically predictable hormone profiles which have been confirmed empirically using both dyes and ^{125}I-labeled LH

Isolated follicles were perifused with a high (100 ng/ml) or low (10 ng/ml) dose of ^{125}I-labeled or unlabeled LH. In all cases, follicles were perifused with plain medium for 30 min prior to the delivery of hormone. Controls were perifused with medium alone. At selected time-points during a perifusion, follicles were removed from the tissue chambers and placed in saline-IBMX (4°C) and subjected to one of the following treatments: (a) whole follicles exposed to ^{125}I-labeled LH were fixed and processed for autoradiography; (b) whole follicles were ground and assayed for cAMP; (c) whole follicles were separated into their component cell groups: cumulus-oocyte complex (COC), granulosa cells, and theca cells; these were assayed for cAMP (2). Dissected thecal shells contained some unavoidable interstitial contamination. In some experiments, follicles were perifused with medium alone or LH for a total of 4 h or 6 h. Initiation of maturation in follicle-enclosed oocytes was then determined in fixed and stained denuded oocytes as described previously (4).

Experimental values (mean ± SEM) were considered to be significantly different from each other at a level of $P<0.05$.

Results

Cell types that bound LH in the presence of high and low doses of LH are shown in Figure 1. Grain counts/unit area at 30 min represent those present in the absence of exposure to ^{125}I LH (controls). When follicles were perifused with the high dose of ^{125}I LH, grain counts in the theca layer increased more than eightfold by 60 min to a level 18 times background by 105 min. Grain counts also rose in the mural granulosa and cumulus cells but were delayed until 60 min in the granulosa and 75 min in the cumulus cells. In addition, the rate of increase was markedly lower for the granulosa and cumulus cells (Fig. 1A). When follicles were perifused with the low dose of LH, grain counts in the theca did not rise significantly above background until 90 min when they reached a peak of 8 times background. Granulosal counts rose twofold by 90 min and no significant change was seen in the cumulus cells (Fig. 1B).

When follicles were exposed to the high dose of LH (Fig. 2A), intracellular cAMP rose significantly at 75 min, reached a peak at 90 min and then declined. When follicles were exposed to the low dose of LH (Fig. 2B), cAMP levels did not rise significantly until 90 min.

In a third series of experiments, follicles were subjected to the same high and low concentration patterns of LH as before and then were separated into their component cell groups. An LH plateau of 100 ng/ml increased cAMP significantly in the theca between 60 and 75 min (Fig. 3A). In the granulosal compartment, cyclic AMP rose significantly by 45 min and remained elevated for the remainder of the perifusion (Fig. 3B). By contrast, 10

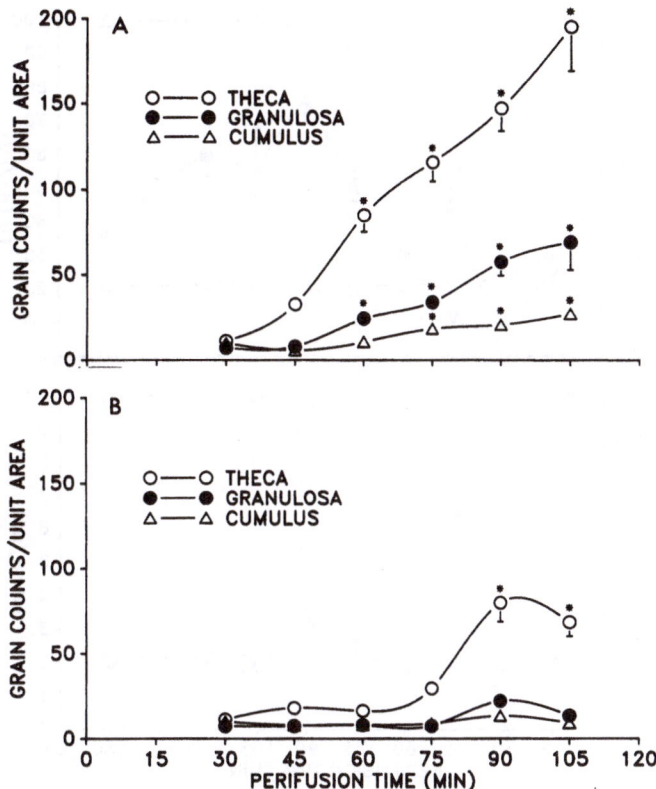

Fig. 1. Differential changes in binding (grain counts/unit area) over time from whole follicles perifused with a high (A) or low (B) dose of $[^{125}I]$I LH. Values marked by asterisk are significantly different from background values at 30 min (n=3).

ng/ml of LH significantly increased cAMP by 90 min only in the granulosal compartment (Fig. 3B). Interestingly, both the theca and granulosal cells from all treatment groups exhibited sinusoidal patterns of cAMP change whose high and low points appeared to depend upon the concentration of LH used (or lack of LH in control groups). Cyclic AMP changes in the COCs were essentially no different from the controls (data not shown).

When follicles were perifused with high or low LH for a total of 4 or 6 h, the percentage of oocytes induced to mature was directly proportional to the concentration of LH used. Each group was significantly different from the other with 100 ng/ml of LH initiating the highest percentage of maturation (100 ng/ml [61%, 4 h; 69%, 6 h] > 10 ng/ml [42%, 4 h; 48%, 6 h] > controls [11%, 4 h; 25%, 6 h]).

Discussion

Previous autoradiographic analyses of LH binding have generally employed either direct application of $[^{125}I]$I-labeled LH to tissue sections (3) or injection of large doses of labeled

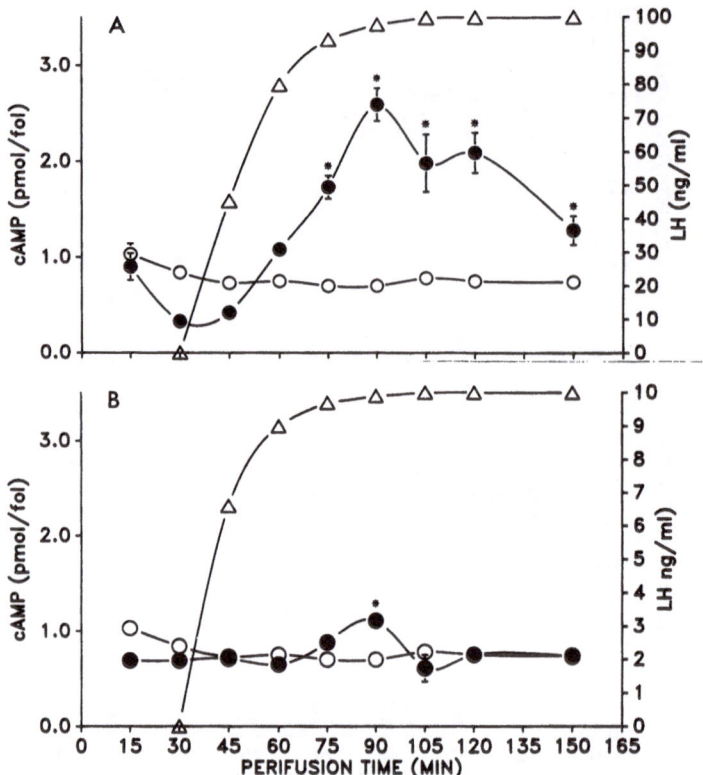

Fig. 2. Changes in cAMP levels (pmol/follicle; closed circles) from whole follicles perifused with a high (A) or low (B) dose of LH (open triangles). Values marked by an asterisk are significantly different from control values (open circles) at identical time-points (n=3).

LH into the whole animal (5). In the present study, intact follicles were exposed to physiological concentrations of either unlabeled or [^{125}I]-labeled LH in a perifusion system. The time-dependent delay in hormone binding by the cell groups exposed to the low dose of LH may be due to reduced LH exposure in the cells internal to the basement membrane. Since LH is normally delivered in a pulsatile manner in vivo, plasma LH may rise and fall before it can reach the inside of the follicle. Recent studies in the rat indicate that during an endogenous pulse of LH, LH levels in the follicular fluid never exceed 20% of peak plasma values (6). In hamster follicles, available LH-binding sites have been reported primarily in the theca and mural granulosa with little or no detectable sites found over the cumulus oophorus and oocyte (3). However, in the present study some LH binding to the cumulus cells appears to exist. Since the greater number of LH receptor sites are found on the theca and mural granulosa cells, it is conceivable that induction of maturation begins in one of these two compartments. This signal may be propagated toward the interior of the follicle and oocyte via gap junctions between the mural granulosa and cumulus cells. However, the

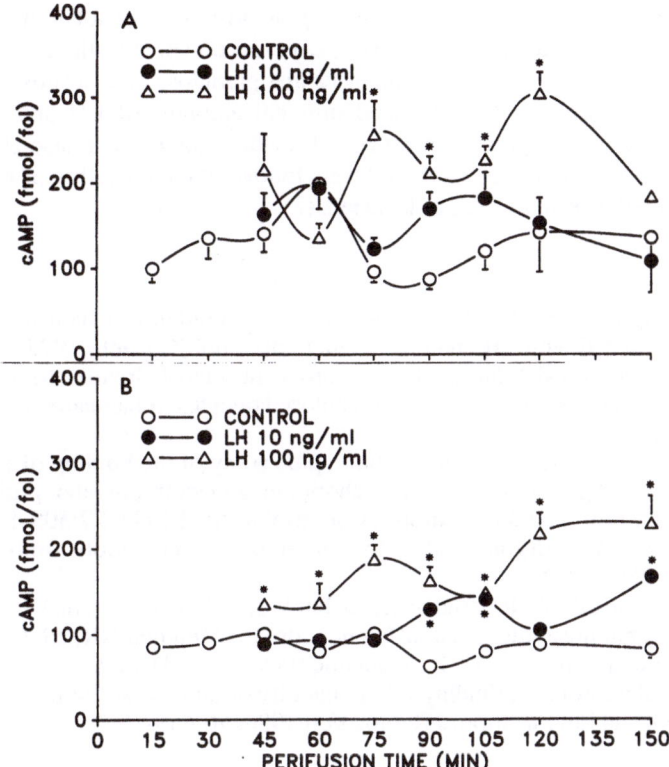

Fig. 3. Differential changes in cAMP levels (fmol/follicle) over time in the theca layer (A) and granulosa layer (B) from whole follicles perifused with a high or low dose of LH. Values marked by an asterisk are significantly different from control values at identical time-points (n=4).

high-dose LH groups showed some LH binding to the COCs; therefore, a direct effect of LH on the COC cannot be ruled out.

The cAMP changes seen in whole follicles following exposure to a high dose of LH appear to reflect a response by both the theca and granulosal compartments. By contrast, whole follicle cAMP changes following exposure to the low dose of LH appear to be mediated by the granulosa cells. Therefore, while the low dose of LH initiated significant binding in the theca layer, the numbers of LH receptors bound may not have been sufficient to appreciably increase adenylate cyclase activity. The granulosal cells, which bound less LH than the theca, may actually be more sensitive to LH stimulation.

The mechanism by which the LH surge initiates maturation in follicle-enclosed oocytes has not yet been determined. However, the present study has shown that the relative patterns of LH binding and cAMP change occurring both in the whole follicle and in its component cell groups directly correlate with the percentage of follicle-enclosed oocytes which were initiated to resume meiosis. Whether the theca is a contributor to the meiotic process is unclear at this time since it is separated from the granulosa by a basal lamina. However, to initiate maturation in follicle-enclosed oocytes, LH must effectively stimulate cells with an adequate number of LH receptors, i.e., the theca and granulosa. The results of the present study, which has shown that COCs bound minimal amounts of LH and produced no significant rise in cAMP, support this concept. Previous studies have also shown that no significant change occurs in oocyte cAMP levels following the induction of meiosis in the follicle-enclosed oocytes and COCs of hamsters (2).

References

1. Makris A, Ryan K. Cyclic AMP and cyclic GMP accumulation in hamster preovulatory follicles stimulated with LH and FSH. Acta Endocrinol (Copenh) 1978; 87:158-63.
2. Hubbard C. Cyclic AMP changes in the component cells of Graafian follicles: possible influences on maturation in the follicle-enclosed oocytes of hamsters. Dev Biol 1986; 118:343-51.
3. Oxberry B, Greenwald G. An autoradiographic study of the binding of ^{125}I-labeled follicle-stimulating hormone, human chorionic gonadotropin and prolactin to the hamster ovary throughout the estrous cycle. Biol Reprod 1982; 27:505-16.
4. Tarkowski A. An air-drying method for chromosome preparations from mouse eggs. Cytogenet 1966; 1:391.
5. Midgley A, Zeleznik A, Rajanjemi H, Richards J, Reichert L. Gonadotropin receptor activity and granulosa luteal cell differentiation. In: Moudgal NR, ed. Gonadotropins and gonadal function. New York: Academic Press, 1974:416-29.
6. Carson R, Salamonsen L, Findlay J. Permeability of rat ovarian follicles to LH during development and luteinization. J Reprod Fert 1986; 76:663-76.

41

The Rat Cholesterol Side-Chain Cleavage Cytochrome P450 (P450scc) Gene: cAMP-Dependent and -Independent Regulation in Ovarian Cells

Ria B. Oonk,[1] Ruud Jansen,[1,2] Gerard J. Hickey,[1] Wanda G. Beattie,[1] and JoAnne S. Richards[1]

[1]Department of Cell Biology, [2]Howard Hughes Medical Institute, Baylor College of Medicine, One Baylor Plaza Houston, TX 77030

Summary

Using a 5′ human P450scc cDNA probe and a human 57-mer oligonucleotide probe, 2 rat P450scc cDNA clones were identified and isolated from combined granulosa cell and luteal cell λgt11 cDNA expression libraries. One 350 bp clone contained the start codon. The other 750 bp clone overlapped on the 5′ end with the 350 bp clone and on the 3′ end with a previously isolated 1.2 kb cDNA clone (1), which contains a poly(A) tail, suggesting that the complete cDNA sequence for rat P450scc is encoded in these 3 cDNA clones. Using the same 5′ human P450scc probes, we have isolated a rat genomic P450scc clone from a rat liver genomic library. The genomic clone contained 3 distinct Bam HI fragments, 3.7, 4.0 and approximately 14 kb in size. The 3.7 and 4.0 kb Bam HI fragments hybridized to the 1.2 kb cDNA and appear to contain 3′ located exons. After subcloning, the 14 kb fragment yielded several transformants with inserts ranging from 8 to 0.5 kb in size. Hybridization with the rat cDNA clones revealed that the 8 kb fragment may represent 5′ upstream or intron sequences. A 6 kb fragment contained the first and probably the next 2 exons. Northern blot hybridization with the analysis, using the 750 bp cDNA probe, demonstrated that P450scc mRNA was low in granulosa cells of preovulatory (PO) follicles but could be induced by an ovulatory dose of LH/hCG in vivo or by forskolin added in vitro. Once induced by LH/hCG in vivo, P450scc mRNA and progesterone biosynthesis were constitutively maintained by luteinized cells in vivo or in vitro. Thus, the induction of P450scc mRNA in granulosa cells from developing follicles is hormone and cAMP dependent. In contrast, the expression of P450scc mRNA in luteinized granulosa cells has become cAMP independent.

Introduction

Previous studies have shown that progesterone biosynthesis appears to be regulated in a cAMP-dependent manner in nonluteinized granulosa cells, and in a cAMP-independent manner in luteal cells (2,3). In this study, we have compared the regulation by cAMP of P450scc mRNA with progesterone production in cultured granulosa cells. To study the molecular mechanisms by which hormones and cAMP regulate P450scc gene expression, we have isolated 2 cDNA clones and 1 genomic clone for the rat 450scc gene.

Methods

Cloning Procedures

cDNA Screening. To isolate 5' rat P450scc cDNA clones, combined granulosa and luteal cell λgt11 cDNA expression libraries were screened with a 5' 572 bp Ava I fragment of the complete human P450scc cDNA (kindly provided by Dr. W. L. Miller, Department of Pediatrics, University of California, San Francisco, CA [4]). To confirm the presence of 5' sequences in the detected clones, an oligonucleotide was made complementary to 57 bp in the first exon of the human cDNA. The region chosen for the oligonucleotide showed 95% similarity between human and bovine sequences for P450scc cDNA (4,5) (Fig. 1), and started 30 bp downstream of the putative processing point of the mitochondrial extension peptide (4). Recombinant phage plaques (1×10^6) of the combined libraries were amplified in *E. coli* Y 1090 cells grown on nitrocellulose filters. Two clones appeared consistently positive after rescreening and were plaque purified. The cDNA inserts (350 and 750 bp in size) were amplified to μg quantities by the polymerase chain reaction (6) using Taq I polymerase (7) and 2 oligonucleotides to the λgt11 Eco RI flanking regions. The fragments were subcloned into pGEM3Z and M13mp18 (for sequencing).

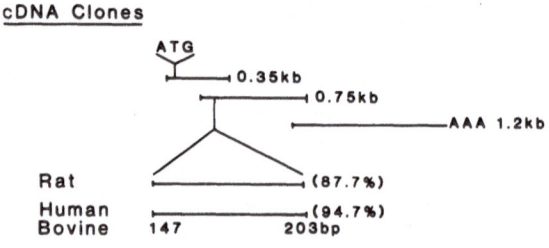

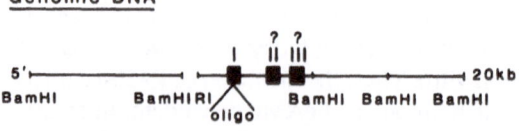

Fig. 1. Schematic of the cDNA clones (upper panel) and genomic clones (lower panel) of P450scc.

Genomic Screening. A rat liver genomic library (Dr. C. B. Kasper, University of Wisconsin, Madison, WI) was screened with the 5′ human Ava I cDNA fragment and the 57-mer oligonucleotide described above. One million recombinant phage plaques (40,000 plaques/150 mm plate) were amplified in *E. coli* K802 cells. The primary screening yielded 23 positive plaques of which one was confirmed positive to both probes after secondary screening. This positive clone (approximately 20 kb in size) was plaque purified, subcloned into pGEM3Z and subjected to restriction mapping.

Animals, Treatments, Cells and Incubations

Granulosa cells from preovulatory (PO) follicles were isolated from 30-day-old intact rats after treatment with a low dose of hCG (0.2 IU twice daily for 2 days). Luteinizing granulosa cells were isolated 7 h after an IV injection of 10 IU hCG (PO+hCG) given after the above described treatment (3). Corpora lutea were isolated from the ovaries of pregnant rats on day 15 of gestation. Granulosa cells were cultured in DMEM:F12 containing 1% fetal bovine serum (FBS). Medium was changed on days 4, 7 and 10. Forskolin (10 μM) was added to half of the cultures on day 7. RNA was extracted using 1% NP-40, as previously described (8), and analyzed by Northern blots using the ^{32}P-labeled 750 bp rat cDNA fragment as probe. A total of 7 μg of total RNA was run in each lane.

Results and Discussion

Isolation of cDNA and Genomic Clones for Rat P450scc

cDNA Clones. To analyze 5′ flanking sequences of the P450scc gene that are presumed to regulate hormone- and tissue-specific transcription of this gene, 5′ cDNA and genomic sequences have been isolated. For this, we used a human 5′ Ava I fragment (4) that contains sequences encoded by the first 3 exons of the human gene (9). To determine if the rat clones possessed sequences of the first exon, we constructed an oligonucleotide to a highly conserved region in the first exon of the human P450scc cDNA as described in Methods. We identified 2 authentic rat P450scc cDNA clones from a mixture of a granulosa cell and a luteal cell cDNA library using the 2 probes described above. The cDNA clones were 350 and 750 bp in size. To obtain substantial amounts of insert DNA, we used the recently described polymerase chain reaction (PCR) that involves exponential amplification of a DNA sequence using DNA polymerase and 2 oligonucleotides (6,7). The PCR method yielded substantial amounts of the cDNA inserts subsequently used for subcloning and sequencing. Preliminary sequence data revealed that the 350 bp fragment contained an ATG initiation codon in a region of 78 bp showing 80% similarity to the human cDNA sequence, plus a region of 200 bp with 84% similarity (Fig. 1). The 750 bp fragment contains 130 bp at the 5′ end which overlap the 350 bp fragment. This overlap region also contains a stretch of 57 bp with 87.7% similarity to the 57-mer oligonucleotide probe. Hybridization analysis further revealed that the 5′ rat 750 bp fragment hybridized to a 3′ rat 1.2 kb fragment (1), which by sequencing analysis has been shown to contain the poly(A) tail. All data together suggest that the 3 rat cDNA clones comprise the complete nucleotide sequence for rat P450scc (Fig. 1).

Genomic Clone. From a rat liver Bam HI genomic library, 1 clone was isolated, plaque purified and the DNA amplified. Bam HI digestion of the clone revealed 3 distinct fragments of 3.7, 4.0 and approximately 14 kb in size. The 3.7 and 4.0 kb fragments could be subcloned in their entirety into pGEM3Z. Both fragments hybridized to the rat 1.2 kb cDNA probe, described above, but did not hybridize to the 5' human 572 bp probe. We conclude that the genomic 3.7 and 4.0 kb sequences may contain the more 3' located exons. After subcloning into pGEM3Z, the large 14 kb genomic fragment (which hybridized to the 5' human 572 bp probe and to the 57-mer oligonucleotide) gave rise to several transformants, the inserts of which ranged in size from 8 to 0.5 kb. The 8 kb fragment did not hybridize to any of our cDNA clones and may therefore represent either a 5' upstream region or a large intron. A number of the other fragments hybridized to the 5' rat 750 bp cDNA, and 2 of these fragments also hybridized to the 57-mer oligonucleotide. The largest of these was 6 kb in size and was selected for further analysis. Restriction mapping and hybridization revealed 3 distinct positive regions in the 6 kb fragment. Based upon comparison with the organization of the human P450scc gene (9), we presume these regions to represent exons 1, 2 and 3 (Fig. 1).

cAMP-Dependent and -Independent Regulation of P450scc in Rat Ovarian Cells

To determine if cAMP-dependent and -independent regulation of progesterone biosynthesis (3) was related to similar regulation of P450scc mRNA levels, granulosa cells from preovulatory (PO) follicles and luteinized granulosa cells from PO follicles isolated 7 h after hCG injection (PO+hCG) were cultured for 1-10 days, as described in Methods (Fig. 2). When granulosa cells from PO follicles were maintained in culture for 7-10 days, the content of P450 mRNA was low. Addition of forskolin markedly induced P450scc mRNA. In contrast, P450scc mRNA content in luteinized granulosa cells isolated from PO+hCG follicles was elevated on days 7 and 10 of culture and did not increase further upon addition of forskolin. In corpora lutea (CL) of pregnancy, a similar high level of P450scc mRNA was present (Figure 2, upper panel). Progesterone biosynthesis by nonluteinized or luteinized granulosa cells showed a pattern that was similar to that for P450scc mRNA content (Fig. 2). In long-term cultures of PO granulosa cells, progesterone levels decreased sharply between 4 and 7 days of culture and continued to decrease at a slower rate during prolonged incubation. Addition of forskolin increased progesterone accumulation with time. In contrast, the amount of progesterone produced by luteinizing granulosa cells was high at day 4, remained elevated on days 7 and 10, and was not further affected by forskolin (Figure 2, lower panel).

The results of these in vitro studies support and extend observations obtained from in vivo studies. Specifically, P450scc enzyme and mRNA contents are low in granulosa and theca cells of small antral and preovulatory follicles, but are rapidly (within 7 h) increased in response to an ovulatory dose of LH/hCG (1,10). Following induction by the LH surge and elevated intracellular concentrations of cAMP, luteinized granulosa and theca cells constitutively maintain elevated amounts of P450scc enzyme and mRNA both in vitro (Fig. 2) and in corpora lutea of gestation and parturition (1,11). Thus, gonadotropic hormones and cAMP are obligatory for the induction of P450scc in preovulatory follicles, whereas maintenance of P450scc enzyme and mRNA contents in luteinized cells appear to be cAMP independent.

To determine the molecular mechanisms that regulate cAMP-dependent and -independent control of P450scc gene expression, we aim to identify specific functional domains

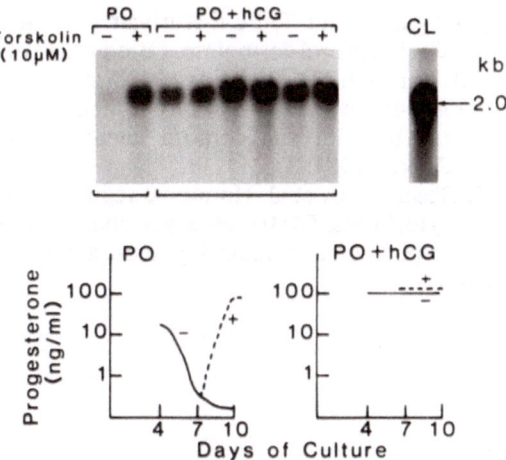

Fig. 2. Induction of P450scc mRNA and progesterone biosynthesis in cultured granulosa cells: effects of forskolin.

in the 5' flanking region of the P450scc gene and the transacting factors that modulate transcription of the P450scc gene in a cAMP-dependent and -independent manner. Accordingly, experiments are in progress to complete the nucleotide sequence of the rat P450scc cDNA clones, to determine the structural organization of the rat P450scc gene, and to identify functional domains in the 5' flanking region to the first exon.

References

1. Goldring NB, Durica JM, Lifka J, et al. Cholesterol side-cleavage P450scc messenger ribonucleic acid: evidence for hormonal regulation in rat ovarian follicles and constitutive expression in corpora lutea. Endocrinology 1987; 120:1942-50.
2. Richards JS, Jahnsen T, Hedin L, et al. Ovarian follicular development: from physiology to molecular biology. Recent Prog Horm Res 1986; 43:231-76.
3. Richards JS, Hedin L, Caston L. Differentiation of rat ovarian thecal cells: evidence for functional luteinization. Endocrinology 1986; 118:1660-8.
4. Chung B, Matteson KJ, Voutilainen R, Mohandas TK, Miller WL. Human cholesterol side-chain cleavage enzyme, P450scc: cDNA cloning, assignment of the gene to chromosome 15, and expression in the placenta. Proc Natl Acad Sci USA 1986; 83:8962-6.
5. Morohashi K, Fujii-Kuriyama Y, Okada Y, et al. Molecular cloning and nucleotide sequence of cDNA for mRNA of mitochondrial cytochrome P-450 (SCC) of bovine adrenal cortex. Proc Natl Acad Sci USA 1984; 81:4647-51.
6. Mullis KB, Faloona FA. Specific synthesis of DNA in vitro via a polymerase-catalyzed chain reaction. Methods Enzymol 1987; 155:335-50.
7. Saiki RK, Gelfand DH, Stoffel S, et al. Primer-directed enzymatic amplification of DNA with a thermostable DNA polymerase. Science 1988; 239:487-91.
8. Pelham HRB. A regulatory upstream promoter element in the Drosophila Hsp 70 heat shock gene. Cell 1982; 40:517-28.

9. Morohashi K, Sogawa K, Omura T, Fujii-Kuriyama Y. Gene structure of human cytochrome P450 (SCC) cholesterol desmolase. J Biochem (Tokyo) 1987; 101:879-87.
10. Hedin L, Rodgers RJ, Simpson ER, Richards JS. Changes in content of cytochrome P450 17α, cytochrome P450scc, and 3-hydroxy-3-methylglutaryl CoA reductase in developing rat ovarian follicles and corpora lutea: correlation with theca cell steroidogenesis. Biol Reprod 1987; 37:211-33.
11. Hickey GJ, Chen S, Besman MJ, et al. Hormonal regulation, tissue distribution, and content of aromatase cytochrome P450 messenger ribonucleic acid and enzyme in rat ovarian follicles and corpora lutea: relationship to estradiol biosynthesis. Endocrinology 1988; 122:1426-36.

42

Inhibitory Coupling Between Protein Kinase C and Cyclic AMP Generation in Swine Granulosa Cells

Matthew B. Wheeler and Johannes D. Veldhuis

University of Virginia School of Medicine
Department of Internal Medicine
Charlottesville, VA 22908

Introduction

The ovarian cyclic AMP (cAMP) effector pathway has been studied extensively with regard to granulosa cell and follicular maturation (1-4). In contrast, the role of the recently described and ubiquitous calcium-sensitive, phospholipid-dependent protein kinase (protein kinase C) effector pathway in ovarian physiology is less well understood. Furthermore, the exact nature of interactions between these two effector systems in the ovary is not known in detail.

In the present study, we have utilized an in vitro system of swine granulosa cells to evaluate the ability of protein kinase C to modulate both receptor- and nonreceptor-mediated cAMP generation.

Materials and Methods

Swine granulosa cells were aspirated aseptically from 1-3 mm porcine ovarian follicles and prepared as previously described (5). Monolayer cultures were established (10^6 cells/ml) in multiwell plates (24 wells/plate) with 2 ml bicarbonate-buffered MEM with 1% fetal calf serum (FCS) and 0.5 mM 3-isobutyl-1-methylxanthine (IBMX). Cultures were maintained at 37°C in a humidified mixture of 95% air:5%CO_2 for varying intervals as indicated. Spent medium was removed every 48 h (or at earlier intervals, as indicated separately in time course experiments) and replenished with fresh medium containing hormones and/or effectors. Time courses were initiated when fresh medium containing hormones and/or effectors was replaced (T=O). At selected intervals, cells were harvested by mechanical scraping and combined with medium, sonicated and assayed for total cAMP content. Cyclic AMP content in granulosa cells was assayed according to the method of Harper and Brooker (6) as modified for ovarian cells (7).

Results were expressed as means ± SEM. Nonlinear, least-squares curve fitting was used to assess dose-response curves to estimate mean half-maximal and maximally effective concentrations of agonist with 67% confidence limits. One- and two-way analysis of variance were performed as indicated, where appropriate. Each experiment was performed at least twice with separate batches of ovaries to confirm reproducibility of the results.

Results

Granulosa cells were incubated with maximally effective concentrations of FSH (200 ng/ml, ovine FSH; NIH oFSH-16), forskolin (100 μM), cholera toxin (3 μg/ml) and/or 12-O-tetradecanoyl phorbol-13-acetate, TPA (30 ng/ml). Forskolin and cholera toxin were used, respectively, to directly activate the catalytic and stimulatory (G_s) subunits of adenylate cyclase independently of the FSH receptor. The presence of TPA in the medium had no significant consistent effect on basal cAMP accumulation (30 min–4 days). TPA did, however, inhibit FSH-, forskolin-, and cholera toxin-stimulated cAMP formation during acute culture (30-60 min; Fig. 1).

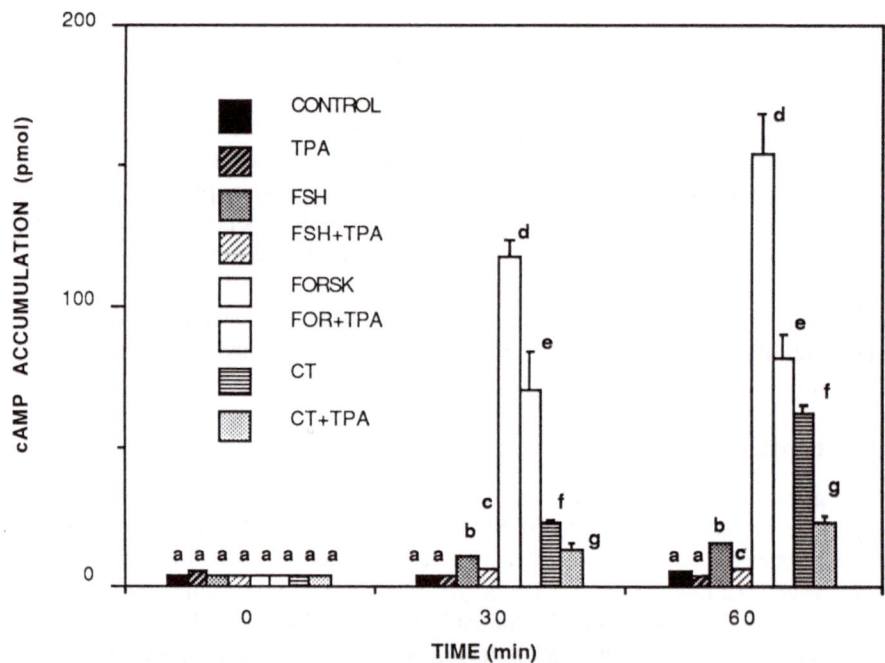

Fig. 1. Time-dependent inhibition by TPA of FSH-, forskolin-, and cholera toxin-stimulated cAMP accumulation in acute (30-60 min) cultures of swine granulosa cells. Cells were preincubated for 48 h (no effectors) and then with or without FSH (200 ng/ml), forskolin (100 μM), or cholera toxin (3 μg/ml) and/or TPA (30 ng/ml). Data are means ± SEM (n=4 determinations) from two independent experiments. [abcdefg] Bars within time-points without common superscripts differ (P<0.05).

The acute inhibition of FSH-mediated cAMP accumulation disappeared at 3 h (FSH, 3.4 ± 0.5 vs. FSH+TPA, 3.8 ± 0.2 pmol) and no inhibition was evident at 7 h (4.0 ± 0.3 vs. 4.4 ± 0.3 pmol), or 24 h (5.3 ± 0.2 vs. 5.1 ± 0.1 pmol). Inhibition was seen again after 48 h (FSH, 15.8 ± 0.3 vs. FSH+TPA, 5.7 ± 0.2; P<0.05) of culture. With longer term culture (2-4 days), TPA inhibited (P<0.05) the FSH- and forskolin-mediated cAMP generation (Fig. 2).

In addition, TPA inhibited the dose-dependent stimulation of cAMP accumulation by cholera toxin on day 2 (Fig. 3). Phorbol ester treatment had minimal effect on the ED_{50} for cholera toxin, *viz.* control 15 ng/ml (67% Confidence Interval: 5.0-24.0) vs. TPA-treated 5.8 ng/ml (3.7-7.5) but decreased the maximal cAMP response from 27 ± 0.9 to 20.6 ± 1 pmol cAMP/48 h (P<0.05) on day 2. On day 4 the action of TPA, ED_{50} for cholera toxin-mediated cAMP generation was unaffected by TPA; i.e., control 37 (33-46) ng/ml vs. TPA-treated 8.7 (2.4-40) ng/ml. The maximal cAMP response was increased by TPA treatment *viz.* control 8.0 ± 0.6 to 11.0 ± pmol cAMP/48 h (P<0.05). Prior exposure of granulosa cells to pertussis toxin (100 ng/ml) for 18 h did not override the inhibitory action of TPA on either receptor-mediated or nonreceptor-mediated cAMP accumulation (data not shown).

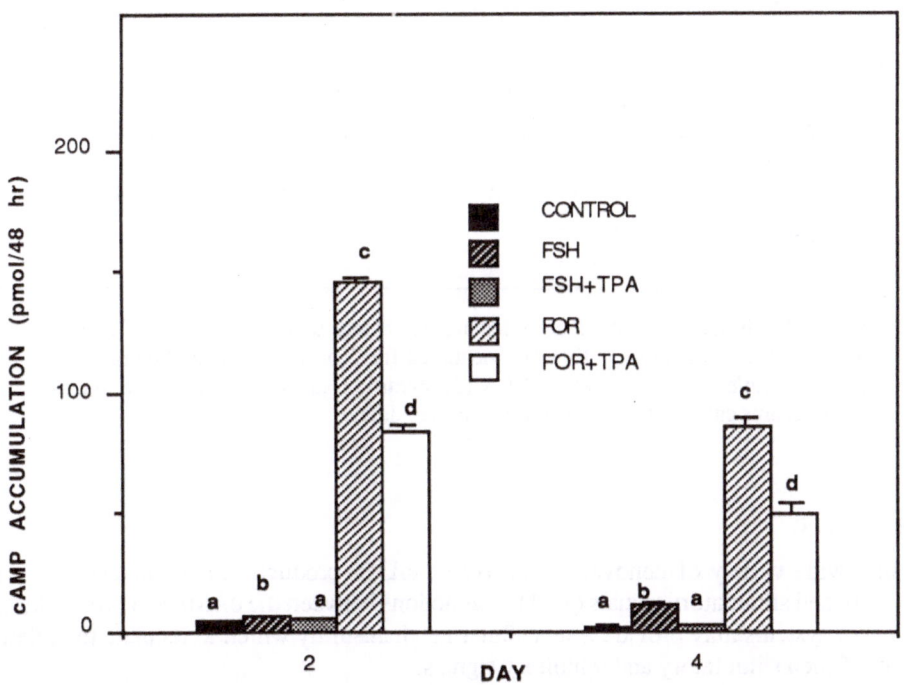

Fig. 2. Time-dependent inhibition by TPA of cAMP accumulation in swine granulosa cells. Monolayer cultures were exposed to FSH (200 ng/ml), forskolin (100 µM) or control (no effectors) and/or TPA (30 ng/ml) for 2 or 4 days. Data are means ± SEM (n=4 determinations) for cAMP accumulation (pmol/48 h) from two independent experiments. [abcd] Bars within time-points without common superscripts differ (P<0.05).

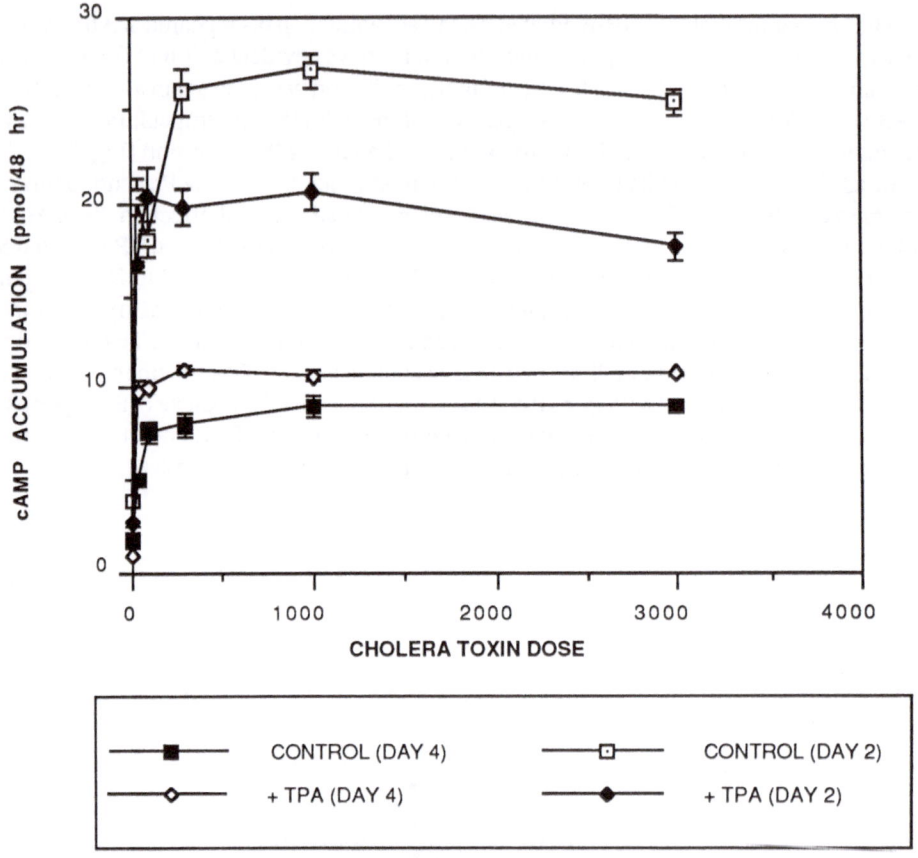

Fig. 3. Inhibition by TPA of dose-dependent cholera toxin stimulation of cAMP accumulation. Granulosa cells were incubated for 2 or 4 days with cholera toxin (30-3000 ng/ml) with or without TPA (30 ng/ml). Data were fit using nonlinear least-squares curve fitting of the untransformed data.

Discussion

In a wide variety of nonovarian cell types, cAMP production is regulated dually by inhibitory and stimulatory signals (8-11). Interactions between the cAMP and protein kinase C effector systems may provide a subcellular mechanism by which to regulate the relative impact of such stimulatory and inhibitory signals.

There are a number of potential sites of protein kinase C interaction with the adenylate cyclase pathway. These include the hormone receptor, the stimulatory (G_s) or inhibitory (G_i) subunits, or the catalytic subunit of adenylate cyclase. In the present study, FSH-stimulated cAMP production was inhibited in a biphasic time course with an acute inhibiting effect of TPA on cAMP accumulation which appears within 30-60 min, disappears by 7 h and reappears again after 48 h of culture. Although the basis for this biphasic temporal pattern is not known, mechanisms may involve inhibition at the level of the FSH receptor, and/or decreased synthesis or function of the adenylate cyclase enzyme as suggested by others (12).

We used cholera toxin to probe alterations in G_s function. In the present study, cholera toxin-stimulated cAMP accumulation was inhibited acutely (30-60 min) as well as on day 2 by activation of protein kinase C. However, on day 4, the effect of phorbol ester on adenylate cyclase enzyme as suggested by others (12).

We used cholera toxin to probe alterations in G_s function. In the present study, cholera toxin-stimulated cAMP accumulation was inhibited acutely (30-60 min) as well as on day 2 by activation of protein kinase C. However, on day 4, the effect of phorbol ester on cholera toxin-mediated cAMP accumulation became stimulatory, in contrast to its previously inhibitory influence. One potential explanation for the reversal of TPA's effects is that granulosa cells exposed to cholera toxin for 48 h form LH receptors that are coupled to an LH-mediated adenylate cyclase system (13). The latter appears to respond in a facilitative fashion to protein kinase C activation (14).

Pertussis toxin was used to examine alterations in G_i function. Our results indicate that the inhibitory action of protein kinase C is not mediated through a pertussis toxin-sensitive mechanism.

An additional site of protein kinase C's modulation of cAMP production in granulosa cells may be the catalytic subunit of adenylate cyclase itself (with or without any changes in the function or amount of guanine nucleotide regulatory proteins). This type of critical regulatory action is supported by the present data in which protein kinase C activation inhibited acute and long-term stimulation of cAMP accumulation by forskolin. Such observations are consistent with functional alterations in the catalytic subunit of adenylate cyclase.

In conclusion, an inhibitory coupling between protein kinase C and cAMP-generating systems exists in swine granulosa cells and is enacted, in part, at the level of the catalytic subunit of adenylate cyclase.

Acknowledgments

We thank Paula Azimi, Diana Juchter-Berry and Jim Garmey for technical assistance, and the Gwaltney-Smithfield Packing Corp. for providing the swine ovaries. This work was supported by NSRA HD 07025 to MBW and RCDA HD00634 and NIH HD16806 to JDV.

References

1. Marsh JM, Mills TM, LaMarie J. Preovulatory changes in the synthesis of cyclic AMP by rabbit Graffian follicles. Biochim Biophys Acta 1973; 304:197-202.
2. Marsh JM. The role of cyclic AMP in gonadal steroidogenesis. Biol Reprod 1976; 14:30-53.
3. Channing CP, Tsafriri A. Mechanisms of action of luteinizing hormone and follicle stimulating hormone on the ovary in vitro. Metabolism 1977; 26:413-68.
4. Lindsey AM, Channing CP. Comparison of the stimulatory effects of ovine and human luteinizing hormone on the accumulation of cyclic AMP by porcine granulosa cells. J Endocrinol 1979; 80:9-20.
5. Veldhuis JD, Klase PA, Strauss JF III, Hammond JM. The role of estradiol as a biological amplifier of the actions of follicle stimulating hormone: in vitro studies in swine granulosa cells. Endocrinology 1982; 111:144-51.

6. Harper JF, Brooker G. Femtomole-sensitive radioimmunoassay for cyclic AMP and cyclic GMP after 2'0 acetylation by acetic anhydride in aqueous solution. J Cyclic Nucleotide Res 1975; 1:207-18.

7. Veldhuis JD, Klase PA. Mechanisms by which calcium ions regulate the steroidogenic actions of luteinizing hormone in isolated ovarian cells in vitro. Endocrinology 1982; 111:1-6.

8. Katada K, Ui M. Direct modification of the membrane adenylate cyclase system by islet-activating protein due to ADP-ribosylation of a membrane protein. Proc Natl Acad Sci USA 1982; 79:3129-33.

9. Cronin MJ, Myers GA, MacLeod RM, Hewlett EL. Pertussis toxin actions on the pituitary-derived 235-1 clone: effects of PGE_1, cholera toxin, and forskolin on cyclic AMP metabolism and prolactin release. J Cyclic Nucleotide Protein Phosphor Res 1983; 9:245-58.

10. Gilman AG. G proteins and dual control of adenylate cyclase. Cell 1984; 36:577-9.

11. Summers ST, Cronin MJ. Phorbol esters enhance basal and stimulated adenylate cyclase activity in a pituitary cell line. Biochem Biophys Res Commun 1986; 135:276-81.

12. Chang FH, Bourne HR. Dexamethazone increases adenylyl cyclase activity and expression of the alpha-subunit of G_s in GH_3 cells. Endocrinology 1987; 1711-5.

13. Knecht M, Catt KJ. Epidermal growth factor and gonadotropin-releasing hormone inhibit cyclic AMP-dependent luteinizing hormone receptor formation in ovarian granulosa cells. J Cell Biochem 1983; 21:209-17.

14. Wheeler MB, unpublished.

43

Luteinizing Hormone (LH)-Like Activity and Follicle-Stimulating Hormone (FSH) Are Sufficient for the Induction of Cystic Ovaries in Hypophysectomized Rats

Katryna Bogovich

Department of Obstetrics and Gynecology, University of South Carolina School of Medicine, Columbia, SC 29208

Introduction

Direct evidence for the role of specific peptides in the induction of ovarian cysts has been difficult to obtain. We have shown that chronic stimulation by human chorionic gonadotropin (hCG) induces cysts in intact immature and pregnant rats but *not* in hypophysectomized (HYPXD) rats (1). Therefore, LH may require at least one other pituitary hormone to induce ovarian cysts. Serum hormone profiles emphasize the complexity of the cystic state (2-4). Yet both women and animals with ovarian cysts display chronically low or normal serum FSH. This study was performed to determine if chronic stimulation by FSH and LH-like activity is sufficient to induce ovarian cysts in HYPXD rats.

Materials and Methods

Immature rats, HYPXD at 21 days of age, were obtained from Charles River, given oranges and 10% sucrose-water in addition to rat chow, and divided into 4 groups receiving: (1) no hormone (controls); (2) 0.5 IU hCG (4000 IU/mg, Sigma Chemical Co.) twice daily for 12 days beginning on day 27; (3) 2 μg ovine FSH (20 U/mg; NIADDK-oFSH-17; less than 0.04 x NIH-LH-S1) daily for 13 days beginning on day 26; or, (4) FSH+hCG beginning on days 26 and 27, respectively. Between 0800-0900 h on the days indicated, 3-4 rats from the appropriate treatment groups were decapitated; blood was collected; and ovaries were excised. At least one ovary from each group was processed for light microscopy. The largest follicles from the remaining ovaries were incubated individually for 4 h at 37°C in Medium 199 containing 10 mM HEPES, pH 7.2, ± 1 mM 8-bromo cAMP (cAMP). Progesterone (P) and androstenedione (A) content was determined by radioimmunoassay (RIA) as previously described (5). Only data from completely HYPXD rats were included in the analyses.

Significant differences between and among groups were determined by analysis of variance and Student's *t* test.

Results

The effects of chronic gonadotropin stimulation on ovarian follicles in HYPXD rats are illustrated in Figure 1. Ovaries from control animals (Fig. 1A) were small, possessing only primordial and preantral follicles. Figure 1B shows that 12 days of treatment with hCG failed to induce cystic ovaries in HYPXD rats although the cross-sectional area of these ovaries was twice that of controls. These data agree with our previous work (1). Ovaries from FSH-treated HYPXD rats (Fig. 1C) possessed many atretic small antral follicles by the morning of day 14 of treatment. Although the cross-sectional area of these ovaries was 4 times that of ovaries from control HYPXD rats, neither thecal nor stromal-interstitial tissue was hypertrophied. Therefore, it is highly unlikely that these follicles were "minicysts" that developed as a result of the residual LH activity in this preparation of FSH. In contrast to all other groups, ovaries from FSH+hCG-treated HYPXD rats (Fig. 1D) possessed cysts up to 3 mm in diameter on the morning of day 13 of combined treatment (day 14 of FSH treatment). Cysts were first observed in these ovaries on day 9 of combined treatment which agrees with the time frame needed to induce ovarian cysts with 0.5 IU hCG in intact immature rats (1). In addition, the cross-sectional area of these ovaries was 9 times that of ovaries from control HYPXD rats.

It is now possible, using these models, to determine the specific effects of chronic FSH and LH-like stimulation on individual follicular functions as follicles develop into ovarian cysts. For example, Figure 2 (left panel) illustrates that follicles from hCG-, FSH-, and FSH+hCG-treated HYPXD rats initially accumulated more P in medium alone than follicles from control animals. After 2 days of treatment, however, P accumulation by follicles from hCG-treated rats decreased to that of follicles from control rats. Progesterone accumulation by follicles from FSH-treated HYPXD rats underwent a sharp decline which was associated with the marked loss of granulosa cells by follicles in these ovaries by day 10 of treatment. By day 12, follicles from these rats accumulated as much P as follicles from control and hCG-treated HYPXD animals. In contrast, follicles from FSH+hCG-treated HYPXD rats were able to produce large amounts of P throughout the treatment period. Yet many of these follicles appeared cystic by day 9 of combined treatment (day 10 of FSH treatment). P accumulation by follicles from control, hCG-, and FSH-treated HYPXD rats increased in response to cAMP on each day tested (Fig. 2, right panel). Indeed, follicles from FSH-treated rats accumulated as much P in response to cAMP as follicles from FSH+hCG-treated HYPXD rats in medium alone (Fig. 2, left panel). P accumulation by follicles from FSH+hCG-treated rats was unaffected by cAMP between days 6 and 9 of combined treatment, but did increase in response to cAMP on the other days of treatment.

An accumulation in medium alone by follicles from control and hCG-treated HYPXD rats was highly variable, averaging 0.4 ng/4-h incubation (Fig. 3, left panel). Follicles from FSH-treated HYPXD rats initially accumulated 0.2 ng A in vitro but this decreased markedly between days 4 and 10, parallelling changes in P accumulation by these follicles (Fig. 2, left panel). In contrast, the ability of follicles from FSH+hCG-treated HYPXD rats to accumulate A in medium alone increased from 0.13 ng on day 2 to almost 5 ng by day 13 of combined

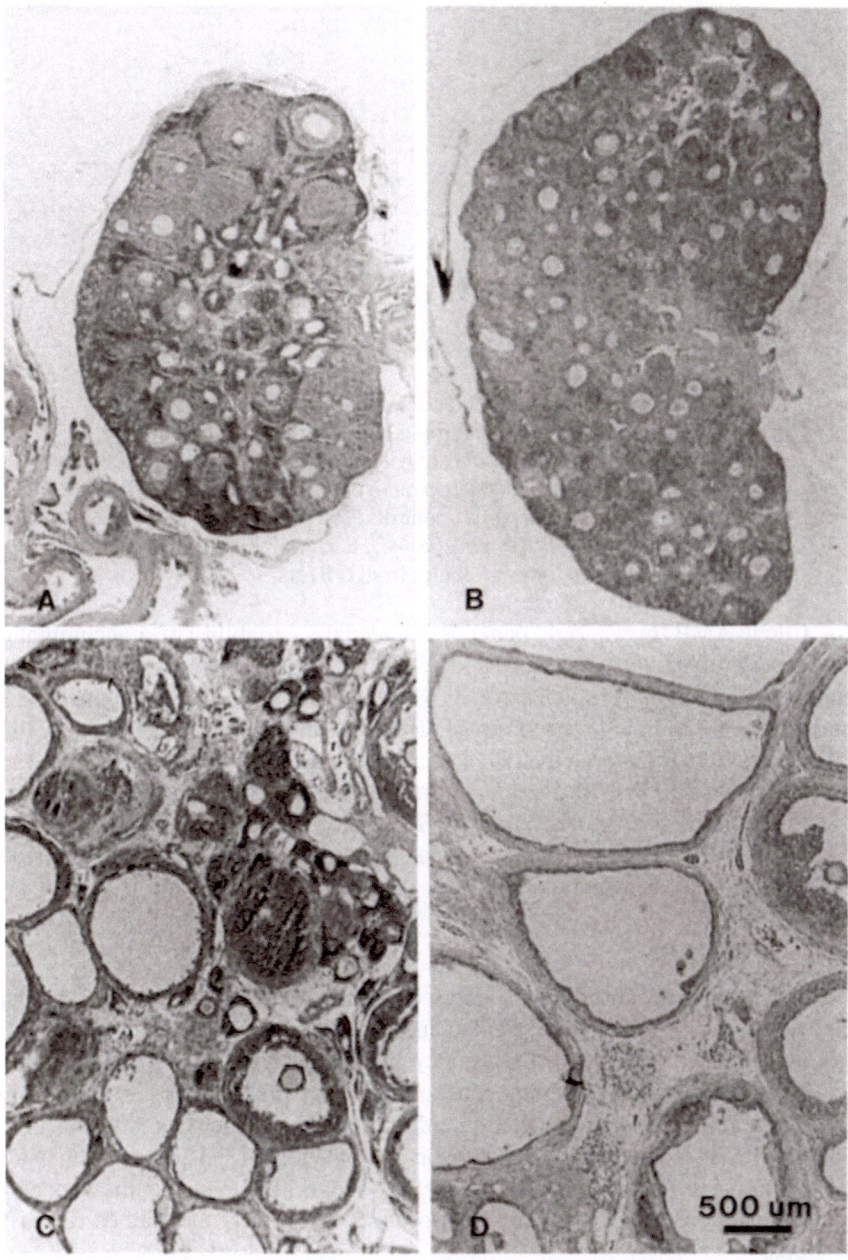

Fig. 1. Effect of chronic gonadotropin stimulation on ovaries of HYPXD rats. Sections depict ovaries on day 39 of life for all groups: (A) control; (B) 0.5 IU hCGx24; (C) 2 μg FSHx13; and, (D) 2 μg FSHx13 + 0.5 IU hCGx24. Photomicrographs were obtained on a Zeiss IM35 microscope at 25x magnification.

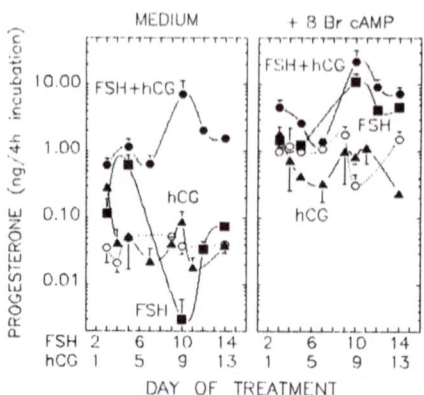

Fig. 2. Changes in follicular P accumulation in vitro in
response to chronic gonadotropin stimulation in vivo. The
largest follicles in the ovaries of each group were incubated
either in medium alone *(left panel)* or in the presence of
8-bromo cAMP *(right panel)*: controls (O—O); hCG (▲—▲);
FSH (■—■); and FSH+hCG (●—●). Each point represents
the mean ± SEM for 6-8 follicles from 6-8 rats.

treatment. Cyclic AMP (Fig. 3, right panel) attenuated the variability of A accumulation in
medium alone for follicles from control and hCG-treated rats. Between days 10 and 14 of
treatment, A accumulation by follicles from FSH-treated rats increased in response to cAMP
to values observed for follicles from control HYPXD rats under these conditions. The limited
ability of follicles from FSH-treated rats to accumulate A supports the concept that the atretic
small antral follicles in these ovaries are *not* "minicysts" which have arisen in response to
the residual LH activity in this preparation of FSH. It is interesting to note that once follicles
from FSH+hCG-treated HYPXD rats take on a cystic appearance, they no longer respond
to cAMP with increased A accumulation.

Discussion

These data provide the first direct evidence of a role for FSH in the induction of ovarian
follicular cysts in the rat. In addition, the data indicate that chronic stimulation by FSH and
LH, alone, is sufficient for the development of cystic ovaries. A role for FSH in the induction
of ovarian cysts is a new and interesting concept. However, this concept is not as surprising
as it might seem at first glance. The literature describing the cystic state indicates that low
or normal serum FSH is a common characteristic for both women and animals with naturally
occurring ovarian cysts (2-4). In addition, to our knowledge, all previous animal models used
to study the induction of cystic ovaries also possess chronically maintained serum FSH
concentrations.

A popular hypothesis regarding the induction of cystic ovaries states that chronic
stimulation by elevated serum LH results in the overproduction of androgens which, in turn,
inhibit the ability of FSH to induce/stimulate granulosa cell functions such as
steroidogenesis—especially aromatase activity. However, the steroidogenic data presented

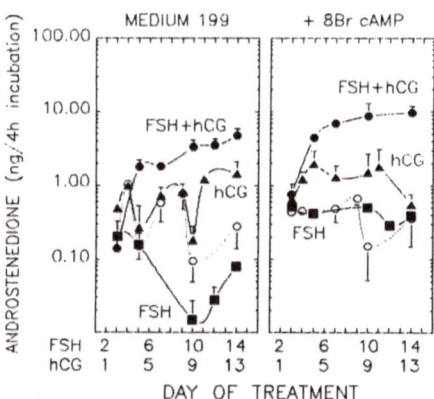

Fig. 3. Changes in follicular A accumulation in vitro in response to chronic gonadotropin stimulation in vivo. The incubates used to determine P accumulation (Fig. 2) also were used to determine A accumulation: controls (o—o); hCG (▲—▲); FSH (■—■); and FSH+hCG (●—●). Each point represents the mean ± SEM of 6-8 follicles from 6-8 rats.

here, and elsewhere (6), by our laboratory strongly suggest that FSH may be needed to stimulate steroid synthesis during the induction of follicular cysts. The hypothesis that ovarian cysts arise because androgens inhibit FSH action was based on observations of follicular function only *after* the cystic state had been established (2-4). Our models suggest that there may be a distinction between the initial development of follicular cysts and the perpetuation of the cystic state. Thus, cysts might develop as a result of chronic, unabated stimulation by LH and FSH in the absence of a gonadotropin surge. However, once cysts have become established, the hormonal milieu produced by these structures might impact both in the ovary and at neuroendocrine sites to perpetuate the cystic state.

References

1. Bogovich K. Induction of follicular cysts in rat ovaries by prolonged administration of human chorionic gonadotropin. In: Mahesh VB, Dhindsa DS, Anderson E, Kalra SP, eds. Regulation of ovarian and testicular function. New York: Plenum Publishing Corp., 1987:659-63.
2. Yen SCC. The polycystic ovary syndrome. Clin Endocrinol (Oxf) 1980; 12:177-208.
3. Coney P-J. Polycystic ovarian disease: current concepts of pathophysiology and therapy. Fertil Steril 1984; 42:667-82.
4. Futterweit W. Polycystic ovary disease. In: Buchsbaum HJ, ed. Clinical perspectives in obstetrics and gynecology. New York: Springer-Verlag, 1984.
5. Bogovich K, Scales LM, Higginbottom E, Ewing LL, Richards JS. Short term androgen production by rat ovarian follicles and long term steroidogenesis by thecal explants in culture. Endocrinology 1986; 118:1379-86.
6. Bogovich K. Induction of ovarian follicular cysts in hypophysectomized rats by gonadotropins: effects on estradiol production and aromatase activity [Abstract]. Biol Reprod 1988; 38(1):173A.

44

Isolation of Steroidogenic Cell Subpopulations in the Follicular Theca of the Ovary in the Domestic Fowl

Enrique Pedernera, Pedro Velazquez,* Yolanda Gomez and
Margarita Gonzalez del Pliego

Departamento de Embriologia, Departamento de Histologia *
Facultad de Medicina, Universidad Nacional Autonoma de
Mexico, Mexico, 04510 DF

The granulosa and the theca of the follicle are the principal source of steroid hormones in the ovary of the domestic fowl. The production of progesterone has been demonstrated in the granulosa layer, while the secretion of 17β-estradiol, testosterone and androstenedione has been found in the theca cells (1-4).

The theca of preovulatory follicles, classified from F1 to F6 in order of decreasing size, represents the 44% of the total aromatase activity of the ovary. The maximal aromatase-specific activity was registered in the F5 follicles (5), and the highest secretion of 17β-estradiol has been found in the theca layer of small (F4 to F6) preovulatory follicles (6,7).

A previous report from our group has demonstrated that, in the immature ovary of the newly hatched chicken, there are two cell subpopulations involved in 17β-estradiol and testosterone secretion. There is a subpopulation of typical steroiodogenic cells that secretes testosterone but does not produce 17β-estradiol, and another subpopulation of relatively undifferentiated epithelial cells involved in 17β-estradiol secretion (8).

In the ovary of the domestic fowl, typical steroidogenic cells and undifferentiated epithelial cells have been described in the theca layer (9). Therefore, it is interesting to elucidate the involvement of cell subpopulations of the theca in the synthesis of steroid hormones in the mature ovary. In the present paper, the separation of subpopulations of theca cell from F5 preovulatory follicles is performed, and the steroidogenic activity of each subpopulation is quantified.

Materials and Methods

Dulbecco's modified Eagle medium (DMEM) and trypsin were obtained from Grand Island Biological Co. (Grand Island, NY), soybean trypsin inhibitor, bovine serum albumin BSA), 1-methyl 3-isobutyl xanthine (MIX), metrizamide, human chorionic gonadotropin (hCG), testosterone and 17β-estradiol were purchased from Sigma Chemical Co. (St. Louis, MO), Sephadex LH-20 was obtained from Pharmacia Fine Chemicals (Uppsala, Sweden). Anti-testosterone and anti 17β-estradiol sera were products from Radioassay Inc. (Carson, CA); [1,2,6,7,-^{3}H]testosterone (94 Ci/mmol) and 17β-[2,4,6,7,-^{3}H]estradiol (92 Ci/mmol) were purchased from Amersham International(Buckinghamshire, England).

Theca Cell Preparation

Adult (46- to 52-week-old) white leghorn hens (Babcock B300) were obtained from the poultry farm of the Veterinary School of the National Autonomous University of Mexico. The birds were maintained in individual cages, and the oviposition controlled. Animals were killed by cervical dislocation 6-8 h after ovulation. The F5 follicle was selected, theca layer was separated from granulosa (10), and released from the adhering connective tissue on the exterior of the follicle. The dissociation of theca was performed by incubation in 0.25% w/v of trypsin in balanced salt solution (Ca^{++}, Mg^{++} free) at 37°C in a shaking bath (90 cycles/min).

Theca cells dispersed after 15 and 30 min of trypsin treatment were recovered from the medium, treated with 0.5% soybean trypsin inhibitor in DMEM with 0.1% BSA, washed with two changes of DMEM-BSA and saved as separated fractions.

In other experiments, the whole theca layer was completely dissociated by trypsin incubation. The isolated cells were treated with trypsin inhibitor, washed with DMEM-BSA, and laid on the top of a continuous metrizamide gradient (0-30%). 30-50 x 10^6 cells in 5 ml of gradient were centrifuged at 4000 x g for 7 min, and 0.5 ml fractions were collected from the top of the centrifuge tube. Fractions containing theca cells were washed with 10 ml of DMEM-BSA. In all cases, the final cell number was counted with the aid of a hemocytometer, and viability was established by the trypan blue exclusion test (11).

Samples (10^6 cells) of isolated theca cells obtained by the two procedures described above were incubated in 1 ml of DMEM with 0.1% of BSA, 0.1 mM of MIX, and 1.0 IU of hCG. The cells were incubated for 120 min at 37°C in a shaking bath (90 cycles/min), under 5% CO_2 and 95% air. Aliquots (50 μl) of the medium were collected; 17β-estradiol and testosterone were directly measured by specific radioimmunoassays that were previously validated (12).

For morphological studies, samples of the theca layer were fixed in 2% glutaraldehyde in 0.15 M phosphate buffer, pH 7.4, postfixed in 1% osmium tetroxide and embedded in plastic resins. Sections of 1 μm thick were stained with toluidine blue for light microscope observations.

Results

The in vitro secretion of 17β-estradiol and testosterone by dissociated cells of the theca obtained after trypsin treatment is shown in Figure 1. The cell dispersion, obtained after 15 min of trypsin incubation, secreted measurable amounts of testosterone; however, secretion of 17β-estradiol was not detected in this fraction. On the other hand, 17β-estradiol secretion was observed in the fraction of theca cells that were dispersed after 30 min of trypsin treatment. In the last fraction, lower level of testosterone was registered compared with the 15-min fraction.

Histological observations of the theca during the trypsin treatment revealed that after 15 min of incubation with the enzyme, almost 80% of cells in the theca interna were dispersed, while in the 30-min fraction, the whole theca was dissociated.

When the isolated cells of the theca were separated in a density gradient (Fig. 2), theca cells collected in fractions of low density secreted testosterone, and no 17β-estradiol secretion was registered in these fractions. The production of 17β-estradiol is at the maximum level in the theca cells that were recovered from the high density fraction of the gradient.

Discussion

In the present study, the in vitro secretion of 17β-estradiol and testosterone by the theca, in the absence of granulosa cells or exogenous precursors, is demonstrated in small (F5) preovulatory follicles, and the existence of two subpopulations of steroidogenic cells in the theca is strongly suggested in the ovary of the domestic fowl.

Since cells that only secreted testosterone could be isolated at 15 min of fractional trypsinization and found in the low-density fraction of the metrizamide gradient, it is proposed that androgen-secreting cells were located at the theca interna because cells of this layer were formerly dispersed by trypsin treatment. Moreover, cells with abundant lipid droplets have been described in the theca interna (13); the results obtained after the isopycnic separation provide additional evidence about the localization of androgen-secreting cells in the theca interna.

On the other hand, cells involved in 17β-estradiol secretion appear to be located in the theca externa because 30 min of trypsin treatment were required to disperse cells of the theca externa and to obtain maximum 17β-estradiol production. These results agree with a previous report that described 17β-estradiol secretion in the theca externa of preovulatory follicles in the ovary of the domestic turkey (14). The identification of estrogen-secreting cells is difficult since several cell types were found in the fraction with the maximal production of 17β-estradiol.

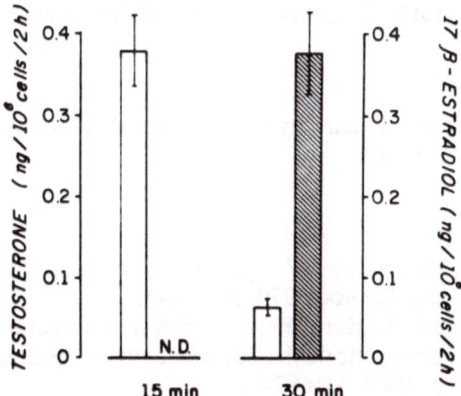

Fig. 1. Testosterone [open] and 17β-estradiol [cross-hatched] secretion in theca cells of preovulatory follicles (F5) in the ovary of the domestic fowl. Cells were obtained after dissociation during 15 and 30 min with trypsin treatment. Values represent mean ± SD.

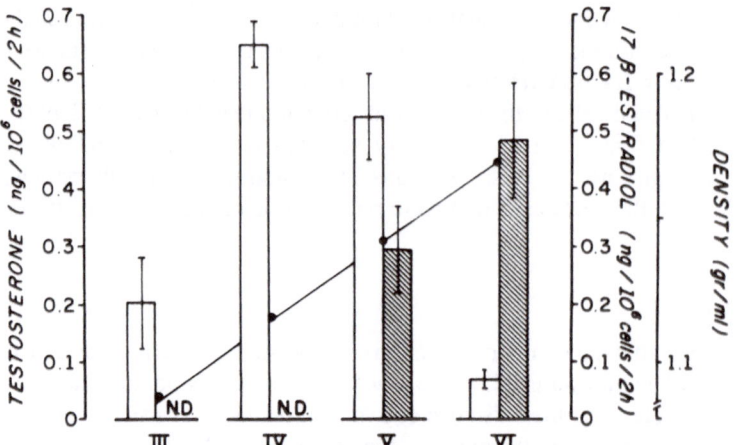

Fig. 2. Secretion in vitro of testosterone [open] and 17β-estradiol [cross-hatched] by the theca cells of preovulatory follicles (F5). Four fractions of dispersed theca cells were recovered from the density gradient. Values represent the mean ± SD.

A pure population of typical steroidogenic cells has been isolated from the ovary of the newly hatched chicken, and secretion of androgens has been demonstrated in these cells. On the other hand, the secretion of 17β-estradiol has been attributed to another subpopulation of relatively undifferentiated epithelial cells (8). The steroidogenic cell subpopulations found in the theca of F5 preovulatory follicle could represent the persistence in the adult ovary of the subpopulations that have been identified in the immature ovary of the newly hatched chicken.

The possibility of a differential regulation by gonadotropins or other hormones of the two subpopulations of steroidogenic cells described in the theca of preovulatory follicles would be a matter of interest in the endocrine study of the avian ovary.

Acknowledgments

This work was supported, in part, by Consejo Nacional de Investigaciones Cientificas y Tecnicas (PCSACNA-050284).

References

1. Huang ES, Kao KJ, Nalbandov AV. Synthesis of sex steroids by cellular components of chicken follicles. Biol Reprod 1979; 20:454-61.
2. Hammond RW, Todd H, Hertelendy F. Effect of mammalian gonadotropins on progesterone release and cyclic nucleotide production by isolated avian granulosa cells. Gen Comp Endocrinol 1980; 41:467-76.
3. Wells JW, Dick HR, Gilbert AB. The biosynthesis of progesterone by fowl granulosa cells in vitro from ^{14}C labeled substrates. J Steroid Biochem 1981; 14:651-6.

4. Marrone BL, Hertelendy F. Decreased androstenedione production with increased follicular maturation in theca cells from the domestic fowl (Gallus domesticus). J Reprod Fertil 1985; 74:543-50.
5. Armstrong DG. Ovarian aromatase activity in the domestic fowl (Gallus domesticus). J Endocrinol 1984; 100:81-6.
6. Marrone BL, Hertelendy F. Steroidogenesis by avian ovarian cells: effects of luteinizing hormone and substrate availability. Am J Physiol (Endocrinol Metab 7) 1983; 244:E487-93.
7. Velazquez P, Gomez Y, Gonzalez del Pliego M, Pedernera E. Cambios en la actividad esteroidogenica de la teca de foliculos preovulatorios de aves [Abstract]. In: Memorias del Congreso Nacional de Ciencias Fisiologicas. Queretaro 1988:95.
8. Pedernera E, Gomez Y, Velazquez P, Juarez-Oropeza MA, Gonzalez del Pliego M. Identification of steroidogenic cell subpopulations in the ovary of the newly hatched chicken. Gen Comp Endocrinol 1988 (in press).
9. Dahl E. Studies of the fine structure of ovarian interstitial tissue 2. The ultrastructure of the thecal gland of the domestic fowl. Z Zellforsch 1970; 109:195-211.
10. Gilbert AB, Evans AJ, Perry MM, Davidson MH. A method for separating the granulosa cells, the basal lamina and the theca of the preovulatory ovarian follicle of the domestic fowl (Gallus domesticus). J Reprod Fertil 1977; 50:179-81.
11. Tennant JR. Evaluation of trypan blue technique for the determination of cell viability. Transplantation 1964; 2:685-94.
12. Pedernera E, Gomar Y. Onset of the response to chorionic gonadotropin in the chick embryo testis. Gen Comp Endocrinol 1984; 54:344-9.
13. Dahl E. Studies of the fine structure of ovarian interstitial tissue 1. A comparative study of the fine structure of the ovarian interstitial tissue in the rat and the domestic fowl. J Anat 1971; 108:275-90.
14. Porter TE, El Halawani ME. Differential steroidogenesis between theca interna and theca externa layers of preovulatory follicles in the domestic turkey [Abstract]. Biol Reprod 1987; 36(suppl 1):92.

45

Evidence for an Endogenous Activator of Inositol Phospholipid Phospholipase C in Intact Rat Corpora Lutea

John S. Davis, Leigh A. West, and Laura L. Weakland

Departments of Internal Medicine and Pharmacology
and Therapeutics, University of South Florida and
J. A. Haley Veterans Hospital, Tampa, FL 33612

Introduction

The inositol phospholipid-phospholipase C transmembrane signalling system provides second messengers that regulate cellular differentiation as well as metabolic and secretory activities (reviewed in references 1,2). These cellular events are presumably mediated by increases in inositol 1,4,5-trisphosphate and diacylglycerol, the two immediate products of phosphatidylinositol 4,5-bisphosphate hydrolysis. Both products contribute to the cellular activity by regulating intracellular calcium mobilization and the activities of protein kinases.

The maturation of the rat corpus luteum (CL) is accompanied by an increased rate of inositol phospholipid turnover (3). Recent reports by Leung and co-workers (4,5) and our laboratory (6,7) have demonstrated that $PGF_{2\alpha}$ and GnRH increase the levels of inositol phospholipid-derived second messengers in rat ovarian tissues. The following experiments were performed (1) to examine the effects of $PGF_{2\alpha}$ and GnRH on inositol phospholipid metabolism in young (day-2) and mature (day-7) rat CL; and, (2) to test whether endogenous prostaglandins or GnRH-like factors could account for the increased level of inositol phospholipid-phospholipase C activity in intact mature CL.

Materials and Methods

PMSG and ovine LH (NIH-oLH-23) were supplied by the NIH. Synthetic GnRH and the GnRH agonist [D-Ala^6, des-Gly^{10}]GnRH ethylamide (GnRHa) were purchased from Beckman. The GnRH antagonist [Ac-Δ^3Pro^1,p-F-D-Phe^2,D-Trp^{3,6}]GnRH (GnRH ANTAG) was purchased from Bachem. Immature (28-day-old) Sprague-Dawley rats (Charles River) were injected subcutaneously with 8 IU PMSG at 0900-1000 a.m. (7). Rats carrying 2- or 7-day-old CL were sacrificed and the ovaries were placed in incubation medium (medium 199 containing 25 mM HEPES and 0.1% BSA, pH 7.4). Isolated single CL were halved and the CL were prelabeled in incubation medium for 3 h with 50 µCi/ml of myo[2-^{3}H]inositol under an atmosphere of 95% O_2, 5% CO_2 at 37°C. Corpora lutea (2-4 per tube) were then preincubated in 0.5 ml of incubation medium for 15 min with or without 10 mM LiCl prior to the addition of hormones. In other experiments, day-7 CL were isolated from surrounding ovarian tissue and dispersed with collagenase as described by Luborsky and Behrman (8). Isolated luteal cells were prelabeled with myo[2-^{3}H]inositol as described above. Incubations with intact CL were terminated in an ice bath, by rinsing with 1 ml ice-cold saline and adding 1 ml ice-cold 10% trichloroacetic acid (TCA). Incubations of isolated cells were terminated by the addition of 10% TCA. Following homogenization, the sample was sedimented by centrifugation (1200 x g, 10 min), and the acid-soluble supernatant was extracted with ether prior to analysis of [^{3}H]inositol phosphates and cAMP. The protein content of the acid insoluble pellet was determined by the method of Lowry et al. (9). [^{3}H]Inositol phosphates were isolated by ion exchange chromatography as previously described (6). cAMP was measured by radioimmunoassay (10).

Results

Figure 1 shows that isolated intact (day-2) CL respond to $PGF_{2\alpha}$ and GnRHa with an increase in inositol phospholipid-phospholipase C activity. $PGF_{2\alpha}$ (10 µM) and GnRHa (100 ng/ml) provoked large increases in the accumulation of inositol mono-, bis- and trisphosphates in the presence of 10 mM LiCl (Fig. 1). Treatment with 10 mM LiCl did not alter basal levels of inositol phosphates. The increases in inositol phosphate accumulation in $PGF_{2\alpha}$ and GnRHa-treated CL were rapid and continuous throughout 15 min of incubation (not shown). LH did not significantly increase inositol phosphate accumulation but did increase cAMP in these incubations (Fig. 1). When compared to day-2 CL, the control levels of all inositol phosphates were increased in day-7 CL (Fig. 1). In addition, $PGF_{2\alpha}$, GnRHa and LH had no effect on accumulation of inositol phosphates in mature CL (Fig. 1). Incubations of day-7 CL with 10 mM LiCl alone exhibited tenfold increases in inositol monophosphate accumulation and approximately twofold increases in the accumulation of inositol bis- and trisphosphates (Table 1). Thus, day-7 CL had a high basal rate of inositol phospholipid metabolism.

To examine whether the enhanced inositol phospholipid metabolism observed in mature CL was due to the presence of endogenous prostaglandins or a GnRH-like compound (11), intact day-7 CL were preincubated for 3 h with 1 µM indomethacin or 100 ng/ml GnRH ANTAG. Basal inositol phosphate accumulation in indomethacin-treated CL was unchanged. Similarly, pretreatment with indomethacin did not alter inositol phosphate accumulation in the presence or absence of $PGF_{2\alpha}$ and GnRH. However, pretreatment with GnRH ANTAG for 3 h resulted in a 56% reduction in basal inositol phosphate accumulation in subsequent incubations with LiCl. Furthermore, the GnRH ANTAG pretreated CL were rendered responsive to exogenous hormones. GnRH (100 ng/ml) and $PGF_{2\alpha}$ (10 µM) provoked 2.1- and 1.7-fold increases in inositol phosphate accumulation in 15-min incubations. Co-incubation of GnRH and the GnRH ANTAG resulted in a 60% reduction of the stimulatory effect of GnRH.

In contrast to intact CL, isolated luteal cells from mature CL were responsive to treatment with LH, $PGF_{2\alpha}$ and GnRHa. Figure 2 shows that $PGF_{2\alpha}$ (1 µM) and GnRHa (100 ng/ml)

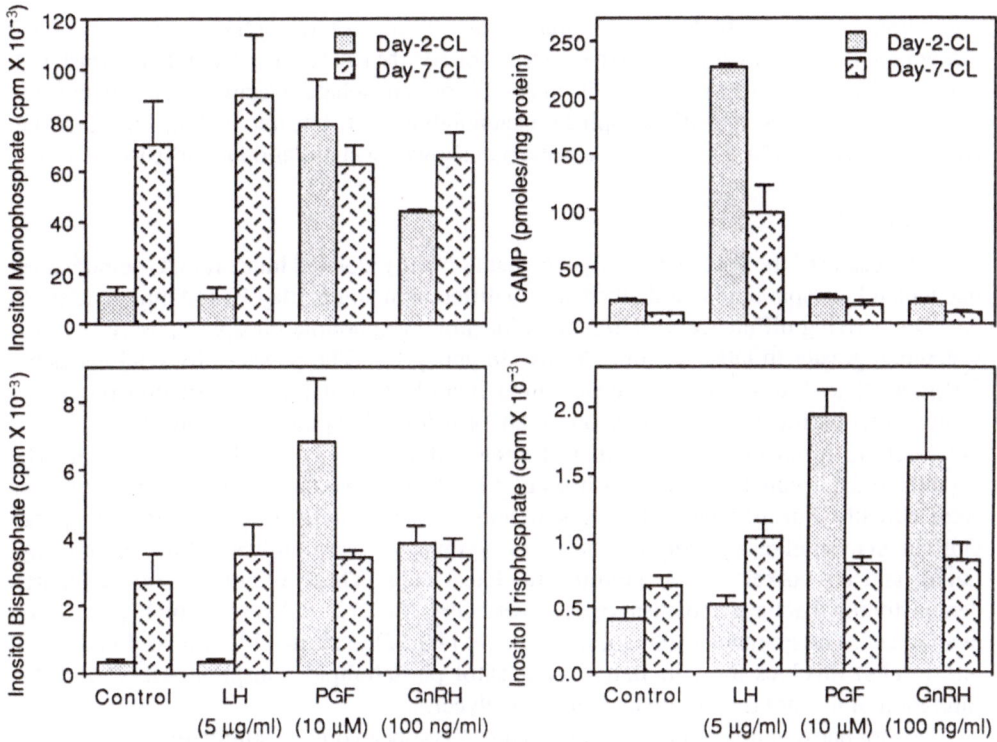

Fig. 1. Inositol phosphate accumulation in 2- and 7-day-old rat CL. After preincubation for 15 min with 10 mM LiCl, CL were incubated for 15 min with control media, LH (5 μg/ml), $PGF_{2\alpha}$ (10 μM) or GnRHa (100 ng/ml). Results are means ± SE of the averages from triplicate incubations in a representative experiment (adapted from reference 6).

provoked 6.2- and 4.6-fold increases in the accumulation of total inositol phosphates. Similar increases were observed in inositol mono-, bis- and trisphosphates in 30-min incubations. Maximal stimulatory effects on inositol phosphate accumulation were observed with 1-10 μM $PGF_{2\alpha}$ and 10-100 ng/ml GnRHa. The effects of $PGF_{2\alpha}$ and GnRH were rapid and

Table 1. Effects of LiCl on inositol phosphate accumulation
in isolated intact day-7 rat CL in vitro

[³H]inositol phosphates	-LiCl	cpm/mg protein* 10 mM LiCl	% increase
inositol monophosphate	5,374 ± 551	54,426 ± 9,643	1,013
inositol bisphosphate	509 ± 94	1,282 ± 207	252
inositol trisphosphate	267 ± 42	440 ± 77	165

Intact mature (day-7) CL were incubated for 30 min in the absence or presence of 10 mM LiCl. *Results are means ± SE of triplicate incubations (adapted from reference 6).

continuous increases in the accumulation of all inositol phosphates were observed throughout a 30-min incubation in the presence of 10 mM LiCl (not shown). In contrast, LH stimulated a small (45%) increase in inositol monophosphate accumulation but did not increase inositol bis- and trisphosphate accumulation. LH, but not $PGF_{2\alpha}$ and GnRHa, stimulated cAMP (Fig. 2) and progesterone (not shown) accumulation in these incubations.

Discussion

The results of the present investigation using freshly isolated intact rat CL demonstrate that inositol phospholipid metabolism is very different in young (day-2) and mature (day-7) CL. One striking difference was that basal inositol phospholipid phospholipase C activity was much greater in intact mature CL than in young CL. The present observations using [^{3}H]inositol to follow inositol phospholipid hydrolysis and [^{3}H]inositol phosphate accumulation confirmed our previous observations using $^{32}PO_4$ incorporation as an index of phospholipid turnover (3,7). Another striking difference was that $PGF_{2\alpha}$ and GnRHa stimulated the accumulation of [^{3}H]inositol phosphates in young CL, whereas mature CL were virtually unresponsive to hormone treatment. The stimulatory effects of $PGF_{2\alpha}$ and GnRHa on inositol phospholipid metabolism in young CL were similar to those reported by Leung and co-workers (4) in cultured rat luteal cells. These findings confirm reports demonstrating that the mechanism of action of $PGF_{2\alpha}$ (4,7,12,14-16) and GnRH (4-6,13) in ovarian cells (rat granulosa cells [5,6,13] and rat [4,7,12], porcine [14] and bovine [15,16] luteal cells) involves the stimulation of inositol phospholipid phospholipase C and the formation of inositol trisphosphate and diacylglycerol.

Inositol phospholipid metabolism in mature CL appeared to be stimulated as a result of hormonal effects in vivo which persisted in vitro. Our present results suggest that an endogenous GnRH-like compound may be responsible, at least in part, for the observed increase in phospholipase C activity. Whether the GnRH ANTAG used in these studies

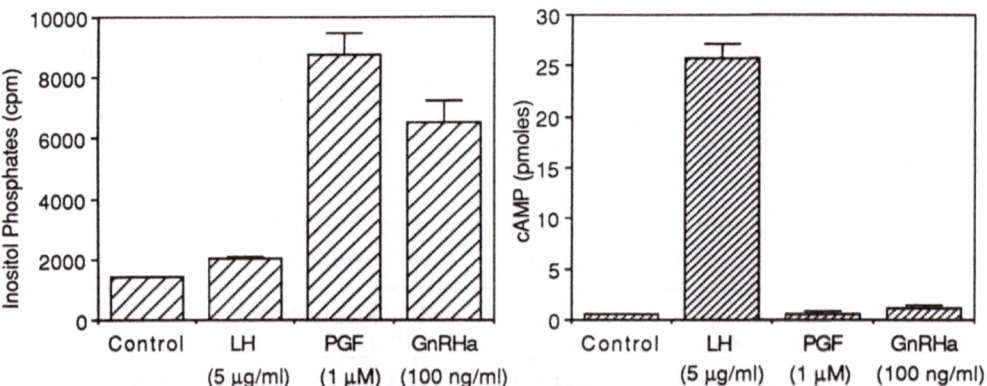

Fig. 2. Inositol phosphate and cAMP accumulation in isolated cells prepared from mature (day-7) CL. Luteal cells (3 x 10^5 cells) were preincubated for 15 min in the presence of 10 mM LiCl and further incubated for 30 min in the absence (control) or presence of LH (5 μg/ml), $PGF_{2\alpha}$ (1 μM) or GnRHa (100 ng/ml). Results are means ± SE from triplicate incubations in a representative experiment. Similar results were observed in four other experiments.

specifically blocks the action of an endogenous rat ovarian GnRH-like compound (11) remains to be established. Such a demonstration would provide strong evidence for a paracrine role of GnRH-like factors in the regulation of CL function. In contrast, the increased inositol phospholipid metabolism in mature CL did not appear to be the result of endogenous prostaglandin production. Further support for the presence of an endogenous activator of inositol phospholipid phospholipase C was provided in studies using preparations of dispersed cells from mature CL. Unlike intact mature CL, dispersed CL cell preparations responded to $PGF_{2\alpha}$ and GnRH with large increases in inositol phosphate accumulation. Additionally, LH stimulated slight increases in inositol phosphate accumulation. The process of dispersing luteal cells with collagenase presumably removed a factor(s) which was responsible for maintaining the high rate of inositol phospholipid turnover. Thus, the enhanced phospholipase C activity in mature CL may represent the ongoing response to factors which are produced in and remain within the intact CL. It also seems likely that other factors which control luteal development and function in the rat (e.g., prolactin, estrogen, insulin) may contribute to the observed changes.

The lack of effect of $PGF_{2\alpha}$ and GnRHa on inositol phospholipid metabolism in isolated mature rat CL suggests that the luteolytic actions of $PGF_{2\alpha}$ and GnRH may involve additional, as yet unidentified, mechanisms. This suggestion is supported by recent studies demonstrating that calcium mobilization (17) and protein kinase C activation (12) are not always associated with luteolytic effects in rat luteal tissues. The enhanced rate of inositol phospholipid metabolism may be related more to the high rate of steroid secretion in mature CL or to increased secretion of peptides. Alternatively, the regulation of cellular differentiation and growth are often associated with increases in inositol phospholipid metabolism (1,2) and the present changes may be an index of CL maturation.

Acknowledgments

This work was supported in part by NIH HD22248 and the Research Service of the Veterans Administration. The authors gratefully acknowledge Linda Sagun for preparation of the manuscript.

References

1. Berridge MJ. Inositol trisphosphate and diacylglycerol: two interacting second messengers. Annu Rev Biochem 1987; 56:159-93.
2. Berridge MJ. Oncogenes, inositol lipids and cellular proliferation. Bio/technology 1984; 2:541-6.
3. Davis JS. Protein kinase activity and phospholipid metabolism in rat CL during pseudopregnancy. In: Toft DO, Ryan RJ, eds. Proceedings of the Fifth Ovarian Workshop. Ovarian Workshops, Champaign, IL, 1985:409-14.
4. Leung PCK, Minegishi T, Ma F, Zhou F, Ho-Yuen B. Induction of polyphosphoinositide breakdown in rat CL by prostaglandin $F_{2\alpha}$. Endocrinology 1986; 119:12-8.
5. Ma F, Leung PCK. Luteinizing hormone-releasing hormone enhances polyphosphoinositide breakdown in rat granulosa cells. Biochem Biophys Res Commun 1985; 130:1201-8.

6. Davis JS, West LA, Farese RV. Gonadotropin-releasing hormone (GnRH) rapidly stimulates the formation of inositol phosphates and diacylglycerol in rat granulosa cells: further evidence for the involvement of Ca^{2+} and protein kinase C in the action of GnRH. Endocrinology 1986; 118:2561-71.

7. Lahav M, West LA, Davis JS. Effects of prostaglandin $F_{2\alpha}$ and a gonadotropin-releasing hormone agonist on inositol phospholipid metabolism in isolated rat CL of various ages. Endocrinology 1988; 123:1044-52.

8. Luborsky JL, Behrman HR. Isolation and functional aspects of free luteal cells. Methods Enzymol 1985; 109:298-316.

9. Lowry OH, Rosebrough NJ, Farr AL, Randall RJ. Protein measurement with the Folin phenol reagent. J Biol Chem 1951; 193:265-75.

10. Davis JS, Weakland LL, Farese RV, West LA. Luteinizing hormone increases inositol trisphosphate and cytosolic free Ca^{2+} in isolated bovine luteal cells. J Biol Chem 1987; 262:8515-21.

11. Aten RF, Williams AT, Behrman HR. Ovarian gonadotropin-releasing hormone-like protein(s): demonstration and characterization. Endocrinology 1986; 118:961-7.

12. Lahav M, Davis JS, Rennert H. Mechanism of the luteolytic action of prostaglandin $F_{2\alpha}$ in the rat. J Reprod Fertil (in press).

13. Davis JS, Weakland LL, West LA, Farese RV. Luteinizing hormone stimulates the formation of inositol trisphosphate and cyclic AMP in rat granulosa cells. Biochem J 1986; 238:597-604.

14. Veldhuis JD. Prostaglandin $F_{2\alpha}$ initiates polyphoshatidylinositol hydrolysis and membrane translocation of protein kinase C in swine ovarian cells. Biochem Biophys Res Commun 1987; 149:112-7.

15. Davis JS, Weakland LL, Weiland DA, Farese RV, West LA. Prostaglandin $F_{2\alpha}$ stimulates phosphatidylinositol 4,5-bisphosphate hydrolysis and mobilizes intracellular Ca^{2+} in bovine luteal cells. Proc Natl Acad Sci USA 1987; 84:3728-32.

16. Davis JS, Alila HW, West LA, Corradino RA, Hansel W. Acute effects of prostaglandin $F_{2\alpha}$ on inositol phospholipid hydrolysis in the large and small cells of the bovine CL. Mol Cell Endocrinol 1988 (in press).

17. Pepperell JR, Behrman HR. Evidence that mobilization of intracellular calcium is not the sole mediator of $PGF_{2\alpha}$ in rat luteal cells. Biol Reprod 1988; 38(suppl 1):103.

46

Estradiol-Induced Synthesis and Translation of Specific Proteins in the Corpus Luteum

M. P. McLean, I. Khan, T. K. Puryear, and G. Gibori

Department of Physiology and Biophysics, University of Illinois
College of Medicine, Chicago, IL 60612

Introduction

Throughout pregnancy in the rat, several hormones control luteal cell function (1). Following nidation, locally formed estradiol becomes essential for the activation of the steps necessary for optimal steroid production and for the growth and survival of the corpus luteum (1). Estradiol stimulation of luteal growth is accompanied by a remarkable proliferation of vascular endothelial cells. However, in contrast to its effect on other target cells, estradiol does not elicit luteal cell multiplication but rather cell hypertrophy and a marked increase in protein synthesis. Although the action of estradiol on overall protein synthesis is dramatic, its effect on such diverse parameters as steroidogenesis and vascularization strongly suggests that this steroid may stimulate specific proteins which mediate its broad spectrum of action.

The aim of this investigation was to examine whether estradiol induces the synthesis of specific proteins in luteal cell subcellular fractions and to examine these estradiol-regulated translational products.

Materials and Methods

Pregnant Sprague-Dawley rats (Holtzman Co., Madison, WI) were hypophysectomized and hysterectomized on day 12 of pregnancy as previously described (2). Rats were treated with or without a 1 cm estradiol implant at the time of surgery, and 72 h later corpora lutea were removed. For the radiolabelling experiments, minced luteal tissue (50-100 mg) was incubated in 2 ml RPMI 1640 medium (Flow Laboratories, McLean, VA) containing 1/10 the normal methionine concentration supplemented with 100 μCi/ml ^{35}S-methionine (Trans-label ^{35}S-Met, ICN Radiochemicals, Irvine, CA). Incubation at 37°C in 95% O_2-5% CO_2 was stopped after 8 h and the tissue and medium were separated. Luteal tissue was homogenized in 20 volumes buffer containing 250 mM sucrose, 50 mM HEPES, 2 mM EDTA, 1 mM PMSF and 1 mM DTT (pH 7.4), and subcellular fractions were isolated by differential centrifugation (5). Radiolabelled proteins were quantified by trichloroacetic acid precipitation (6) and separated on 7.5-15% gradient SDS-polyacrylamide gels (7). Gels were infiltrated with 1 M sodium salicylate (8) and, following fluorography, quantified by densitometry. Nonlabelled luteal proteins were quantified (9) and examined by SDS-polyacrylamide gel electrophoresis (SDS-PAGE). For the in vitro translation experiment, total RNA was extracted using the method of Chirgwin (10) from corpora lutea of hypophysectomized and hysterectomized rats treated with or without estradiol for 3 days. RNA was translated using a reticulocyte lysate kit (Promega, Madison, WI) and ^{35}S-methionine (Amersham, Arlington Heights, IL). Radiolabelled translated proteins were separated by SDS-PAGE for fluorography.

Results

Corpora lutea exposed to estradiol in vivo hypertrophied, as noted by the increase in luteal weight (4.1 ± 0.14 mg vs. 2.2 ± 0.06 mg in nonestradiol-treated rats). Estradiol treatment in vivo also increased luteal incorporation of ^{35}S-methionine (26.2 ± 6.2% vs. 12.7 ± 1.8% for nonestradiol-treated rats). Although no differences in nuclear synthesized proteins were found, estradiol increased specific luteal protein synthesis in all other cellular compartments (Fig. 1).

Estradiol stimulated the synthesis of 3 mitochondrial proteins with molecular weights of 80, 50, and 32 kd (Figures 1 and 2). The 80 kd and 32 kd mitochondrial proteins were 2.1- and 2.5-fold higher in luteal cells of rats treated with estradiol. The 50 kd protein was noted mainly in the Coomassie blue stained gels (Fig. 1). In the microsomal fraction, estradiol enhanced 100, 80, and 32 kd proteins (Fig. 1, 2). These proteins were elevated 2.3-, 1.6-, and 1.9-fold, respectively. Estradiol stimulated the production of luteal proteins with molecular weights of 60, 50 and 14 kd in the cytosolic fraction (Fig. 1, 2). This hormone also affected markedly the secretion of newly synthesized proteins with molecular weights of 60, 50 and 14 kd (Fig. 1). These proteins were stimulated 1.7-, 1.6- and 1.3-fold by estradiol treatment. Luteal tissue not exposed to estradiol displayed a significant enhancement in a cytosolic 38 kd protein, suggesting that estradiol may prevent the induction of this protein.

Changes in RNA populations in response to estradiol were assayed by in vitro translation and subsequent gel electrophoresis of samples containing equivalent amounts of incorporated radioactivity. Estradiol increased the RNA encoding 3 specific proteins (50, 48 and 32 kd; Fig. 3) by 1.8-, 1.7- and 2.5-fold, respectively.

Discussion

As expected, estradiol enhanced overall luteal protein synthesis as reflected in the increased luteal weight and amino acid incorporation. In addition, estradiol stimulated the synthesis of several specific proteins which were localized within several luteal subcellular compartments or secreted into the incubation medium. Estradiol treatment in vivo did not appear to alter protein synthesis localized to the nuclear compartment, while all other luteal fractions contained estradiol-induced newly synthesized proteins. The precise biological function for these estradiol-induced proteins have yet to be determined. However, it is quite likely that these proteins are related to estradiol's action on luteal cell growth, vascularization and/or steroidogenesis.

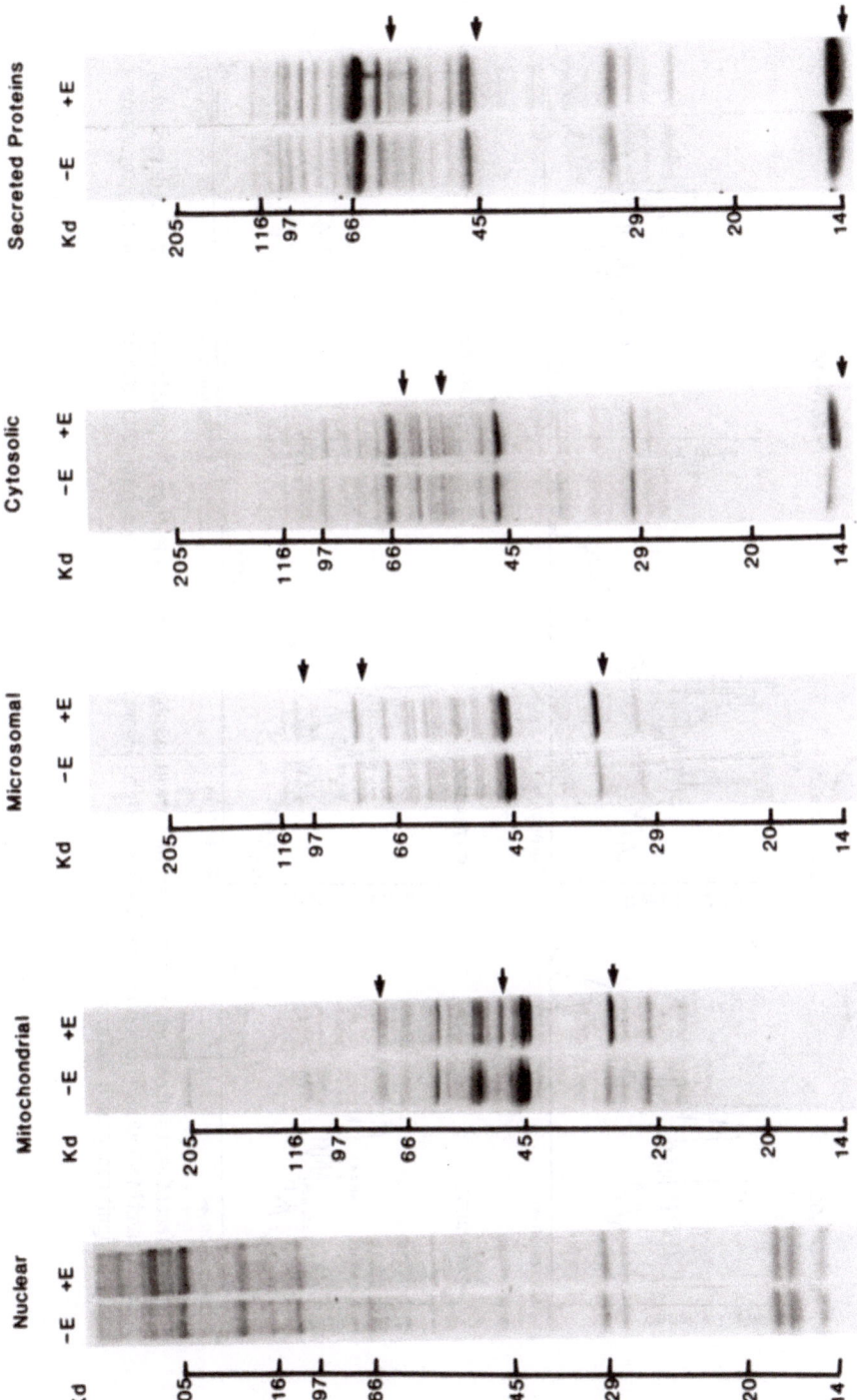

Fig. 1. Effect of estradiol on the luteal subcellular protein profile. Corpora lutea were obtained from rats treated as described. Nuclear, mitochondrial, microsomal and cytosolic compartments were separated by differential centrifugation. Luteal proteins, either 50 µg or 100,000 cpm-secreted proteins, were separated by SDS-PAGE (7.5-15% gradient gel) and stained with Coomassie blue. Arrows indicate the estradiol-enhanced proteins.

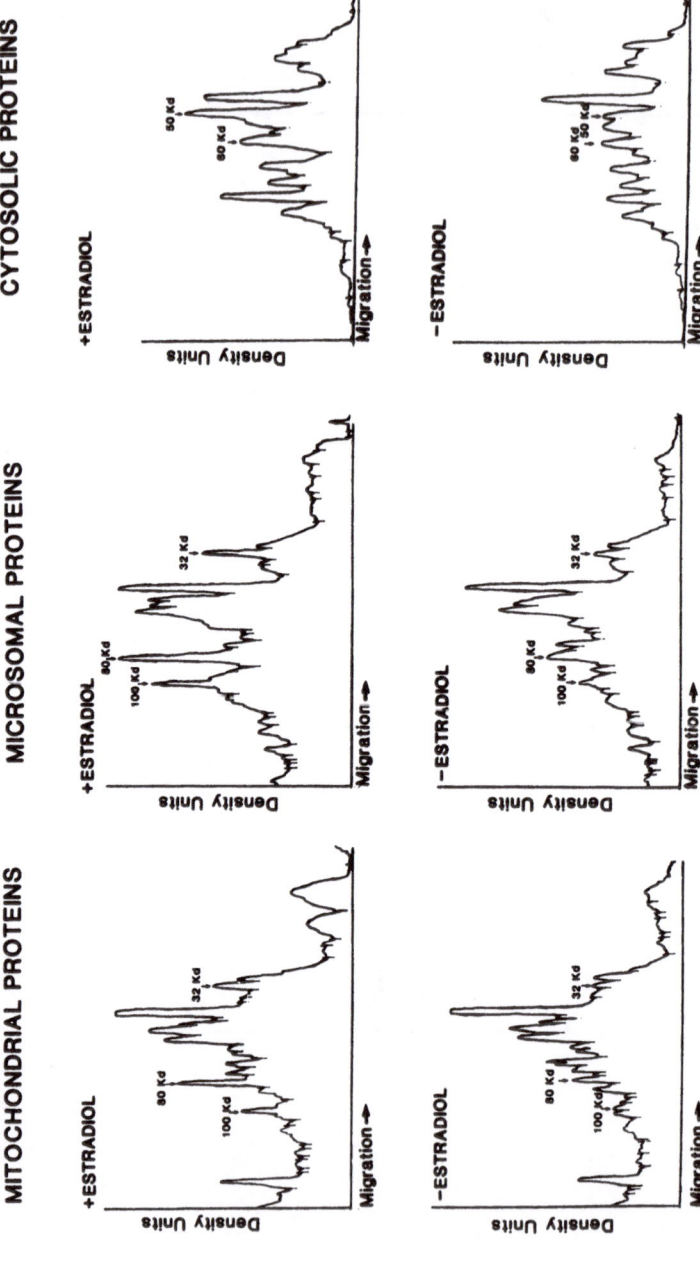

Fig. 2. Effect of estradiol on luteal synthesized proteins within subcellular compartmenys. Corpora lutea were treated as described in Materials and Methods. Radiolabelled proteins (100,000 cpm) were identified by fluorography and quantified by densitometry. Arrows indicate significant protein differences.

TRANSLATED PROTEINS

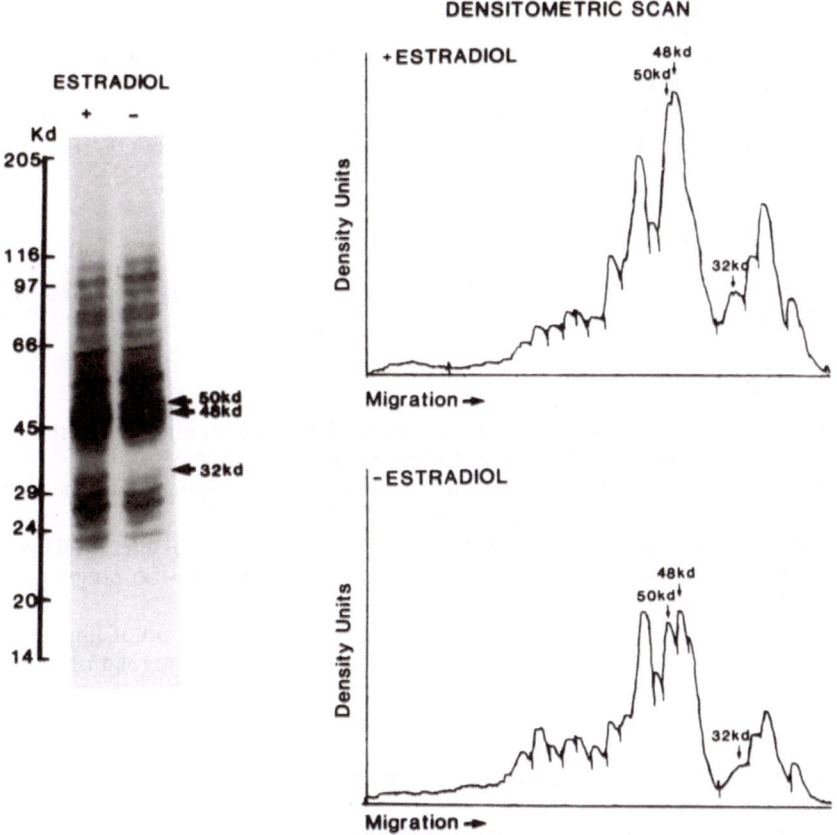

Fig. 3. Comparison of protein synthesis in vitro by luteal total RNA isolated from rats treated for 3 days with estradiol or vehicle.

In MCF-7 human breast cancer cells, estradiol has been reported to increase both a 52 kd (11) and a 32 kd protein (12). The 52 kd-secreted glycoprotein is believed to have either autocrine or paracrine growth-stimulating action in MCF-7 cells (11), while no function has been assigned to the 32 kd protein (12). It is not known whether these proteins are similar to the 50 kd mitochondrial and 32 kd microsomal luteal proteins reported in the present study. The 32 kd microsomal protein appeared as the major estradiol-induced protein in the corpus luteum. This increase within the mitochondrial fraction was variable and may be due to contamination by microsomal proteins. A marked increase in the synthesis of this protein was observed in both ^{35}S-methionine incorporation and in vitro MRNA translation. This protein may, therefore, represent a protein marker for the action of estradiol in the corpus luteum. Of great interest was the finding that estradiol enhances both the synthesis and secretion of a 14 kd protein. Recent investigations in our laboratory suggest that the radical vascular changes that take place in the capillary wreath of the corpus luteum after estradiol treatment appear to be mediated by basic fibroblast growth factor (bFGF). Estradiol treatment dramatically enhances immunosayable 14 kd bFGF in the luteal cell. Whether the 14 kd protein whose synthesis is markedly affected by estradiol is bFGF remains to be investigated.

Acknowledgments

This research was supported by NIH grant HD 11119. MPM was supported by NRSA fellowship HD 6982.

References

1. Gibori G, Khan I, Warshaw ML, et al. Placental derived regulators and the complex control of luteal cell function. Recent Prog Horm Res 1988; 44:377-429.
2. Gibori G, Keyes PL. Role of intraluteal estrogen in the regulation of the rat corpus luteum during pregnancy. Endocrinology 1978; 102:1176-82.
3. Gibori G, Chen Y-DI, Khan I, Azhar S, Reaven GM. Regulation of luteal cell lipoprotein receptors, sterol contents, and steroidogenesis by estradiol in the pregnant rat. Endocrinology 1984; 114:607-17.
4. Khan I, Sridaran R, Johnson DC, Gibori G. Selective stimulation of luteal androgen biosynthesis by luteinizing hormone: comparison of hormonal regulation of $P450_{17\alpha}$ in corpora lutea and follicles. Endocrinology 1987; 121:1312-9.
5. Fleischner S, Kervina M. Subcellular fractionation of rat liver. Methods Enzymol 1974; 3:6-41.
6. Hubbard AL, Cohn ZA. Externally disposed plasma membrane proteins. J Cell Biol 1975; 64:438-60.
7. Laemmli UK. Cleavage of structural proteins during the assembly of the head of bacteriophage T_4. Nature 1970; 227:680-5.
8. Chamberlain JP. Fluorographic detection of radioactivity in polyacrylamide gels with the water-soluble fluor, sodium salicylate. Anal Biochem 1979; 95:132-5.
9. Bradford MN. A rapid and sensitive method for the quantitation of microgram quantities of protein utilizing the principle of protein-dye binding. Anal Biochem 1976; 72:248-54.
10. Chirgwin JM, Przbyla AC, MacDonald RJ, Rutter WJ. Isolation of biologically active ribonucleic acid from sources enriched in ribonuclease. Biochemistry 1979; 18:5294-9.
11. Vignon F, Capony F, Chambon M, Freiss G, Garcia M, Rochefort H. Autocrine growth stimulation of the MCF-7 breast cancer cells by estrogen-regulated 52 K protein. Endocrinology 1986; 118:1537-45.
12. Sheen YY, Katzenellenbogen BS. Antiestrogen stimulation of the production of a 37,000 molecular weight secreted protein and estrogen stimulation of the production of a 32,000 molecular weight secreted protein in MCF-7 human breast cancer cells. Endocrinology 1987; 120:1140-51.

47

Dual Activation of Adenylate Cyclase and Phospholipase C by Prostaglandins of the E and I Series in Bovine Luteal Cells

Leigh A. West, Laura L. Weakland, Robert A. Duncan, and John S. Davis

Departments of Internal Medicine and Pharmacology and Therapeutics, University of South Florida and J. A. Haley Veterans Hospital, Tampa, FL 33612

Introduction

Maintenance of the corpus luteum (CL) is dependent on a balance between a number of luteotropic and luteolytic factors (recently reviewed in references 1 and 2). Prostaglandins (PG) are important paracrine and endocrine factors which control CL function. Prostaglandins of the E and I series stimulate steroidogenesis in bovine luteal tissues (2-4), presumably via their ability to activate adenylate cyclase (4,5). Thus, their actions are analogous to the stimulatory actions of luteinizing hormone (LH) on adenylate cyclase and progesterone synthesis. Although $PGF_{2\alpha}$ has a luteolytic effect in vivo, $PGF_{2\alpha}$ also stimulates progesterone synthesis in incubations of cells (2) or slices (3,6) of bovine luteal tissue in vitro. This luteotropic action of $PGF_{2\alpha}$, however, does not involve the activation of adenylate cyclase (4) or an increase in cAMP (4,7) in bovine luteal tissue. Instead, $PGF_{2\alpha}$ stimulates the inositol phospholipid-phospholipase C transmembrane signalling system (7-10). This system is coupled to increases in intracellular calcium and protein kinase C activation (8,10,11). Recent studies also show that LH activates the inositol phospholipid-phospholipase C signalling system in bovine luteal cells (12,13). The present studies were performed to examine whether the luteotropic prostaglandins of the E and I series also activate this transmembrane signalling system.

Materials and Methods

Corpora lutea were obtained from cows during early pregnancy, sliced, and dispersed with collagenase as previously described (13). Luteal cell preparations (1-1.5 x 10^7 cells/ml) were preincubated for 3 h in medium containing (50 µCi/ml) myo[2-^{3}H]inositol under an atmosphere of 95% O_2/5% CO_2 at 37°C. After this relabeling period, the cells were washed and incubations were performed in triplicate with 10^6 viable cells, in a final volume of 0.5 ml of medium 199 containing 25 mM Hepes and 0.1% bovine serum albumin under an atmosphere of 95% O_2/5% CO_2, at 37°C. After a 15-min preincubation with 10 mM LiCl, control media or hormones were added and the incubations were continued for up to 30 min. Incubations were terminated by the addition of 0.5 ml ice-cold 10% trichloroacetic acid. [^{3}H]Inositol phosphates were purified on columns of BioRad AG 1-X8 ion-exchange resin (13) or high performance liquid chromatography employing a Partisil SAX column and a linear gradient (0.01-1 M) of ammonium phosphate buffered with phosphoric acid to pH 3.8 (14). In other experiments for measurement of progesterone and cAMP levels, incubations of luteal cells (10^5 cells) lasted 2 h. Isobutylmethylxanthine (100 μM) was included in incubations for cAMP measurements but was omitted from incubations for progesterone since preliminary experiments indicated that isobutylmethylxanthine blocked the stimulatory effects of prostaglandins on progesterone accumulation. Progesterone and cAMP were measured by radioimmunoassay (13).

Results

Table 1 shows that $PGF_{2\alpha}$ and $PGF_{1\alpha}$ stimulate the accumulation of inositol mono-, bis- and trisphosphates in bovine luteal cells. Maximal stimulatory effects of $PGF_{2\alpha}$ on inositol phosphate accumulation were observed at 1-10 μM while maximal effects of $PGF_{1\alpha}$ were observed at 10-100 μM. Analysis of various isomers of inositol phosphates by high performance liquid chromatography revealed the presence of inositol 1,4,5- and 1,3,4-tris-phosphates, inositol 1,3,4,5-tetrakisphosphate, inositol 1,3- and 1,4-bisphosphates and inositol 1- and 4-monophosphates (14). Inositol 1,4,5-trisphosphate was the initial product formed after addition of $PGF_{2\alpha}$. Inositol 1,4,5-trisphosphate was formed continually over 30 min of incubation but the 1,3,4-trisphosphate isomer was the [^{3}H]inositol trisphosphate that accumulated in $PGF_{2\alpha}$-stimulated luteal cells.

Tables 1 and 2 show that the luteotropic prostaglandins PGE_1, PGE_2 and carba-prostacyclin (PGI_2, Cayman Chemical) stimulate accumulation of inositol mono-, bis- and trisphosphates in isolated bovine luteal cells. The actions of this group of prostaglandins were also rapid and continuous over 30 min of incubation (not shown). Maximal stimulatory effects of PGE_2 and PGE_1 were observed with prostaglandin concentrations of 10-100 μM and 500 μM, respectively. The maximal response to PGI_2 was observed at 10-100 μM. However, at maximally effective concentrations, PGI_2 was only 70% as effective as $PGF_{2\alpha}$ or PGE_2. While the concentration response relationships between prostaglandins were different, the concentration response relationships for inositol mono-, bis-, and trisphosphate accumulation in response to a given prostaglandin were similar.

Figure 1 shows the effects of prostaglandins on cAMP and progesterone accumulation in 2-h incubations of isolated bovine luteal cells. $PGF_{2\alpha}$ had no effect on cAMP accumulation at concentrations of 0.01-10 μM, but slight increases were observed at 100 μM. $PGF_{2\alpha}$ also stimulated twofold increases in progesterone accumulation. $PGF_{1\alpha}$ slightly increased progesterone at high concentrations (100 μM) but had little effect on cAMP accumulation. PGE_2 (100 μM) stimulated a 47-fold increase in cAMP accumulation and a 3.2-fold increase in progesterone synthesis. In comparison, PGE_1 was slightly less effective than PGE_2, provoking 42-fold and 2.7-fold increases in cAMP and progesterone accumulation, respectively. PGI_2 also increased cAMP (22-fold increase) and progesterone (1.9-fold increase) in

Table 1. Effects of LH and $PGF_{2\alpha}$, $PGF_{1\alpha}$ and PGE_1 on inositol phosphate accumulation in bovine luteal cells

Treatment	[^{3}H]Inositol Phosphates (cpm/10^6 cells)*		
	Inositol Monophosphate	Inositol Bisphosphate	Inositol Trisphosphate
Control	6,316 (109)	365 (10)	239 (9)
LH (1 µg/ml)	11,817 (120)	1,711 (42)	553 (20)
$PGF_{2\alpha}$ (10 µM)	17,879 (160)	1,573 (34)	677 (25)
$PGF_{1\alpha}$ (100 µM)	17,210 (211)	1,575 (20)	784 (37)
PGE_1 (100 µM)	14,088 (875)	835 (34)	475 (13)

Isolated bovine luteal cells were preincubated for 15 min in 0.5 ml of Medium 199 containing 0.1% bovine serum albumin and 10 mM LiCl. Control media or treatments were added and the incubations were continued for an additional 30 min. *These values are the means (SE), n=3.

bovine luteal cells. In contrast to the effects of prostaglandins in these incubations, LH (1 µg/ml) provoked large increases in cAMP accumulation (1800-fold) and a 4.8-fold increase in progesterone accumulation.

Discussion

The results of this study demonstrate that the luteotropic prostaglandins PGE_2, PGE_1, and PGI_2 stimulate the inositol phospholipid-phospholipase C and the adenylate cyclase transmembrane signalling systems in bovine luteal cells. The rank order for the stimulatory action of prostaglandins on inositol phosphate accumulation was $PGF_{2\alpha} > PGF_{1\alpha} > PGE_2 > PGI_2 > PGE_1$. The rank order for the stimulatory actions on cAMP accumulation was $PGE_2 > PGE_1 > PGI_2 > PGF_{2\alpha} > PGF_{1\alpha}$. The rank order for the stimulatory actions of pros-

Table 2. Effects of LH and $PGF_{2\alpha}$, PGE_2 and PGI_2 on inositol phosphate accumulation in bovine luteal cells

Treatment	[^{3}H]Inositol Phosphates (cpm/10^6 cells)*		
	Inositol Monophosphate	Inositol Bisphosphate	Inositol Trisphosphate
Control	4,205 (344)	199 (7)	140 (8)
LH (1 µg/ml)	17,846 (369)	2,712 (127)	1,155 (151)
$PGF_{2\alpha}$ (10 µM)	23,085 (460)	2,509 (127)	1,414 (84)
PGE_2 (100 µM)	22,908 (437)	1,776 (216)	937 (21)
PGI_2 (100 µM)	16,875 (227)	1,393 (37)	745 (39)

Isolated bovine luteal cells were incubated as described in Table 1. *These values are the means (SE), n=3.

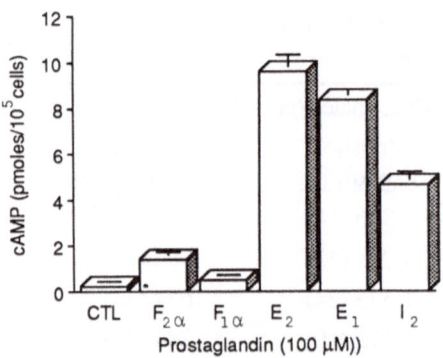 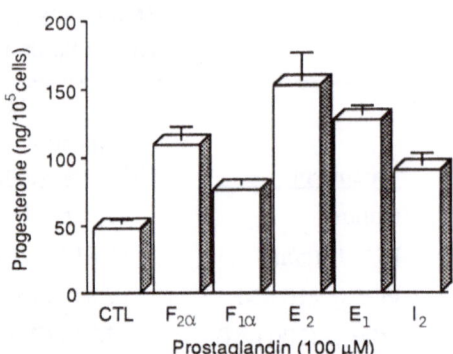

Fig. 1. Effects of LH and prostaglandins on cAMP and progesterone accumulation in bovine luteal cells. Bovine luteal cells were incubated for 2 h in the presence of control medium, LH or a variety of prostaglandins. Incubations for cAMP measurements contained 100 μM isobutylmethylxanthine. These values are the means (SE) of triplicate incubations in a representative experiment.

taglandins on progesterone accumulation was similar to that observed for cAMP accumulation. This observation is in keeping with the well-known stimulatory effects of cAMP on steroid synthesis in the CL. Activation of protein kinase C can also stimulate progesterone secretion alone (2,15) or augment the steroidogenic response to suboptimal concentrations of LH (15). The augmentation of steroidogenesis in the presence of small increases in cAMP (as observed for PGE_2 and PGI_2) may be an important response to hormones which activate the inositol phospholipid-phospholipase C transmembrane signalling system.

In addition to their stimulatory effects on steroid secretion, prostaglandins stimulate the secretion of protein hormones from the CL. Taylor and Clark have shown that $PGF_{2\alpha}$ (16), PGE_2 (16) and PGI_2 (17) stimulate relaxin release from porcine luteal cells. Abdelgadir et al. (18) recently reported that $PGF_{2\alpha}$ simulates the release of oxytocin from slices of bovine CL. Secretory events are closely coupled to calcium mobilization and protein kinase C activation in many tissues (11). It seems likely that the effects of prostaglandins on protein hormone secretion are mediated by the inositol phospholipid-phospholipase C transmembrane signalling system.

The results of these studies suggest that the ability of prostaglandins, $PGF_{2\alpha}$ in particular, to induce functional luteolysis requires more than the activation of phospholipase C and associated increases in intracellular calcium. Each of the prostaglandins examined stimulated the formation of inositol trisphosphate and mobilization of intracellular calcium (not shown). These responses were associated with increases in progesterone secretion in isolated bovine luteal cells. Recent studies by Pepperell and Behrman (19) and Lahav et al. (20,21) also suggest that phospholipase C activation and calcium mobilization are not sufficient to explain the luteolytic action of $PGF_{2\alpha}$ in the rat CL.

Acknowledgments

This work was supported, in part, by NIH HD22248 and the Research Service of the Veterans Administration. The authors gratefully acknowledge Linda Sagun for preparation of the manuscript.

References

1. Niswender GD, Schwall RH, Fitz TA, Farin CE, Sawyer HR. Regulation of luteal function in domestic ruminants: new concepts. Recent Prog Horm Res 1985; 141:101-51.
2. Hansel W, Dowd JP. New concepts on the control of the corpus luteum function. J Reprod Fertil 1986; 78:755-68.
3. Speroff L, Ramwell PW. Prostaglandin stimulation of in vitro progesterone synthesis. J Clin Endocrinology 1970; 30:345-50.
4. Marsh JM. The effect of prostaglandins on the adenyl cyclase of the bovine corpus luteum. Ann NY Acad Sci 1970; 180:416-25.
5. Abramowitz J, Birnbaumer L. Prostacyclin activation of adenylyl cyclase in rabbit corpus luteum membranes: comparison with 6-keto prostaglandin $F_{1\alpha}$ and prostaglandin E_1. Biol Reprod 1979; 21:609-16.
6. Hixon JE, Hansel W. Effects of prostaglandin $F_{-2\alpha}$, estradiol and luteinizing hormone in dispersed cell preparations of bovine corpora lutea. In: Channing CP, Marsh JM, eds. Ovarian follicular and corpus luteum function, 1979:613-20.
7. Davis JS, Alila HW, West LA, Corradino RA, Hansel W. Acute effects of prostaglandin $F_{2\alpha}$ on inositol phospholipid hydrolysis in the large and small cells of the bovine CL. Mol Cell Endocrinol 1988; 85:43-50.
8. Davis JS, Weakland LL, Weiland DA, Farese RV, West LA. Prostaglandin $F_{2\alpha}$ stimulates phosphatidylinositol 4,5-bisphosphate hydrolysis and mobilizes intracellular Ca^{2+} in bovine luteal cells. Proc Natl Acad Sci USA 1987; 84:3728-32.
9. Leung PCK, Minegishi T, Ma F, Zhou F, Ho-Yuen B. Induction of polyphosphoinositide breakdown in rat CL by prostaglandin $F_{2\alpha}$. Endocrinology 1986; 119:12-8.
10. Veldhuis JD. Prostaglandin $F_{2\alpha}$ initiates polyphosphatidylinositol hydrolysis and membrane translocation of protein kinase C in swine ovarian cells. Biochem Biophy Res Commun 1987; 149:112-7.
11. Berridge MJ. Inositol trisphosphate and diacylglycerol: two interacting second messengers. Annu Rev Biochem 1987; 56:159-93.
12. Davis JS, Farese RV, March JM. Stimulation of phospholipid labeling and steroidogenesis by luteinizing hormone in isolated bovine luteal cells. Endocrinology 1981; 109:469-75.
13. Davis JS, Weakland LL, Farese RV, West LA. Luteinizing hormone increases inositol trisphosphate and cytosolic free Ca^{2+} in isolated bovine luteal cells. J Biol Chem 1987; 262:8515-21.
14. Duncan RA, West LA, Weakland LL, Davis JS. Rapid increases in inositol 1,4,5-trisphosphate and inositol 1,3,4,5-tetrakisphosphate in agonist-stimulated bovine luteal cells: effects of $PGF_{2\alpha}$ [Abstract]. Abstract 951, Proceedings of the 70th Annual Meeting of the Endocrine Society, 1988; 258.
15. Brunswig B, Mukhopadhyay AK, Budnick LT, Bohnet HG, Leidenberger FA. Phorbol ester stimulates progesterone production by isolated bovine luteal cells. Endocrinology 1936; 118:743-9.
16. Taylor MJ, Clark CL. Detection of relaxin release by porcine luteal cells using a reverse hemolytic plaque assay: effect of prostaglandins E_2 and $F_{2\alpha}$, human chorionic gonadotropin and oxytocin. Biol Reprod 1987; 37:377-84.
17. Taylor MJ, Clark CL. Prostacyclin stimulates relaxin release from cultured porcine luteal cells. Biol Reprod 1987; 37:1241-7.

18. Abdelgadir SE, Swanson LV, Oldfield JE, Stormshak F. Prostaglandin $F_{2\alpha}$-induced release of oxytocin from bovine corpora lutea in vitro. Biol Reprod 1987; 37:550-5.

19. Pepperell JR, Behrman HR. Evidence that mobilization of intracellular calcium is not the sole mediator of $PGF_{2\alpha}$ in rat luteal cells. Biol Reprod 1988; 38(suppl 1):103.

20. Lahav M, Davis JS, Rennert H. Mechanism of the luteolytic action of prostaglandin $F_{2\alpha}$ in the rat. J Reprod Fertil (in press).

21. Lahav M, West LA, Davis JS. Effects of prostaglandin $F_{2\alpha}$ and a gonadotropin-releasing hormone agonist on inositol phospholipid metabolism in isolated rat CL of various ages. Endocrinology 1988; 123:1044-52.

48

The Steroidogenic Response of Large and Small Luteal Cells to Dibutyryl cAMP and 25-OH-Cholesterol

Carol J. Smith and R. Sridaran

Department of Physiology, Morehouse School of Medicine
Atlanta, Georgia 30310

Abstract. The mammalian corpus luteum consists of two major types of steroidogenic cells based upon size and histological characteristics. In this study, large (>22 μ) and small (12-21 μ) luteal cells from day 8 pregnant rats were separated by elutriation after enzyme dissociation. Aliquots of cells were incubated for 4 h at 37°C in Medium 199 (control), medium plus dibutyryl cAMP (cAMP) at 0.5 mM or 5 mM, or medium plus 10 μg/ml 25-OH-cholesterol. Production of progesterone, testosterone, and estradiol was measured by radioimmunoassay (RIA). Both cell types showed an increase in progesterone and estradiol synthesis when incubated with cAMP; however, the large luteal cells responded to a tenfold lower dose (0.5 mM) of cAMP than did the small cells which required 5 mM for stimulation. CAMP (5 mM) also resulted in an increase of testosterone release from small luteal cells. Progesterone synthesis was enhanced by 25-OH-cholesterol in the large luteal cells. These results suggest that the two cell types differ functionally with respect to steroidogenesis during pregnancy, and that the large luteal cells may be a major source of progesterone production.

Introduction

During early pregnancy, the corpus luteum of the rat produces testosterone in response to luteinizing hormone (LH) (1). Testosterone is then aromatized within the corpus luteum to estradiol (2), and estradiol enhances progesterone synthesis (3,4). Progesterone is necessary for the maintenance of pregnancy (5).

The corpus luteum of the pregnant rat consists of two types of steroidogenic cells based upon size and histological features (6). Small luteal cells are characterized by a size of 12-21 μ and an irregularly shaped nucleus with dense heterochromatin lining the periphery of the nucleus (6,7). Large luteal cells are >22 μ and possess a rounded nucleus with dispersed chromatin (6,7). Both large and small luteal cells contain steroidogenic organelles.

One study utilizing the pregnant rat (6) and several other studies using domestic ruminants (5) have indicated that the two types of luteal cells may differ functionally as well as histologically. In this study, we examined how each type of luteal cell in the pregnant rat responds to substrates and the secretagogue, dibutyryl cAMP, in the production of steroid hormones.

Materials and Methods

Timed-pregnant Sprague-Dawley rats were obtained from Holtzman Co. (Madison, WI), and housed at 23-25°C with a 14-h light/10-h dark photoperiod. On day 8 of pregnancy (with day 1 as day of insemination), the ovaries were dissected out while the rats were under ether anesthesia. The corpora lutea were removed, cleaned of any adhering follicles with fine-tipped forceps and placed in Medium 199 (GIBCO) gassed with 95% O_2/5% CO_2. After all of the corpora lutea were removed, the incubation medium was changed to Hank's Balanced Salt Solution without Ca^{++}, Mg^{++}, to which collagenase (50 U/ml), dispase (2.4 U/ml), and DNase (200 U/ml) were added.

The methodology employed for enzyme incubation and tissue dissociation followed the basic procedures by Nelson and Khan (6). After the tissues were dissociated into cells, the cells were separated by elutriation using the same parameters as used by Fitz et al. (8). For each cell type, cells were counted with a hemacytometer and viability determined after incubation in 0.4% trypan blue. Aliquots of approximately 10^5 cells were incubated as cell suspensions for 4 h at 37°C in Medium 199. Synthesis of progesterone and testosterone was measured by RIA as previously described (4,1). Estradiol-17β was measured by a double-antibody RIA kit produced by Diagnostic Products Corp. (Los Angeles, CA). The sensitivities of the assays were as follows: progesterone, 0.025 ng/, testosterone, 5 pg/, estradiol 5 pg/assay tube.

Results

In large luteal cells, progesterone synthesis was enhanced by 0.5 mM dibutyryl CAMP or 10 µg/ml 25-OH-cholesterol (Fig. 1). Estradiol production also increased when large luteal cells were incubated with 0.5 mM dibutyryl CAMP (Fig. 2).

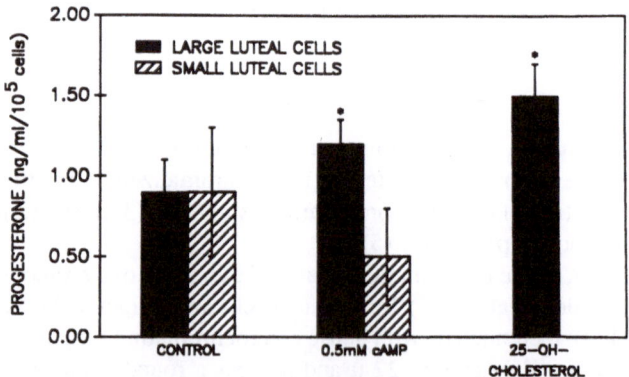

Fig. 1. Progesterone synthesis by separated large and small luteal cells after incubation with 0.5 mM cAMP or 10 µg/ml 25-OH-cholesterol. Shown are means ± SEM.

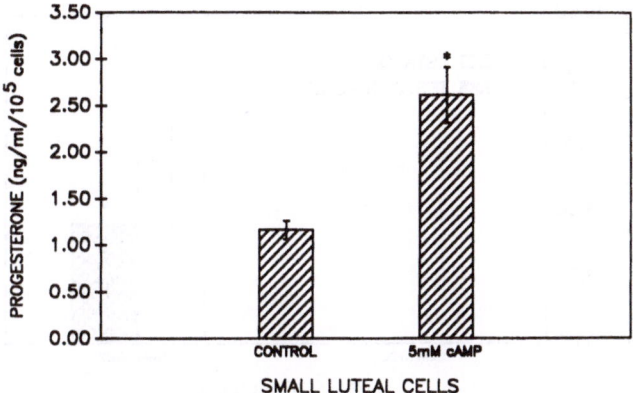

Fig. 2. Estradiol and testosterone production by large luteal cells after incubation with 0.5 mM cAMP. Shown are means ± SEM.

Small luteal cells did not respond to 0.5 mM dibutyryl cAMP (Fig. 1). However, production of progesterone and estradiol was stimulated with a tenfold higher dose of dibutyryl cAMP (5 mM) (Fig. 3 and 4).

While 0.5 mM dibutyryl cAMP did not stimulate testosterone release in either cell type, a dose of 5 mM resulted in an increase in testosterone secretion in small luteal cells (Fig. 4).

Discussion

Although both cell types appear steroidogenic, the role each plays in the production of testosterone, estradiol, and progesterone may vary. Dibutyryl cAMP stimulates estradiol and progesterone production in both cell types, but the large luteal cells respond to a tenfold lower dose. Testosterone levels in the media containing small luteal cells were also elevated after incubation with a stimulatory dose of dibutyryl cAMP. In large luteal cells, elevated

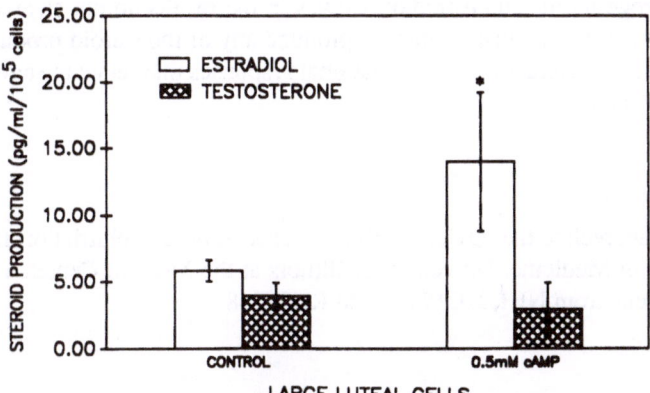

Fig. 3. Progesterone production by small luteal cells after treatment with 5 mM cAMP. Shown are means ± SEM.

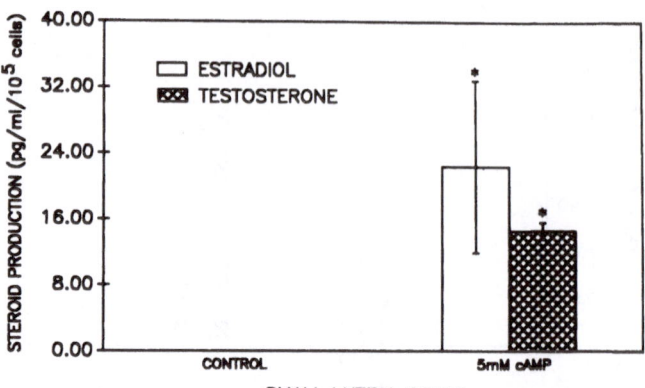

Fig. 4. Estradiol and testosterone synthesis by small luteal cells after incubation with 5 mM cAMP. Shown are means ± SEM.

testosterone levels were not seen after incubation with 0.5 mM dibutyryl cAMP, the same dose that stimulated estradiol and progesterone production. This suggests that both cell types are capable of testosterone synthesis, but aromatization occurs rapidly in the large luteal cells. Since LH acts on the corpus luteum at this stage of pregnancy to stimulate testosterone synthesis (1), it would be of interest to know which cell type would respond to LH in vitro, and whether a response to LH would parallel that seen with dibutyryl cAMP.

Progesterone production depends, in part, upon the availability of cholesterol (9). In addition, corpora luteal tissue from pregnant rats shows a dose-response increase in progesterone synthesis to high-density lipoproteins (HDL) concentrations (10). In this study, 25-OH-cholesterol enhanced progesterone production in the large luteal cells, suggesting that the large luteal cells are an important source of progesterone production in the corpus luteum.

These reported functional differences between the two luteal cell types indicate that the large luteal cells from day 8 pregnant rats possess a greater steroidogenic capacity for the production of progesterone and estradiol. However, the results do not clearly demonstrate whether the two cell types must interact to produce any of the steroid products, and more studies are necessary to examine other functional responses that relate to steroidogenesis in the rat corpus luteum.

Acknowledgments

We greatly appreciate the advice on tissue dissociation and elutriation from Dr. Scott Nelson, College of Medicine, University of Illinois at the Medical Center. This work was supported by grants from NIH, HD17867 and RR08248.

References

1. Sridaran R, Basuray R, Gibori G. Source and regulation of testosterone secretion in pregnant and pseudopregnant rats. Endocrinology 1981; 108:855-61.

2. Elbaum D, Keyes L. Synthesis of 17β-estradiol by isolated ovarian tissues of the pregnant rat: aromatization in the corpus luteum. Endocrinology 1976; 99:573-9.
3. Takayama M, Greenwald GS. Direct luteotropic action of estrogen in the hypophysectomized hysterectomized rat. Endocrinology 1973; 92:1405-13.
4. Gibori G, Antczak E, Rothchild I. The role of estrogen in the regulation of luteal progesterone secretion in the rat after day 12 of pregnancy. Endocrinology 1977; 100:1483-95.
5. Niswender GD, Schwall RH, Fitz TA, Farin CE, Sawyer HR. Regulation of luteal function in domestic ruminants: new concepts. Recent Prog Horm Res 1985; 41:101-51.
6. Nelson S, Khan I. Estradiol biosynthesis in the corpus luteum of the pregnant rat involves two different luteal cell populations [Abstract]. The Endocrine Society Meeting, Indianapolis, 1987:216.
7. Hansel W, Dowd JP. New concepts of the control of corpus luteum function. J Reprod Fertil 1986; 78:755-68.
8. Fitz TA, Mayan MH, Sawyer HR, Niswender GD. Characterization of two steroidogenic cell types in the ovine corpus luteum. Biol Reprod 1982; 27:703-11.
9. Savard K. The biochemistry of the corpus luteum. Biol Reprod 1973; 8:183-202.
10. Khan I, Gibori G, Belanger A, Chen Y-DI. Steroid effect on lipoprotein utilization in luteal cell steroidogenesis. In: Strauss JF, Menon KMJ, eds. Lipoprotein and cholesterol metabolism in steroidogenic tissues. Philadelphia: GF Stickley, 1985:155-8.

49

Steroidal Regulation of Sterol Carrier Protein-2 and P450$_{SCC}$ Expression in the Corpus Luteum

M. P. McLean, T. K. Puryear, I. Khan, J. T. Billheimer,[1] J. Orly,[2] and G. Gibori

Department of Physiology and Biophysics, University of Illinois College of Medicine, Chicago, IL 60612; [1]DuPont Experimental Station Wilmington, DE 19898; [2]Department of Biological Chemistry Hebrew University, Jerusalem, Israel

Summary

A primary action of estradiol in the corpus luteum of the pregnant rat is to increase the supply of cholesterol substrate for progesterone production by stimulating cholesterol synthesis, uptake and mobilization (1-3). To determine whether estradiol also affects cholesterol processing, its action of the expression of sterol carrier protein (SCP$_2$) and cytochrome P450$_{scc}$, proteins involved in the transport and cleavage of cholesterol, respectively, were investigated. Although mitochondria isolated from luteal cells of estradiol-treated rats secreted significantly more progestagen than the luteal mitochondria from control animals, data presented here indicate that estradiol's action does not involve stimulation of either the P450$_{scc}$ message or its content. Whereas estradiol had no effect on P450$_{scc}$, it caused a marked (threefold) increase in the mitochondrial content of SCP$_2$ as estimated by densitometry of the labelled immune complex on Western blots. The bulk of SCP$_2$ was associated with the mitochondrial fraction of corpora lutea from estradiol-treated rats. In conclusion, increased luteal cell progestagen synthesis by estradiol appears to be directly associated with an increase in mitochondrial SCP$_2$, an effect independent of either luteal P450$_{scc}$ content or message.

Introduction

Cholesterol is the obligatory precursor of progesterone biosynthesis in the corpus luteum of the rat, and changes in either its concentration or metabolism would be expected to directly affect progesterone production. In the rat luteal cell, cholesterol has been shown to be both produced de novo (2) and transported in via plasma high density lipoproteins (3). However, the essential step in steroid biosynthesis is not dependent on cholesterol availability but, rather on the conversion of cholesterol to pregnenolone. This occurs on the inner mitochondrial membrane where the cytochrome P450 side-chain cleavage enzyme ($P450_{scc}$) which is responsible for cleaving the side-chain of cholesterol, is located (4). Cholesterol is quite insoluble and is transported to the $P450_{scc}$ enzyme bound to a carrier protein. Recently, sterol carrier protein-2 (SCP_2) has been found to transport cholesterol (5). Since estradiol enhances both cholesterol availability and progesterone biosynthesis, it became of interest to determine whether it also affects $P450_{scc}$ and SCP_2 expression in luteal cells.

Materials and Methods

Pregnant Sprague-Dawley rats were hysterectomized and hypophysectomized on day 12 as previously described (6) and treated with or without a 1 cm estradiol or testosterone implant. Seventy-two h later, corpora lutea were moved, processed as previously described (7) and fractionated by differential ultracentrifugation (8) to obtain the various subcellular compartments. Subcellular protein content was estimated (9) and proteins were separated by SDS-polyacrylamide gel electrophoresis (SDS-PAGE) (10).

Mitochondrial fractions were prepared and assayed for $P450_{scc}$ enzyme activity (11) in the presence or absence of 25-OH cholesterol (50 µg/ml). Enzyme activity was expressed as the amount of C_{21}-sterols formed per minute per mg protein.

To examine $P450_{scc}$ content, separated proteins were transferred to nitrocellulose (12) and immunoblotting was performed by blocking nonspecific binding with 5% nonfat milk; $P450_{scc}$ was identified using a polyclonal antibody to $P450_{scc}$ (13) complexed with an ^{125}I-labelled second antibody.

Luteal cell SCP_2 content was examined by immunoblotting using the method described above with the following changes. Nonspecific binding was blocked with 5% gelatin and SCP_2 was identified using a highly specific polyclonal SCP_2 antibody (14). The SCP_2 antibody was complexed to ^{125}I-protein A and visualized by autoradiography.

RNA was extracted (15) from corpora lutea of hypophysectomized and hysterectomized rats treated for 3 days with or without estradiol. Total RNA was separated by agarose electrophoresis and transferred to Gene Screen (DuPont, Boston, MA). Northern blots were hybridized to a random oligonucleotide ^{32}P-labelled $P450_{scc}$ cDNA (kindly provided by Dr. Joanne Richards) and the hybrid complex was visualized by autoradiography.

Results

The effect of steroid treatment on mitochondrial cytochrome $P450_{scc}$ enzyme activity was measured in the presence and absence of 25-OH cholesterol. In the absence of exogenous cholesterol (Table 1), mitochondria isolated from corpora lutea of estradiol- and testosterone-treated rats produced more C_{21}-steroids than mitochondria from nonsteroid-treated animals. In the presence of 25-OH cholesterol, this difference was eliminated, indicating that substrate availability rather than $P450_{scc}$ enzyme activity was affected by steroid treatment.

Immunoblotting of $P450_{scc}$ (Fig. 1) indicated that estradiol had no stimulatory effect on the amount of enzyme protein present in the corpus luteum. The level of $P450_{scc}$ mRNA, determined by Northern blotting with a cDNA probe for P450scc, was also not increased by in vivo estradiol treatment (Fig. 1).

Table 1. Effect of estradiol or testosterone on luteal
side-chain cleavage enzyme activity

Treatment	Side-chain cleavage activity C_{21}-Steroids (Pmol.min.$^{-1}$mg Protein^{-1})	
	-25-OH Cholesterol	+25-OH Cholesterol
Vehicle	57.0 ± 7.0	973.0 ± 31.0
Estradiol	147.0 ± 18.0	993.0 ± 67.0
Testosterone	119.0 ± 19.0	900.0 ± 95.0

Rats were treated as described in Materials and Methods. On day 15, corpora lutea were isolated and side-chain cleavage enzyme activity measured in mitochondria in the absence or presence of 25-OH cholesterol (50 μg/ml).

In the rat corpus luteum, the bulk of SCP_2 is found to be associated with the membranous compartments (mitochondrial, microsomal) rather than the cytosolic fraction (data not shown). When animals were treated with estradiol, mitochondrial SCP_2 content increased

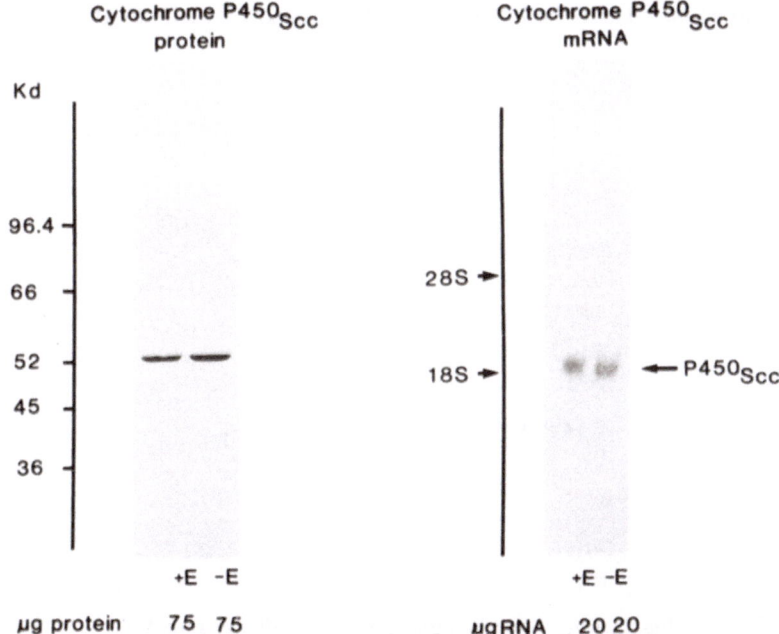

Fig. 1. Effect of estradiol on $P450_{scc}$ content and $P450_{scc}$ mRNA in luteal cells. Corpora lutea were obtained from rats treated as described in Materials and Methods. Soluble mitochondrial extracts were analyzed by immunoblotting using a specific $P450_{scc}$ antibody (13). Total RNA was extracted and subjected to Northern analysis using ^{32}P-labelled $P450_{scc}$ cDNA.

threefold (Fig. 2). Concomitant with this increase in mitochondrial SCP_2, a reduction in cytosolic SCP_2 content was observed. This suggests that estradiol enhanced both the translocation and luteal content of SCP_2.

Discussion

The results of this investigation indicate that mitochondria isolated from corpora lutea of rats treated with either estradiol or with aromatizable androgen produced greater quantities of progestins. However, results of the present investigation indicate that estradiol accomplishes this by not affecting the activity or the content of $P450_{scc}$ enzyme protein. First, the difference in C_{21}-steroids synthesized by mitochondria isolated from rats treated with or without estradiol was abolished when 25-OH cholesterol was added to the incubation. Secondly, Western blotting of mitochondrial $P450_{scc}$ protein indicated that estradiol had no effect on enzyme content. Lastly, estradiol had no effect on $P450_{scc}$ mRNA, as determined by Northern blot analysis. These results suggest that progesterone production was dependent on delivery of the cholesterol substrate to the $P450_{scc}$ enzyme rather than on a change in this enzyme proper. These data are consistent with other reports suggesting that after luteinization occurs, $P450_{scc}$ is no longer affected by hormones and both the $P450_{scc}$ content and mRNA remain constant throughout gestation (16).

This report is the first to demonstrate that increased steroid synthesis can be directly correlated with an increase in the luteal cholesterol transport protein, SCP_2. The threefold

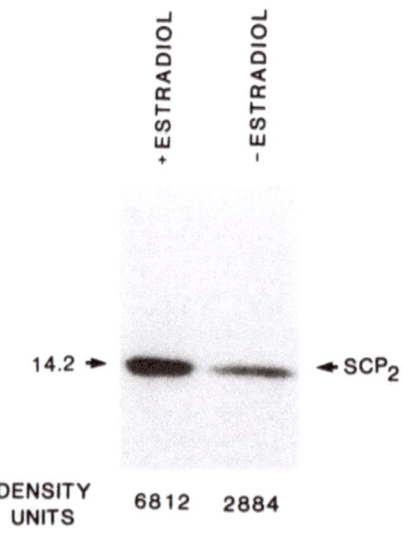

Fig. 2. Mitochondrial content of SCP_2 after estradiol administration. Mitochondria were isolated from corpora lutea of rats treated as described in Materials and Methods. Mitochondrial proteins (50 μg) were separated by SDS-Page analyzed by immunoblotting using a specific SCP_2 antibody (14). Labelled immune complexes were estimated by densitometry.

increase in mitochondrial SCP_2 content by estradiol treatment occurred in absence of any effect of estradiol on the $P450_{scc}$ enzyme. This suggests that estradiol may regulate the intracellular transport of cholesterol from the outer to inner mitochondrial membrane (5) by increasing luteal SCP_2 content. Estradiol, in addition to increasing luteal SCP_2 content, also appeared to increase translocation of the SCP_2 from the cytosol to the mitochondria. However, this was far less dramatic since the majority of the SCP_2 was associated with the membranous compartments.

In conclusion, data presented here suggest that in addition to estradiol increasing cholesterol biosynthesis (2), uptake and mobilization (3), this hormone may stimulate cholesterol transport to the inner mitochondrial membrane increasing luteal SCP_2 content and translocation. The results further demonstrate that the stimulatory action of estradiol on luteal cell progesterone biosynthesis occurs without any changes in $P450_{scc}$ activity, content or mRNA level.

Acknowledgments

This research was supported by NIH grant HD 11119. MPM was supported by a NRSA fellowship HD 6982.

References

1. Gibori G, Chen Y-DI, Khan I, Azhar S, Reaven GM. Regulation of luteal cell lipoprotein receptors, sterol contents, and steroidogenesis by estradiol in the pregnant rat. Endocrinology 1984; 114:609-17.
2. Azhar S, Khan I, Chen Y-DI, Reaven GM, Gibori G. Regulation of luteal cell 3-hydroxy-3-methylglutaryl coenzyme A reductase activity by estradiol. Biol Reprod 1985; 32:333-41.
3. Khan I, Belanger A, Chen Y-DI, Gibori G. Influence of high density lipoprotein on estradiol stimulation of luteal steroidogenesis. Biol Reprod 1985; 32:96-104.
4. Yogo N, Kobayaski S, Sekiyama S, et al. Further studies on the submitochondrial localization of cholesterol side chain-cleaving enzyme system in hog adrenal cortex by sonic treatment. J Biochem (Tokyo) 1970; 68:775-83.
5. Scallen TJ, Noland BJ, Garvey KL, et al. Sterol carrier protein 2 and fatty acid-binding protein. J Biol Chem 1985; 260:4733-9.
6. Gibori G, Keyes PL. Role of intraluteal estrogen in the regulation of the rat corpus luteum during pregnancy. Endocrinology 1978; 102:1176-82.
7. McLean MP, Khan I, Puryear TK, Gibori G. Estradiol induced synthesis and translation of specific proteins in the corpus luteum. In: Hirshfield A, ed. Paracrine communication in the ovary—ontogenesis and growth factors. New York: Plenum (in press).
8. Fleischner S, Kervina M. Subcellular fractionation of rat liver. Methods Enzymol 1974; 31:6-41.
9. Bradford MN. A rapid and sensitive method for the quantitation of microgram quantities of protein utilizing the principle of protein-dye binding. Anal Biochem 1976; 72:248-54.
10. Laemmli UK. Cleavage of structural proteins during the assembly of the head of bacteriophage T_4. Nature 1970; 227:680-5.
11. Mori M, Marsh JM. The site of luteinizing hormone stimulation of steroidogenesis in mitochondria of the rat corpus luteum. J Biol Chem 1982; 257:6178-83.

12. Towbin H, Staehelin T, Gordon J. Electrophoretic transfer of proteins from polyacrylamide gels to nitrocellulose sheets: procedure and some applications. Proc Natl Acad Sci USA 1979; 76:4350-4.

13. Zlotkin T, Farkash Y, Orly J. Cell-specific expression of immunoreactive cholesterol side-chain cleavage cytochrome P-450 during follicular development in the rat ovary. Endocrinology 1986; 119:2809-20.

14. Billheimer JT, Gaylor JL. Cytosolic modulators of activities of microsomal enzymes of cholesterol biosynthesis. J Biol Chem 1980; 255:8128-35.

15. Chirgwin JM, Pryzbyla AE, MacDonald RJ, Rutter WJ. Isolation of biologically active ribonucleic acid from sources enriched in ribonuclease. Biochemistry 1979; 18:5294-9.

16. Richards JS, Jahnson T, Hedin L, et al. Ovarian follicular development: from physiology to molecular biology. Recent Prog Hormone Res 1987; 43:231-76.

50

Regulation of HMG-CoA Reductase Gene Expression in the Corpus Luteum: Role of Estradiol

T. K. Puryear, I. Khan, and G. Gibori

Department of Physiology and Biophysics, University of Illinois College of Medicine, Chicago, IL 60612

Introduction

HMG-CoA reductase, the rate limiting enzyme in cholesterol biosynthesis, is regulated in both steroidogenic and nonsteroidogenic cells via negative feedback mechanism by either sterols or their metabolites. Steroidogenic tissues have, in addition, another mode of enzyme regulation due to their marked need for cholesterol substrate. We have previously demonstrated that estradiol enhances markedly and specifically the activity of this enzyme in the corpus luteum of the pregnant rat. The observation that estradiol stimulates hMG-CoA reductase activity without changing the phosphorylation/dephosphorylation state of the enzyme led us to hypothesize that estradiol acts to specifically increase hMG-CoA reductase synthesis by increasing mRNA levels encoding this protein. This hypothesis has been directly tested using a cDNA and an antibody for hMG-CoA reductase message and protein, respectively. In addition, since a decrease in cellular sterol upregulates the level of hMG-CoA reductase mRNA, we examined the possibility that estradiol's action on hMG-CoA reductase activity, content and mRNA is mediated by estradiol depletion of cholesterol storage.

Materials and Methods

The animal model was essentially prepared as described previously (1). Briefly, pregnant rats of Sprague-Dawley strain were hypophysectomized and hysterectomized on day 12 of pregnancy and were treated with or without a 1-cm estradiol implant. Corpora lutea were isolated 72 h later. In this rat model, corpora lutea are exquisitely responsive to estradiol which causes a dramatic increase in both luteal growth and progesterone biosynthesis (2).

To measure hMG-CoA reductase activity, corpora lutea were homogenized in 100 mM potassium phosphate buffer pH 7.4 containing 10 mM EDTA, 5 mM dithiothreitol and 0.25 M sucrose. To obtain microsomal fractions, homogenates were centrifuged first at 10,000 x g for 20 min. The supernatant fractions were then centrifuged at 105,000 x g for 1 h. The sedimented microsomal pellets were washed twice and hMG-CoA reductase activity was determined as previously described (3).

Luteal and serum cholesterol were extracted and separated by silicic acid/celite column chromatography after saponification in alcoholic KOH, cholesteryl esters were quantitated as described previously (4).

To isolate RNA, corpora lutea were suspended in 4 vol/w of 4 M guanidine isothiocyanate. Tissue was rapidly homogenized and centrifuged at 150,000 g x through a 5.7-ml cesium chloride cushion for 16 h at 15°C. The resultant pellet was washed twice with 100% ethanol (-20°C), dried, resuspended in an appropriate volume of sterile diethyl pyrocarbonate-treated water and quantitated by spectrophotometry at 260 nM. Equal amounts of RNA from each treatment were size fractionated on 1% agarose formaldehyde gels and transferred to Gene Screen Plus (DuPont, NEN) via capillary action. Nucleic acid size was determined using a synthetic RNA size ladder (Bethesda Research Labs). A plasmid containing 4.5 Kb cDNA insert for the hMG-CoA reductase, the sequence of which was reported by Chin et al. (5), was obtained through American Type Culture Collection. The full length insert was isolated from low melting point agarose gel. HMG-CoA reductase cDNA was labelled to high specific activity (10^7-10^8 cpm/µg) using the random oligonucleotide-primed method (6). Blots were prehybridized at 42°C overnight in a solution containing 50% formamide, 6 x SCC (0.9 M NaCl, 0.09 M Na citrate), 50 mM $NaPO_4$ (pH 6.5), 1% SDS, 100 µg/ml yeast RNA, 1 µg/ml poly U. Hybridization was carried out overnight in the same solution containing 1-5 x 10^6 cpm/ml of hMG-CoA reductase cDNA. Samples for dot blotting were prepared as recommended by the manufacturer and blots were then processed in the same way as Northern blots.

To examine hMG-CoA reductase protein content, microsomal proteins were separated by SDS-PAGE and transferred to nitrocellulose. The blots were blocked in a buffer containing 5% nonfat milk for 1 h at room temperature and then exposed to hMG-CoA reductase monoclonal antibody (7) for 1 h. Blots were then exposed to [12]I-labelled second antibody for 1 h at room temperature, washed extensively and autoradiographed.

Results

The ability of estradiol treatment to upregulate luteal hMG-CoA reductase is shown in Figure 1. The data on the left indicate that estradiol caused a two- to threefold increase in enzyme activity in the rat corpus luteum. This change in activity was accompanied by an increase in hMG-CoA reductase protein content (middle panel). Although less dramatic, the pattern of change was similar to that observed for hMG-CoA reductase activity. Estradiol treatment caused a twofold increase in enzyme content over the vehicle-treated group. The estradiol effect on hMG-CoA reductase protein was specific since the content of $P450_{scc}$, another enzyme involved in the steroidogenic pathway, was not affected by estradiol treatment (data not shown).

We next examined whether estradiol affects luteal cell content of hMG-CoA reductase mRNA. As shown in Figure 1, right panel, hMG-CoA reductase cDNA hybridized with a band of approximately 4.2 kb. This RNA band is the expected size of the hMG-CoA mRNA of rat liver (5). Luteal hMG-CoA mRNA content was increased by more than twofold after 72 h of sustained estradiol treatment.

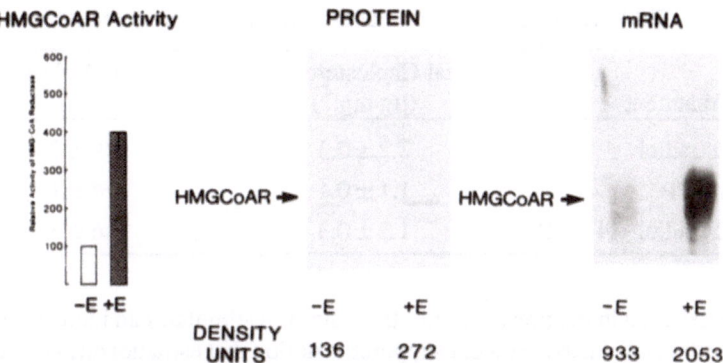

Fig. 1. Estradiol action on luteal hMG-CoA reductase activity, enzyme
protein and mRNA levels. HMG-CoA reductase protein was analyzed by
Western blot and hMG-CoA reductase mRNA by Northern blot.

Since decrease in cellular sterol upregulates mRNA levels for this reductase (8) and since
estradiol depletes cholesterol storage in the luteal cell (9), it was of interest to determine
whether estradiol's action on hMG-CoA reductase mRNA was mediated primarily by
changes in the cellular content of cholesterol. This was accomplished by examining the
separate and combined action of estradiol and 4-APP. 4-APP is known to lower the cellular
content of cholesterol ester and increase hMG-CoA reductase activity (3). Indeed, 4-APP
caused a marked decrease in circulating cholesterol and luteal cell cell content of sterol ester.
Although addition of estradiol to 4-APP treatment did not further reduce the 4-APP induced
decrease in luteal sterol content (Table 1), it markedly increased both the hMG-CoA
reductase activity and the level of its message (Fig. 2), indicating that the increase in
hMG-CoA reductase expression induced by estradiol is not simply a consequence of cellular
sterol depletion.

Discussion

The present investigation was undertaken to gain a fuller understanding of the molecular
mechanisms of regulation of steroidogenesis in rat luteal cells. Our previous studies have
raised the possibility that modulation of intracellular sterol synthesis and metabolism is
involved in the process by which estradiol or androgen precursor stimulates steroidogenesis
in the rat corpus luteum (9,10). Estradiol enhances markedly and specifically the activity of
the rate limiting enzyme in cholesterol biosynthesis, hMG-CoA reductase, in the corpus
luteum of pregnant rat (3). Changes in hMG-CoA reductase activity can be due to changes
at the level of enzyme content or catalytic efficiency. Mechanisms involving control at the
level of existing enzyme have been proposed to explain the in vivo changes in the activity
of hMG-CoA reductase through a direct modulation (12). One of these mechanisms entails
covalent modification of the enzyme by a cycle of phosphorylation and dephosphorylation
associated with the modulation of activity (13). However, our findings indicate that hMG-
CoA reductase is present to a large extent in an inactive phosphorylated form in the luteal
cells of pregnant rat and that estradiol-induced activation was not due to changes in the
phosphorylation state of the enzyme (11).

Table 1. Effect of estradiol and/or 4APP on sterol content

Treatment	Luteal Cholesterol Ester ($\mu g \cdot mg^{-1}$)	Serum Cholesterol ($mg \cdot dl^{-1}$)
Estradiol	2.2 ± 0.3	49 ± 2
4-APP	1.1 ± 0.1	14 ± 1
Estradiol + 4-APP	1.2 ± 0.3	16 ± 3

The observation in the present report that estradiol stimulates an increase in hMG-CoA reductase protein and mRNA content support the notion that estradiol does not alter the state of activation of already present enzyme but rather enhances the availability of luteal hMG-CoA reductase. The results further demonstrate the molecular basis for the hormonal regulation of hMG-CoA reductase synthesis and activity in luteal cells.

In nonsteroidogenic cells, hMG-CoA reductase is upregulated when luteal sterol content is suppressed (8). A similar sterol negative feedback system and hMG-CoA reductase regulation appears to be operative in rat luteal cells. In view of the fact that sterol ester content of the corpus luteum falls in response to estradiol (9), the rise in hMG-CoA reductase could be viewed as a simple consequence of cellular sterol depletion. However, results of this

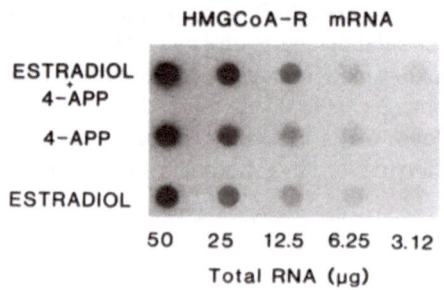

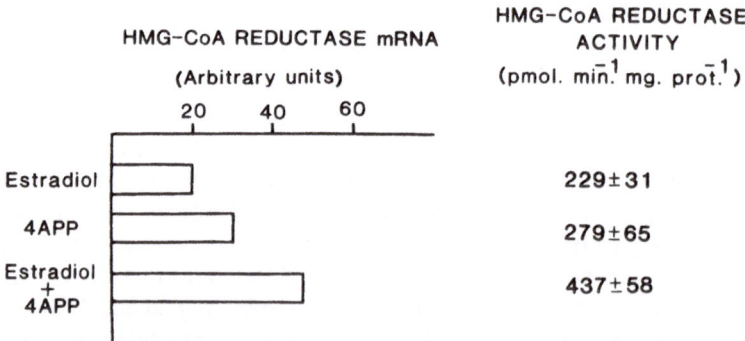

Fig. 2. Estradiol and/or 4APP effect on hMG-CoA reductase activity and mRNA levels hMG-CoA mRNA was analyzed by dot-blot hybridization and quantitated by densitometry.

investigation indicate that estradiol modulation of hMG-CoA reductase is not entirely due to a decrease in cellular sterol levels and that estrogen regulates hMG-CoA reductase expression by a separate mechanism. We, therefore, conclude that corpora lutea of pregnant rat possess an estradiol-mediated mechanism for increasing hMG-CoA reductase mRNA level, which is distinct from the cholesterol negative feedback regulation of hMG-CoA gene expression.

Acknowledgments

The authors wish to thank Dr. David Shapiro for the generous supply of hMG-CoA reductase monoclonal antibody. This research was supported by NIH grant HD 11119.

References

1. Gibori G, Keyes PL. Role of intraluteal estrogen in the regulation of the rat corpus luteum during pregnancy. Endocrinology 1978; 102:1176-82.
2. Khan I, Glaser LA, Gibori G. Reactivation of regressing corpora lutea by estradiol in pregnant rat: dependence on placental lactogen. Biol Reprod 1987; 37:1083-8.
3. Azhar S, Chen Y-DI, Reaven GM. Gonadotropin modulation of 3-hydroxy-3-methylglutaryl coenzyme A reductase activity in desensitized luteinized rat ovary. Biochemistry 1984; 23:4533-8.
4. Vershoor-Klostwyk AH, Vershoor L, Azhar S, Reaven GM. Role of exogenous cholesterol in regulation of adrenal steroidogenesis in the rat. J Biol Chem 1982; 257:7666-71.
5. Chin DJ, Gil G, Russel DW, et al. Nucleotide sequence of 3-hydroxy-3-methylglutaryl coenzyme A reductase, a glycoprotein of endoplasmic reticulum. Nature 1984; 308:613-7.
6. Feinberg AP, Vogelstein B. A technique for radiolabelling DNA restriction endonuclease fragments to a high specific activity. Anal Biochem 1983 132:6-13.
7. Clark RE, Martin GG, Barton MC, Shapiro DJ. Production and characterization of monoclonal antibodies to rat liver microsomal 3-hydroxy-3-methylglutaryl coenzyme A reductase. Proc Natl Acad Sci USA 1982; 79:3734-8.
8. Liscum L, Luskey KL, Chin DJ, Ho YK, Goldstein JL, Brown MS. Regulation of 3-hydroxy-3-methylglutaryl coenzyme A reductase and its mRNA in rat liver as studied with a monoclonal antibody and cDNA probe. J Biol Chem 1985; 32:333-41.
9. Gibori G, Chen Y-DI, Khan I, Azhar S, Reaven GM. Regulation of luteal cell lipoprotein receptors. Endocrinology 1984; 114:609-14.
10. Khan I, Belanger A, Chen Y-DI, Gibori G. Influence of high density lipoprotein on estradiol stimulation of luteal steroidogenesis. Biol Reprod 1985; 32:96-104.
11. Azhar S, Khan I, Chen Y-DI, Reaven GM, Gibori G. Regulation of luteal cell 3-hydroxy-3-methylglutaryl coenzyme A reductase activity by estradiol. Biol Reprod 1985; 32:333-41.
12. Beg ZH, Stonik JA, Brewer HB Jr. Phosphorylation and modulation of the enzyme activity of native and protease cleaved purified hepatic 3-hydroxy-3-methylglutaryl coenzyme A reductase by a calcium/calmodulin-dependent protein kinase. J Biol Chem 1987; 262:13228-32.
13. Kenelly PJ, Rodwell VW. Regulation of 3-hydroxy-3-methylglutaryl coenzyme A reductase by reversible phosphorylation-dephosphorylation. J Lipid Res 1985; 26:903-8.

51

Pertussis Toxin Uncouples Enkephalin-Mediated Inhibition of Rabbit Luteal Adenylyl Cyclase

Joel Abramowitz and Bhanu P. Jena

Department of Zoology, Iowa State University of Science
and Technology, Ames, Iowa 50011-3223

Hormonally responsive adenylyl cyclases are membrane-bound enzyme systems which consist of at least five distinct components: receptors for stimulatory and inhibitory hormones; transducing proteins called Gs and Gi, respectively, which mediate the effects of hormone-occupied receptor and function in a guanine nucleotide- and Mg ion-dependent fashion; and a catalytic component, which produces cAMP (for review on the component nature of adenylyl cyclases, see 1). Previous studies from our laboratory indicate that rabbit corpora lutea contain an adenylyl cyclase system that, in addition to being stimulated by gonadotropin and catecholamines (2,3), is attenuated by guanine nucleotides and enkephalin (4,5) suggesting the presence of Gi. As first demonstrated by Katada and Ui (6,7), one method to substantiate the existence of Gi in a given tissue is to treat the tissue with pertussis toxin and a [^{32}P]NAD, demonstrate the [^{32}P]ADP-ribosylation of a membrane protein with an Mr of 40-41,000 daltons and show that this treatment uncouples inhibitory receptors linked to adenylyl cyclase. In this study we present such data establishing the existence of Gi in the rabbit corpus luteum.

Materials and Methods

Materials, treatment of animals, preparation of membranes, procedures for the adenylyl cyclase assays, [^{32}P]ADP-ribosylation, sodium dodecyl sulfate polyacrylamide gel electrophoresis (SDS-PAGE) and protein determination were as previously described (4,5,8). In addition, pertussis toxin was from List Biological Laboratories (Campbell, CA). All experiments were repeated a minimum of three times with similar results and representative experiments are presented.

Results and Discussion

Effects on ADP-Ribosylation

Autoradiographic analysis of luteal membranes subjected to SDS-PAGE after treatment with [^{32}P]NAD, ATP and GTP in the presence and absence of pertussis or cholera toxins revealed that pertussis toxin treatment resulted in the specific [^{32}P]ADP-ribosylation of a protein that migrates with an Mr value of 40,000 (Fig. 1). This value is in good agreement with the reported Mr value of the *alpha* subunit of the major pertussis toxin substrate, presumably Gi, purified from rabbit liver (9) and human erythrocytes (10). Cholera toxin treatment resulted in the specific [^{32}P]ADP-ribosylation of two proteins with Mr values of 42,000 and 46,000 (Fig. 1). Under optimal exposure conditions, the higher Mr cholera toxin substrate migrates as a doublet. Previous studies from our laboratory have shown that the proteins with Mr values of 42,000 and 46,000 labeled by cholera toxin in the rabbit corpus luteum correspond to *alpha* subunits of Gs (8). In order to determine whether cholera and pertussis toxins truly ADP-ribosylate different proteins, rabbit luteal membranes were incubated in the presence of 5 mM NAD in the presence and absence of 40 μg/ml cholera toxin or 20 μg/ml pertussis toxin for 20 min, washed twice and subjected to toxin treatment using [^{32}P]NAD. Prior treatment of rabbit luteal membranes with cholera toxin and un-labeled NAD prevented subsequent labeling with cholera toxin and [^{32}P]NAD but not labeling with pertussis toxin and [^{32}P]NAD. Treatment of membranes with pertussis toxin and unlabeled NAD did not prevent subsequent labeling with cholera toxin and [^{32}P]NAD and reduced labeling with pertussis toxin and [^{32}P]NAD demonstrating that distinct proteins are labeled by pertussis and cholera toxins. Incubation of luteal membranes in the presence of 25 μg/ml pertussis toxin and 5 mM NAD for up to 4 h did not prevent subsequent labeling in the presence of [^{32}P]NAD and 2.5 μg/ml pertussis toxin for 10 min, suggesting that Gi is

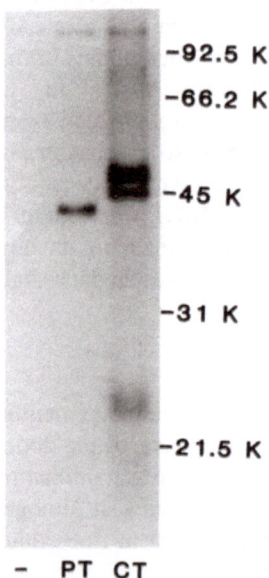

−   PT CT

Fig. 1. Pertussis and cholera toxin-mediated [^{32}P]ADP-ribosyla-tion of rabbit luteal membrane proteins. Luteal membranes (150 μg) were incubated in the absence (–) or presence of 2.5 μg/ml pertussis toxin (PT) or 40 μg/ml cholera toxin (CT) in a volume of 100 μl in the presence of [^{32}P]NAD; then 75 μg of membrane protein was subjected to SDS-PAGE.

present in excess of Gs in the rabbit corpus luteum as has been suggested in several other tissues (11).

Pertussis toxin-mediated [^{32}P]ADP-ribosylation was time-dependent and dependent upon the concentration of pertussis toxin and membrane present during the incubation. Guanine and adenine nucleotides both modify the extent to which pertussis toxin can ADP-ribosylate its substrate. Removing GTP from the incubation or replacing it with GMP-P(NH)P decreased pertussis toxin-specific labeling by 90% and 85%, respectively. GDPβS, GTPαS and NaF were capable of supporting pertussis toxin-mediated ADP-ribosylation. However, GTPαS and NaF were 40-60% less effective in supporting ADP-ribosylation than GTP. Furthermore, removing ATP from the incubation or substituting AMP reduced pertussis toxin-mediated labeling 70%. ADP and AMP-P(NH)P were able to support pertussis toxin-specific ADP-ribosylation but only to 45-50%, the extent seen with ATP. These actions of guanine and adenine nucleotides on pertussis toxin-mediated ADP-ribosylation are in agreement with previously published studies (12-14). The actions of both adenine and guanine nucleotides on enhancing pertussis toxin-mediated ADP-ribosylation are complex and reflect different potential sites of nucleotide action. One is to stabilize the pertussis toxin substrate itself (12,14). The second is to bind to the toxin and activate the toxin by promoting dissociation of the pertussis toxin subunits (13-15). However, whether the enhanced ADP-ribosylation by pertussis toxin in the presence of NaF is due to a direct effect on the toxin or stabilization of the pertussis toxin substrate must await further study. Interestingly, we have also observed enhanced ADP-ribosylation by cholera toxin in the presence of NaF (8).

Effects on Adenylyl Cyclase Activity

In the presence of 25 μM forskolin, GTP and GMP-P(NH)P inhibited luteal adenylyl cyclase activity by 15% and 35%, respectively (Table 1). The further addition of 8 μM [D-ala^2, met^5]enkephalin amide (Da-ENK) caused an additional 25% inhibition of adenylyl cyclase activity in the presence of GTP plus forskolin, but did not alter enzymatic activity in the presence of forskolin alone or forskolin plus GMP-P(NH)P. Treatment of luteal membranes, with 5 μg/ml pertussis toxin, 5 mM NAD and 2.5 mM ATP, completely reversed the inhibitory action of GTP and GTP plus Da-ENK on the forskolin-stimulated enzyme but did not reverse the inhibitory action of GMP-P(NH)P. Pertussis toxin treatment did not alter forskolin-stimulated adenylyl cyclase activity. Using the criteria established by Katada and Ui (6,7), these findings clearly demonstrate for the first time that the inhibitory actions of guanine nucleotide and enkephalin on luteal adenylyl cyclase activity are mediated via Gi. The lack of an effect of pertussis toxin treatment on GMP-P(NH)P-mediated inhibition of forskolin-stimulated luteal adenylyl cyclase activity is in agreement with studies demonstrating a similar lack of an effect of pertussis toxin treatment on GMP-P(NH)P-mediated inhibition of adenylyl cyclase activity in S49 mouse lymphoma cyc cells (16) and rat pars intermedia (17). It should be noted that in order to observe pertussis toxin reversal of GTP and GTP plus Da-ENK-mediated inhibition of forskolin stimulated adenylyl cyclase activity, it was necessary to have high concentrations of ATP present during toxin treatment. Thus, when toxin treatment was performed in the presence of 0.1 mM ATP, instead of 2.5 mM ATP, we were not able to demonstrate pertussis toxin-mediated changes in rabbit luteal adenylyl cyclase activity. This requirement for high ATP levels during pertussis toxin treatment of

Table 1. Effects of pertussis toxin treatment on
rabbit luteal adenylyl cyclase activity *

Additions to Assay	Control	Pertussis Toxin Treated
	Adenylyl Cyclase Activities (pmol/min/mg)	
None	183 ± 9	186 ± 5
GTP	159 ± 5	193 ± 8
GMP-P(NH)P	124 ± 6	123 ± 8
Da-ENK	180 ± 10	186 ± 8
Da-ENK plus GTP	116 ± 8	195 ± 11
Da-ENK plus GMP-P(NH)P	115 ± 10	126 ± 9

*Luteal membranes were incubated for 30 min at 32.5°C in medium containing 2.5 mM ATP, 5 mM NAD and a nucleotide triphosphate regenerating system in the absence (control) and presence of 5 µg/ml pertussis toxin. The incubation mixture was diluted fivefold prior to assessment of adenylyl cyclase activity. Adenylyl cyclase activity was determined as described in (5) the presence of 0.1 mM ATP, 3.0 mM $MgCl_2$ and 25 µM forskolin. When present, GTP and GMP-P(NH)P were 25 µM and Da-ENK was 8 µM. The membrane protein content was 4 µg/50-µl cyclase assay. Values represent the mean ± SD of triplicate determinations.

luteal membranes in order to uncouple inhibitory input to adenylyl cyclase is probably due to the activating effect of ATP on pertussis toxin (12,14,15).

In summary, we have shown that the rabbit corpus luteum contains a single pertussis toxin substrate with an Mr of 40,000 daltons. This pertussis toxin substrate appears to represent the *alpha* subunit of Gi as pertussis toxin treatment of rabbit luteal membranes uncouples enkephalin-mediated inhibition of adenylyl cyclase activity. In light of the findings that the corpus luteum contains opioid peptides (18,19) and that the ovary contains mRNA for both proenkephalin (20) and proopiomelanocortin (21), it appears that a paracrine or autocrine mechanism is present in the ovary to negatively regulate adenylyl cyclase via Gi and thus modify cAMP-mediated processes in the ovary.

Acknowledgment

This work was supported in part by Grant HD-22058 from the NIH.

References

1. Birnbaumer L, Codina J, Mattera R. Regulation of hormone receptors and adenylyl cyclases by guanine nucleotide binding N proteins. Recent Prog Horm Res 1985; 41:41-99.
2. Birnbaumer L, Yang PC, Hunzicker-Dunn M, Bockaert J, Duran JM. Adenylyl cyclase activities in ovarian tissues. I. Homogenization and conditions of assay in Graffian

follicles and corpora lutea of rabbits, rats, and pigs: regulation by ATP and some comparative properties. Endocrinology 1976; 99:163-84.

3. Abramowitz J, Birnbaumer L. Properties of the hormonally responsive rabbit luteal adenylyl cyclase: effects of guanine nucleotides and magnesium ion on stimulation by gonadotropin and catecholamines. Endocrinology 1982; 110:773-81.

4. Abramowitz J, Campbell AR. Enkephalin-mediated inhibition of forskolin-stimulated rabbit luteal adenylyl cyclase activity. Biochem Biophys Res Commun 1983; 116:574-80.

5. Abramowitz J, Campbell AR. Effects of guanine nucleotides and divalent cations on forskolin activation of rabbit luteal adenylyl cyclase: evidence for the existence of an inhibitory guanine nucleotide-binding regulatory component. Endocrinology 1984; 114:1955-62.

6. Katada T, Ui M. Islet-activating protein. A modifier of receptor-mediated regulation of rat islet adenylate cyclase. J Biol Chem 1981; 256:8310-7.

7. Katada T, Ui M. Direct modification of the membrane adenylate cyclase system by islet-activating protein due to ADP-ribosylation of a membrane protein. Proc Natl Acad Sci USA 1982; 79:3129-33.

8. Abramowitz J, Campbell AR. Cholera toxin action on rabbit corpus luteum membranes: effects on adenylyl cyclase activity and adenosine diphospho-ribosylation of the stimulatory guanine nucleotide-binding regulatory component. Biol Reprod 1985; 32:463-74.

9. Bokoch GM, Katada T, Northup JK, Ui M, Gilman AG. Purification and properties of the inhibitory guanine nucleotide-binding regulatory component of adenylate cyclase. J Biol Chem 1984; 259:3560-7.

10. Codina J, Hildebrandt J, Sekura RD. N_s and N_i, the stimulatory and inhibitory regulatory components of adenylyl cyclases. Purification of the human erythrocyte proteins without the use of activating regulatory ligands. J Biol Chem 1984; 259:5871-86.

11. Gilman AG. G proteins: transducers of receptor-generated signals. Annu Rev Biochem 1987; 56:615-49.

12. Tsai SC, Adamik R, Kanaho Y, Hewlett EL, Moss J. Effects on guanine nucleotides and rhodopsin on ADP-ribosylation of the inhibitory GTP-binding component of adenylate cyclase by pertussis toxin. J Biol Chem 1984; 259:15320-3.

13. Lim LK, Sekura RD, Kaslow HR. Adenine nucleotides directly stimulate pertussis toxin. J Biol Chem 1985; 260:2585-8.

14. Mattera R, Codina J, Sekura RD, Birnbaumer L. The interaction of nucleotides with pertussis toxin. Direct evidence for a nucleotide binding site on the toxin regulating the rate of ADP-ribosylation of N_i, the inhibitory regulatory component of adenylyl cyclase. J Biol Chem 1986; 261:11173-9.

15. Burns DL, Manclark CR. Adenine nucleotides promote dissociation of pertussis toxin subunits. J Biol Chem 1986; 261:4324-7.

16. Hildebrandt JD, Sekura RD, Codina J, Iyengar R, Manclark CR, Birnbaumer L. Stimulation and inhibition of adenylyl cyclases mediated by distinct regulatory proteins. Nature 1983; 302:706-9.

17. Cote TE, Frey EA, Sekura RD. Altered activity of the inhibitory guanyl nucleotide-binding component (N_i) induced by pertussis toxin. Uncoupling of N_i from receptor with continued coupling of N_i to the catalytic unit. J Biol Chem 1984; 259;8693-8.

18. Tsong SD, Phillips DM, Halmi N, Kreiger DT, Bardin CW. β-Endorphin is present in the male reproductive tract of five species. Biol Reprod 1982; 27:755-64.

19. Shaha C, Margioris A, Liotta AS, Kreiger DT, Bardin CW. Demonstration of im-
    munoreactive β-endorphin- and α_3-melanocyte-stimulating hormone-related peptides
    in the ovaries of neonatal, cyclic and pregnant mice. Endocrinology 1984; 115:378-84.
20. Kilpatrick DL, Rosenthal JL. The proenkephalin gene is widely expressed within the
    male and female reproductive systems of the rat and hamster. Endocrinology 1986;
    119:370-4.
21. Melner MH, Young SL, Czerwiec FS, et al. The regulation of granulosa cell
    proopiomelanocortin messenger ribonucleic acid by androgens and gonadotropins.
    Endocrinology 1986; 119:2082-8.

52

Attenuated In Vivo Progesterone Secretion by Ovine Corpora Lutea After Exposure to Luteinizing Hormone

Ov Slayden and Fredrick Stormshak

Department of Animal Science, Oregon State University
Corvallis, OR 97331

Introduction

Exogenous gonadotropin releasing hormone (GnRH) and its agonistic analogs appear to display a marked antigonadotropic activity, interfering with luteinizing hormone (LH)-induced synthesis of progesterone by the developing corpus luteum in a variety of species (1). In cattle, administration of GnRH has been shown to reduce serum progesterone concentrations during the estrous cycle without causing luteal regression (2,3). This action of GnRH appears to be linked to the downregulation of luteal LH receptors (3). Loss of LH receptors and subsequent gonadal desensitization following treatment with GnRH was initially attributed to GnRH-induced release of LH (4). However, the presence of high-affinity binding sites for GnRH in the ovaries of the rat (5) and the antisteroidogenic effect of this decapeptide in hypophysectomized rats (6) has implicated a possible direct action of GnRH on the mammalian ovary. Recently, an ovarian protein (GLOH) which binds to rat GnRH receptors has been isolated from the ovaries of the ewe and the cow (7). While gonadal GnRH receptors have been identified in the rat, specific binding sites for this decapeptide have not been found in domestic species (8). Therefore, the mechanism by which GnRH reduces luteal steroidogenesis in domestic species remains enigmatic.

The objective of this research was to compare the effects of LH and GnRH administered on day 2 of the estrous cycle on progesterone secretion by the ovine corpus luteum.

Materials and Methods

Experiment 1

Ten western range ewes were assigned in replicate to a control (n=5) and treatment group (n=5) and checked twice daily with 2 vasectomized rams for estrous behavior. Ewes in each group were laparotomized on day 2 of the cycle (detected estrus = day 0 of the cycle), and ewes with developing corpora lutea in both ovaries were subjected to unilateral ovariectomy. Treatment consisted of an injection of 25 µg GnRH directly into the artery supplying the ovary bearing the remaining corpus luteum. Controls were injected with an equal volume of physiological saline only. Jugular blood was collected from all ewes at time 0, 15, 30, 45 and 60 min after injection for LH radioimmunoassay following the procedure of McCarthy and Swanson (9) and on day 3, 5, 7, 9 and 11 of the cycle for progesterone analysis by radioimmunoassay (10).

Experiment 2

Ten range ewes were assigned to control (n=5) and treatment groups (n=5), checked for estrous behavior and laparotomized following the procedure described in experiment 1. Treatment consisted of an injection of 50 ng GnRH directly into the artery supplying the corpus luteum. Controls were injected with an equal volume of saline only. Jugular blood was collected from all ewes at time 0, 15, 30, 45 and 60 min after injection for LH analysis and on day 4, 6, 8 and 10 of the cycle for progesterone analysis by radioimmunoassay.

Experiment 3

Twelve range ewes were assigned at random to a control (n=6) and treatment group (n=6). Treatment consisted of an IV injection (jugular) with 100 µg oLH (time = 0) and 50 µg oLH at time = 15, 30 and 45 min. Controls were injected with an equal volume of saline only. Jugular blood was collected for LH analysis following each injection and at 15-min intervals for 1 h following the last injection. Jugular blood was also collected on day 4, 6, 8 and 10 of the cycle for progesterone radioimmunoassay.

Statistical Analysis

There was no effect of number of corpora lutea in laparotomized ewes on serum concentrations of progesterone as determined by analysis of covariance. Thus, data on serum concentrations of LH and progesterone were analyzed by split-plot analysis of variance and differences among means tested for significance by use of Fishers Protected Least Significant Difference.

Results and Discussion

Treatment with 25 µg GnRH increased serum LH levels at 15, 30, 45 and 60 min (P<0.001) and reduced serum progesterone levels on day 7 through 11 of the cycle (treatment x day interaction; P<0.005). Mean peak levels of LH (ng/ml) in control and treated ewes were 4.93 and 19.16, respectively; common estimate of SE = 1.37. Mean levels of progesterone (ng/ml) in control and treated ewes on day 3, 5, 7, 9 and 11 were: control, 0.30, 0.62, 1.34, 1.60, 1.83 vs. treated, 0.25, 0.61, 0.91, 1.26, and 1.53, respectively; common estimate of SE = 0.21.

Treatment of ewes with 50 ng GnRH resulted in a slight rise in serum LH at time = 15 min (mean ± SE; control vs. treated ewes: 2.47 ± 1.18 vs. 6.03 ± 2.55 ng/ml). There was no significant treatment effect of 50 ng GnRH on serum progesterone levels on day 4 through day 10 of the cycle.

Injection of ewes with LH resulted in an increase in serum LH concentration which peaked time = 15 min. This dose of gonadotropin was intentionally pharmacological and resulted in peak serum LH concentrations of 44.35 ± 2.49 ng/ml (control = 3.71 ± 0.56 ng/ml) which began to decline 30 min following the last injection and averaged 9.72 ± 1.83 ng/ml at time = 105 min (control = $4.24 \pm .31$ ng/ml). Treatment of ewes with LH reduced serum progesterone levels on day 6 and 8 of the cycle (treatment x day interaction; $P<0.01$). Mean serum concentrations of progesterone (ng/ml) in control and treated ewes on day 4, 6, 8 and 10 were: control, 0.52, 1.43, 1.60, 1.95 vs. treated, 0.47, 0.94, 1.18, and 1.87, respectively; common estimate of SE = 0.31.

Results of these experiments indicate that exposure of the developing corpus luteum to elevated levels of LH on day 2 impairs subsequent development or ability of luteal cells to synthesize and (or) secrete progesterone early in the cycle. Injection of 50 ng GnRH which did not result in a concomitant surge of LH also did not result in an antigonadotropic response. These data suggest that the antisteroidogenic effect of GnRH is mediated through LH in the ewe rather than directly on the ovary as has been reported to occur in the rat. However, a single injection of 50 ng GnRH may also be subthreshold to a dose which will induce a gonadal effect.

Luteal development involves both an increase in the number and size of the luteal cells (11). Injection of ewes with LH or human chorionic gonadotropin in mid-cycle results in an increase in the proportion of large to small steroidogenic luteal cells (12). However, luteal receptor concentrations have been shown to decrease following administration of non-physiologically high levels of LH to ewes (13) and after GnRH treatment in cattle (3). Therefore, GnRH administered on day 2 may act by inducing secretion of LH that causes downregulation of LH receptors with a consequent reduction in the recruitment of large steroidogenic cells and, hence, suppression of progesterone secretion during the first half of the cycle.

Summary

Our results indicate that administration of 25 µg GnRH via the ovarian artery and the concomitant increase in endogenous secretion of LH as well as injection of high doses of LH on day 2 impairs subsequent ability of the ovine corpus luteum to synthesize and (or) secrete progesterone on day 4 through 9 of the cycle. Low doses of GnRH (50 ng) did not suppress serum progesterone concentrations. These data suggest that the antisteroidogenic action of GnRH is mediated through endogenous LH release but do not exclude possible functions of this peptide in the ovary.

Acknowledgment

This research was supported, in part, by a grant from CEVA Laboratories.

References

1. Hsueh AJW, Jones PBC. Extrapituitary actions of gonadotropin-releasing hormone. Endocr Rev 1981; 2:437-61.
2. Lucy MC, Stevenson JS. Gonadotropin-releasing hormone at estrus: luteinizing hormone, estradiol and progesterone during the periestrual and postinsemination periods in dairy cattle. Biol Reprod 1986; 35:300-11.

3. Rodger LD, Stormshak F. Gonadotropin-releasing hormone induced alteration of bovine corpus luteum function. Biol Reprod 1986; 35:149-56.

4. Cusan L, Auclair C, Belanger A, et al. Inhibitory effects of long term treatment with a luteinizing hormone-releasing hormone agonist on the pituitary-gonadal axis in male and female rats. Endocrinology 1979; 104:1369-76.

5. Clayton RN, Harwood JP, Catt KJ. Gonadotropin-releasing hormone analogue binds to luteal cells and inhibits progesterone production. Nature 1979; 282:90-3.

6. Hsueh AJW, Erickson GF. Extrapituitary action of gonadotropin-releasing hormone: direct inhibition of ovarian steroidogenesis. Science 1979; 204:854-5.

7. Aten RF, Ireland JJ, Weems CW, Behrman HR. Presence of gonadotropin-releasing hormone-like proteins in bovine and ovine ovaries. Endocrinology 1987; 120:727-33.

8. Brown JL, Reeves JJ. Absence of specific luteinizing hormone releasing hormone receptors in ovine, bovine and porcine ovaries. Biol Reprod 1983; 29:1179-82.

9. McCarthy MS, Swanson LV. Serum LH concentration following castration, steroid hormone and gonadotropin releasing hormone treatment in the male bovine. J Anim Sci 1976; 43:151-8.

10. Koligian KB, Stormshak F. Progesterone synthesis by ovine fetal cotyledons in vitro. J Anim Sci 1976; 42:439-43.

11. Schwall RH, Gamboni F, Mayan M, Niswender GD. Changes in the distribution of sizes of ovine luteal cells during the estrous cycle. Biol Reprod 1986; 34:911-8.

12. Farin CE, Moeller CL, Mayan H, Gamboni F, Sawyer HR, Niswender GD. Effect of luteinizing hormone and human chorionic gonadotropin on cell populations in the ovine corpus luteum. Biol Reprod 1988; 38:413-21.

13. Suter DE, Fletcher PW, Sluss P, Reichert LE Jr, Niswender GD. Alterations in the number of ovine luteal receptors for LH and progesterone secretion induced by homologous hormone. Biol Reprod 1980; 22:205-10.

53

Comparison of Gonadotropin- and Catecholamine-Induced Alterations of the Adenylyl Cyclase G-Proteins in Rabbit Corpora Lutea

Bhanu P. Jena and Joel Abramowitz

Department of Zoology, Iowa State University of Science and Technology, Ames, Iowa 50011

It is well established that the corpus luteum in rabbits contains an adenylyl cyclase that is responsive to both LH/hCG and catecholamines (1-4), and that both these hormones activate the same adenylyl cyclase (3,4). Earlier studies have shown that exposure of corpora lutea or ovarian tissues to either LH/hCG or catecholamines leads to refractoriness of the adenylyl cyclase in these tissues (5,6), and that this refractoriness is in part reflective of changes and/or loss in receptor function (7,8). Guanine nucleotide-binding regulatory proteins (G-proteins) transduce hormone-receptor occupancy to the catalytic subunit of adenylyl cyclase, hence playing a crucial role in signal transduction (9). Therefore, the present study was undertaken to assess changes in luteal adenylyl cyclase activity and G-protein function, after injection of either hCG or epinephrine (EPI) to pseudopregnant female rabbits. In this study, we present data that show alterations in G-proteins of the rabbit luteal adenylyl cyclase system after hormone treatment.

Materials and Methods

The source of materials for the adenylyl cyclase assay has been published earlier (10). S49 cyc- murine lymphoma cell lines were grown in our laboratory, and plasma membranes prepared as published (11). New Zealand White rabbits (3-4 kg) were used. Pseudopregnancy was initiated with 0.3 IU pFSH, sc, twice daily for 3 days followed by 100 IU hCG, IV, on day 4. On day 7 after hCG injection, rabbits were injected either IV, with 100 IU hCG, or sc, with EPI (2.5 mg/kg), and euthanized at different times after injection. Control animals were injected similarly, but with 0.9% saline instead of the hormone. Four control and 4 hormone-treated animals were taken for each time-point. Dissected rabbit corpora lutea from each animal were homogenized separately and membrane particles prepared and adenylyl cyclase assays were performed as previously described (1). Luteal Gs (the stimulatory

G-protein of adenylyl cyclase) activity in both control and treated rabbits was assessed by the ability of luteal cholate extracts to reconstitute NaF- and ISO-stimulated adenylyl cyclase activity in S49 cyc- membranes as described (12).

Results and Discussion

In control luteal membranes, there was no significant change in basal, oLH-, isoproterenol- (ISO-), sodium fluoride- (NaF-) and forskolin-stimulable adenylyl cyclase. In addition, no significant changes in NaF- and ISO-reconstituted adenylyl cyclase activities were seen in cholate extracts from control membranes (Table 1). In contrast, both hCG and EPI treatment depressed adenylyl cyclase activity and altered G-protein function.

HCG treatment resulted in a 2.5-fold increase in basal adenylyl cyclase activity over control levels after 3 h, and returned to control levels by 24 h (Fig. 1). This high basal adenylyl cyclase activity could be due to irreversibly bound hCG to membrane receptors (13). Similar results have been reported from earlier studies in pregnant and pseudopregnant rabbits (14). HCG treatment resulted in a 41% decrease in LH-stimulable adenylyl cyclase activity at 6

Table 1. Summary of ISO- and NaF-reconstituted adenylyl cyclase activity in control, hCG- and EPI-treated rabbits

Time After Treatment	Control		hCG Treated	
	NaF	ISO	NaF	ISO
		(pmol cAMP/mg/20 min)		
3 h	1072 ± 59	403 ± 10	758 ± 75*	235 ± 18**
6 h	787 ± 105	350 ± 94	1300 ± 66**	619 ± 13**
12 h	996 ± 70	403 ± 5	1049 ± 200	125 ± 41**
24 h	894 ± 35	359 ± 13	409 ± 40**	124 ± 14**
48 h	655 ± 130	226 ± 19	355 ± 51*	70 ± 14**
	Control		EPI Treated	
1.5 h	1007 ± 103	282 ± 4	333 ± 12**	32 ± 2**
3 h	1113 ± 136	252 ± 23	379 ± 77**	97 ± 13**
6 h	1104 ± 136	257 ± 18	398 ± 79**	92 ± 18**
12 h	687 ± 126	224 ± 96	660 ± 67	217 ± 52
24 h	795 ± 28	217 ± 54	845 ± 59	243 ± 36
48 h	795 ± 19	232 ± 47	849 ± 70	257 ± 40

Cholate extracts of luteal membranes were prepared from 4 control and 4 hormone-treated animals for each time-point. Cholate extracts were then reconstituted into S49 cyc-membranes and their ISO- and NaF-stimulable adenylyl cyclase activity assayed, as previously described (12). Values are mean $\pm$ SD of 3 separate assays, each assay done in triplicate. *Significantly different from controls (P<0.01). **Significantly different from controls (P<0.0001).

h, whereas no change in ISO-stimulable activity was observed until 12 h. This indicates that until 12 h, desensitization was homologous after which desensitization was heterologous. HCG treatment also resulted in altered NaF- and forskolin-stimulable adenylyl cyclase activity. There was a 25% depression of NaF-stimulable adenylyl cyclase at 3 h after which NaF-stimulable activity increased, prior to a time-dependent decrease. In contrast, forskolin-stimulable adenylyl cyclase remained elevated for 12 h, prior to a time-dependent decrease. After EPI treatment, similar changes in LH-, ISO-, NaF- and forskolin-stimulated adenylyl cyclase activities were observed in luteal membranes, indicating heterologous desensitization (Fig. 1). At 1.5 h, stimulable adenylyl cyclase activities were depressed by 24-30% and continued to decline until 6 h, when stimulable adenylyl cyclase activities were depressed by 45-52%. Stimulable adenylyl cyclase activities then increased such that by 24 h, values were at control levels. Therefore, in EPI-treated animals, recovery of the cyclase system from its refractory state is seen within 24 to 48 h, whereas the depressed state is maintained even after 48 h in hCG-treated animals. These studies indicate that loss in luteal adenylyl cyclase activity upon hCG treatment is permanent but slower in onset than the loss in adenylyl cyclase upon EPI treatment.

HCG treatment resulted in a 25% decrease in NaF-reconstituted activity at 3 h, a 75% increase at 6 h and a return to control levels at 12 h, that was followed by a 55% decrease at 24 and 48 h. These changes in NaF-reconstituted activity parallel changes in NaF-stimulated adenylyl cyclase activity, suggesting that changes in Gs may be responsible for altered response of the adenylyl cyclase system to NaF. Similar changes were observed in ISO-reconstituted activity at 3 and 6 h following hCG treatment. At 12 h, ISO-reconstituted activity was depressed by 65% and remained at this level for the remainder of the study

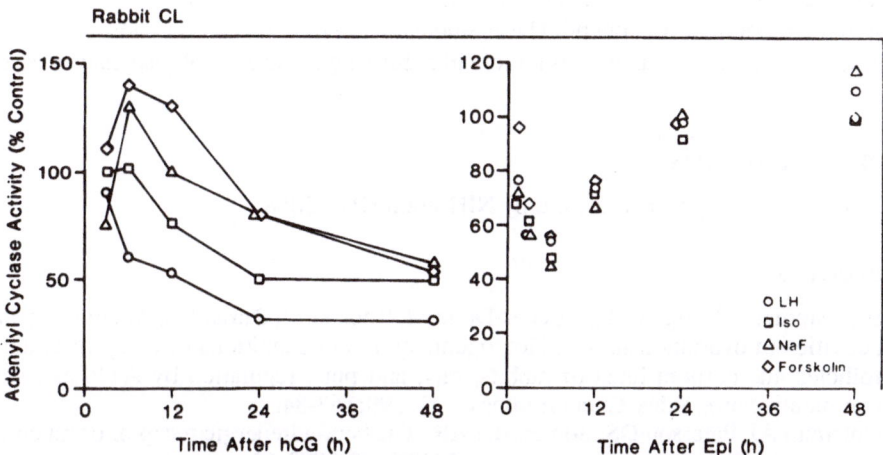

Fig. 1. Effect of hCG- and EPI-treatment on luteal adenylyl cyclase activity. Assays were performed for 10 min under standard assay conditions as described (1), in the presence or absence of 10 μg/ml oLH, 0.1 mM ISO, 10 mM NaF and 0.1 mM forskolin. The membrane protein concentration was 6-10 μg/5Oμl assay. Values were calculated by dividing the mean adenylyl cyclase activity from treated animals by the mean adenylyl cyclase activity from control animals and multiplied by 100.

period. There is clearly a dissociation of the NaF- and ISO-reconstituted activity 12 h following hCG treatment. This finding is supportive of the fact that Gs has different sites for NaF-stimulation and receptor coupling, and that in this case, the *beta*-adrenergic receptor coupling domain of Gs is altered prior to alteration of the NaF stimulating domain (9). Earlier studies in highly luteinized rat ovaries show that hCG-induced heterologous desensitization of adenylyl cyclase results in attenuation Gs activity by approximately 35% as assessed by cyc- reconstitution regardless of the stimulatory ligands used (15). In contrast, NaF- and ISO-reconstituted Gs activities were depressed by 60-65%, 1.5 h after EPI treatment and remained at this level for 6 h. After this point, NaF- and ISO-reconstituted Gs activities increased such that by 24 h they were at control levels (Table 1). On the other hand, studies on catecholamine-induced desensitization of turkey erythrocytes show that after 4 h of treatment there is a significant loss of ISO- but not NaF-reconstituting activity (16). In the present study, the correspondence of depressed NaF-stimulated adenylyl cyclase activity and NaF-reconstituting activity up to 6 h following EPI treatment further suggests that changes in Gs may be responsible for altered response of the adenylyl cyclase system to NaF. The similar pattern of depression of ISO- and NaF-reconstituted activity suggests alterations in both the catalytic and receptor coupling domains of Gs. Therefore, these studies indicate that loss in responsiveness of adenylyl cyclase in luteal tissue, due to hormone treatment, is due in part to altered G-protein function.

In summary, the injection of 100 IU hCG or 2.5 mg/kg EPI to pseudopregnant rabbits resulted in depressed adenylyl cyclase activity and altered G-protein in luteal membranes. The similarity in the pattern of G-protein alteration and changes in the adenylyl cyclase activity on hormone treatment indicates that alteration in G-proteins is in part responsible for the loss in adenylyl cyclase activity seen. This study demonstrates that the receptor-coupling domain and the NaF-stimulatory sites on Gs are separate, and that those two domains are altered on hormone treatment. These studies also show that in addition to hormone receptors, G-proteins play an important role in regulating the hormonal responsiveness of a tissue.

Acknowledgments

This work was supported, in part, by NIH grant HD-22058.

References

1. Birnbaumer L, Yang PC, Hunzicker-Dunn M, Bockaert J, Duran JM. Adenylyl cyclase activities in ovarian tissues. I. Homogenization and conditions of assay in Graafian follicles and corpora lutea of rabbits, rats, and pigs: regulation by ATP, and some comparative properties. Endocrinology 1976; 99:163-84.
2. Coleman AJ, Paterson DS, Somerville AR. The beta-adrenergic receptor of rat corpus luteum membranes. Biochem Pharmacol 1979; 28:1003-13.
3. Abramowitz J, Birnbaumer L. Properties of the hormonally responsive rabbit luteal adenylyl cyclase: effects of guanine nucleotides and magnesium ion on stimulation by gonadotropin and catecholamines. Endocrinology 1982; 110:773-81.
4. Abramowitz J, Iyengar R, Birnbaumer L. Guanine nucleotide and magnesium ion regulation of the interaction of gonadotropic and beta-adrenergic receptors with their

hormones: a comparative study using a single membrane system. Endocrinology 1982; 110:336-46.

5. Stormshak F, Casida LE. Effects of LH and ovarian hormones on corpora lutea of pseudopregnant and pregnant rabbits. Endocrinology 1965; 77:337-42.

6. Harwood JP, Dufau ML, Catt KJ. Differing specificities in the desensitization of ovarian adenylyl cyclase by epinephrine and human chorionic gonadotropin. Mol Pharmacol 1979; 15:439-44.

7. Catt KJ, Harwood JP, Richert ND, Conn PM, Conti M, Dufau ML. Luteal desensitization: hormonal regulation of LH receptors, adenylate cyclase and steroidogenic responses in the luteal cell. Adv Exp Med Biol 1979; 112:647-62.

8. Sibley DR, Lefkowitz RJ. Molecular mechanisms of receptor desensitization using the beta-adrenergic receptor-coupled adenylate cyclase system as a model. Nature 1985; 317:124-9.

9. Gilman AG. G proteins: transducers of receptor-generated signals. Annu Rev Biochem 1987; 56:615-49.

10. Sigafoos JF, Abramowitz J. Comparison of the ability of seven gonadotropin preparations from different mammalian sources to interact with the adenylyl cyclase system in corpora lutea from rabbits and rats. Comp Biochem Physiol 1987; 86A:453-60.

11. Iyengar R, Abramowitz J, Bordelon-Riser ME, Blume AJ, Birnbaumer L. Regulation of hormone-receptor coupling to adenylyl cyclase. Effects of GTP and GDP. J Biol Chem 1980; 255:10312-21.

12. Sigafoos JF, Abramowitz J. Effects of N-ethylmaleimide on gonadotropin and beta-adrenergic receptor function coupled to rabbit luteal adenylyl cyclase. Endocrinology 1986; 119:1432-8.

13. Abramowitz J, Birnbaumer L. Temporal characteristics of gonadotropin interaction with rabbit luteal receptors and activation of adenylyl cyclase: comparison to the mode of activation of catecholamine receptors. Endocrinology 1982; 111:970-6.

14. Hunzicker-Dunn M, Birnbaumer L. Adenylyl cyclase activities in ovarian tissues. II. Regulation of responsiveness to LH, FSH, and PGE1 in the rabbit. Endocrinology 1976; 99:185-97.

15. Kirchick JH, Iyengar R, Birnbaumer L. Human chorionic gonadotropin-induced heterologous desensitization of adenylyl cyclase from highly luteinized rat ovaries: attenuation of regulatory N component activity. Endocrinology 1983; 113:1638-46.

16. Briggs MM, Stadel JM, Iyengar I, Lefkowitz RJ. Functional modification of the guanine nucleotide regulatory protein after desensitization of turkey erythrocytes by catecholamines. Arch Biochem Biophys 1983; 142-51.

54

Immunohistochemical and Morphological Observations of Macrophages in the Human Ovary

H. Katabuchi, Y. Fukumatsu, and H. Okamura

Department of Obstetrics and Gynecology, Kumamoto University
Medical School, 1-1-1 Honjo, Kumamoto 860, Japan

Introduction

Macrophages have been identified within the corpus luteum of several species, including human (1-3). In addition to their well recognized phagocytic property, macrophages have been shown to exert other influences in luteal tissue. Recently, Kirsch et al. reported that macrophages secrete substances that stimulate luteal cell progesterone production in the mouse corpus luteum (4), and Halme et al. suggested that peritoneal macrophages may exert luteotropic effects on human granulosa-luteal cells (5).

The present study was undertaken to examine the distribution and morphological changes of macrophages within human ovaries and to discuss a possible role of macrophages in ovarian cells.

Materials and Methods

Materials

Seven ovaries were obtained from 7 women who underwent laparotomy for reasons other than the presence of malignancy. The women's ages ranged from 28 to 43 years.

Light Microscopy

Tissue specimens were fixed in 10% buffered formalin for making routine paraffin sections, which were stained with hematoxylin and eosin (HE).

Immunohistochemistry

Immediately after removal, ovarian tissue specimens were excised from the walls of follicles, capsules of corpus luteum or corpus albicans, depending on the condition of the ovaries and cut into small pieces of blocks. These blocks were fixed in 4% periodate-lysine and 2% paraformaldehyde (PLP) fixative for 4 h at 4°C, and cryostat sections were prepared according to the method described elsewhere (6). These sections were incubated with two monoclonal antibodies; HLe-1 (Becton Dickinson, USA) specific for human leukocytes and FMC 32 (Australian Monoclonal Development, Australia) specific for human monocyte-macrophages according to the avidin-biotin PO complex (ABC) method. For immunohistochemical detection of human chorionic gonadotropin (hCG), we performed the PO anti-PO (PAP) method using polyclonal antisera against hCG (DAKO, Denmark). PO activity was visualized by incubating the sections for 5-10 min with 3,3′-diaminobenzidine in 0.5 mg/ml of tris-HCl buffer (pH 7.6) containing 0.01% H_2O_2.

Electron Microscopy

Small pieces of fresh ovarian tissue specimens obtained in the same way were fixed in a chilled 2.5% glutaraldehyde for 2 h, and postfixed by the routine procedures. The 1 μ-thick sections were stained with a toluidine blue solution for light microscopic survey. The ultrathin sections were stained with lead citrate and uranyl acetate, and observed by an electron microscope (Hitachi 12A).

Results

At the resting stage of the ovarian follicles, both the ovarian cortex and the medulla were made up of a stromal or interstitial tissue, which was composed of collagenous fibers and spindle-shaped cells. Many of these cells displayed ultrastructural characteristics typical of both fibroblasts and smooth muscle cells, but neither lymphocytes nor macrophages were identified. Immunohistochemical observation also showed that any ovarian cells had no reactivity with HLe-1 and FMC 32 antibodies at this stage. With the development of follicles, the stromal cells tended to become concentrically arranged outside the follicles. HLe-1 positive cells appeared in the stroma and gradually increased in number, but FMC 32 positive cells had a smaller cell population. They were frequently encountered near the perifollicular capillaries of the stroma (Fig. 1). However, when the development of ovarian follicles was interrupted, FMC 32 positive cells were mainly observed in the cavity of follicles (Fig. 2). In accordance with immunohistochemical findings, macrophages were observed mainly near the capillaries on electron microscopy (Fig. 3). These macrophages had large polygonal nuclei and extended their pseudopodia from the cell surface. They had few cytoplasmic vacuoles and granules, but contained lysosomes of various sizes (Fig. 4).

With the luteinization of follicles, the granulosa cells and the theca interna cells hypertrophied and gradually developed into a corpus luteum, both cell types accumulated lipid droplets and granules in their cytoplasm. On electron microscopy, the lipid droplets varied in size and electron density, and were dispersed throughout the cytoplasm singly or in clusters. The ultrastructural architecture of the granules showed their lysosomal nature. FMC 32 positive cells as well as HLe-1 positive cells were observed inside and outside of the corpus luteum, and their total number increased further in comparison to the stage of the folliculogenesis (Fig. 5). Some of FMC 32 positive cells, which existed near the capillaries of the stroma and lined up in one or two files around the corpus luteum, were also positive for hCG (Fig. 6). In mature corpora lutea, those macrophages were ultrastructurally characterized by the presence of many electron-dense lysosomal granules and phagocytic granules of variable configuration and structure throughout their cytoplasm (Fig. 7). In addition to

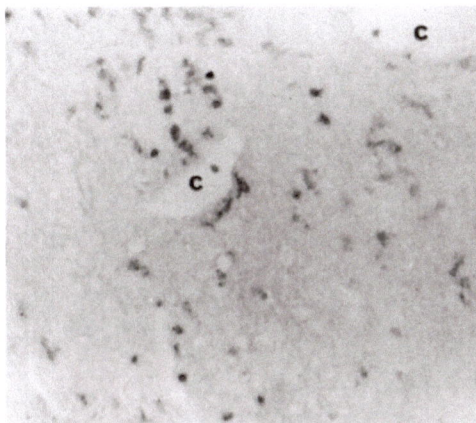

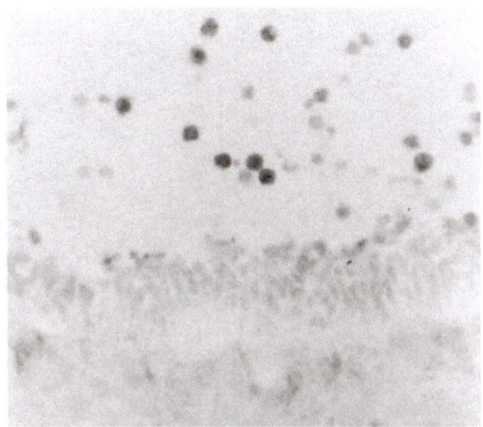

Fig. 1. FMC 32 positive cells near the perifollicular capillaries in a developing follicle. c, capillary. x 200.

Fig. 2. FMC 32 positive cells in the cavity of an atretic follicle. x 650.

these organelles, many lipid droplets and cholesterol crystals with figures of long squares were also found in regressing corpora lutea (Fig. 8).

Discussion

On the period of structural luteolysis, macrophages contain many lipid droplets and cholesterol crystals throughout their cytoplasm. This finding implies a picture of phagocytosis and degradation in lysosomes of damaged luteal cells by macrophages. It is the most recognized phagocytic property of macrophages in the ovary.

On the other hand, the mononuclear cells with the morphological features of macrophages were first present in the stroma of ovary with the maturation of follicles, and their

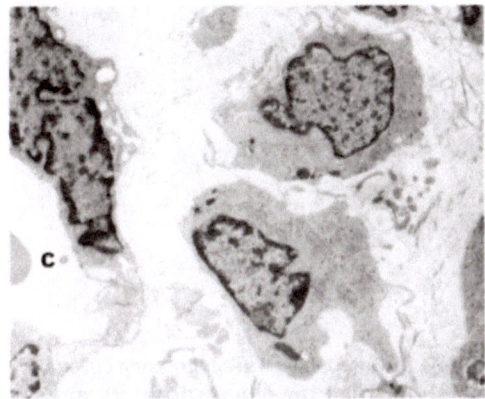

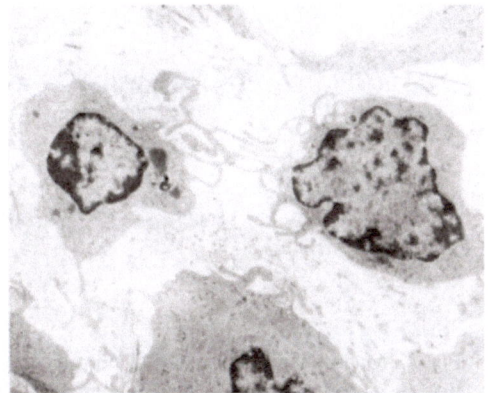

Fig. 3. Macrophages in developing follicles, situated close by the perifollicular capillaries. c, capillary. x 5,100.

Fig. 4. Macrophages in developing follicles, containing lysosomes of various sizes. x 6,200.

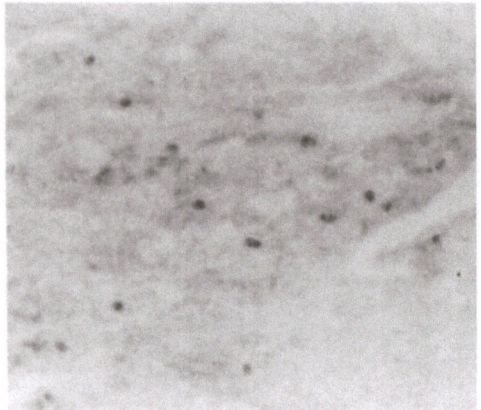

Fig. 5. FMC 32 positive cells inside and outside of the corpus luteum at the stage of luteinization. x 250.

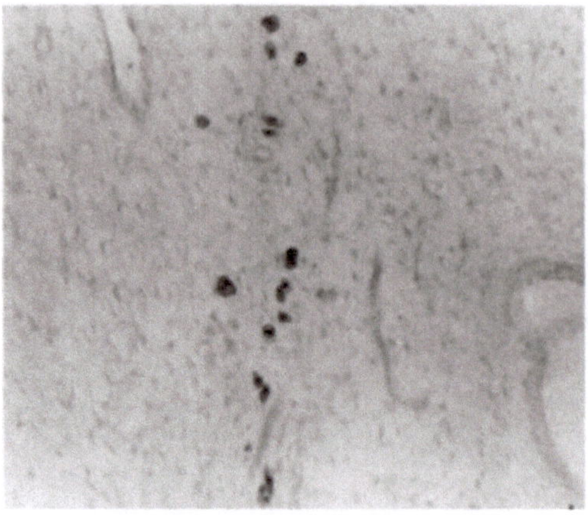

Fig. 6. HCG positive macrophages lined up in one or two files around the corpus luteum at the stage of luteinization. x 150.

intracellular organelles were developed without cytoplasmic vacuoles or granules. Recently, it was pointed out that fibroblast growth factor and epidermal growth factor are mitogenic for human granulosa cells (7). Macrophages also have been shown to secrete interleukin-1 and macrophage-derived growth factor and promote the proliferation of fibroblasts. Thus, it would appear that macrophages may play an indirect role in the control of human granulosa cell proliferation. Of particular interest is our observation that some macrophages stained positive for hCG during the luteinization. It is suggested that macrophages may regulate the

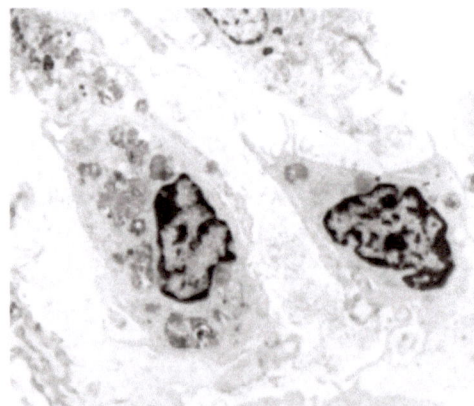

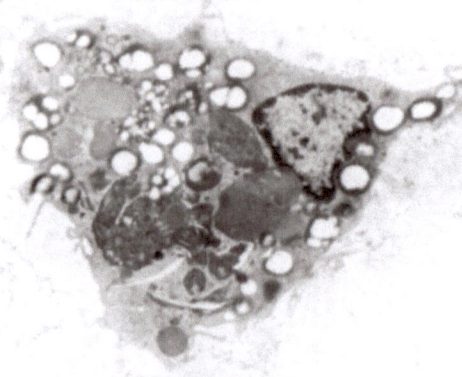

Fig. 7. Macrophages in a mature corpus luteum, having many electron-dense lysosomal granules and phagocytic granules of variable configuration and structure in the cytoplasm. x 4,000.

Fig. 8. Macrophages in a regressing corpus luteum, having many droplets and cholesterol crystals with figures of long squares in the cytoplasm. x 5,000.

concentration of luteotropic/luteolytic complex by secreting growth factors and/or ingesting gonadotropin.

In conclusion, we suggest that macrophages can be responsible for human granulosa cell proliferation and progesterone production in each respective stage of folliculogenesis and luteinization.

References

1. Bulmer D. The histochemistry of ovarian macrophages in the rat. J Anat 1964; 98:313-9.
2. Gillim SW, Christensen KA, McLennan CE. Fine structure of the human menstrual corpus luteum at its stage of maximum secretory activity. Am J Anat 1969; 126:409-28.
3. Paavola LG. The corpus luteum of the guinea pig. Fine structure at the time of maximum secretion and during regression. Am J Anat 1977; 150:565-604.
4. Kirsch TM, Friedman AC, Vogel RL, Flickinger GL. Macrophages in corpora lutea of mice: characterization and effects on steroid secretion. Biol Reprod 1981; 25:629-38.
5. Halme J, Hammond MG, Syrop CH, Tolbert LM. Peritoneal macrophages modulate human granulosa-luteal cell progesterone production. J Clin Endocrinol Metab 1985; 61:912-6.
6. Takeya M, Hsiao L, Takahashi K. A new monoclonal antibody TRPM-3, binds specifically to certain rat macrophage populations: immunohistochemical and immunoelectron microscopic analysis. J Leukocyte Biol 1987; 41:187-95.
7. Tapanainen J, Leinonen PJ, Tapanainen P, Yamamoto M, Jaffe RB. Regulation of human granulosa-luteal cell progesterone production and proliferation by gonadotropins and growth factors. Fertil Steril 1987; 48:576-80.

55

Phosphorylation of Sterol Carrier Protein 2 by Protein Kinase C

A. Steinschneider, M. P. McLean, J. T. Billheimer,[1]
H. C. Palfrey,[2] and G. Gibori

Department of Physiology and Biophysics, University of Illinois
College of Medicine, Chicago, IL 60612; [1]DuPont Experimental Station
Wilmington, DE 19898; [2]University of Chicago, Chicago, IL 60637

Introduction

Ca^{++} has been implicated in the regulation of the steroidogenic response to tropic hormones (1-3), including the transport of cholesterol to the mitochondrial site of side-chain cleavage, a step that may also involve sterol carrier protein 2 (SCP_2) (4). SCP_2 is a cholesterol carrier that facilitates the intracellular transfer of cholesterol to cytochrome $P450_{scc}$, the rate-limiting enzyme in the steroidogenic process, located in the inner mitochondrial membrane. Thus, changes in the content and/or activity of SCP_2 may be expected to play a key role in cholesterol transport and, therefore, in steroidogenesis (5). SCP_2 is present in nonsteroidogenic and steroidogenic tissues, including the ovary (6,7). Ovarian SCP_2 closely resembles hepatic SCP_2 in its amino acid composition (7) and, presumably, in its overall structure.

Since one of the principal calcium-mediated events is the alteration of the phosphorylation state of cellular proteins, and regulation of their activities, it became of interest to explore whether SCP_2 is a potential control point for phosphorylation-mediated hormonal regulation. As a first step, we investigated whether SCP_2 is a substrate for purified, major type, Ca^{++}- and non-Ca^{++}-dependent protein kinases.

Materials and Methods

Materials

Highly purified SCP_2 was prepared from rat liver (8), dialyzed in the cold against 10 mM Tris pH 7.4, 5 mM β-mercaptoethanol (ME) and stored frozen at -80°C. Purified protein kinase C (PKC) from calf brain and calmodulin kinase II (CaM-PK II) and synapsin I from rat brain were used. Myosin light chain kinase (MLCK) and myosin light chains (MLC) from turkey gizzard were kindly provided by Dr. P. De Lanerolle. Other materials were obtained from commercial sources.

Phosphorylation Assays

Following preequilibration for 2 min at 30°C, reactions were initiated by addition of 1 μCi or more ATP-[γ-^{32}P]. After incubation for 15 min at 30°C, phosphate transfer was terminated by the addition of one-third volume 20% glycerol, 9% SDS, 10% β-ME, 0.125 M Tris pH 6.8, 3 mM EDTA and 0.02% bromophenol blue. Samples were chilled rapidly on ice and then denatured at 85-90°C for 10 min. The products were subjected to SDS-PAGE using 7.5-18% linear gradient polyacrylamide gel slabs, stained with Coomassie blue R250 and visualized by autoradiography.

Results

To investigate whether purified protein kinases employ SCP$_2$ as substrate, phosphate transfer from ATP-[γ-^{32}P] was monitored under optimal conditions. The limit of detection on a molar basis was estimated at 10^{-5} or less phosphate/SCP$_2$. As shown in Figures 1 and 2, cAMP-dependent protein kinase (PKA), CaM-PK II, MLCK and PKC effectively catalyzed the radiolabelling of histone IIa, synapsin I, MLC and histone III, respectively, known substrates for these kinases used as positive controls (Fig. 1, 2). Autophosphorylation of the kinases and labelling of other attending proteins were also evident. However, only calf or rabbit brain PKC catalyzed the phosphorylation of a Mr 14,000 protein(s) that migrated like SCP$_2$ (Fig. 2) and reacted with SCP$_2$-specific antiserum (Western blot, not shown). A second Mr 16,000 protein that frequently accompanies SCP$_2$ (5,8) was also a substrate (Fig. 2). Direct counting of Mr 14,000 phosphoprotein(s), excised from the same gel, indicated that approximately 5×10^{-4} and 2×10^{-4} moles phosphate/mole SCP$_2$ had been incorporated using the calf brain enzyme, 1 μM SCP$_2$ as acceptor and 38 μM or 3.7 μM ATP, respectively, as phosphate donor.

To establish further that SCP$_2$ is a substrate for PKC, phosphorylation studies were performed in the presence of polymyxin B, a PKC inhibitor (9,10). Figure 3 shows that phosphate transfer was stimulated by Ca^{++} and phospholipid (PL) and blocked by inhibitory concentrations of polymyxin B. Other experiments indicated that neither Ca^{++} alone, Ca^{++} and CaM nor cAMP stimulated phosphate transfer into SCP$_2$ by the partially purified PKC preparation used here (not shown).

Discussion

Phosphorylation studies performed with highly purified SCP$_2$ and Ca^{++}- and cAMP dependent kinases have revealed that SCP$_2$ is a specific substrate for PKC. Thus, phosphorylation by PKC was stimulated by Ca^{++} and phospholipid, PKC cofactors, and was blocked by polymyxin B, a PKC inhibitor. CaM-PKII and MLCK, two other calcium-dependent, major type protein kinases, failed to affect detectable phosphate transfer to SCP$_2$ under conditions allowing for intense phosphorylation of their established substrates, Synapsin I and MLC, respectively. CAMP-dependent kinase also failed to phosphorylate SCP$_2$. This is in agreement with the absence from the published amino acid sequence (11) of the

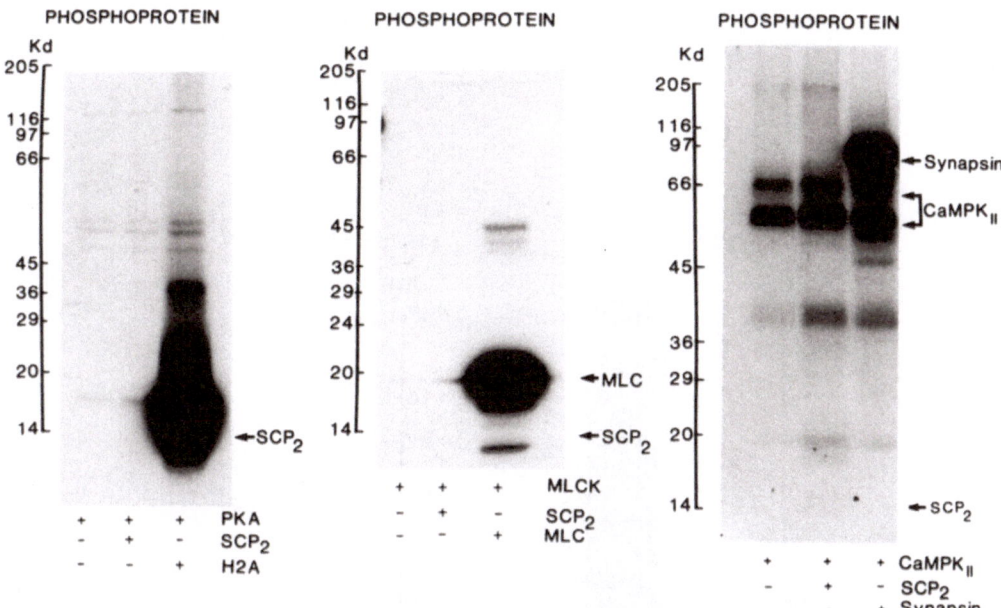

Fig. 1. Phosphorylation by major type protein kinases. ATP-^{32}P, 13.3 µM; SCP$_2$, 5.8 µM. *Left panel:* Tris pH 7.4, 25 mM; MgSO$_4$, 5.5 mM; dithiothreitol (DTT), 1 mM; cAMP, 4 µM; 3-isobutyl-1-methylxanthine (IBMX), 2 µM; bovine heart PKA catalytic subunit (Sigma), 550 pmolar units; histone IIa (Sigma) 30 µg/ml. *Middle panel:* Tris pH 7.4, 25 mM; MgSO$_4$, 6 mM; DTT, 1 mM; CaCl$_2$, 1.5 mM; bovine testis CaM (Boehringer), 10 µg/ml; rat brain CaM protein kinase II, 1.25 µg/ml; rat brain Synapsin I, 6 µg/ml. *Right panel:* Tris pH 7.4, 15 mM; MgSO$_4$, 10 mM; CaCl$_2$, 4 mM; CaM, 10 µg/ml; MLCK, 15 µg/ml; MLC, 70 µg/ml.

consensus sequences that usually accompany the respective phosphate acceptor sites for phosphorylation by cAMP-dependent kinase. Phosphate incorporation was on the order of 10^{-4} moles/mole SCP$_2$. Compared to Histone III, a known substrate for PKC, SCP$_2$ preparations incorporated less phosphate. Possibly high occupancy by phosphate of additional SCP$_2$ harbored acceptor sites, if any, may have precluded further phosphorylation in vitro.

Activation of PKC has been found to promote steroidogenesis by several endocrine glands, including differentiated granulosa and luteal cells (12-14). Our finding that PKC causes SCP$_2$ phosphorylation suggests the possibility that at least one site of action of the calcium, phospholipid-dependent kinase may be the activation of SCP$_2$ and cholesterol transport. The notion that phosphorylation serves to mark SCP$_2$ molecules destined for further intracellular processing (15) is also consistent with our results.

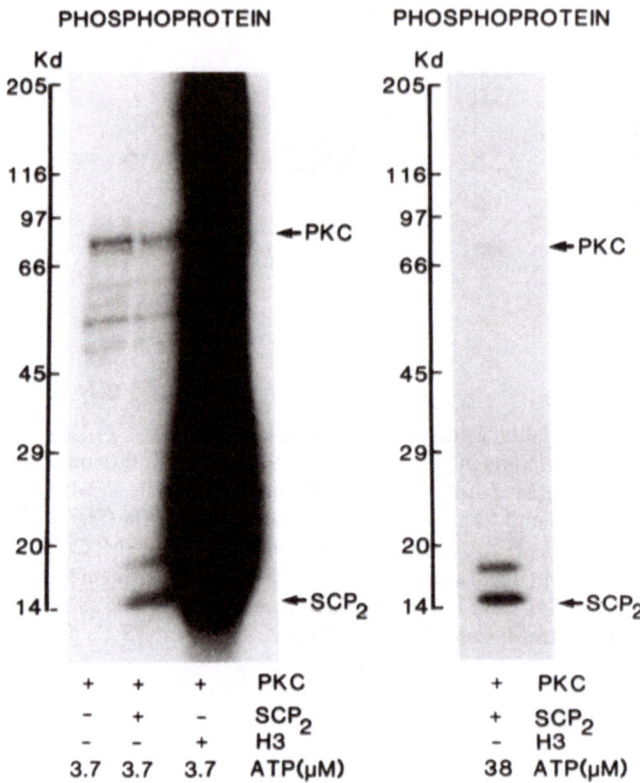

Fig. 2. Phosphorylation of SCP$_2$ by PKC. SCP$_2$, 1 μM; Tris pH 7.4, 25 mM; MgSO$_4$, 6 mM; L-α-phosphatydil-L-serine, 40 μg/ml; 1,2 dioleoyl-rac-glycerol (diolein), 4 μg/ml; CaCl$_2$, 1.5 mM; calf brain PKC; 10 ng/ml protein; histone III (Sigma), 33 μg/ml. PL-phosphatidyl serine, diolein.

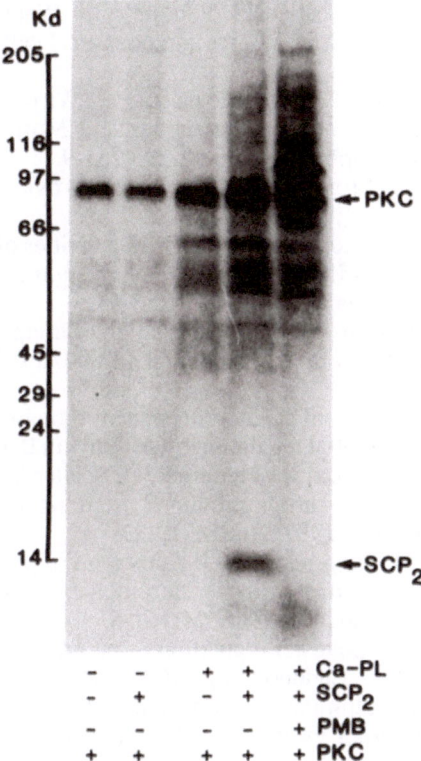

Fig. 3. Effect of Ca^{++}-PL and polymyxin B on the phosphorylation of SCP$_2$ by PKC. As in Figure 2 except 1.6 µM ATP-^{32}P.
Polymyxin B sulfate (Sigma), 5 x 10^{-4} M.

Acknowledgments

This research was supported by NIH Grant HD 11119. MPM was supported by a NRSA Fellowship HD 6982.

References

1. Hall PF, Osawa S, Thomasson C. A role for calmodulin in the regulation of steroidogenesis. J Cell Biol 1981; 90:402-7.
2. Carnegie JA, Tsang BK. The calcium-calmodulin system: participation in the regulation of steroidogenesis at different stages of granulosa cell differentiation. Biol Reprod 1984; 30:515-22.
3. Veldhuis JD, Klase JF, Demers LM, Chafouleas JG. Mechanisms subserving calcium's modulation of luteinizing hormone action in isolated swine granulosa cells. Endocrinology 1984; 114:441-8.
4. Vahouny GV, Chanderbhan R, Kharroubi A, Noland BJ, Pastuszyn A, Scallen TJ. Sterol carrier and lipid transfer proteins. Adv Lipid Res 1987; 22:83-113.

420   A. STEINSCHNEIDER ET AL.

5. Trzeciak WH, Simpson ER, Scallen TJ, Vahouny GV, Waterman MR. Studies on the synthesis of sterol carrier protein-2 in rat adrenocortical cells in monolayer culture. J Biol Chem 1987; 262:3713-7.
6. Teerlink T, Van der Krift TP, Van Heusden PH, Wirtz KWA. Determination of nonspecific lipid transfer protein in rat tissues and Morris hepatomas by enzyme immunoassay. Biochim Biophys Acta 1984; 793:251-9.
7. Tanaka T, Billheimer JT, Strauss JF III. Luteinized rat ovaries contain a sterol carrier protein. Endocrinology 1984; 114:533-40.
8. Trzaskos JM, Gaylor JL. Cytosolic modulators of activities of microsomal enzymes of cholesterol biosynthesis; purification and characterization of a nonspecific lipid-transfer protein. Biochim Biophys Acta 1983; 751:52-65.
9. Steinschneider A, Khan I. In vitro phosphorylation of midpregnant rat luteal proteins in the presence of polymyxin B and compound 48/80 [Abstract]. Endocrine Soc 70th Ann Meeting 1988; 343.
10. Wrenn RW, Wooten MW. Dual calcium dependent protein phosphorylation systems in pancreas and their differential regulation by polymyxin B. Life Sci 1984; 35:267-76.
11. Pastuszyn A, Noland BJ, Bazan JF, Fletterick RJ, Scallen TH. Primary sequence and structural analysis of sterol carrier protein 2 from rat liver: homology with immunoglobulins. J Biol Chem 1987; 262:13219-27.
12. Shinohara O, Knecht M, Feng K, Catt KJ. Activation of protein kinase C potentiates cyclic AMP production and stimulates steroidogenesis in differentiated ovarian granulosa cells. J Steroid Biochem 1985; 24:161-8.
13. Kawai Y, Clark MR. Phorbol ester regulation of rat granulosa cell prostaglandin and progesterone accumulation. Endocrinology 1985; 116:2320-6.
14. Brunswig B, Bohnet HG. Stimulation of progesterone production in bovine luteal cells by mezerin and the phorbol ester PMA. Acta Endocrinol [suppl] (Copenh) 1986; 111:72-3.
15. Gibson DM. Reversible phosphorylation of hepatic HMG-CoA reductase in endocrine and feedback control of cholesterol biosynthesis. In: Preiss B, ed. Regulation of HMG-CoA reductase. Academic Press, 1985:79-132.

56

Histological Assessment of Ovarian Follicle Number in Mice as a Screen for Ovarian Toxicity

J. J. Heindel,[1] P. J. Thomford,[2] and D. R. Mattison[2]

[1]Developmental and Reproductive Toxicology Group,
National Toxicology Program, NIEHS, RTP, NC;
[2]University of Arkansas for Medical Sciences, Little Rock AR
and National Center for Toxicological Research, Jefferson, AR

Introduction

Reproductive processes in both males and females are susceptible to interference from chemical insult (1). While there are biological markers of male reproductive toxicity (2,3), there are few markers for female reproductive toxicity (4,5). In addition, current methods for assessing female reproductive vulnerability to xenobiotics are inadequate. For example, some forms of end-organ toxicity (e.g., ovarian, tubal or uterine) are not addressed. For that reason, subtle disruption of reproductive function is not detected in standard reproductive toxicity protocols.

We are, therefore, investigating alternative endpoints of reproductive or gonadal toxicity in the female. The ovary was chosen as the target organ for our studies because it plays a central role in female reproduction. The process of oogenesis, however, is less amenable to easy measurement than spermatogenesis since the oogonia stop dividing before birth and the mature female rodent produces only about a dozen oocytes per cycle, unlike the male which produces millions of sperm per day (2). Thus, methods of assessing ovarian toxicity cannot depend only on methods which directly count oocyte production and release, but are more likely to be successful if they rely on assessing follicular populations. Therefore, we evaluated ovarian response to toxicants by quantitating follicle number by size. In order to relate ovarian response to an actual measurement of fertility, ovaries were removed from mice undergoing the National Toxicology Program's (NTP) Reproductive Assessment by Continuous Breeding (RACB) protocol (6,7) which assesses both reproductive toxicity and determines the affected sex. This design allows direct comparison of reproductive performance and ovarian follicle populations (8,9) in the same mouse.

The RACB protocol consists of four tasks. Task 1, the dose range finding study, is conducted to determine doses for the continuous breeding phase. The chemical is administered for 14 days and maximum tolerated dose (MTD) is estimated. Task 2, the continuous breeding phase, determines the effect of the MTD and two lower doses on fertility during 98 days of cohabitation. The numbers of litters produced, and the number, sex, and weight of pups/litter are measured as an index of fertility. If fertility is altered, Task 3 (a crossover mating trial) is conducted to determine the affected sex. Task 4 evaluates reproductive performance of the offspring (F1) from the last Task 2 litter (i.e., they are mated within a dose group when they are 74 ± 10 days of age and the number, weight and sex of pups is determined). The F0 animals after Task 3 (positive study) and Task 2 (negative study) and the F1 adults are necropsied and reproductive organ weights and sperm parameters are assessed. For the purpose of this evaluation, the ovaries were removed at necropsy from mice in 15 RACB studies in order to test the possibility of using differential follicle counts as a marker of reproductive toxicity. Of the 15 chemicals tested, 7 were negative in the RACB protocol (i.e., showed no reproductive toxicity), 3 were positive but the affected sex could not be accurately determined, 4 were toxic to both males and females and 1 was only toxic to the female.

Materials and Methods

For RACB studies, CD-1 mice were obtained, treated and housed as previously described (6,7). Reproductive performance of F0 mice was assessed in Task 2. The affected sex was determined in a crossover mating study during Task 3. Reproductive performance of F1 mice was assessed in Task 4.

At the conclusion of Task 3 or 4, ovaries were removed at necropsy, fixed in Bouin's medium for 12-24 h, stored in 70% ethanol, dehydrated, embedded, serially sectioned at 6 μm, mounted and stained with hematoxylin and eosin. The number of small, growing, and antral follicles were counted in every 10th section (8,9). Ovaries from at least 10 animals were analyzed for each treatment group.

Results and Discussion

We initially assessed inter-animal variability by pooling control follicle counts from all the studies (n=120). Table 1 shows the mean number $\pm$ SD of small growing and antral follicles from the control ovaries from Task 3 and Task 4 necropsies. Note that the Task 4 (F1 adults) are younger (74 ± 10 days of age) than the Task 3 mice (238 ± 10 days of age) and therefore have more small and growing follicles per ovary. In order to determine the chance of detecting a significant decrease in the number of follicles, the statistical power was calculated (Table 1). This analysis revealed that among Task 3 CD-1 mice, a change in the number of small, growing and antral follicles of 47%, 39% or 67% would be necessary in order to detect a statistically significant difference at P<0.05.

When ovaries from the treated animals were compared to their respective controls (Table 2), there were no alterations in the differential follicle counts in nine of the RACB studies which were either negative, when only male reproduction was altered or when the affected sex could not be determined (bisphenol A, ethanol, propantheline bromide, propylene glycol,

Table 1. Statistical power analysis for decreases in
ovarian follicle counts in CD-1 mice *

	Mean	SD	Approximate power for detecting a decrease of . . .		
			20%	30%	40%
Task 3					
Small	236.3	94.1	<<70%	~65%	87%
Growing	62.7	20.8	<70%	80%	96%
Antral	5.5	3.2	<<70%	<<70%	<70%
Task 4					
Small	408.3	114.9	<70%	90%	>99%
Growing	107.0	28.2	~65%	94%	>99%
Antral	10.9	4.7	>>70%	>70%	81%

*These power calculations assume: (1) one dosed and one control group; (2) sample size of 20 per group; (3) underlying normality of data; (4) significance at $P<0.05$; and, (5) treatment does not alter underlying standard deviation.

9-aminoacridine, triethylene glycol diacetate, propylene glycol monomethyl ether, trichloroethylene, oxalic acid).

Three of the five xenobiotics which impaired female reproduction showed reduced numbers of small and growing follicles compared to their concurrent controls (2,2-bis,bromomethyl-1,3-propanediol, ethylene glycol monomethyl ether, and methoxyacetic acid). Note the dose-related effect on follicle number in the Task 4–2,2-Bis(bromoethyl)-1,3-propanediol study. Also note that ovarian toxicity was evident in the younger (Task 4) animals treated with methoxyacetic acid since conception, while no effect was evident in the Task 3 animals when treatment commenced in adulthood. There were no significant differences in follicle counts in the di-N-hexyl phthalate or the tricresyl phosphate-treated mice.

Thus, not all reproductive toxicants which impair female reproduction are identified by changes in follicle counts. This is consistent with toxicity at other sites. In this study, no false positives were identified; that is, no ovarian changes were seen with chemicals which did not impair female reproduction (Table 3). Therefore, as suggested by earlier studies (10,11), quantitation of follicle number may be a valuable indicator of ovarian toxicity.

Table 2. Summary of follicle counts in treated animals *

Chemical	Task	Dose	Small	Follicle Count Growing	Antral	RACB Result
Ethanol (ETH)						
	T4	0%	543 ± 161	96 ± 33	14 ± 8	Neg
		15%	605 ± 192	95 ± 35	12 ± 4	
Trichloroethylene (TCE)						
	T3	0%	250 ± 66	70 ± 15	1 ± 1	Pos
		0.6%	286 ± 85	70 ± 14	1 ± 1	
	T4	0%	490 ± 120	118 ± 24	3 ± 2	
		0.6%	476 ± 180	108 ± 31	1 ± 1	
Tricresyl Phosphate (TCP)						
	T3	0%	238 ± 97	69 ± 25	3 ± 2	M&F
		0.2%	201 ± 107	56 ± 24	2 ± 2	
	T4	0%	438 ± 109	113 ± 17	5 ± 4	
		0.1%	406 ± 113	103 ± 33	2 ± 2	
2,2-Bis(bromoethyl)-1,3-propanediol (BPD)						
	T3	0%	163 ± 103	58 ± 23	6 ± 3	F
		0.4%	33 ± 23**	14 ± 12**	2 ± 2*	
	T4	0%	356 ± 137	98 ± 26	12 ± 8	
		0.1%	224 ± 103*	80 ± 27	12 ± 5	
		0.2%	118 ± 67**	53 ± 22	8 ± 4	
		0.4%	31 ± 24**	26 ± 18*	7 ± 5	
Ethylene glycol (EG)						
	T3	0%	201 ± 81	69 ± 25	3 ± 2	Pos
		1.5%	267 ± 83	69 ± 22	3 ± 3	
	T4	0%	354 ± 81	99 ± 28	1 ± 1	
		1.5%	299 ± 39	69 ± 22	1 ± 1	
Ethylene glycol monomethyl ether (EGMME)						
	T3	0%	212 ± 67	105 ± 30	11 ± 5	M&F
		0.1%	110 ± 85**	63 ± 32**	4 ± 3**	
	T4	0%	124 ± 73	53 ± 23	7 ± 4	
		0.3%	113 ± 52	51 ± 23	10 ± 6	
Oxalic acid (OA)						
	T4	0%	283 ± 115	93 ± 31	3 ± 3	Pos
		0.2%	303 ± 135	115 ± 45	2 ± 2	
Propantheline bromide (PB)						
	T2	0%	238 ± 115	49 ± 15	6 ± 5	Neg
		0.5%	262 ± 51	45 ± 8	4 ± 3	
	T4	0%	423 ± 152	83 ± 25	6 ± 5	
		0.5%	394 ± 115	69 ± 17	7 ± 3	

*(Table 2 is continued on next page.)

Table 2. Summary of follicle counts in treated animals *(continued)*

Chemical	Task	Dose	Small	Follicle Count Growing	Antral	RACB Result
Propylene glycol (PG)						
	T4	0%	432 ± 112	112 ± 31	27 ± 6	Neg
		5.0%	326 ± 104	86 ± 21	24 ± 7	
Propylene glycol monomethyl ether (PGME)						
	T4	0%	378 ± 135	96 ± 21	21 ± 9	Neg
		2.0%	303 ± 72	83 ± 17	23 ± 7	
9-Aminoacridine (9AA)						
	T4	0%	282 ± 112	92 ± 33	4 ± 4	Neg
		0.05%	250 ± 105	83 ± 26	4 ± 4	
Triethylene glycol diacetate (TGD)						
	T4	0%	488 ± 104	131 ± 42	3 ± 2	Neg
		3.0%	515 ± 103	144 ± 32	4 ± 3	
Bisphenol A (BA)						
	T3	0%	284 ± 78	43 ± 12	7 ± 4	Neg
		1.0%	263 ± 73	68 ± 5	4 ± 3	
	T4	0%	458 ± 90	122 ± 23	3 ± 3	
		1.0%	419 ± 89	16 ± 36	8 ± 5	
Di-N-Hexyl phthalate (NHP)						
	T3	0%	227 ± 103	62 ± 28	12 ± 6	M&F
		1.2%	273 ± 96	56 ± 13	11 ± 4	
Methoxyacetic acid (MAA)						
	T3	0%	259 ± 139	64 ± 23	3 ± 4	M&F
		0.4%	221 ± 90	53 ± 24	3 ± 2	
	T4	0%	547 ± 140	129 ± 24	37 ± 11	
		0.1%	304 ± 173**	83 ± 19**	19 ± 5*	

*P<0.05, **P<0.01. Pos = Reproductive toxicant with sex not identified. Neg = No evidence of reproductive toxicity in RACB. M or F = Evidence of reproductive toxicity in male or female

Table 3. Summary of results from reproductive assessment and ovarian follicle counts

Ovarian Follicle Counts	Reproductive Assessment by Continuous Breeding	
	Female Toxicant	No Effect/Male Only
Decreased	BPD, EGMME, MAA	
No Change	NHP, TCP	ETH, TCE, EG, PGME, OA, PB, PG, 9AA, TGD, BA

References

1. Mattison DR, ed. Reproductive toxicology. New York: Alan R. Liss, Inc., 1983.
2. Aman RP. Use of animal models for detecting specific alterations in reproduction. Fundam Appl Toxicol 1982; 2:13-26.
3. Committee on Biological Markers of the National Research Council. Biological markers in environmental health research. Environ Health Perspect 1987; 74:3-9.
4. Hatch M. Introduction: biological assessments in female reproductive toxicology. Environ Health Perspect 1987; 75:55-6.
5. Miller RK. Biomarkers of toxicity during pregnancy. Environ Health Perspect 1987; 74:77-80.
6. Lamb JC IV. Reproductive toxicity testing: evaluating and developing new testing systems. J Am Coll Toxicol 1985; 4:163-71.
7. Reel JR, Lawton AD, Wolkowski-tyl R, Davis GW, Lamb JC IV. Evaluation of a new reproductive toxicology protocol using diethylstilbestrol as a positive control compound. J Am Coll Toxicol 1985; 4:147-62.
8. Takizawa K, Yagi H, Jerina DM, Mattison DR. Experimental ovarian toxicity following intraovarian injection of benzo(a)pyrene or its metabolites in mice and rats. In: Dixon RL, ed. Target organ toxicity: gonads (reproductive and genetic toxicology). New York: Raven Press, 1985:69-94.
9. Pedersen T, Peters H. Proposal for a classification of oocytes and follicles in the mouse ovary. J Reprod Fertil 1968; 17:555-7.
10. Kastenbaum MA, Hoel DG, Bowman KO. Sample size requirements: one-way analysis of variance. Biometrika 1970; 57:421-30.
11. Mattison DR, Nightingale MS. Oocyte destruction by polycyclic aromatic hydrocarbons is not linked to the inducibility of ovarian aryl hydrocarbon (benzo(a)pyrene) hydroxylase activity in (DBA/2N x C57BL/6N)Fl x DBA/2N backcross mice. Pediatr Pharmacol (New York) 1982; 2:11-21.
12. Takizawa K, Yagi H, Jerina DM, Mattison DR. Murine strain differences in ovotoxicity following intraovarian injection with benzo(a)pyrene,(+)-(7R,8S), (-)-(7R,8S)-dihydrodiol, or (+)-(7R,8S)-diol(9S,10r)-epoxide-2. Cancer Res 1984; 44:2571-6.

57

Ovarian Morphometric Changes following Cyclophosphamide Treatment

David R. Plowchalk and Donald R. Mattison

University of Arkansas for Medical Sciences, Little Rock, AR,
and the National Center Toxicological Research, Jefferson, AR

Cyclophosphamide (CP) is a bifunctional alkylating agent routinely used in the treatment of a wide variety of malignancies and immunological disorders. Although CP can be quite effective in the management of these diseases, it also causes several adverse side effects. Observations by a number of investigators show that CP acts as a potent toxicant in the female reproductive system, capable of producing transient amenorrhea or complete ovarian failure (1-3). These side effects are accompanied by a reduction in serum estrogen and progesterone levels and an increase in FSH and LH, suggesting toxicity at the level of the ovary and not at the level of the hypothalamus or pituitary (4). Indeed, many animal studies demonstrate that CP produces a time-, dose-, strain-, and species-dependent destruction of oocytes and follicles (5-7). These data, collected in rodents, suggest that primordial follicles are most sensitive to CP insult, followed by growing and antral follicles. Although such changes in follicle pools are well defined, quicker and more sensitive assays are needed to assess earlier changes occurring in the follicle complex itself and other ovarian components that may be indicative signs of ovarian toxicity. Given the dynamic nature of follicle growth and replacement, it is possible that growing and antral follicles are equally or more sensitive than primordial follicles.

The primary objectives of this study were to (1) reexamine the dose response and time course of follicle and oocyte destruction by CP using differential follicle counts; (2) establish whether changes in total ovarian, growing follicle, antral follicle and corpus luteum volumes occur in response to CP treatment; and, (3) appraise the usefulness of these morphometric measurements as biomarkers of ovarian toxicity.

Materials and Methods

Animals

Seven- to 8-week-old female C57BL/6N mice were given a single ip injection of either 0, 75, 200, or 500 mg/kg cyclophosphamide (Sigma, St. Louis, MO) dissolved in 1 ml of normal saline. The mice were then killed by cervical dislocation at 1, 3, or 7 days posttreatment. The ovaries were removed, placed in Bouin's fixative for 24 h, transferred to 70% ethanol, dehydrated, embedded, serially sectioned (0.006 mm), and stained with hematoxylin and eosin.

Follicle Counts

Differential follicle classifications were made using a modification of the method by Pedersen and Peters (8), where primordial follicles, growing follicles and antral follicles were types I-III, types IV-V, and types VI-VIII, respectively. Total follicle counts were calculated by summing the follicle counts obtained from every 10th section; therefore, the numbers reported are not absolute follicle numbers, but are instead relative to the counting procedure.

Volume Measurements

All volume measurements were made using a Bioquant IV morphometric system (R & M Biometrics, Inc., Nashville, TN). Total ovarian volume was calculated by measuring every 10th section and using the following equation:

$$\text{Ovarian Volume (mm}^3) = \Sigma \text{ [Section Area mm}^2 \times 0.006 \text{ mm} \times 10].$$

Volume measurements of corpora lutea, antral follicles, and growing follicles represent the total volume (mm^3) occupied by each component. These volumes were calculated by measuring every 5th section and using the following equation:

$$\text{Component Volume (mm}^3) = \Sigma \text{ [Component Area mm}^2 \times 0.006 \text{ mm} \times 5].$$

Due to the small size of individual ovarian components relative to total ovarian volume, every 5th section rather than every 10th section was measured in order to obtain a better estimation of volume. Interstitial volume simply refers to all ovarian tissues not included in the other volume measurements and was calculated by subtracting the sum of the ovarian component volumes from the total ovarian volume. Analysis of ovarian component volumes was performed only on the 500 mg/kg dose group.

Results

Differential Follicle Counts

Primordial follicle numbers were significantly reduced at all doses and time-points (Fig. 1A). Virtually all follicles were destroyed by 3 days in the high-dose group. The estimated ED_{50} for primordial follicle destruction at 72 h was 105 mg/kg. Antral follicles were also destroyed in a time- and dose-dependent fashion. At 500 mg/kg, antral follicles were reduced to a minimum at 3 days (7% control) before rebounding to 62% of control at 7 days. Similarly, at a dose of 200 mg/kg, antral follicle numbers fell to 52% of control in 1 day, but quickly recovered to normal levels for the duration of the experiment (Fig. 1C).

The growing follicle pool was relatively unaffected by CP, showing a significant reduction only in the high-dose group at 7 days (Fig. 1B).

Morphometric Analysis

Significant reductions in ovarian volume (41%) occurred within 24 h of treatment with 500 mg/kg CP and remained depressed for 7 days (Fig. 1D). Although the other treatment groups appeared to have slight decreases in ovarian volumes, they were not significantly different from controls.

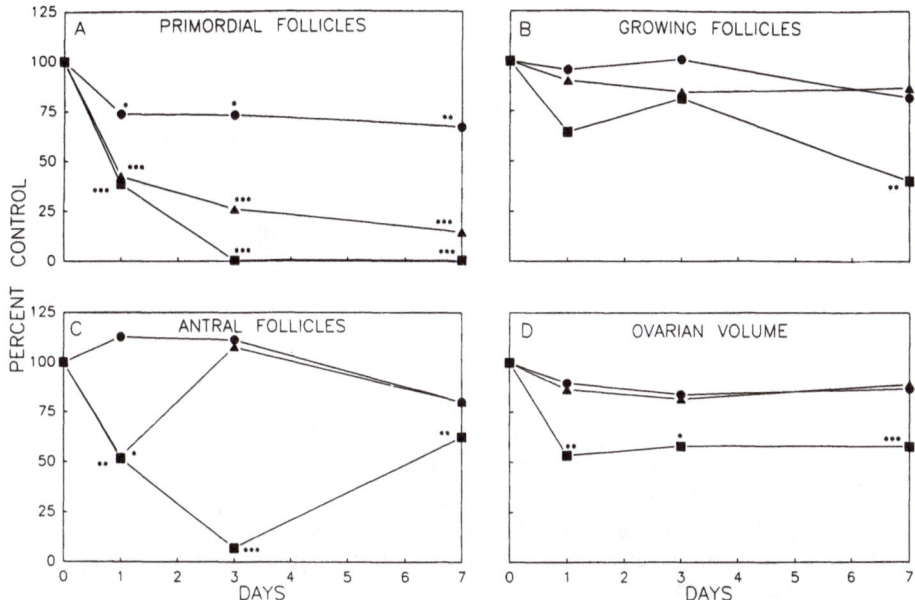

Fig. 1. Time course of primordial (A), growing (B), and antral (C) follicle destruction by 75 (circles), 200 (triangles), and 500 mg/kg (squares) cyclophosphamide. Each time-point represents the mean ovarian follicle numbers or ovarian volume (D) of 4-5 mice, represented as percent saline controls. (*P<0.05, **P<0.01, ***P<0.001.)

Figure 2 is a graphic representation of volume changes observed in specific ovarian components of mice treated with 500 mg/kg CP. Alterations in total antral follicle volume directly reflected those changes exhibited by antral follicle counts. A 54, 81, and 38% reduction in total antral follicle volume occurred at 1, 3, and 7 days, respectively (Table 1). This reduction accounted for most (19.6%) of the ovarian volume loss at 3 days, and approximately a third of the volume loss at 1 and 7 days. While interstitial area and growing follicle volumes were unaltered and antral volume was recovering at 7 days, corpora lutea volume fell to zero, accounting for about 17% of the total ovarian volume loss.

Discussion

Differential follicle counting has proven to be a very useful technique for assessing the ovarian toxicity of a number of xenobiotics, including cyclophosphamide (5,6,9). Morphometric analysis also appears to be a promising method for further defining dynamic changes in the ovary in response to xenobiotics. Ovarian volume measurements reflect gross alterations occurring in the ovary that are a culmination of changes in a number of ovarian components. In this study, volume measurements of specific components in ovaries of the high-dose group revealed that, indeed, the total ovarian volume loss was a dynamic process. At 1 day after treatment, the total volume loss was mainly due to interstitial area and antral follicle volume loss, while at 7 days the volume loss could be attributed to the disappearance

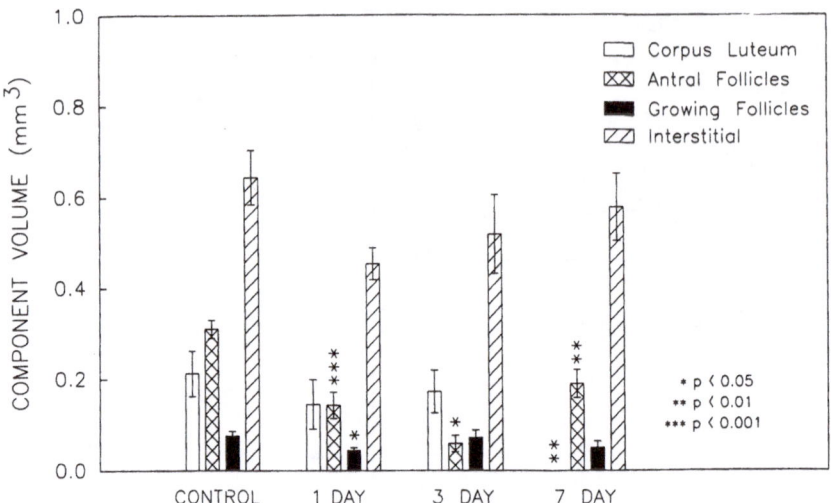

Fig. 2. Changes in total corpus luteum, antral follicle, growing follicle, and interstitial tissue volumes 1, 3, and 7 days after treatment with 500 mg/kg cyclophosphamide.

of corpora lutea. Given that the estrous cycle of the mouse is 4-5 days, the absence of corpora lutea at 7 days is probably due to the earlier destruction of antral follicles which is seen at 1 and 3 days following treatment.

Growing follicle counts were reduced only in the high-dose group at 7 days (Fig. 1B); however morphometric measurement at Day 1 showed there to be a significant reduction in growing follicle volume. This indicates that although follicle counts are normal, analysis of volume can determine early structural changes in the follicle complex. A reduction in volume may represent inhibition of granulosa cell proliferation or oocyte growth or the beginnings of follicular atresia. The information gained from this study suggests morphometric analysis

Table 1. Effect of cyclophosphamide (500 mg/kg) on the volume of specific ovarian components and total ovarian volume

Ovarian Component	Day 1 % Loss Comp.*	Day 1 % Loss TOV**	Day 3 % Loss Comp.	Day 3 % Loss TOV	Day 7 % Loss Comp.	Day 7 % Loss TOV
Corpus luteum	32.0	5.3	18.4	3.0	100.0	16.6
Antral follicle	54.0	13.1	80.9	19.6	38.0	9.3
Growing follicle	42.0	2.5	2.6	0.1	32.0	1.8
Interstitial	30.0	15.1	19.4	9.8	10.2	5.1
Ovary	–	36.0	–	32.5	–	32.8

*Percent loss in component volume compared to saline controls. **Percent loss in Total Ovarian Volume accounted for by the loss in component volume.

has potential usefulness as a screen for ovarian toxicity by revealing modifications in the ovary not discovered by follicle counting.

References

1. Warne GL, Fairley KF, Hobbs JB, Martin FR. Cyclophosphamide-induced ovarian failure. N Engl J Med 1973; 289:1159-62.
2. Koyama H, Wada T, Nishizawa Y, et al. Cyclophosphamide-induced ovarian failure and its therapeutic significance in patients with breast cancer. Cancer 1977; 39:1403-9.
3. Kumar R, McEvoy J, Biggart JD, McGeown MG. Cyclophosphamide and reproductive function. Lancet 1972; June 3:1212-4.
4. Dnistrian AM, Schwartz MK, Fracchia AA, et al. Endocrine consequences of CMF adjuvant therapy in premenopausal and postmenopausal breast cancer patients. Cancer 1983; 51:803-7.
5. Shiromizu K, Thorgeirsson S, Mattison DR. Effect of cyclophosphamide on oocyte and follicle number in Sprague-Dawley rats, C57BL/6N and DBA/2n mice. Pediatr Pharmacol (New York) 1984; 4:213-21.
6. Mattison DR, Chang L, Thorgeirsson SS, Shiromizu K. The effects of cyclophosphamide, azathioprine, and 6-mercaptopurine on oocyte and follicle number in C57BL/6N mice. Res Commun Chem Pathol Pharmacol 1981; 31:155-61.
7. Jarrel J, Young Lai EV, Barr R, McMahon A, Belbeck L, O'Connell G. Ovarian toxicity of cyclophosphamide alone and in combination with ovarian irradiation in the rat. Cancer Res 1987; 47:2340-3.
8. Pedersen T, Peters H. Proposal for a classification of oocytes and follicles in the mouse ovary. J Reprod Fertil 1968; 17:555-7.
9. Mattison DR, Shiromizu K, Nightingale MS. Oocyte destruction by polycyclic aromatic hydrocarbons. Am J Ind Med 1983; 4:191-202.

58

Heparin, But Not N-Desulfated Heparin, Enhances Cumulus Expansion of Mouse and Cow Oocytes in Serum-Free Medium

S. E. Bollig-Fenton, D. J. Miller, M. E. Bellin, and
R. L. Ax

Endocrinology-Reproductive Physiology Program
University of Wisconsin-Madison, 53706

Introduction

Glycosaminoglycans (GAGs) are follicular constituents that have been implicated as regulators of several cellular processes in ovarian follicles. In a dose-dependent manner, commercially available GAGs inhibited cumulus mass expansion in the presence of FSH and serum (6) and inhibited gonadotropin binding to granulosa cells (1,2). In the same manner, follicular GAGs inhibited LDL degradation and progesterone production (3) and zona pellucida hardening in vitro (4). Heparin, one type of GAG, inhibits those cellular processes and is the most "potent" inhibitor of the chemical classes of GAGs tested (1-4). Heparin has O- and N-substituted sulfate groups and is the most highly sulfated of the GAGs (5). The ability of GAGs to affect FSH-induced expansion of cumulus cells is related to degree of GAG sulfation (6). GAGs containing less sulfate, such as the chondroitin sulfates and hyaluronic acid, were less effective at inhibiting FSH-induced cumulus mass expansion (6). This suggested importance of sulfation in the ability of GAGs to inhibit FSH-induced cumulus cell expansion, but there are also other structural differences between those classes of GAGs (1). It is not known if GAGs affect cumulus mass expansion in cultures lacking FSH. Desulfation of heparin affects its interactions with many cells. For example, desulfation of heparin reduced its ability to inhibit LDL degradation and progesterone production by granulosa cells (3).

The objectives of this study were (1) to determine the effect of heparin on FSH-stimulated and spontaneous cumulus cell expansion in cow and mouse oocytes; and, (2) to investigate the effect of N-desulfation of heparin on its ability to regulate cumulus mass expansion.

Materials and Methods

Oocyte Collection and Handling

Twenty-two-day-old, female, random-bred Swiss Webster mice were injected with 5 IU of pregnant mare serum gonadotropin (Sigma Chemical Co., St. Louis, MO) and killed 48 h later by cervical dislocation. Ovaries were transferred to a modified Tyrode's medium (TALP 7,8) lacking fetal bovine serum and hypotaurine. Oocyte-cumulus complexes (OCCs) were released from ovaries by puncturing the follicles with a 25 g needle. Bovine ovaries were obtained from a local abattoir and transported to the laboratory in 0.9% NaCl at 39°C. Ovaries were washed with 70% EtOH. The follicular fluid was aspirated from small follicles (1-5 mm) by use of a 22 g needle and 3 ml syringe, within 3 h of ovary collection. Complexes were allowed to settle in a test tube for 20 min and were transferred to a 60 x 15 mm dish (Falcon, Oxnard, CA) containing TALP. Bovine and murine OCCs were then treated similarly. OCCs were collected with a micropipette and washed by transferring them serially between 3 dishes containing TALP. Only viable complexes as assessed by 0.2% trypan blue exclusion were used. Three to six complexes were placed in each 40 μl droplet of medium. Droplets containing OCCs were incubated for 48 h at 39°C (9) with 5% CO_2 at 100% humidity, under paraffin oil.

Heparin and FSH Treatments

Treatments were added immediately after washing the complexes and consisted of heparin (Calbiochem, San Diego, CA), FSH (Sigma Chemical Co., St. Louis, MO), heparin and FSH, N-desulfated heparin, or N-desulfated heparin and FSH. Concentrations of the heparins utilized were 0, .01, .1, 1.0 or 10.0 mg/ml and concentrations of FSH were 0 or 10.0 μg/ml. The total sulfate content of the N-desulfated heparin was reduced from approximately 17% to 6% by incubating the pyridinium salt of heparin with 95% DMSO at 50°C for 1.5 h (10).

After 24 and 48 h of culture, complexes were visually rated 1 (compact, unexpanded complexes) to 4 (fully expanded complexes), based on a previous report (11). OCCs whose outer cumulus cells were slightly expanded were rated 2, and when outer and inner cumulus cells were slightly expanded the OCC was scored 3.

Statistical Analysis

Experiments were factorial in design and evaluated by analysis of variance with main effects of heparin type and concentration, FSH concentrations, culture time and species. Differences between specific treatments were detected by Tukey's Studentized Range Test (12). On a replicate day, at least 15 oocytes were assigned to each of 12 different treatments. Experiments were replicated 3 times with mouse OCCs and 9 times for bovine OCCs.

Results

Totals of 1918 oocytes from cattle and 528 oocytes from mice were examined for cumulus expansion. Expansion scores for individual oocytes were similar at 24 and 48 h (P>.10). Therefore, scores for 48 h are discussed.

Heparin, but not N-desulfated heparin, enhanced expansion of cumulus complexes in a dose-dependent manner (P<.001). As the dose of heparin increased (0, .01, to .1 mg/ml), the mean expansion score for bovine and mouse OCCs significantly increased (P<.01, Fig. 1). OCCs incubated with N-desulfated heparin failed to exhibit significant cumulus mass expansion. OCCs cultured in the presence of 0, .01, .1, 1.0 or 10.0 mg/ml of N-desulfated heparin exhibited mean expansion scores of 1.7, 1.5, 1.5, 1.7 and 1.6, respectively. Analysis of variance detected an overall difference in species in regard to OCC expansion scores across doses of heparin (P<.001). The basis for the differences was that .01 mg/ml heparin stimulated expansion of bovine OCCs to a greater degree than mouse OCCs (P<.01, Fig. 1).

FSH did not facilitate mouse and bovine cumulus cell expansion, but expansion was enhanced when heparin was added to cultures. At 48 h of culture, the mean expansion scores for bovine OCCs exposed to FSH (10 μg/ml) or heparin (.01 mg/ml) were $1.7 \pm .09$ (n=420) and $3.2 \pm .20$ (n=330), respectively. Mean 48-h expansion scores for the mouse OCCs exposed to FSH (10 μg/ml) or heparin (.01 mg/ml) were $1.7 \pm .07$ (n=51) and $2.4 \pm .08$ (n=62), respectively. Expansion scores of OCCs obtained from cultures containing 10 μg/ml FSH with each dose of heparin or N-desulfated heparin did not differ from results obtained from cultures using heparin or N-desulfated heparin without FSH (P=.90 at 48 h, data not shown).

Discussion

Heparin has been shown to affect cellular processes in a dose-dependent manner. Heparin binds to granulosa cells (13) and is a potent inhibitor of progesterone secretion and LDL degradation by granulosa cells (3). The degree of N-sulfation of heparin is important for its ability to exert its effects on cellular processes because chemical N-desulfation of heparin negates binding to granulosa cells (13) and other cellular effects (3). This study

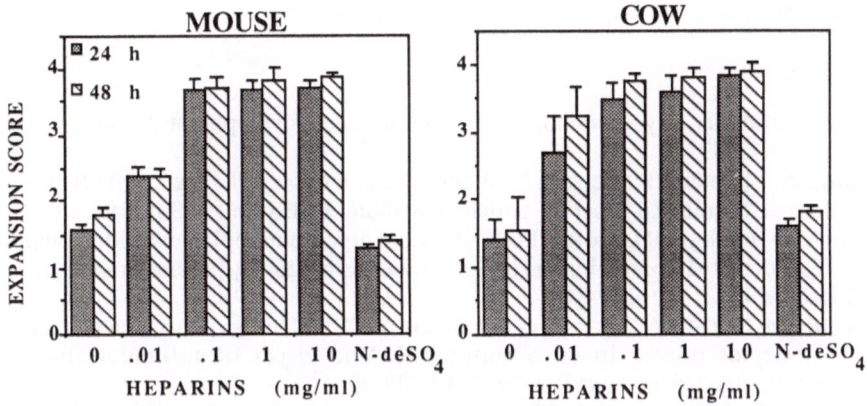

Fig. 1. Comparisons of mean OCC expansion scores for the various heparin doses at 24 h and 48 h. Scores shown are means pooled across all FSH concentrations since there was no effect upon addition of FSH to cultures. N-deSO$_4$ represents the mean of all expansion scores of OCCs that were cultured with all doses of N-desulfated heparin. Average expansion scores of all OCCs cultured with doses of N-desulfated heparin were not significantly different from the controls (P>.05).

showed that heparin enhanced cumulus mass expansion in the absence of fetal bovine serum and FSH. However, when heparin was chemically N-desulfated, it lost its ability to affect cumulus expansion. This study utilized doses of heparin in the same range as studies in which heparin inhibited cumulus expansion in the presence of FSH and serum (6).

This study supports a previous report (14) indicating that in the absence of fetal bovine serum, FSH did not stimulate cumulus expansion. In this study, when FSH and heparin were combined in OCC cultures there was no additive effect on expansion of the cumulus cells. FSH stimulated mouse cumulus cell expansion in the presence of fetal bovine serum (15,16). Cumulus expansion was accompanied by synthesis of hyaluronic acid, an unsulfated GAG, in the mouse (16) and bovine (17). In the presence of serum, the hyaluronic acid was retained within the cumulus cell matrix but without serum the hyaluronic acid was released into the medium and expansion did not occur (14). FSH and serum did not seem to be obligatory for cumulus mass expansion because heparin alone effectively substituted for FSH and serum to facilitate cumulus expansion in these experiments.

The mechanism of heparin to enhance cumulus expansion is not known. Heparin binds to granulosa cells, and that binding requires N-sulfates (13). Since heparin, but not its N-desulfated derivative, enhanced cumulus expansion in these studies, we propose that the ability of heparin to evoke expansion follows binding to cumulus cells. GAGs have been shown to stimulate plasminogen activator release (18), to bind to phospholipases and growth factors (19,20), and to modulate production of other GAGs (20). Therefore, a single locus, or multiple loci, may exist where heparin can exert its effect to regulate cumulus expansion.

Acknowledgments

Thanks are extended to Brad Haley for obtaining bovine ovaries from Peck's Meat Packing, Milwaukee, WI. This research was supported by the University of Wisconsin College of Agricultural and Life Sciences and NIH Grant HD-13964.

References

1. Ax RL, Bellin ME. Glycosaminoglycans and follicular development. J Anim Sci 1988; 66(suppl 2):32-49.
2. Nimrod A, Lindner HR. Heparin facilitates the induction of LH receptors by FSH in granulosa cells cultured in serum-enriched medium. FEBS Lett 1980; 119:155-7.
3. Bellin ME, Veldhuis JD, Ax RL. Follicular fluid glycosaminoglycans inhibit degradation of low density lipoproteins and progesterone production by porcine granulosa cells. Biol Reprod 1987; 37:1179-84.
4. De Felici M, Salustri A, Siracusa G. "Spontaneous" hardening of the zona pellucida of mouse oocytes during in vitro culture. II. The effect of follicular fluid and glycosaminoglycans. Gamete Res 1985; 12:227-35.
5. Gallagher JT, Walker A. Molecular distinctions between heparan sulfate and heparin. Biochem J 1985; 230:665-74.
6. Eppig JJ. Ovarian glycosaminoglycans: evidence for a role in regulating the response of the oocyte-cumulus cell complex to FSH. Endocrinology 1981; 108:1992-4.
7. Bavister BD, Yanagimachi R. The effects of sperm extract and energy sources on the motility and acrosome reaction of hamster sperm in vitro. Biol Reprod 1977; 16:228-37.

8. Parrish JJ, Susko-Parrish J, Winer MN, First NL. Capacitation of bovine sperm by heparin. Biol Reprod 1988; 38:1171-80.
9. Lenz RW, Ball GD, Leibfried ML, Ax RL, First NL. In vitro maturation and fertilization of bovine oocytes are temperature-dependent processes. Biol Reprod 1983; 29:173-9.
10. Inoue Y, Nagasawa K. Selective N-desulfation of heparin with dimethyl sulfoxide containing water or methanol. Carbohydr Res 1976; 46:87-95.
11. Ball GD, Ax RL, First NL. Mucopolysaccharide synthesis accompanies expansion of bovine cumulus-oocyte complexes in vitro. In: Mahesh VB, Muldoon TG, Saxena BB, Sadler WA, eds. Functional correlates of hormone receptors in reproduction. New York: Elsevier-North Holland, 1980:561-3.
12. Neter J, Wasserman W. Analysis of factor effects. In: Applied linear statistical models. Homewood: RD Irwin, 1974:473-7.
13. Bellin ME, Wentworth BC, Ax RL. Comparisons of the ability of follicular fluid glycosaminoglycans and chemically desulfated heparin to compete for heparin-binding sites on granulosa cells. Biol Reprod 1987; 37:293-300.
14. Eppig JJ. Role of serum in FSH-stimulated cumulus expansion by mouse oocyte-cumulus cell complexes in vitro. Biol Reprod 1980; 22:629-33.
15. Eppig JJ. Gonadotropin stimulation of the expansion of cumulus oophori isolated from mice: general conditions for expansion in vitro. J Exp Zool 1979; 208:111-20.
16. Eppig JJ. FSH stimulates hyaluronic acid synthesis by oocyte-cumulus cell complexes for mouse preovulatory follicles. Nature 1979; 281:483-4.
17. Ball GD, Bellin ME, Ax RL, First NL. Glycosaminoglycans in bovine oocyte-cumulus complexes: morphology and chemistry. Mol Cell Endocrinol 1982; 28:113-22.
18. Abbadini M, Zhu GJ, Maggi A, Pangrazzi J. Dermatan sulfate induces plasminogen activator release in the perfused rat hindquarters. Blood 1987; 70:1858-60.
19. Horigome K, Hayakawa M, Inoue K, Nojima S. Purification and characterization of phospholipase A2 released from rat platelets. J Biochem (Tokyo) 1987; 101:625-31.
20. Lindahl U, Hook M. Glycosaminoglycans and their binding to biological macro-molecules. Annu Rev Biochem 1978; 47:385-417.

59

A Fibronectin Receptor Competitive Blocker Inhibits GnRH Induced Meiosis in Follicle-Enclosed Oocytes

M. Yemini, R. Tomur, and T. T. Hung

Division of Reproductive Endocrinology and REPSCEND Laboratory
Department of Obstetrics and Gynecology, University of Miami
School of Medicine, Miami, FL 33101

Introduction

Mammalian oocytes are arrested at the diplotene stage of the first meiotic division before ovulation and the preovulatory surge of gonadotropin initiates resumption of meiosis (1). Oocyte maturation can also be effectively induced by gonadotropin releasing hormone (GnRH) or GnRH agonist (2). The process which leads to oocyte maturation is probably mediated by follicular components and is not the result of a direct interaction between the female gamete and the hormone (3,4). During the process of follicular growth, a complex sequence of changes occur, including granulosa cells (GCs) differentiation, extracellular matrix (ECM) interaction with the GCs affecting the differentiation as well as the cytoplas-matic and nuclear maturation of the oocyte (1,5). Fibronectin (Fn) is a major component of the ECM and has been implicated in a wide variety of cellular properties, particularly those involving the interaction of cells with ECM (6). Recently, it has been demonstrated that GCs can synthesize and secrete Fn (7,8), and cytodifferentiation of GCs was induced by GnRH which, in turn, promoted Fn secretion (9).

Altogether, this evidence has led us to study the possible involvement of Fn in GnRH regulation of oocyte maturation by using an in vitro culturing system of rats' preovulatory antral follicles. GnRH agonist and two synthetic peptide probes, one is a specific inhibitor and the other is a noninhibitor to Fn function, were added to the culture medium in order to evaluate their effects on oocyte maturation.

Material and Methods

Isolation of Preovulatory Follicles

Immature 21-day-old Sprague-Dawley rats (Charles River, Wilmington, MA) were sent to our lab and were kept in a controlled environment with respect to temperature and light.

Pregnant mare's serum was administered subcutaneously on day 26-27 of age at a dose of 10 IU and the rats were sacrificed 48 h later. The ovaries were excised and preovulatory follicles were isolated with the help of a dissecting microscope.

Incubation Procedure

Follicles were incubated (10 per dish) in 0.9 ml of Ham's F-10 (pH-7.4) and supplemented with penicillin (50 μ/ml) and streptomycin (50 μG/ml). The agents to be tested were added at the start of incubation. All experiments were carried out under a humidified atmosphere of 5% CO_2 in air at 37°C. During several individual experiments, follicles from each rat were divided among 2-3 dishes with different agents to be tested, one of them a negative or positive control (negative control = no agent was added; positive control = only GnRH analog was added to the Ham's F-10). After 4 h of incubation, the follicles were incised and the cumulus/oocyte complexes were recovered.

Hormones and Chemicals

PMSG and GnRH analog (GnRH ethylamide-pGlu-His-Trp-Ser-Try-im-Bzl-d-His-Leu-Arg-Pro-NHEt) were purchased from Sigma Company, St. Louis, MO, and GnRH analog was examined at the concentration of 10 and 100 ng/ml. The synthetic oligopeptide GRGDS (Gly-Arg-Gly-Asp-Ser) was purchased from Peninsula Lab, Belmont, CA and GRGESP (Gly-Arg-Gly-Glu-Ser-Pro) from Telios, Inc., San Diego, CA and was examined at the concentration of 100 and 500 μM. Ham's F-10, penicillin and streptomycin were purchased from Gibco Lab, Grand Island, NY.

Examination of Oocytes

Oocytes were examined with Nomarski interference contrast microscopy (400 x magnification). Oocytes with intact germinal vesicle were considered immature, and those with germinal vesicle breakdown (GVB) were considered maturing. The fraction of GVB for individual experiments was calculated and the results are reported as the mean ⊥ standard deviation of several experiments with the same treatment. The results were analyzed statistically by using Student's t test.

Results

The effect of various concentrations of the two synthetic peptide probes on the meiosis inducing effect of the GnRH analog during 4 h of incubation is depicted in Table 1. GRGDS inhibits the GnRH analog-induced meiosis. The degree of inhibition (as well as the degree of statistical significance) was dependent on both the GnRH analog and GRGDS concentration. GRGDS alone has no effect on oocyte maturation and there was no statistical difference from the negative control. In contrast to GRGDS, GRGESP has no effect on meiosis induced by GnRH analog.

Discussion

We have been able to demonstrate in this study that the stimulatory effects of GnRH analog on meiosis in preovulatory rat follicles are effectively blocked by the synthetic peptide GRGDS. This peptide contained the sequence Arg-Gly-Asp (RGD), a key structural element for cell attachment and activity of Fn, making it possible to specifically inhibit the cell

Table 1. Effect of synthetic oligopeptides on the meiosis-inducing effect of
GnRH analog on follicle-enclosed oocytes incubated for 4 h

Treatment				
GnRHa ng/ml	GRGDS μM	GRGESP μM	No. of Oocytes	% of GVB
10			120	51.1 ± 11.3
100			117	72.9 ± 11.6
			90	13.0 ± 3.9
10	100		60	34.1 ± 12.7
10	500		47	22.8 ± 12.1
100	100		56	48.8 ± 10.8
100	500		50	41.1 ± 5.9
10		100	34	51.2 ± 3.3
10		500	36	55.5 ± 7.8
	100		19	15.3 ± 0.6
	500		22	13.6 ± 1.7

P<0.005
P<0.02
P<0.001
P<0.01
P<0.001

GnRHa = Gonadotropin Releasing Hormone Analog. GRGDS = Gly-Arg-Gly-Asp-Ser.
GRGESP = Gly-Arg-Gly-Glu-Ser-Pro. GVB= Germinal Vesicle Breakdown.

attachment function of Fn in a noncytotoxic manner (10,11). In contrast, GRGESP, a peptide which contains no cell-binding sequence, did not show any inhibitory effect on GnRH analog-induced meiosis. These findings emphasize the specificity of GRGDS effect which is likely to be a competitive blocker of receptor for cell-binding domain for Fn. As previously reported, GnRH promotes Fn secretion and cytodifferentiation of GCs (9). The function of Fn secretion by GCs remains to be determined. It is proposed that Fn secretion may provide the proper extracellular environment for the follicle, the GCs or the oocyte during the process of maturation and by this may effect meiosis.

Previous studies have shown that the extracellular matrix components including Fn appear to affect GCs differentiation, resulting in various biochemical and structural characteristics which are important for the process of ovulation and meiotic maturation (1,5,12,13). A previously published paper (14) has indicated that human follicular fluid Fn/protein ratio seems to correlate with oocyte maturity and fertilization. These findings agree with our results which indicate that Fn-follicle interaction is crucial for rat oocyte GnRH-induced meiosis. Further study needs to be performed in order to elucidate the exact role model as well as its physiological significance in an in vivo condition.

Acknowledgments

The authors would like to thank Mrs. Lottie MacFarlane for her diligent preparation of this manuscript, and Dr. William J. LeMaire for his timely suggestions.

References

1. Yoshimura Y, Wallach EE. Studies of the mechanism(s) of mammalian ovulation. Fertil Steril 1987; 47:22-34.
2. Hillensjo T, LeMaire WJ. Gonadotropin releasing hormone agonists stimulate meiotic maturation of follicle-enclosed rat oocytes in vitro. Nature 1980; 287:145-6.
3. Dekel N, Beers WH. Development of the rat oocyte in vitro inhibition of maturation in the presence or absence of the cumulus oophorus. Dev Biol 1980; 75:247-54.
4. Lawrence TS, Dekel N, Beers WH. Binding of hCG by rat cumuli oophori and granulosa cells. A comparative study. Endocrinology 1980; 106:1114-8.
5. Amsterdam A, Rotmensch S. Structure-function relationships during granulosa cell differentiation. Endocr Rev 1987; 8:309-37.
6. Hynes RO. Fibronectin and its relation to cellular structure and behavior. In: Hay ED, ed. Cell biology of extracellular matrix. New York: Plenum Press, 1981:295-334.
7. Skinner MK, McKeracher HL, Dorrington JH. Fibronectin as a marker of granulosa cell cytodifferentiation. Endocrinology 1985; 117:886-92.
8. Lobb DK, Dorrington JH. Human granulosa and thecal cells secrete distinct protein profiles. Fertil Steril 1987; 48:243-8.
9. Dorrington JH, Skinner MK. Cytodifferentiation of granulosa cells induced by gonadotropin-releasing hormone promotes fibronectin secretion. Endocrinology 1986; 118:2065-71.
10. Pierschbacher MO, Ruoslahti E. Cell attachment activity of fibronectin can be duplicated by small synthetic fragments of the molecule. Nature 1984; 309:30-4.
11. Pierschbacher MO, Ruoslahti E. Variants of the cell recognition site of fibronectin that retain attachment-promoting activity. Proc Natl Acad Sci USA 1984; 81:5985-8.
12. Ben-Ze'ev A, Amsterdam A. In vitro regulation of granulosa cell differentiation. J Biol Chem 1987; 262:5366-76.
13. Ben-Ze'ev A, Amsterdam A. Regulation of cytoskeletal proteins involved in cell contact formation during differentiation of granulosa cells on extracellular matrix. Proc Natl Acad Sci 1986; 83:2894-8.
14. Tsuiki A, Preyer J, Hung TT. Fibronectin and glycosaminoglycans in human preovulatory follicular fluid and their correlation to follicular maturation. Hum Reprod; 3:425-9.

Author Index

Subject Index